Applied Spatial Statistics for
Public Health Data

WILEY SERIES IN PROBABILITY AND STATISTICS

Established by WALTER A. SHEWHART and SAMUEL S. WILKS

A complete list of the titles in this series appears at the end of this volume.

Applied Spatial Statistics for Public Health Data

LANCE A. WALLER

Emory University
Department of Biostatistics
Atlanta, Georgia

CAROL A. GOTWAY

National Center for Environmental Health
Centers for Disease Control and Prevention
Atlanta, Georgia

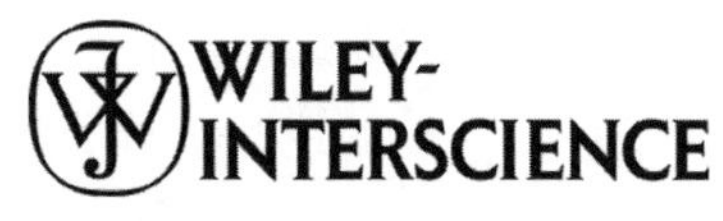

A JOHN WILEY & SONS, INC., PUBLICATION

Published by John Wiley & Sons, Inc., Hoboken, New Jersey.
Published simultaneously in Canada.

Library of Congress Cataloging-in-Publication Data:

Waller, Lance A., 1965–
Applied spatial statistics for public health data / Lance A. Waller, Carol A. Gotway.
p. cm.—(Wiley series in probability and statistics)
Includes bibliographical references and index.
ISBN 0-471-38771-1 (coth)
1. Public health—Statistical methods. 2. Spatial analysis (Statistics) I. Gotway, Carol A., 1961– II. Title. III. Series.

RA440.85.W34 2004
614′.07′27—dc22

2003066065

Printed in the United States of America.

10 9 8 7 6 5 4

Statistics, too, have supplied us with a new and powerful means of testing medical truth....

Dr. Benjamin Babbinton
President of the London Epidemiological Society, 1850
Lancet, Volume 2, p. 641

Dedicated with love to

Dr. Alisha A. Waller
Allyn, Matthew, and Adrian Waller
Dr. Clement A. and Mrs. Patricia L. Gotway

Contents

Preface

> Spatial statistical analysis has never been in the mainstream of statistical theory. However, there is a growing interest both for epidemiologic studies, and in analyzing disease processes.

The above is a quote one of us (L.A.W.) received on a grant review in 1997, and it outlines succinctly our motivation for this book. Topics in spatial statistics are usually offered only as special-topic elective courses, if they are offered at all. However, there is growing interest in statistical methods for the analysis of spatially referenced data in a wide variety of fields, including the analysis of public health data. Yet, there are few introductory, application-oriented texts on spatial statistics. For practicing public health researchers with a general background in applied statistics seeking to learn about spatial data analysis and how it might play a role in their work, there are few places to turn.

Our goal is to provide a text that moves from a basic understanding of multiple linear regression (including matrix notation) to an application-oriented introduction to statistical methods used to analyze spatially referenced health data. This book is less an effort to push the methodological frontier than an effort to gather and consolidate spatial statistical ideas developed in a broad variety of areas and discuss them in the context of routinely occurring spatial questions in public health. A complication in this effort is the wide variety of backgrounds among this interest group: epidemiologists, biostatisticians, medical geographers, human geographers, social scientists, environmental scientists, ecologists, political scientists, and public health practitioners (among others). In an effort to provide some common background, in Chapters 1 to 3 we provide an overview of spatial issues in public health, an introduction to typical (nonspatial) analytic methods in epidemiology (for geographers who may not have encountered them previously), and an introduction to basic issues in geography, geodesy, and cartography (for statisticians and epidemiologists who may not have encountered them previously). In Chapter 4 we merge ideas of geography and statistics through exploration of the methods, challenges, and approaches associated with mapping disease data. In Chapter 5 we provide an introduction to statistical methods for the analysis of spatial point patterns, and in Chapters 6 and 7 we extend these to the particular issue of identifying disease clusters, which is often of interest in public health. In Chapter 8 we explore statistical methods for mapping environmental exposures and provide an introduction to the field of geostatistics. Finally, in Chapter 9 we outline modeling methods used to link spatially referenced exposure and disease data.

Throughout, we provide "data breaks" or brief applications designed to illustrate the use (and in some cases, misuse) of the methods described in the text. Some sequences of data breaks follow the same data set, providing bits and pieces of a broader analysis to illustrate the steps along the way, or simply to contrast the different sorts of insights provided by different methods. In general, we collect methods and ideas around central questions of inquiry, then explore the particular manner in which each method addresses the question at hand. We also include several case studies, wherein we provide a start-to-finish look at a particular data set and address the components of analysis illustrated through the data breaks in a new (and often more involved) setting.

Finally, since spatial statistics is often out of the mainstream of statistical theory, it is often also out of the mainstream of statistical software. Most of the analyses in this book utilized routines in SAS (Littell et al. 1996), the S+SpatialStats module for S-plus (Kaluzny et al. 1998), and various libraries in the freely available R (Ihaka and Gentleman 1996) language. For particular applications, we made use of the freely available software packages WinBUGS (Spiegelhalter et al. 1999), SaTScan (Kulldorff and International Management Services, Inc. 2002), and DMAP (Rushton and Lolonis 1996), and used the geographic information system (GIS) packages ArcGIS and ArcView (Environmental Systems Research Institute 1999, including the spatial autocorrelation scripts for ArcView by Lee and Wong 2001). Regarding Internet addresses, we decided to provide references and detailed descriptions of particular data sets and software packages since links often shift and go out of date. However, we do post related links, the tabulated data sets, and most of our R and SAS codes relating to the data breaks on the book's Web site, linked from *www.wiley.com*. This code should allow readers to duplicate (and hopefully expand!) many of the analyses appearing throughout the book, and perhaps provide a launching point for the analyses of their own data.

L. A. WALLER
C. A. GOTWAY CRAWFORD

Atlanta, Georgia

Acknowledgments

To begin at the beginning, we have to go back to 1999. Owen Devine had substantial input into the original outline and we wish he had been able to continue with us to the end. Brad Carlin, Linda Young, and Ray Waller provided good advice on choosing a publisher and defining the contract terms. Graduate students at the University of Minnesota and Emory University heard the early rumblings of some of the material here and their reactions, frustrations, and enthusiasm drove much of the layout and structure of the text.

Particular individuals provided very helpful review comments on certain chapters. Linda Pickle provided valuable suggestions updating our original ideas on visualization in Chapter 4, and Dan Carr constructed the linked micromap example and suggested several references on current research in cartographic visualization. Felix Rogers was nice enough to let us play with his data on very low birthweights that we used extensively in Chapter 4 and then again in Chapter 9. Owen Devine gave us many editorial suggestions on Chapter 4 which improved our writing. Aila Särkkä provided very thoughtful comments improving the original presentation of point process material in Chapter 5. In 1997, Richard Wright provided Lance with one of his all-time favorite data sets, the medieval grave site data that are featured predominately in Chapters 5 and 6. Dick Hoskins, Bob McMaster, Gerry Rushton, Dan Griffith, and Luc Anselin gamely entertained off-the-cuff questions in a patient and helpful manner. Betsy Hill, Traci Leong, DeMarc Hickson, and Monica Jackson all provided valuable comments regarding Chapters 6 and 7. David Olson, Ricardo Olea, and Konstantin Krivoruchko provided detailed reviews of Chapter 8, and many of their suggestions greatly improved this chapter. Brad Carlin and Alan Gelfand provided valuable insight and a great sounding board for the section on Bayesian models for disease mapping in Chapter 9. Eric Tassone expertly implemented multiple versions of the hierarchical Bayesian Poisson regression model, providing the conclusion to the series of New York leukemia data breaks. Andy Barclay deserves mention for his encouragement and example. We have yet to find a statistical computation that he can't decipher or improve. Throughout, Steve Quigley at Wiley offered patient encouragement by often noting that completed texts tended to sell better than works in progress.

Noel Cressie merits special mention. In particular, this book would not be a Wiley book if not for his unconditional support of the project. He has been there for us in many ways throughout our careers, and with respect to this endeavor, he convinced Wiley to take us on as authors, provided suggestions on the original table of contents, and reviewed a draft of the entire book. His review of the entire book was especially important to us. We needed someone objective, yet knowledgeable, to check on the overall flow and vision. His specific comments on Chapter 9 helped us focus this chapter and better link it to the earlier material. We are very grateful for his help and very lucky to be able to count on him.

On the production side, we thank Connie Woodall for her wonderful help with some of our complex graphics. We are very thankful to David Olson for his ability to buffer Carol from the noise at work and allow her time to write. Charlie Crawford provided excellent technical writing advice, and we thank Charlie, Kevin Jones, and Blackstone and Cullen, Inc. for our ftp site, which was very helpful in allowing us to exchange files easily. Alisha Waller did us a tremendous favor by technically editing the entire book just before it was submitted for publication. Alisha and Charlie were both more than wonderful during the entire process, but especially toward the end, when finishing this book became the focus of our lives. We appreciate their support more than we can say. We also appreciate the support and understanding of our friends and colleagues (most notably Linda Pickle and the other coauthors on the "best practices in spatial statistics" guide, Oli Schabenberger, and Linda Young) as we greatly delayed joint work with them while we were working on this book. We thank the staff at the Caribou Coffee, LaVista at North Druid Hills, Atlanta, Georgia, for their hospitality and the gallons of coffee and wonderful lattes we've enjoyed over the last five years while we met to discuss the book.

All of the people listed above provided comments that improved the presentation of the material found here, but we ultimately retain the final responsibility for any errors, typos, or muddy descriptions that remain.

Finally, we owe a debt of gratitude to each other. At one point in the final months of writing, Lance remarked,"It's a miracle we don't hate each other yet!" While we knew we shared a similar philosophy on applied statistics, we have different backgrounds and different research areas. Thus, we needed to blend our ideas into something of which we could both be proud. Through our collaboration, the book contains far more details than if Lance wrote it alone, and far fewer than if Carol wrote it alone, yielding a balance we hope is much better for the readers than anything either of us could have produced without the other.

L. A. W.
C. A. G. C.

CHAPTER 1

Introduction

Time, space, and causality are only metaphors of knowledge, with which we explain things to ourselves.

Friedrich Nietzsche (1844–1900)

It is part of human nature to try to discover patterns from a seemingly arbitrary set of events. We are taught from an early age to "connect the dots," learning that if we connect the right dots in the right way, a meaningful picture will emerge. People around the world look to the night sky and create patterns among the stars. These patterns allow navigation and provide a setting for a rich variety of mythologies and world views. In scientific studies, formalized methods for "connecting the dots" provide powerful tools for identifying associations and patterns between outcomes and their putative causes. In public health, identification and quantification of patterns in disease occurrence provide the first steps toward increased understanding and possibly, control of that particular disease.

As a component of the pattern observed, the location *where* an event happens may provide some indication as to *why* that particular event occurs. Spatial statistical methods offer a means for us to use such locational information to detect and quantify patterns in public health data and to investigate the degree of association between potential risk factors and disease. In the nine chapters of this book, we review, define, discuss, and apply a wide variety of statistical tools to investigate spatial patterns among data relating to public health.

1.1 WHY SPATIAL DATA IN PUBLIC HEALTH?

The literature uses the phrases *geographical epidemiology*, *spatial epidemiology*, and *medical geography* to describe a dynamic body of theory and analytic methods concerned with the study of spatial patterns of disease incidence and mortality. Interest in spatial epidemiology began with the recognition of maps as useful tools for illuminating potential "causes" of disease.

Applied Spatial Statistics for Public Health Data, by Lance A. Waller and Carol A. Gotway
ISBN 0-471-38771-1

Dr. John Snow's study of London's cholera epidemic in 1854 provides one of the most famous examples of spatial epidemiology. Snow believed that cholera was transmitted through drinking water, but at the time, this theory was met with extreme skepticism (Snow 1855; Frerichs 2000). Although the cholera deaths appeared to be clustered around the Broad Street public water pump, Snow could not find any evidence of contamination at that particular pump. His contemporary critics noted that people tended to live close to public drinking water supplies, so the clustering observed could simply have been due to the population distribution: outbreaks occur where people are. However, by considering a few carefully selected controls (i.e., people nearby that did not have cholera) and by interviewing surviving members of almost every household experiencing a cholera death, Snow eventually gathered support for his theory. Brody et al. (2000) provide a detailed history of the role of maps (by Snow and others) in the investigation of the 1854 outbreak.

Other early examples of spatial epidemiology include the study of rickets made by Palm (1890), who used maps to delineate the geographical distribution of rickets. Palm observed the greatest incidence in industrial urban areas that had a cold and wet climate. Today we know that rickets is caused by a vitamin D deficiency, which in turn can be caused by a lack of ultraviolet radiation. In a related but more recent study, Blum (1948) surmised sunlight as a causal factor for skin cancer, again based primarily on the geographical distribution of disease cases observed.

Clearly, where people live can be of great importance in identifying patterns of disease. However, spatial analyses in public health need not pertain solely to *geographical distributions* of *disease*. The spatial distributions of the sociodemographic structure, occupational patterns, and environmental exposures of a population are also of particular interest.

1.2 WHY STATISTICAL METHODS FOR SPATIAL DATA?

Although best known among spatial analysts for the Broad Street maps, it was Dr. Snow's careful case definition and analysis of cholera deaths in a wider area of London that placed him among the founders of epidemiology rather than from his maps per se (Lilienfeld and Stolley 1984, pp. 28–29; Hertz-Picciotto 1998, pp. 563–564; Rothman and Greenland 1998, p. 73). Central to this analysis was Snow's "natural experiment," wherein he categorized cholera deaths by two water companies, one drawing water upstream from London (and its sewage), the other downstream. The water company service was so intermingled that "in many cases a single house has a supply different from that on either side" (Snow 1936, p. 75). Thus, in addition to maps, study design and simple statistics were important tools in Snow's analysis.

The analysis of spatial public health data involves more than just maps and visual inference. Medical science provides insight into some specific causes of disease (e.g., biological mechanisms of transmission and identification of infectious agents); however, much remains unknown. Furthermore, not all persons experiencing a suspected causal exposure contract the disease. As a result, the analysis of public health data often builds from the statistical notion of each person having a *risk* or probability of contracting a disease. The analytic goal involves identification and quantification of any exposures, behaviors, and characteristics that may modify a person's risk. The central role of probabilities motivates the use of *statistical methods* to analyze public health data and the use of *spatial statistical methods* to (1) evaluate differences in rates observed from different geographic areas, (2) separate pattern from noise, (3) identify disease "clusters," and (4) assess the significance of potential exposures. These methods also allow us to quantify *uncertainty* in our estimates, predictions, and maps and provide the foundations for statistical inference with spatial data. Some spatial statistical methods are adaptations of familiar nonspatial methods (e.g., regression). However, other methods will most likely be new as we learn how to visualize spatial data, make meaningful maps, and detect spatial patterns.

Applying statistical methods in a spatial setting raises several challenges. Geographer and statistician Waldo Tobler summarized a key component affecting any analysis of spatially referenced data through his widely quoted and paraphrased *first law of geography*: "Everything is related to everything else, but near things are more related than far things" (Tobler 1970). This law succinctly defines the statistical notion of (positive) *spatial autocorrelation*, in which pairs of observations taken nearby are more alike than those taken farther apart. Weakening the usual assumption of independent observations in statistical analysis has far-reaching consequences. First, with independent observations, any spatial patterns are the result of a spatial *trend* in the probabilistic expected values of each observation. By allowing spatial correlation between observations, observed spatial similarity in observations may be due to a spatial trend, spatial autocorrelation, or both. Second, a set of correlated observations contains less statistical information than the same number of independent observations. Cressie (1993, pp. 14–15) provides an example of the reduction in *effective sample size* induced by increasing spatial autocorrelation. The result is a reduction in statistical precision in estimation and prediction from a given sample size of correlated data compared to what we would see in the same sample size of independent observations (e.g., confidence intervals based on independent observations are too narrow to reflect the appropriate uncertainty associated with positively correlated data). Ultimately, all statistical methods for spatial data have to take the spatial arrangement, and the resulting correlations, of the observations into consideration in order to provide accurate, meaningful conclusions.

1.3 INTERSECTION OF THREE FIELDS OF STUDY

We focus this book on statistical methods and assume that our readers have a familiarity with basic probabilistic concepts (e.g., expectation, variance, covariance, and distributions) and with statistical methods such as linear and logistic regression (including multivariate regression). Most of the methods presented in the book

Table 1.1 Representative List of Journals That Regularly Contain Articles on Spatial Statistical Methods Useful in the Analysis of Public Health Data

Field of Study	Journals
Statistics/Biostatistics	*Applied Statistics* *Biometrics* *Biometrika* *Environmetrics* *Journal of the American Statistical Association* *Journal of the Royal Statistical Society, Series A* *Journal of the Royal Statistical Society, Series B* *Statistics in Medicine* *Statistical Methods in Medical Research*
Epidemiology	*American Journal of Epidemiology* *Epidemiology* *International Journal of Epidemiology* *Journal of Epidemiology and Community Health*
Geography/Geology	*Annals of the Association of American Geographers* *Environment and Planning A* *Health and Place* *International Journal of Geographic Information Science* *Journal of Geographical Systems* *Mathematical Geology* *Social Science and Medicine*

build from these concepts and extend them as needed to address non-Gaussian distributions, transformations, and correlation assumptions.

Even though our focus is on statistical methods, we recognize that the analysis of spatially referenced public health data involves the intersection of at least three traditionally separate academic disciplines: statistics, epidemiology, and geography. Each field offers key insights into the spatial analysis of public health data, and as a result, the literature spans a wide variety of journals within each subject area. Table 1.1 lists several journals that regularly contain articles relating to the spatial analysis of health data.

Although by no means exhaustive, the journals listed in Table 1.1 provide a convenient entry point to the relevant literature. In our experience, journal articles tend to reference within a subject area more often than between subject areas, so searches across disciplines will probably reveal a wider variety of related articles than searches conducted on journals within a single discipline.

At times, the relationship between statistics and the fields of both epidemiology and geography is less than cordial. Often, a backlash occurs when statisticians attempt to transfer a family of methods wholesale into a new area of application without input from the subject-matter experts regarding the appropriateness of assumptions, the availability of requisite data, and even the basic questions of interest. We refer readers interested in such debates to Bennett and Haining (1985),

Openshaw (1990), and Rothman and Greenland (1998, Chapters 2 and 12). As always, there are two sides to the story. An equal amount of criticism also occurs when epidemiologists and geographers use and extend statistical methods without fully appreciating the assumptions behind them or the theoretical foundations on which their validity is based. Often, this just results in inefficiency (and underutilized and annoyed statisticians!) but there are times when it also produces strange inconsistencies in analytical results and erroneous or unsubstantiated conclusions. As applied spatial statisticians, we appreciate both sides and attempt to walk a fine line between emphasizing important assumptions and theoretical results and focusing on practical applications and meaningful research questions of interest.

1.4 ORGANIZATION OF THE BOOK

Many spatial statistics books (e.g., Upton and Fingleton 1985; Cressie 1993; Bailey and Gatrell 1995) organize methods based on the type of spatial data available. Thus, they tend to have chapters devoted to the analysis of spatially continuous data (e.g., elevation and temperature, where we can potentially observe a point anywhere on Earth), chapters devoted to statistical methods for analyzing random locations of events (e.g., disease cases), and chapters devoted to the analysis of *lattice data*, a term used for data that are spatially discrete (e.g., county-specific mortality rates, population data).

Although the data type does determine the applicable methods, our focus on health data suggests an alternative organization. Due to the variety of disciplines interested in the spatial analysis of public health data, we organize our chapters based on particular questions of interest. In order to provide some common ground for readers from different fields of study, we begin with brief introductions to epidemiologic phrases and concepts, components and sources of spatial data, and mapping and cartography. As statisticians, we focus on reviews of statistical methods, taking care to provide ongoing illustrations of underlying concepts through *data breaks* (brief applications of methods to common data sets within the chapters outlining methodologies). We organize the methods in Chapters 2–9 based on the underlying questions of interest:

- *Chapter 2*: introduction to public health concepts and basic analytic tools (*What are the key elements of epidemiologic analysis?*)
- *Chapter 3*: background on spatial data, basic cartographic issues, and geographic information systems (*What are the sources and components of spatial data, and how are these managed?*)
- *Chapter 4*: visualization of spatial data and introductory mapping concepts (*How do we map data effectively to explore patterns and communicate results?*)
- *Chapter 5*: introduction to the underlying mathematics for spatial point patterns (*How do we describe patterns mathematically in spatially random events?*)

- *Chapter 6*: methods for assessing unusual spatial clustering of disease in point data (*How do we tests for clusters in collections of point locations for disease cases?*)
- *Chapter 7*: methods for assessing spatial clustering in regional count data (*How do we test for clusters in counts of disease cases from geographically defined areas?*)
- *Chapter 8*: methods for exposure assessment and the analysis of environmental data (*How do we spatially interpolate measurements taken at given locations to predict measurements at nonmeasured locations?*)
- *Chapter 9*: methods for regression modeling using spatially referenced data (*How do we quantify associations between spatially referenced health outcomes and exposures?*)

Collectively, we hope these questions and the methodology described and illustrated in each chapter will provide the reader with a good introduction to applied spatial analysis of public health data.

CHAPTER 2

Analyzing Public Health Data

Disease generally begins that equality which death completes.
Samuel Johnson (London, September 1, 1750),
quoted in the *Columbia Encyclopedia*

Any important disease whose causality is murky, and for which treatment is ineffectual, tends to be awash in significance.
Susan Sontag, *Illness as Metaphor*, 1979, Vintage Books, Ch. 8

The results of studies of health and related risk factors permeate the public health literature and the popular press. We often read of associations between particular diseases (e.g., cancers, asthma) and various "exposures" ranging from levels of various environmental pollutants, to lifestyle factors such as diet, to the socioeconomic status of persons at risk. Although some studies involve carefully controlled experiments with random assignment of exposures to individuals, many involve *observational* data, where we observe disease outcomes and exposures among a subset of the population and want to draw inferences based on the patterns observed.

The analysis of public health data typically involves the concepts and tools of *epidemiology*, defined by MacMahon and Pugh (1970) as the study of the distribution and determinants of disease frequency. In this chapter we provide a brief review of assumptions and features of public health data, provide an outline of the basic toolbox for epidemiological analysis, and indicate several inferential challenges involved in the statistical analysis of such data.

2.1 OBSERVATIONAL VS. EXPERIMENTAL DATA

In most cases, epidemiological analyses are based on observations of disease occurrence in a population of people "at risk." Typically, we want to relate occurrence patterns between collections of people experiencing different levels of exposure to some factor having a putative impact on a person's risk of disease. Such *observational studies* differ in several important ways from *experimental studies* common in other fields of scientific inquiry. First, experimental studies attempt to control all factors that may modify the association under study, while observational studies

Applied Spatial Statistics for Public Health Data, by Lance A. Waller and Carol A. Gotway
ISBN 0-471-38771-1

cannot. Second, most experimental studies randomize assignment of the factors of interest to experimental units to minimize the impact of any noncontrolled concomitant variables that may affect the relationship under study. Observational studies step in where experimental studies are infeasible due to expense or ethical concerns. For example, studying a very rare disease experimentally often involves huge recruitment costs; withholding a treatment with measurable impact often violates ethical research standards. Whereas controlled randomization of assignment of a potential treatment within the confines of a clinical trial may be a justifiable use of human experimentation, random assignment of exposure to a suspected carcinogen for the purposes of determining toxicity is not.

The presence of controlled environments and randomization in experimental studies aims to focus interpretation on a particular association while limiting the impact of alternative causes and explanations. Observational studies require more care in analysis and interpretation, since controlled environments and randomization often are not possible. Consequently, observational studies involve potential for a wide variety of misinterpretation. The nature of observational studies, particularly of epidemiological studies in the investigation of determinants of disease, provides a framework for interpretation for most spatial analyses of public health data. Central to this framework is the quantification of patterns in the frequency of disease occurrence among members of the population under observation.

2.2 RISK AND RATES

The study of disease in a population begins by addressing the occurrence of a particular outcome in a particular population over a particular time. A common goal of an epidemiological study is to determine associations between patterns of disease occurrence and patterns of exposure to hypothesized risk factors. Due to the central nature of disease occurrence summaries in epidemiology, the related literature contains very specific nomenclature for such summaries. We outline the basic ideas here, referring interested readers to epidemiology texts such as Selvin (1991, Chapter 1) or Rothman and Greenland (1998, Chapter 3) and the references therein for more detailed discussion.

2.2.1 Incidence and Prevalence

The first distinction contrasts disease incidence and disease prevalence. *Incidence* refers to the occurrence of *new* cases within a specified time frame and provides a view of onset within a relatively narrow window of time. *Prevalence* refers to the total number of *existing* cases over a specific time frame and provides a summary of the current burden of the disease under study within the population. For a given disease, incidence and prevalence differ when diseased individuals survive for long periods of time, so that prevalent cases include people who recently contracted the disease (incident cases) and people who contracted the disease some time ago. For diseases with a high likelihood of subsequent mortality in a relatively short time span, incidence and prevalence will be similar. Most epidemiological applications favor incidence over prevalence as an outcome in order to assess factors influencing disease onset, since both onset and duration influence prevalence. However, in cases where onset is difficult to ascertain (e.g., congenital malformations, infection with HIV), researchers may use prevalence coupled with assumptions regarding disease duration as a surrogate for incidence (Rothman and Greenland 1998, pp. 44–45).

2.2.2 Risk

The *risk* of contracting a disease represents the probability of a person contracting the disease within a specified period. We stress that in this context, risk is an attribute of a person, determined and modified by characteristics such as age, gender, occupation, and diet, among other *risk factors*. Risk is an unobserved and dynamic quantity that we, the researchers, wish to estimate. A primary goal of an epidemiological study is to summarize the level of risk of a particular disease in a particular population at a particular time. Associated with this goal is that of identifying factors influencing risk, and quantifying their impact, through observation of disease occurrence within a study population. The statistical question becomes one of estimating risk and related interpretable quantities from observations taken across this study population.

2.2.3 Estimating Risk: Rates and Proportions

In general use the term *rate* defines the number of occurrences of some defined event per unit time. However, application to disease incidence raises some complications, and the epidemiologic literature is quite specific in definitions of disease rates (Elandt-Johnson 1975; Rothman and Greenland 1998, pp. 31–37). Unfortunately, the literature on spatial data analysis applied to health data is not similarly specific, resulting in some potential for misunderstanding and misinterpretation. Although we review relevant issues here, our use of the term *disease rate* in this book falls somewhere between the strict epidemiologic definition(s), and the general use in the spatial epidemiological literature, for reasons outlined below.

In an observational setting, subjects under study may not be at risk for identical times. People move from the study area, are lost to follow-up, or die of causes unrelated to the disease under study. As a result, the epidemiological definition of *incidence rate* is the number of incident (new) cases observed in the study population during the study period divided by the sum of each person's observation time. We often refer to the denominator as a measure of *person-time*, reflecting the summation of times over the persons under observation. Rothman and Greenland (1998, p. 31) note that person-time differs from calendar time in that person-time reflects time summed over several people during the same calendar time rather than a sequential observation of people. In epidemiological studies of chronic, nonrecurring diseases, a person's contribution to person-time ends at onset, since at that point, the person is no longer among the population of people at risk for contracting the disease.

Under the person-time definition, a disease rate is not an estimate of disease risk. In fact, the person-time rate is expressed in inverse time units (often written as "cases/person-year") and, technically, has no upper limit. Although a population of 100 persons can only experience 100 cases of a nonrecurring disease, these cases could happen within any person-time period (e.g., 10, 100, or 10,000 person-years), affecting the magnitude of the incidence rate.

In contrast to the precise epidemiological use of *rate*, the spatial epidemiology literature (including journals in statistics, biostatistics, and geography) tends to use *disease rate* to refer to the number of incident cases expected per *person* rather than per unit of *person-time*. That is, this use of *disease rate* refers to the total number of cases observed divided by the total number of people at risk, both within a fixed time interval. Technically, this usage corresponds to a incidence *proportion* rather than a *rate*, but is very common because this incidence proportion is a population-based estimate of (average) individual risk within the study population. We note that the time interval provides critical context to interpretation of an incidence proportion, as we expect very different values from data collected over a single year and that collected over a decade (since the numerator of the ratio increases each year but the number at risk is fairly stable and often assumed constant).

The primary differences between the incidence proportion and the incidence rate lie in assumptions regarding each person's contribution to the denominator of the ratio under consideration. In a closed population (no people added to or removed from the at-risk population during the study period) where all subjects contribute the same observation time, the incidence proportion would be equal to the incidence rate multiplied by the length of the (common) observation time for each person. Some difference between the two quantities always remains since a person stops contributing person-time to the denominator of the incidence rate the moment that person contracts the disease. However, this difference between the incidence rate and incidence proportion diminishes with rare diseases in the population at risk and/or short observation time per person (i.e., with less loss of observed person-time per diseased person). This feature represents one of several instances outlined in this chapter where the assumption of a *rare disease* (disease with low individual risk) provides convenient numerical approximations. (See the exercises at the end of this chapter to assess the impact of the precise rarity of a disease on the performance of some approximations.)

For the remainder of the book we take care to clarify our use of the term *disease rate* in any given instance. In most cases we follow the spatial literature in using the term to refer to incidence proportion and appeal to an assumption of a rare disease to justify this use for most of our examples. However, applications of the spatial statistical techniques outlined in subsequent chapters to more common diseases require a more careful wording and interpretation of results.

2.2.4 Relative and Attributable Risks

Incidence proportions provide an estimate of the average disease risk experienced by members of a study population. Often, analytic interest centers around comparing risks between individuals with and without a certain exposure. We define the term *exposure* broadly to include both doses of a particular substance and general lifestyle patterns (e.g., age, smoking, a certain type of occupation, number of children). For simplicity, we discuss the impact of a binary exposure, so we partition our study population into exposed and nonexposed subgroups. Two common methods for comparing risk estimates between these two subgroups are to compare *risk differences* or *risk ratios*, defined as their names suggest. These two quantities address the additive and multiplicative impact of exposure, respectively. The literature often refers to the risk difference as the *attributable risk* since it defines the (additive) impact to a person's total risk that is attributable to the exposure under study. Similarly, risk ratios define the *relative risk* or the multiplicative impact of the exposure on a person's risk of disease. The epidemiologic and public health literature, as well as the press, tends to favor reporting relative risk estimates due to ease of communication (e.g., "a 0.000567 increase in risk" versus "a 22% increase in risk") and due to ease of estimation, as outlined in the sections below.

2.3 MAKING RATES COMPARABLE: STANDARDIZED RATES

Most diseases affect people of certain ages disproportionately. In general, there is an increasing incidence of cancer with age, with marked increases for ages greater than 40 years. Since incidence proportions reflect estimated average risks for a study population, populations containing more people in higher age ranges will have higher summary incidence proportions and rates than those of younger populations. As a result, the incidence proportion for two regions may appear different, but this difference may be due entirely to the different age distributions within the regions rather than to a difference in the underlying age-specific risk of disease. *Rate standardization* offers a mechanism to adjust summary rates to remove the effect of known risk factors (such as age) and make rates from different populations comparable.

As an example of the need for rate standardization, consider the population proportions for two hypothetical counties shown in Figure 2.1. We use the same age-specific disease rates for both counties. The age-specific rates on leukemia incidence correspond to those reported by the U.S. National Cancer Institute through the Surveillance Epidemiology and End Results (SEER) cancer registries (Horm et al. 1984), but the age distributions are entirely hypothetical. If both counties have 10,000 residents but different age distributions, we expect more cases for the county represented in the lower plot since this county has more residents in the higher-age (and higher-risk) categories.

The number of cases expected in a region is clearly a function of the age distribution of the population at risk. The question then becomes: How do we compare observed rates from regions with different age distributions?

A common option is *rate standardization*, a method by which analysts select a *standard population* and adjust observed rates to reflect the age distribution within

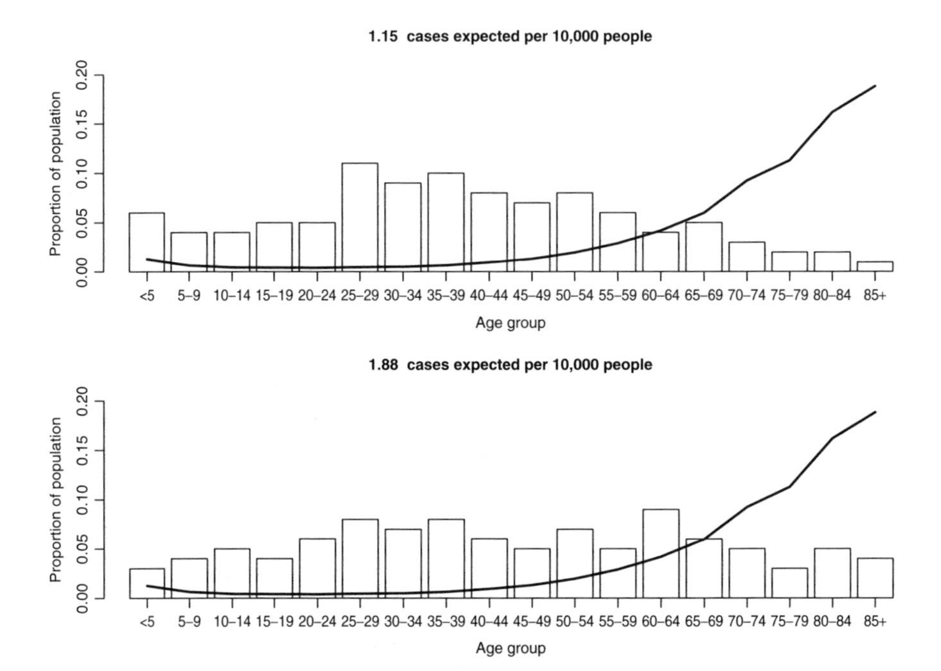

FIG. 2.1 Hypothetical example illustrating the impact of different age distributions on the number of cases expected based on age-specific incidence proportions. Bar heights represent population proportions, and the black line is proportional to the age-specific incidence of leukemia (all types) observed in the Surveillance Epidemiology and End Results (SEER) study from 1978–1981 (see text).

the standard population. Possible standard populations include a superpopulation containing the study population (e.g., the population reported by a national census) and the total subpopulation (if we are interested in standardizing some subset of individuals, for example, from a particular region within the study area). In the United States, researchers often use the 1940, the 1970, and increasingly, the 2000 decennial census values to represent a standard population.

Statistically, rate standardization amounts to taking a weighted average of observed age group–specific rates where the weights relate the age distribution in the study population to that in the standard population. Standardization typically involves adjusting observed rates to reflect rates and counts that we would observe if either the observed age-specific rates (proportions) applied to the standard population or the population standard's age-specific rates (proportions) applied to the study population. The literature refers to the former approach as *direct age standardization* (we apply the observed age-specific rates *directly* to the standard population) and to the latter approach as *indirect age standardization* (we use age-specific rates from the standard population to estimate *indirectly* the numbers of cases expected in each age group in the study population observed).

We detail direct and indirect age standardization in the following two sections. To set notation, suppose that we have J age groups. Let y_j and n_j denote the number of cases and the number of people at risk in age group j for the *study population observed*, respectively, where $j = 1, \ldots, J$. Define $r_j = y_j/n_j$ to be the observed incidence proportion in age group j. Similarly, let $y_j^{(s)}$, $n_j^{(s)}$, and $r_j^{(s)}$ denote the number of cases, number of people at risk in age group j, and the observed incidence proportion for the *standard population*. Finally, let

$$y_+ = \sum_{j=1}^{J} y_j$$

$$y_+^{(s)} = \sum_{j=1}^{J} y_j^{(s)}$$

$$n_+ = \sum_{j=1}^{J} n_j$$

and

$$n_+^{(s)} = \sum_{j=1}^{J} n_j^{(s)}.$$

2.3.1 Direct Standardization

Direct standardization seeks to answer the question: How many cases would we observe in the standard population if the observed age-specific rates of disease applied? (Mausner and Kramer 1985, p. 339). That is, we seek to translate the observed incidence to what would be observed in our standard set of persons at risk. Direct standardization requires the following data (Inskip 1998, p. 4239):

- Age-specific rates (incidence proportions) for the study population observed, $r_j = y_j/n_j$, $j = 1, \ldots, J$
- Number of people at risk in the standard population, $n_j^{(s)}$
- Total number of cases observed in the standard population, $y_+^{(s)}$

Applying the age-specific rates from the observed study population to the numbers of people at risk in the standard population gives the age-specific number of cases expected in the standard population, denoted

$$E_j^{(s)} = r_j n_j^{(s)} = \frac{y_j}{n_j} n_j^{(s)}$$

for $j = 1, \ldots, J$. Therefore, the overall expected rate in the standard population is

$$\frac{\sum_{j=1}^{J} E_j^{(s)}}{n_+^{(s)}} = \frac{\sum_{j=1}^{J} r_j n_j^{(s)}}{n_+^{(s)}} = \frac{\sum_{j=1}^{J} (y_j/n_j) n_j^{(s)}}{n_+^{(s)}}. \tag{2.1}$$

Note that equation (2.1) corresponds directly to a weighted average of the age-specific rates observed in the study population, where the weights correspond to the numbers at risk in each age group within the standard population.

In addition to the directly standardized rate defined in equation (2.1), we could compare the number of cases expected in the standard population ($\sum_j E_j^{(s)}$) to the number observed ($y_+^{(s)}$). Their ratio defines the *comparative mortality figure* (CMF) (Inskip 1998, pp. 4239–4240):

$$\text{CMF} = \frac{\sum_j E_j^{(s)}}{y_+^{(s)}}.$$

Note that the directly standardized rate is simply the crude incidence proportion in the standard population multiplied by the CMF, since

$$\text{CMF}\frac{y_+^{(s)}}{n_+^{(s)}} = \frac{\sum_j E_j^{(s)}}{n_+^{(s)}}.$$

Direct standardization requires accurate assessment of the age-specific incidence proportions for the study population observed. For rare diseases, the incidence proportions observed, $r_j = y_j/n_j$, may be statistically unstable, particularly if n_j is small, in that the addition or deletion of a single case within a particular age group could drastically change the value of r_j. Often, the standard population is much larger and the values $r_j^{(s)} = y_j^{(s)}/n_j^{(s)}$ may provide more stable estimates of age-specific incidence proportions. In addition, age-specific incidence counts ($y_j, j = 1, \ldots, J$) may not be as readily available as the total observed incidence count (y_+) and the age-specific population counts ($n_j, j = 1, \ldots, J$) within the study population observed, due to confidentiality issues or simply due to data limitations. In such cases, direct standardization is not available and we turn to indirect methods.

2.3.2 Indirect Standardization

Indirect standardization reverses the roles of the study population observed and the standard population and seeks to answer the question: What would be the number of cases expected in the study population if people in the study population contracted the disease at the same rate as people in the standard population? (Mausner and Kramer 1985, p. 341). As a mirror image of direct standardization, indirect standardization requires data reversing the roles of the study population observed and the standard population (Inskip 1998, p. 4239):

- Age-specific rates (incidence proportions) for the standard population, $r_j^{(s)} = y_j^{(s)}/n_j^{(s)}, j = 1, \ldots, J$
- Number of people at risk in the study population observed, n_j
- Total number of cases observed in the study population observed, y_+

The first two items allow calculation of the number of cases expected in age group j in the study population observed when the age-specific incidence proportions apply:

$$E_j = r_j^{(s)} n_j = \frac{y_j^{(s)}}{n_j^{(s)}} n_j$$

for $j = 1, \ldots, J$. Then the total number of cases expected in the study population observed (using the age-specific rates from the standard population) is

$$E_+ = \sum_{j=1}^{J} E_j = \sum_{j=1}^{J} r_j^{(s)} n_j = \sum_{j=1}^{J} \frac{y_j^{(s)}}{n_j^{(s)}} n_j.$$

The most common application of indirect standardization compares the number of cases observed in the study population, y_+, to the number of cases expected using age-specific rates from the standard population, E_+, through the *standardized mortality ratio* (SMR), where

$$\text{SMR} = y_+/E_+.$$

Some texts refer to the *standardized incidence ratio* (SIR) when referring to incidence rather than mortality, but the term *SMR* is widely used for both mortality and morbidity (including incidence), and we use SMR throughout the remainder of the text. SMR values greater than 1.0 indicate more cases observed in the observed study population than expected based on the age-specific incidence proportions from the standard population. Often, analysts report the SMR in percentage units by multiplying the ratio by 100.

Multiplication of the SMR and the crude rate in the standard population provides the standardized rate indirectly:

$$\text{SMR} \frac{y_+^{(s)}}{n_+^{(s)}}.$$

Note that by convention and due to the alternating roles of the observed study population and the standard population, the SMR has observed totals in the numerator, and (indirectly) standardized expectations in the denominator, but the CMF has observed totals in the denominator and (directly) standardized expectations in the numerator.

2.3.3 Direct or Indirect?

The statistical and epidemiologic literature contains many discussions of the relative merits of direct and indirect standardization [see Fleiss (1981, Chapter 14), Tukey (1988), and Selvin (1991, pp. 29–35) for discussion and related references]. To better see the underlying difference between direct and indirect standardized rates, Pickle and White (1995) suggest rewriting the indirectly standardized rate as follows:

$$\text{SMR}\ \frac{y_+^{(s)}}{n_+^{(s)}} = \frac{\sum_{j=1}^{J}(y_j/n_j)n_j \Big/ \sum_{j=1}^{J} n_j}{\sum_{j=1}^{J}(y_j^{(s)}/n_j^{(s)})n_j \Big/ \sum_{j=1}^{J} n_j} \ \frac{\sum_{j=1}^{J}(y_j^{(s)}/n_j^{(s)})n_j^{(s)}}{\sum_{j=1}^{J} n_j^{(s)}}.$$

The expansion of the SMR (left-hand component on the right-hand side of the equation) reflects a ratio of weighted averages where the crude rates in both the observed study population and the standard population are weighted by the observed study population's age structure. The right-hand component is a weighted average of the crude rate in the standard population with weights based on the age structure of the standard population. The reexpression of the SMR implies that weights differ for each study population considered, unlike directly standardized rates, where the weights depend on the standard population.

The dependence of indirect standardization on the age structure of the study population raises the question of the comparability between indirectly standardized rates calculated for different study populations (e.g., for different geographic regions). Pickle and White (1995, pp. 617–618) outline the following conditions under any one of which direct and indirect standardization produce identical (or at least proportional) results:

1. If the proportional population distribution of the study population is identical to that of the standard population (i.e., $n_j/n_+ = n_j^{(s)}/n_+^{(s)}$, for $j = 1, \ldots, J$).
2. If the age-specific rates in the study population are identical to those in the standard population (i.e., $r_j = r_j^{(s)}$ for $j = 1, \ldots, J$). In this case, both direct and indirect standardized rates reduce to the crude rates from the study population.
3. If the age-specific rates are proportional to those in the standard population (i.e., $r_j = \alpha r_j^{(s)}$ for some constant α), the indirectly standardized rate equals the crude rate in the standard population times α.

Conditions 1 and 2 reflect rather idealized situations and most applications of indirectly standardized rates appeal to condition 3. As an illustration, suppose that we wish to compare indirectly standardized rates from two counties, where we use the same standard population for each county. Under condition 3 we assume that the age-specific rates within the study population of each county are multiples of the corresponding rates in the (common) standard population. While the constant of proportionality (α) may differ between counties, it remains constant across age categories within each county. That is, if the incidence proportion for ages 0–5 years was 1.5 times that of the standard population for the same age group for the first county, we assume that the incidence proportion for all other age groups in that county are 1.5 times the corresponding rate in the standard population. If we also assume that age-specific incidence proportions for the second county are proportional to those in the standard population (perhaps by a constant of proportionality other than 1.5), we may safely compare the two counties' indirectly standardized rates.

Condition 3 is termed the *product model* (cf. Breslow and Day 1975; Gail 1978) and often motivates the use of an *internal standard population* consisting of age-specific rates from a superpopulation containing the regions (e.g., counties) to compare rather than an *external standard* based on individuals from an entirely separate population. In particular, if we wish to compare indirectly standardized rates between counties within the same state, we may wish to use data from the entire state as the standard population to obtain a standardized rate for each county. Note that proportionality is not guaranteed by the use of an internal standard (Freeman and Holford 1980, p. 198), for instance, if a county has a higher incidence rate than the standard population for a few but not all age groups. Gail (1978) offers statistical tests of the multiplicity assumption in condition 3. Gail (1978, p. 226) also suggests a graphical test of the proportionality assumption. If r_{ij} denotes the incidence proportion observed in age group j for region i ($i = 1, \ldots, I$ and $j = 1, \ldots, J$), plot j versus $\ln(r_{ij})$ and connect all points corresponding to each $i, i = 1, \ldots, I$. Under condition 3 (the product model), the curves corresponding to each region i should be parallel to each other and to the curve corresponding to $\ln(r_j^{(s)})$, subject to some random variability.

In practice, the choice between direct or indirect standardization often reduces to the type of data available. If age-specific incidence counts are unavailable for the study population but age-specific rates are available for a standard population, indirect standardization offers the only option available.

2.3.4 Standardizing to What Standard?

The analyst must also choose a population standard. As mentioned in the preceding section, one often uses marginal (aggregate) standards in indirect standardization and assumes proportionality to obtain comparable indirectly standardized rates. The inherent comparability of directly standardized rates offers us a wider choice in standards, but increased choice does not mean decreased dependence on the choice of standard. Krieger and Williams (2001) comment on the impact of changing from the 1940 standard population to the 2000 standard population in reference to measures of health disparities and inequalities between sociodemographic subgroups. In a related commentary, Pamuk (2001) provides a brief but thorough history and overview of the use of standardization in reporting summaries of vital statistics (particularly mortality data) and raises several important points. Foremost among these is the trade-off between the simplicity of summarizing information across age groups and the implicitly associated loss of information (i.e., we give up age-specific information in order to provide an age-standardized statistic summarizing across age categories).

In addition to age standardization, we could also standardize rates to compensate for other risk strata (e.g., gender, race, and/or ethnicity). Although examples of such standardization exist, the most common applications of rate standardization involve adjustments for age.

2.3.5 Cautions with Standardized Rates

As illustrated above, the goal of standardizing rates is to provide summaries across groups adjusted for known variations in risk within the structure of the population of interest. Although we illustrate standardization with respect to a single risk factor, the idea extends readily to any collection of risk factors as long as we have the appropriate reference rates and population sizes for each distinct risk category. Standardization seeks to remove variations in summary measures (rates or proportions) due solely to these known risk factors, so any remaining differences suggest risk differences other than those adjusted for.

This said, it is important to note that standardized rates represent *summaries* across population strata experiencing differing risks. As summaries, standardized rates may mask important differences occurring at the stratum level. Fleiss (1981, pp. 239–240) reviews several valid critiques of the use of standardized rates, particularly for violations of the proportionality assumption of condition 3 above. While acknowledging that standardization does not provide a substitute for examining the age (or other stratum-specific) group's specific rates themselves, Fleiss (1981, p. 240) offers three primary reasons for standardization:

1. Comparing single summaries between several study populations (e.g., regions such as counties) rather than comparing tables of age-specific rates is relatively easy.
2. When some age groups contain very small numbers at risk, the age-specific estimates may be too imprecise (statistically unstable) for accurate comparisons.
3. For some subpopulations of particular interest (e.g., members of racial or ethnic minorities), accurate age-specific rates may not exist.

2.4 BASIC EPIDEMIOLOGICAL STUDY DESIGNS

Standardization provides a commonly reported means of "adjusting" observed proportions and rates for the presence of known risk factors. Statistical modeling of epidemiological data extends such ideas, allowing estimation of the impact of particular risk factors and their interactions with observed incidence (or prevalence) counts. We next consider the types of data collected in epidemiological studies, followed by a description of the analytical approaches often used to quantify such associations.

At their most basic level, most epidemiological studies seek to quantify the impact of a certain exposure on a certain disease. The simplest case involves a binary exposure and binary disease, where we classify study subjects as either "exposed" or "unexposed" (denoted E^+ or E^-, respectively), and "diseased" or "not diseased" (denoted D^+ or D^-, respectively). The classifications allow construction of the contingency table shown in Table 2.1.

The *design* of the epidemiological study reflects the manner in which we observe individuals in order to fill in n_{++}, n_{-+}, n_{+-}, and n_{--} in Table 2.1. As mentioned

Table 2.1 Basic Epidemiological Contingency Table Cross-Classifying the Study Population

	E^+	E^-
D^+	n_{++}	n_{-+}
D^-	n_{+-}	n_{--}

above, most epidemiological studies are *observational* rather than *experimental*, in that the researcher observes rather than assigns the exposures of interest (often for ethical reasons).

2.4.1 Prospective Cohort Studies

The *cohort study* is the observational analog to an experiment where the researcher defines two groups, or *cohorts*, of disease-free individuals similar in all respects except for exposure status, then follows the groups over time (i.e., *prospectively*, or forward through time) and observes disease status among subjects within each group. Note that the only difference between such a *prospective cohort study* and a large experimental clinical trial is that in the former the researcher has no control over assignment into exposure groups. Also note that a prospective cohort study fixes the marginal total numbers in groups E^+ and E^- ($n_{++} + n_{+-}$ and $n_{-+} + n_{--}$, respectively), allowing us to estimate relative or attributable risks by comparing incidence proportions between the two groups using

$$\frac{n_{++}}{n_{++} + n_{+-}} \quad \text{and} \quad \frac{n_{-+}}{n_{-+} + n_{--}}.$$

Note that for rare diseases we may need very large numbers of exposed and unexposed subjects to observe even a single case, let alone enough to provide statistical stability in estimating the underlying disease incidence via the incidence proportions observed in each group. In addition, if we suspect a long lag period between exposure and disease onset, we may need to follow our cohort for an extended period. Since rare diseases (e.g., cancers) are often of interest in epidemiological studies, alternative approaches for filling in the cells in Table 2.1 may prove more time- and cost-efficient.

2.4.2 Retrospective Case–Control Studies

A common alternative to prospective cohort studies are *case–control studies*, where we choose a sample of ($n_{-+} + n_{++}$) diseased persons (*cases*), then choose a sample of ($n_{--} + n_{+-}$) nondiseased persons (*controls*) similar to the cases in risk factors not of primary interest (e.g., age), and classify the cases and controls by each person's past (i.e., *retrospective*) exposure status. In contrast to the cohort study, where we fixed the total number exposed and unexposed, in case–control studies we fix the number of diseased and nondiseased (i.e., we fix a different set of marginal totals in Table 2.1 under each design).

Note that under the case–control design, we can determine the proportions exposed among cases and controls directly, but not the incidence proportions for exposed and unexposed. We can, however, estimate relative measures of incidence between exposed and unexposed subjects, as outlined in Section 2.5.

2.4.3 Other Types of Epidemiological Studies

Prospective cohort and retrospective case–control studies provide the basis for the large majority of epidemiological studies. However, there are many variations on these themes. For example, we could define a *retrospective cohort* design based on cohorts identified in the past and followed to the present. Such studies frequently occur in occupational settings where cohorts of workers and company medical records provide relevant documentation.

In addition to prospective and retrospective designs, there are also *cross-sectional designs* where we determine disease and exposure status at a single time. Such studies provide estimates of disease prevalence rather than incidence and can be biased toward the prevalence of long-lasting cases rather than all cases (since people surviving with the disease longer have a greater chance of being selected at any given point in time than people experiencing a short time between diagnosis and death). In cross-sectional studies, neither the total number of diseased and nondiseased nor the total number of exposed and unexposed is considered fixed.

For our purposes, the notions of prospective cohort and retrospective case–control studies provide a basis for analysis of observational epidemiological data. The data sets in this book reflect both sorts of study designs and some cross-sectional data as well. See Rothman and Greenland (1998, Chapters 5–7) for a fuller discussion of the advantages and limitations of these and other types of epidemiological studies, as well as additional references to the relevant literature.

2.5 BASIC ANALYTIC TOOL: THE ODDS RATIO

The analytic purpose of an epidemiologic study is to quantify any observable difference in disease risk between the exposed and unexposed subjects in the study. As mentioned in Section 2.2.4, a common measure of risk difference is the *relative risk* or ratio of disease risk in the exposed population at risk to the disease risk in the unexposed population. A prospective cohort design allows us to estimate both the attributable risk (the risk difference) and the relative risk (the multiplicative increase or decrease in risk) associated with exposure, using incidence proportions as estimates of risk based on the rare disease assumption. However, accurate statistical estimation of incidence proportions (and associated asymptotic normality of the estimators) for rare diseases can require very large sample sizes.

In comparison, case–control studies allow direct frequency-based estimation of the probability of exposure given disease status [Pr(exposure|disease)] rather then the quantity of interest (i.e., the probability of disease status given exposure [Pr(disease|exposure)]). As above, we denote the presence and absence of disease and the presence and absence of exposure by D^+, D^-, E^+, and E^-, respectively. We could use Bayes' theorem to reverse the order of the conditional probability:

$$\Pr(D^+|E^+) = \frac{\Pr(E^+|D^+)\Pr(D^+)}{\Pr(E^+)},$$

but this requires accurate estimates of the marginal probabilities of disease and of exposure in the population for which we wish to draw inference [$\Pr(D^+)$ and $\Pr(E^+)$, respectively]. We may have estimates of the former from national health surveys or disease registries, but such estimates of the latter are rarely available.

However, a case–control study readily provide estimates of $\Pr(E^+|D^+)$ and $\Pr(E^+|D^-)$, so expanding $\Pr(E^+)$ via the law of total probability yields

$$\Pr(D^+|E^+) = \frac{\Pr(E^+|D^+)\Pr(D^+)}{\Pr(E^+|D^+)\Pr(D^+) + \Pr(E^+|D^-)\Pr(D^-)},$$

and similarly,

$$\Pr(D^+|E^-) = \frac{\Pr(E^-|D^+)\Pr(D^+)}{\Pr(E^-|D^+)\Pr(D^+) + \Pr(E^-|D^-)\Pr(D^-)}$$

(Neutra and Drolette 1978; Kleinbaum et al. 1982, p. 146). Given an estimate of $\Pr(D^+)$, we have the necessary components to build an estimate of the relative risk, RR, by substituting estimates for each component in

$$\begin{aligned}\text{RR} &= \frac{\Pr(D^+|E^+)}{\Pr(D^+|E^-)}\\ &= \frac{\Pr(E^+|D^+)}{\Pr(E^-|D^+)}\,\frac{\Pr(E^-|D^+)\Pr(D^+) + \Pr(E^-|D^-)\Pr(D^-)}{\Pr(E^+|D^+)\Pr(D^+) + \Pr(E^+|D^-)\Pr(D^-)}.\end{aligned}$$

For a very rare disease, $\Pr(D^+) \approx 0$, $\Pr(D^-) \approx 1$, and

$$\begin{aligned}\text{RR} &\approx \frac{\Pr(E^+|D^+)}{\Pr(E^-|D^+)}\,\frac{\Pr(E^-|D^-)}{\Pr(E^+|D^-)}\\ &= \frac{\Pr(E^+|D^+)/\Pr(E^-|D^+)}{\Pr(E^+|D^-)/\Pr(E^-|D^-)},\end{aligned}$$

which defines the *exposure odds ratio*, the ratio of the *odds* of exposure in the disease population to the odds of exposure in the nondiseased population. (Recall that the *odds* of an event equals the ratio of the probability of the event occurring divided by the probability of the event not occurring.) The exposure odds ratio observed results from inserting the frequency-based estimates of each conditional probability based on Table 2.1:

$$\frac{\dfrac{n_{++}}{(n_{++}+n_{-+})}\left(1-\dfrac{n_{++}}{n_{++}+n_{-+}}\right)}{\dfrac{n_{+-}}{(n_{+-}+n_{--})}\left(1-\dfrac{n_{+-}}{n_{+-}+n_{--}}\right)}=\frac{n_{++}n_{--}}{n_{+-}n_{-+}},$$

recalling that the first subscript of n denotes the exposure status (+ or −), and the second, disease status.

Next, consider the *risk odds ratio observed* from a cohort study based on frequency-based estimates of probabilities $\Pr(D^+|E^+)$ and $\Pr(D^+|E^-)$: namely, estimating

$$\frac{\Pr(D^+|E^+)/\Pr(D^-|E^+)}{\Pr(D^+|E^-)/\Pr(D^-|E^-)}$$

via

$$\frac{\dfrac{n_{++}}{n_{++}+n_{+-}}\left(1-\dfrac{n_{++}}{n_{++}+n_{+-}}\right)}{\dfrac{n_{-+}}{n_{-+}+n_{--}}\left(1-\dfrac{n_{-+}}{n_{-+}+n_{--}}\right)}=\frac{n_{++}n_{--}}{n_{+-}n_{-+}}.$$

Since the exposure odds ratio observed from case–control studies is algebraically equivalent to the risk odds ratio observed from cohort studies, we simply refer to the *odds ratio*, regardless of study type. The similarity between the odds ratio and the risk ratio for rare diseases, and the invariance of the odds ratio observed to the underlying study type, motivate its use as a single, easily calculated quantity summarizing associations between exposure and disease for both prospective cohort and retrospective case–control studies.

See Somes and O'Brien (1985) and Rothman and Greenland (1998, pp. 95–96, 242) for further details regarding calculation and interpretation of the odds ratio in epidemiologic studies.

2.6 MODELING COUNTS AND RATES

Linear regression offers a broad framework for fitting models to data and investigating associations between outcome and any number of explanatory variables, assuming independent error terms, each following an identical Gaussian distribution. Texts such as Neter et al. (1996) and Draper and Smith (1998) provide overviews of applied regression analysis, and we assume familiarity with linear models at this level.

Most analyses of public health data involve disease counts, proportions, or rates as outcome variables rather than the continuous outcomes familiar in linear regression. Whereas large counts or rates may roughly follow the assumptions of linear models, spatial analyses often focus on counts from small areas with relatively few subjects at risk and few cases expected during the study period. Such instances require models appropriate for count or rate outcomes.

2.6.1 Generalized Linear Models

The family of *generalized linear models* (GLMs) provides a collection of models extending basic concepts from linear regression to applications where error terms follow any of a wide variety of distributions, including the binomial and Poisson families for modeling count data.

GLMs consist of a *random component* defining the distribution of error terms, a *systematic component* defining the linear combination of explanatory variables, and a *link function* defining the relationship between the systematic and random components. We define each component here briefly, closely following Agresti (1990, Section 4.1), in order to introduce *logistic regression* and *Poisson regression*, two approaches widely used to model count outcomes in epidemiologic research.

The random component comprises independent outcomes (denoted Y_i for $i = 1, \ldots, n$) from a distribution within the *exponential family* (Cox and Hinkley 1974, pp. 28–29); that is, the probability density or mass function may be expressed in the form

$$f(y_i; \boldsymbol{\theta}_i) = \exp[a(\boldsymbol{\theta}_i) + b(y_i) + y_i Q(\boldsymbol{\theta}_i)],$$

where $a(\cdot)$, $b(\cdot)$, and $Q(\cdot)$ represent arbitrary functions of distributional parameters $\boldsymbol{\theta}_i$, or observed values y_i, as noted. For a vector of independent observed values from the exponential family, we have

$$f(y_1, \ldots, y_n; \boldsymbol{\theta}_1, \ldots, \boldsymbol{\theta}_n) = \exp\left[\sum_{i=1}^{n} a(\boldsymbol{\theta}_i) + \sum_{i=1}^{n} b(y_i) + \sum_{i=1}^{n} y_i Q(\boldsymbol{\theta}_i)\right]. \quad (2.2)$$

Most of the well-known distributional families (e.g., Gaussian, binomial, Poisson, and gamma) fall into the exponential family, so the class of error structures supported within GLMs is quite broad.

The systematic component of the GLM corresponds to $\mathbf{X}\boldsymbol{\beta}$, where $\mathbf{X}$ denotes the design matrix, with each row listing the values of covariates observed corresponding to the observation of y_i, and $\boldsymbol{\beta}$ denotes the vector of model parameters.

The link function $g(\cdot)$ provides a functional connection between the systematic component $X\boldsymbol{\beta}$ and $E(\mathbf{Y})$, the expected value of $\mathbf{Y} = (Y_1, \ldots, Y_n)'$. Specifically,

$$g\,[E(\mathbf{Y})] = \mathbf{X}\boldsymbol{\beta}.$$

The mean, $E(\mathbf{Y})$, is often among the distributional parameters $\boldsymbol{\theta}$ for members of the exponential family, so $Q(\boldsymbol{\theta}_i)$ is often a function of $E(y_i)$. Setting $Q(\boldsymbol{\theta}_i) = \mathbf{X}_i\boldsymbol{\beta}$ (where $\mathbf{X}_i$ denotes row i of the design matrix) results in the *canonical link* for a particular distribution family.

Obtaining estimates (maximum likelihood and otherwise) for GLM parameters ($\boldsymbol{\beta}$) generally requires iterative procedures rather than closed-form solutions for linear models (cf. McCullagh and Nelder 1989, pp. 115–117; Dobson 1990, pp. 39–42). We do not detail these methods here; however, most modern statistical software packages contain routines for fitting GLMs, particularly logistic and Poisson regression. These two families of generalized linear models see wide application in the epidemiological literature. We review logistic and Poisson regression models below and extend them to spatial models in subsequent chapters.

For additional details regarding GLMs, Dobson (1990) provides a general introduction and McCullagh and Nelder (1989) a thorough treatment of the theory and application of GLMs. In addition, O'Brien (1992) describes the use of GLMs in geography.

2.6.2 Logistic Regression

Suppose that we observe binary outcomes y_i, where $y_i = 1$ indicates the presence of the disease of interest in subject i and $y_i = 0$ denotes its absence. Let π denote the (unknown) probability of disease prevalence in the population under study. (We refer to prevalence rather than incidence since we are concerned with presence or absence in this simple example.) The random variable Y_i follows a Bernoulli distribution with probability of disease π. The joint probability associated with the observed data $y_1, \ldots, y_n$ is

$$f(y_1, \ldots, y_n; \pi) = \prod_{i=1}^{n} \pi^{y_i}(1-\pi)^{1-y_i},$$

which may be rewritten as

$$f(y_1, \ldots, y_n; \pi) = \exp\left[\sum_{i=1}^{n} \log(1-\pi) + \sum_{i=1}^{n} y_i \log\left(\frac{\pi}{1-\pi}\right)\right],$$

which, by comparison with equation (2.2), is a member of an exponential family with $\boldsymbol{\theta}_i = \pi$, $a(\boldsymbol{\theta}_i) = \log(1-\pi)$, $b(y_i) = 0$, and $Q(\boldsymbol{\theta}_i) = \log\left[\pi/(1-\pi)\right]$. Here, since $E(Y_i) = \pi$, the canonical link is

$$g(E(y_i)) = g(\pi) = \log[\pi/(1-\pi)],$$

known as the *logit link.*

Logistic regression represents the GLM based on a Bernoulli random component and the logit link; that is, for covariates $x_1, \ldots, x_p$,

$$\begin{aligned} \log[\pi/(1-\pi)] &= \beta_0 + \beta_1 x_1 + \cdots + \beta_p x_p \\ &= \mathbf{X}\boldsymbol{\beta}. \end{aligned} \tag{2.3}$$

We often recast equation (2.3) as

$$E(y_i) = \pi = \frac{\exp(\mathbf{X}\boldsymbol{\beta})}{1+\exp(\mathbf{X}\boldsymbol{\beta})},$$

describing the expected value of the outcome as a function of model covariates.

Note that β_k represents the expected change in the log odds of $Y_i = 1$ associated with a unit increase in x_k (holding all other covariate values constant). For a binary covariate x_k (e.g., the presence or absence of a particular exposure indicated by $x_k = 1$ or 0, respectively), $\exp(\beta_k)$ represents the odds ratio of Y_i with respect to exposure x_k, since the odds ratio equals the ratio of the exponentiated right-hand side of equation (2.3) for $x_k = 1$ and $x_k = 0$, and

$$\frac{\exp(\beta_0 + \cdots + \beta_k + \cdots + \beta_p x_p)}{\exp(\beta_0 + \cdots + \beta_{k-1}x_{k-1} + \beta_{k+1}x_{k+1} + \cdots + \beta_p x_p)} = \exp\beta_k.$$

The connection between logistic regression parameters and the odds ratio combined with the properties of the odds ratio described in Section 2.5 implies that logistic regression is appropriate for the analysis of both prospective and retrospective studies. McCullagh and Nelder (1989, pp. 111–114) note that the logit link is unique in this respect among link functions proposed for the analysis of binary data, including the *probit link* common in bioassay (cf. Finney 1971).

Logistic regression also provides an analytic tool for binomial observations where each observation y_i denotes the *number* of people with a particular condition among n_i at risk. For example, suppose that we observe y_i the number of people contracting the disease under investigation among the n_i at risk in geographic region i, where $i = 1, \ldots, I$. Note that in this setting i indexes a *collection* of people rather than each person, as was the case in the Bernoulli model above. As a simple probabilistic model of disease occurrence, suppose that the y_i represent observations of binomially distributed random variables where each person is subject to the same risk of disease, π:

$$Y_i \sim \text{binomial}(n_i, \pi),$$

so $E(Y_i) = n_i\pi$ and $\text{Var}(Y_i) = n_i\pi(1-\pi)$. In addition, suppose that we also observe a set of p covariates $x_{i1}, \ldots, x_{ip}$ in region i and wish to model the disease probability π as a function of these (regional) covariates.

The binomial distribution (corresponding to random variables representing sums of independent Bernoulli observations) is also in the exponential family (Bickel and Doksum 1977, pp. 68–69), also with the logit as its canonical link function. As with the Bernoulli (0/1) case, we model the unknown individual probability of disease incidence, π, where $E(Y_i) = n_i\pi$ and

$$\log\left(\frac{\pi}{1-\pi}\right) = \mathbf{X}\boldsymbol{\beta}.$$

For binary exposure covariates, estimated model parameters again represent the odds ratio associated with the exposure.

2.6.3 Poisson Regression

For rare diseases we often use the Poisson approximation to the binomial distribution in modeling count data. The Poisson distribution also arises from modeling observed point locations as random events, as we will see in Chapter 5. The Poisson distribution is also a member of the exponential family with the natural logarithm as the canonical link function. For regional counts $Y_1, \ldots, Y_I$ independently and identically distributed as Poisson random variables with mean and variance equal to $E(Y_i)$, a *Poisson regression* approach models the expected value as a function of regional covariates:

$$\log[E(Y_i)] = \mathbf{X}\boldsymbol{\beta} \tag{2.4}$$
$$E(Y_i) = \exp(\mathbf{X}\boldsymbol{\beta}).$$

As with logistic regression, β_k represents the increase in log odds associated with a unit increase in x_{ik}, holding all other covariates fixed.

This concludes a very basic overview of generalized linear models. Kleinbaum et al. (1982) and Rothman and Greenland (1998, Chapters 20 and 21) provide much more detail on particular aspects of applying such models in the analysis of observational public health data, and McCullagh and Nelder (1989) give a thorough review of GLMs in general.

2.7 CHALLENGES IN THE ANALYSIS OF OBSERVATIONAL DATA

Linear and generalized linear models provide valuable analytical tools for the analysis of both experimental and observational data. However, special concerns arise in the observational setting that are often not covered in introductory courses and texts on statistical modeling, which often assume an experimental setting in model development and interpretation. We review two issues common in epidemiological analysis but often not addressed in introductory courses in statistical modeling: bias and confounding.

2.7.1 Bias

In an experimental setting, researchers control experimental conditions that could influence the observed associations between treatment and outcome, and assume that the randomized assignment of treatments to experimental subjects (*randomization*) allows unbiased estimation of any uncontrolled conditions affecting the association of interest. That is, by randomly assigning treatments, the experimenter removes (or at least averages out) any potential bias in the estimation due to different levels of some uncontrolled factor. For example, consider a hypothetical clinical study of the treatment of the common cold by a new experimental treatment, compared to "treatment" by a placebo. If we assign the first n patients presenting during an outbreak to the new treatment and the next n to the placebo group, the measured effectiveness of the new treatment could be biased if patients presenting early in the outbreak tended to live healthier lifestyles in general (e.g., more exercise, better diet) than their counterparts who present later in the outbreak. In this case, some unmeasured characteristic (here, lifestyle) affects the composition of the treatment and placebo groups in a manner that will tend to make the treatment appear more effective than it actually is. Contrast the first experimental design to one where patients are randomly allocated to the treatment or control group as they present at the clinic for treatment. In this case, the unmeasured factor (lifestyle) is randomly split between the treatment and control groups and the potential bias disappears with adequate sample size.

Observational studies, by their nature, do not randomize treatment; rather, the researcher observes treatment levels in study participants often for ethical reasons (e.g., it is unethical to randomize subjects to be smokers or nonsmokers, or to participate in occupations with exposures to hazardous materials). As a result, observational studies contain many potential biases in their estimates of associations between treatments (exposures) and outcomes. The epidemiologic literature provides a thorough discussion of many different sources of bias and assigns names to particular types. We review the most common of these and refer readers to Rothman and Greenland (1998, Chapter 8) for more detailed description and discussion.

Selection Bias *Selection bias* results when the relationship between exposure and disease differs for persons participating in the study and those who are theoretically eligible to participate, but do not. Selection bias may result from different exposure–disease associations among subjects who volunteer for a study than among those who do not volunteer. This bias may also result from the *healthy worker effect* (Rothman and Greenland 1998, p. 119), common in occupational studies where exposure–disease associations among workers (who by definition are healthy enough to work) may not accurately reflect those among nonworkers, limiting inference to the study population rather than the population at large. Another form of selection bias results if subjects with certain exposures are more likely to be diagnosed with the outcome of interest than subjects without the exposure.

Recall Bias An example of *recall bias* occurs when diseased subjects are more likely than healthy subjects to recall past exposures. For example, families of childhood leukemia patients may present more detailed recollections of household chemical use than do families of nondiseased children. Recall bias can occur in both case–control studies (the preceding example) and prospective cohort studies (e.g., exposed subjects present more detailed recollection of disease episodes than do unexposed subjects).

Misclassification Bias Incorrect assignment of disease or exposure status for study participants may result in *misclassification bias*. The bias is lessened if misclassification occurs at random between disease and exposure classes, but may be appreciable if misclassification occurs at different rates for different classes. We note some overlap with selection bias and recall bias.

2.7.2 Confounding

Confounding is a central notion in epidemiology, defined as "a distortion in the estimated exposure effect that results from differences in risk between the exposed and unexposed that are not due to exposure" (Rothman and Greenland 1998, p. 255). Confounding involves the biases above, but tends to focus on factors associated with the bias rather than the bias per se. That is, one often refers to *confounding factors* or *confounders* as the source of differential selection, recall, or misclassification. Rothman and Greenland (1998, p. 255) define two necessary conditions for a variable to be a confounder:

1. The variable must be a risk factor for the disease among the unexposed (although it may not cause the disease directly).
2. The variable must be associated with the exposure variable in the population providing study participants.

In our example based on a study of a new treatment for the common cold, with the new treatment assigned to the first n study participants, "healthy lifestyle" acts as a potential confounder since it is a risk factor for the disease (here the "disease" reflects speedy recovery from a cold), and it relates to the assignment of treatment or placebo (the "exposure" of interest).

As another example of confounding, consider the following situation. Suppose that we observe outcomes in subjects experiencing one level of exposure and wish to compare them to unexposed subjects. If the unexposed participants differ from the exposed participants with respect to a factor related to the disease (e.g., age), an estimate of the effect of exposure on outcome by comparisons of outcome proportions in the two exposure groups can (often, will) be different from the true effect (i.e., the estimate is *biased* and *confounded*).

Simple examples based on dichotomous exposures, diseases, and confounders appear in almost any epidemiological textbook (e.g., Kleinbaum et al. 1982; Rothman and Greenland 1998); however, the issue appears in very few statistical texts. One reason for the omission is the traditional focus of statistical texts on experimental design and analysis of randomized experiments rather than observational data. While confounding can arise in randomized designs [e.g., through aliasing, or see Greenland et al. (1999) for other examples], the issue is much more pervasive in the observational setting.

Another reason that statistical texts often omit confounding is the inherent difficulty of formalizing the concept mathematically (cf. Greenland and Robins 1986; Wickramaratne and Holford 1987, 1989, 1990; Greenland 1989, 1998; Holland 1989; Mantel 1989, 1990; Weinberg 1993, 1994; Joffe and Greenland 1994; Greenland et al. 1999). The difficulty arises since the presence or absence of confounding is dependent on the definition of outcome. For instance, Greenland (1998) notes that there are no confounders for the effect of any exposure on 200-year survival. Also, although there are similarities between confounding and the statistical notion of interactions between independent variables, it is possible to have interactions without confounding, confounding without interactions, or confounding with interactions [see Kleinbaum et al. (1982, p. 246) for examples]. Finally, when the outcome, exposure, and potential confounder are categorical variables, confounding is similar to *noncollapsibility* in the analysis of contingency tables. However, the terms are again not equivalent (without further restrictions; see Gail 1986) and it is possible to have either with or without the other [see Greenland and Robins (1986), Greenland (1998), and Greenland et al. (1999) for examples and a more complete discussion].

2.7.3 Effect Modification

If the association between exposure to a putative risk factor and the outcome of interest varies with the level of another variable, we refer to that variable as an *effect modifier*. Effect modification is also referred to as *nonuniformity of effect* and as *heterogeneity of effect*. Kleinbaum et al. (1982, p. 247, Chapter 19) and Rothman and Greenland (1998, p. 254) note that effect modification differs from confounding on several levels. First, confounding represents a bias in effect estimation which we, the analysts, seek to prevent or at least minimize. In contrast, effect modification is a property of the exposure–outcome association under study. Simply put, we seek to control confounding by careful selection and classification of study participants, but we wish to report precisely how an effect modifier changes the association between the exposures and outcome of interest.

2.7.4 Ecological Inference and the Ecological Fallacy

In epidemiology, the term *ecological inference* refers to the process of deducing individual behavior from aggregate data. This term is due to Robinson (1950), who noted that in *ecological studies*, the statistical object is a group of persons. He stressed the difference between ecological and individual correlations, noting that the two are almost certainly not equal, leading him and others to question the results of numerous studies in which conclusions on individual behavior had been drawn from grouped data.

Robinson (1950) provided one very convincing example of the difference between ecological and individual correlations, based on the relationship between nativity and literacy. For each of the lower 48 states in the United States, he measured the percent of the population who were foreign-born and the percent who were literate (based on 1930 data). The correlation based on 48 pairs of points is 0.53. This is an *ecological correlation*, since the unit of analysis is not a person but a group of people—the residents of each state. In reality, however, the association between nativity and literacy is negative: the correlation computed using individuals as the unit of analysis is −0.11. Thus, in this example and in many, if not most, studies based on grouped data, ecological correlations give the wrong individual-level inference. The *ecological fallacy* occurs when analyses based on grouped data lead to conclusions different from those based on individual data (Selvin 1958). The resulting bias is often referred to as *ecological bias* (Richardson 1992; Greenland and Robins 1994), which is comprised of two components: *aggregation bias* due to the grouping of individuals and *specification bias* due to the differential distribution of confounding variables created by grouping (Morgenstern 1982).

Referring back to our basic epidemiological study design in Table 2.1, the contrast between individual and ecological analyses can easily be seen. Individual correlation depends on the internal cell frequencies, n_{++}, n_{-+}, n_{+-}, and n_{--}. Ecological correlation is based on the marginal totals $(n_{++} + n_{-+})$, $(n_{+-} + n_{--})$, $(n_{++} + n_{+-})$, and $(n_{-+} + n_{--})$. The ecological inference problem arises since marginal totals do not uniquely determine the internal cell frequencies: There are many combinations of cell counts that can reproduce the marginal totals. Statistics for individual-level inference, such as risk ratios, odds ratios, and the correlation coefficient (the ϕ coefficient in 2×2 tables), depend on the internal cell counts. Thus, solutions to the ecological inference problem have centered around developing valid methods for reconstructing the internal frequencies from the marginal totals.

One such solution has been called *ecological regression* (Goodman 1959). Suppose that we have I tables like Table 2.1, corresponding to the relationship between exposure and disease in I groups. These groups could be demographic (e.g., race, age) or geographical (e.g., counties, states). A linear regression model relating the proportion of diseased individuals in each group, y_i, to the proportion of people exposed in each group, x_i, may be written as

$$y_i = \beta_0 + \beta_1 x_i + \epsilon, \qquad i = 1, \ldots, I.$$

The parameters β_0 and β_1 can be estimated by least squares (ordinary or weighted). Then the estimate $\hat{\beta}_0$ is an estimate of the proportion of nonexposed persons who contracted the disease: It is the height of the regression equation at $x = 0$, corresponding to groups with no exposed persons. The estimate $\hat{\beta}_0 + \hat{\beta}_1$ (the regression line at $x = 1.0$) is the proportion of exposed persons who contacted the disease. The validity of this model for individual-level inference rests on the implicit assumption the relationship between exposure and disease is constant over the groups, with cell probabilities varying randomly about their expectations.

There are many more recently proposed solutions to the ecological inference problem. One that has received much attention in the literature was proposed by King (1997). He essentially uses linear regression with random coefficients to relax the constancy assumption in Goodman's ecological regression. King's most basic approach is based on the regression model

$$y_i = p_i x_i + q_i(1 - x_i), \qquad i = 1, \ldots, I,$$

where p_i is the proportion of exposed subjects who contracted the disease and q_i is the corresponding proportion for the nonexposed. Assuming that (p_i, q_i) are independent and identically distributed bivariate Gaussian variables, they can be estimated by maximum likelihood. King (1997) has developed more sophisticated models and inferential procedures for more complex problems, and many of these can be implemented using his EI and EZI programs, available from his Web site.

Of course, any solution to the ecological inference problem is only as good as the validity of its assumptions when applied to a given problem. Some assumptions must be made since the data necessary for individual-level inference are simply not available. Freedman et al. (1998) give a comparative overview of several methods for ecological inference and discuss the effect of the assumptions on the estimates and the use of model diagnostics to detect departures from these assumptions.

Ecological analyses can be based on any grouped variables, such as gender, race, or age. However, *geographical correlation studies*, special cases of ecological correlation studies, are concerned with the association between two variables that are averages across geographic regions. Such studies are conducted routinely in the analysis of environmental health data. For example, if we want to study the association between a person's health risk (e.g., thyroid cancer) and exposure to a particular water contaminant (e.g., atrazine from pesticide use), we rarely have the luxury of obtaining individual-level exposure data. It is difficult to measure individual exposures without great expense and inconvenience to the person. Instead, we identify the level of exposure based on average levels in municipal water supplies, estimate the rate of health events in the communities served by the various water supplies, and attempt to link the two on a community-wide, not an individual-level, basis. Inferential problems arise since we have no way to guarantee that the people with thyroid cancer were in fact exposed to the atrazine levels measured from the municipal water supply. We discuss spatial regression models useful in the analysis of geographical correlation studies in Chapter 9. As with all ecological studies, geographical correlation studies also suffer from aggregation bias and specification bias, but the effects of these biases on inference are more complex, due to the spatial nature of the problem. In such cases, ecological inference is then considered to be a special case of the modifiable areal unit problem (MAUP) (Yule and Kendall 1950; Openshaw and Taylor 1979; Openshaw 1984); and the change of support problem (COSP) in spatial statistics (Cressie 1993, 1996). The resulting aggregation bias and specification bias are now related to scale and zoning effects associated with combining regions of different sizes and shapes. We discuss these issues in more detail in Chapter 4.

2.8 ADDITIONAL TOPICS AND FURTHER READING

This chapter is necessarily brief and offers only an outline of epidemiological concepts and analytic tools for the analysis of public health data (admittedly from a statistician's viewpoint). Lilienfeld and Stolley (1984) provide an accessible introduction to the field of epidemiology, and Greenland (1987) contains reprints of several seminal publications from the years 1946–1977 relating to foundations of epidemiological inference. Kleinbaum et al. (1982) illustrate the standard statistical tools of epidemiology, and Rothman and Greenland (1998) provide a comprehensive overview to the concepts and methods associated with modern epidemiological analysis. Causal inference represents a growing area of interest in the analysis of observational data and motivates a growing body of analytical methods. Many of these approaches are beyond the scope of this book and we refer interested readers to an excellent review article by Greenland et al. (1999), a brief interaction between Lindley (2002) and Pearl (2002), and the text by Pearl (2001).

2.9 EXERCISES

2.1 Tukey (1988) presents two examples illustrating the difference between direct and indirect rate standardization. The numbers are hypothetical but effectively illustrate the difference between the approaches. The first example represents a "clean" example, where direct and indirect adjustments are fairly comparable. The second represents a "dirty" example, where the standardized rates are different.

(a) The upper portion of Table 2.2 presents the number at risk in each of five age strata, the number of cases observed in each age stratum, and the rate (incidence proportion) within each stratum. To highlight the different data requirements for direct and indirect standardization, we label as NA (not available) data elements unnecessary for direct standardization

Table 2.2 Hypothetical Observed Data (Top) and Standard Population (Bottom) for the Clean Example of Calculating *Direct* Standardization[a]

Number at Risk in Age Stratum	Cases in Age Stratum	Rate (per 100,000)
10,000	6	60
20,000	15	75
30,000	75	250
40,000	160	400
50,000	300	600

Number at Risk in Age Stratum of Standard Population	Percent in Age Stratum	Cases in Age Stratum of Standard Population	Rate (per 100,000)
12,000,000	12	NA	NA
16,000,000	16	NA	NA
20,000,000	20	NA	NA
24,000,000	24	NA	NA
28,000,000	28	NA	NA

Source: Data from Turkey (1988).

[a]NA, not available (and not needed for direct standardization).

Table 2.3 Hypothetical Observed Data (Top) and Standard Population (Bottom) for the Clean Example of Calculating *Indirect* Standardization[a]

Number at Risk in Age Stratum	Cases in Age Stratum	Rate (per 100,000)
10,000	NA	NA
20,000	NA	NA
30,000	NA	NA
40,000	NA	NA
50,000	NA	NA
	(total = 556)	

Number at Risk in Age Stratum of Standard Population	Percent in Age Stratum	Cases in Age Stratum of Standard Population	Rate (per 100,000)
12,000,000	12	7,200	60
16,000,000	16	16,000	100
20,000,000	20	40,000	200
24,000,000	24	72,000	300
28,000,000	28	140,000	500

Source: Data from Tukey (1988).

[a]NA, not available (and not needed for indirect standardization).

but needed for indirect standardization. Use the information in the lower portion of Table 2.2 to calculate the directly standardized rate of disease.

(b) The upper and lower portions of Table 2.3 present information regarding the data observed and the standard population necessary to calculate the indirectly adjusted rates. We maintain the same format in Tables 2.2 and 2.3 to highlight the different data required for direct and indirect standardization, respectively. Calculate this rate and compare to the directly adjusted rate calculated using the information in Table 2.2. Do you observe any differences between the directly and indirectly standardized rates?

(c) Next, consider the addition of an additional age stratum with very few people at risk and a single observed case, as shown in Table 2.4. Additional and changed information from Table 2.2 appears in boldface (note that population proportions change, due to the addition of the extra stratum). Calculate the directly standardized rate for these data.

(d) Finally, Table 2.5 presents the modified data necessary to calculate the indirectly standardized rate. How do the directly and indirectly

Table 2.4 Hypothetical Observed Data (Top) and Standard Population (Bottom) for the Dirty Example of Calculating *Direct* Standardization[a]

Number at Risk in Age Stratum	Cases in Age Stratum	Rate (per 100,000)
10,000	6	60
20,000	15	75
30,000	75	250
40,000	160	400
50,000	300	600
10	**1**	**10,000**

Number at Risk in Age Stratum of Standard Population	Percent in Age Stratum	Cases in Age Stratum of Standard Population	Rate (per 100,000)
12,000,000	**10.8**	NA	NA
16,000,000	**14.4**	NA	NA
20,000,000	**18.0**	NA	NA
24,000,000	**21.6**	NA	NA
28,000,000	**25.2**	NA	NA
10,000,000	**9.0**	**NA**	**NA**

Source: Data from Tukey (1988).

[a]NA, not available (and not needed for direct standardization). Boldface values represent an additional age stratum not appearing in the clean example.

standardized rates from the dirty example compare? Discuss the difference between the clean and dirty examples.

2.2 Consider the typical epidemiologic 2×2 table cross-classifying disease and exposure (cf. Table 2.1). To see the impact of both sample size and the rarity of the disease on the similarity between the relative risk and the odds ratio, consider a study with 1000 exposed and 1000 nonexposed subjects. Suppose that $\Pr(D^+|E^-) = 0.1$ and the relative risk is 2.0 [i.e., $\Pr(D^+|E^-)/\Pr(D^+|E^-) = 2$].

(a) Given the sample size and probability of disease, define the expected elements of the 2×2 table and calculate the odds ratio.

(b) Repeat the calculation for $\Pr(D^+|E\ \ ) = 0.01$, 0.001, 0.0001, and 0.00001. Discuss the relationship with between the relative risk and the odds ratio.

(c) Repeat for a study with 10,000 exposed and 10,000 unexposed subjects and for a study with 500 exposed and 500 unexposed subjects. Describe

Table 2.5 Hypothetical Observed Data (Top) and Standard Population (Bottom) for the Dirty Example of Calculating *Indirect* Standardization[a]

Number at Risk in Age Stratum	Cases in Age Stratum	Rate (per 100,000)
10,000	NA	NA
20,000	NA	NA
30,000	NA	NA
40,000	NA	NA
50,000	NA	NA
10	NA	NA
	(total = **557**)	

Number at Risk in Age Stratum of Standard Population	Percent in Age Stratum	Cases in Age Stratum of Standard Population	Rate (per 100,000)
12,000,000	**10.8**	7,200	60
16,000,000	**14.4**	16,000	100
20,000,000	**18.0**	40,000	200
24,000,000	**21.6**	72,000	300
28,000,000	**25.2**	140,000	500
10,000,000	**9.0**	**100,000**	**1,000**

Source: Data from Tukey (1988).

[a]NA, not available (and not needed for indirect standardization). Boldface values represent an additional age stratum not appearing in the clean example.

how the relationship between the relative risk and the odds ratio changes with respect to sample size.

2.3 For a count, Y, following a Poisson regression model, show that β_k corresponds to the log odds associated with a unit increase in the covariate x_k, holding all other covariates constant.

2.4 Consider the Scottish lip cancer data described and analyzed in Breslow and Clayton (1993). The data in Table 2.6 are the total number of observed and expected lip cancer cases in males in the 56 districts of Scotland during 1975–1980; the percentage of the district population employed in agriculture, fishing, and forestry (%AFF); and the longitude and latitude coordinate of the center of each district.

(a) Using linear regression, regress the observed number of lip cancer cases on the percentage engaged in agriculture, fishery, or forestry. What do you conclude about the effect of this covariate on the number of lip cancer in males? What are the assumptions of this regression? Are they valid for these data?

(b) Perform the same regression, weighting by the expected number of lip cancer cases. Does this weighted regression help account for the violations in assumptions that you noted earlier? Do your conclusions change?

(c) Use Poisson regression to assess the effect of the percentage engaged in agriculture, fishery, or forestry on the number of lip cancer cases observed. What do you conclude?

(d) Include the latitude coordinate as another covariate in your regressions and adjust both regressions for this covariate. This variables serves as a surrogate for "northernlingless." For the linear regression, be sure to put this covariate in the model first, before %AFF. Do your conclusions change? What does this say about the effects of confounding?

(e) Summarize your conclusions about lip cancer in Scottish males during 1975–1980.

Table 2.6 Scottish Lip Cancer Data[a]

District	Observed	Expected	% AFF	Longitude	Latitude
1	9	1.4	16	57.29	5.50
2	39	8.7	16	57.56	2.36
3	11	3.0	10	58.44	3.90
4	9	2.5	24	55.76	2.40
5	15	4.3	10	57.71	5.09
6	8	2.4	24	59.13	3.25
7	26	8.1	10	57.47	3.30
8	7	2.3	7	60.24	1.43
9	6	2.0	7	56.90	5.42
10	20	6.6	16	57.24	2.60
11	13	4.4	7	58.12	6.80
12	5	1.8	16	58.06	4.64
13	3	1.1	10	57.47	3.98
14	8	3.3	24	54.94	5.00
15	17	7.8	7	56.30	3.10
16	9	4.6	16	57.00	3.00
17	2	1.1	10	57.06	4.09
18	7	4.2	7	55.65	2.88
19	9	5.5	7	57.24	4.73
20	7	4.4	10	55.35	2.90
21	16	10.5	7	56.75	2.98
22	31	22.7	16	57.12	2.20
23	11	8.8	10	56.40	5.27
24	7	5.6	7	55.63	3.96
25	19	15.5	1	56.20	3.30
26	15	12.5	1	56.10	3.60

Table 2.6 (*continued*)

District	Observed	Expected	% AFF	Longitude	Latitude
27	7	6.0	7	55.24	4.09
28	10	9.0	7	55.95	2.80
29	16	14.4	10	56.60	4.09
30	11	10.2	10	55.90	3.80
31	5	4.8	7	55.47	4.55
32	3	2.9	24	55.00	4.36
33	7	7.0	10	55.83	3.20
34	8	8.5	7	56.30	4.73
35	11	12.3	7	55.29	4.98
36	9	10.1	0	55.94	4.95
37	11	12.7	10	55.76	5.02
38	8	9.4	1	55.91	4.18
39	6	7.2	16	56.15	4.99
40	4	5.3	0	56.05	4.91
41	10	18.8	1	55.88	4.82
42	8	15.8	16	56.03	4.00
43	2	4.3	16	56.15	3.96
44	6	14.6	0	55.82	4.09
45	19	50.7	1	55.93	3.40
46	3	8.2	7	55.65	4.75
47	2	5.6	1	55.71	4.45
48	3	9.3	1	55.79	4.27
49	28	88.7	0	55.90	4.55
50	6	19.6	1	56.45	3.20
51	1	3.4	1	56.00	4.27
52	1	3.6	0	56.15	4.64
53	1	5.7	1	55.79	4.70
54	1	7.0	1	55.99	4.45
55	0	4.2	16	55.68	3.38
56	0	1.8	10	55.18	3.40

[a]Data are the district number; the observed and expected numbers of lip cancer cases in males; the percentage of the population engaged in agriculture, fishing, or forestry; and the longitude and latitude coordinates of the center of each district.

CHAPTER 3

Spatial Data

It is impossible not to feel stirred at the thought of the emotions... at certain historic moments of adventure and discovery: Columbus when he first saw the Western shore, Pizarro when he stared at the Pacific Ocean, Franklin when the electric spark came from the string of his kite, Galileo when he first turned his telescope to the heavens. Such moments are also granted to students in the abstract regions of thought, and high among them must be placed the morning when Descartes lay in bed and invented the method of coordinate geometry.

A. N. Whitehead, quoted in Maling (1973)

Spatial information is comprised of data that can be viewed or located in two or three (or more) dimensions. As we have seen in Chapter 1, when the spatial arrangement of the data is important to their understanding, an analysis that explicitly uses spatial information can be very informative. In this chapter we explore the essential features of spatially referenced data, including location, map projections, and support. We also review the types and sources of spatial data pertaining to public health and give an overview of geographic information systems (GISs) that provide computational tools for managing, merging, and displaying spatial data.

3.1 COMPONENTS OF SPATIAL DATA

There are three components to spatial data: *features, supports,* and *attributes.* A *feature* is an object with a specific spatial location and distinct properties. There are several types of spatial features:

1. *Point*: a precise location, $\mathbf{s}$, in space; a dot on a map. For example, a point could be the geographic location of your house or the location of an air monitoring station.

Applied Spatial Statistics for Public Health Data, by Lance A. Waller and Carol A. Gotway
ISBN 0-471-38771-1

2. *Line*: a sequential collection of connected points. Roads, rivers, and geographical boundaries are examples of linear features.
3. *Area*: a region enclosed by lines. Counties, states, and census tracts are all examples of areal spatial objects.
4. *Volume*: a three-dimensional object having height or depth (vertical extent) as well as horizontal extent. The most common examples of volumetric features are geologic formations such as aquifers.

A collection of features of the same type is called a *feature class*. For example, if we know the locations of several air monitoring stations, each station is a point feature and the collection of all locations is a point feature class.

Each feature is of a certain size and shape and has a specific spatial orientation. Taken together, these properties form the *support* of the data. Points, or spatial locations, have the smallest support. They have zero size, no shape, and no orientation. Lines have length and can indicate direction. Regions have area and boundaries that may impose properties on the associated features. For example, a circle and a rectangle are both areal features, yet they are inherently different spatial objects even if they have the same area.

Attributes are observations or measured values associated with features (e.g., the NO_x concentrations recorded at air monitoring stations, the racial composition of counties, the salinity of rivers). Attributes provide the data with which statisticians are most familiar [i.e., most (nonspatial) statistical analyses examine attribute data without regard to location or support]. In any given analysis we may have a single type of attribute of interest, or several types of attributes associated with each feature (e.g., we may have ozone, particulate matter, and sulfur dioxide measurements at each monitoring station; or the percentage of the population in each county self-identifying in each of several race categories). When several types of attributes are associated with the spatial features, the data are called *multivariate*. Some authors do not always distinguish spatial (*location space*) from multivariate (*variable space*), since spatial data can be referenced by two coordinates in the plane that may also be considered "variables." However, statisticians need to distinguish the two terms since the body of methods presented in courses on multivariate statistics is often very different from the multidimensional methods used for spatial data analysis. The distinction is simple if we think in terms of attributes and features. *Multivariate* refers to more than one type of attribute; *multidimensional* refers to more than one coordinate axis in space. Since this book is introductory, our primary focus will be on the analysis of a single type of attribute in two-dimensional space, although we provide references to statistical methods for multivariate and three-dimensional spatial data.

Thus, spatial data consist of features indexed by spatial locations and with specified supports, and attributes associated with those features. Spatial statistical analysis will be based not only on the attribute data, but will also depend on the spatial locations and the features associated with these locations. To get started, we need ways to reference spatial location, as described in the next section.

3.2 AN ODYSSEY INTO GEODESY

Webster's Collegiate Dictionary defines *geodesy* as "a branch of applied mathematics concerned with the determination of the size and shape of the earth and the exact positions of points on its surface." To work with spatial data, we need a way to reference spatial location. We also need methods for measuring distances between locations and for describing complex shapes and their properties. In this section we provide a very brief overview of the science of geodesy, drawing on concepts from geometry and topology.

3.2.1 Measuring Location: Geographical Coordinates

Many different *coordinate systems* have been developed to reference a point uniquely on Earth's surface. Most of these involve approximating Earth by a sphere or ellipsoid in order to use the geometrical properties of these objects to form the basis of the coordinate system. Earth is not a perfect sphere, nor a perfect ellipsoid, and its surface is not smooth, complicating the calculation of precise locations. In this book we make the simplifying assumption that latitude and longitude (a spherical coordinate system described in some detail below) provide enough location accuracy for our purposes, and refer interested readers to the geodesy literature for more detailed discussions (cf. Smith 1997).

The system of latitude and longitude provides a means of uniquely referencing any point on the surface of a sphere (Figure 3.1). Lines of longitude circle the Earth passing through the north and south poles. All places on the same meridian have the same longitude. The line of longitude passing through the Greenwich Observatory in England has the value 0°. Thus, longitude measures the horizontal angle formed between the line drawn from a given point to the center of the sphere and a line drawn from the center of the sphere to the 0° line of longitude (Figure 3.2). Due to its rotational nature, we report longitude in degrees (0° to 180°) east or west from the 0° meridian, with meridians west of 0° longitude termed *west longitude* and those east of 0° termed *east longitude*. Since the surface of Earth curves, the distance between two meridians depends on where we are on Earth: the intermeridian distance is smaller near the poles and larger near the equator.

To reference north–south positions, lines of latitude (called *parallels*) are drawn perpendicular to the lines of longitude, with the equator designated as 0° latitude (the largest circle defined by a plane perpendicular to the axis of Earth's rotation). Latitudes in the northern hemisphere are termed *north latitudes* and those in the southern hemisphere are called *south latitudes* (see Figure 3.1). Thus, on a spherical Earth, latitude measures the vertical angle (in degrees) between two line segments: one going from the location of interest to the center of the sphere, the other joining the equator with the center of the sphere. Figure 3.2 indicates that on a spherical Earth, these segments intersect at the center of the Earth, but since Earth is actually flattened somewhat at the poles, the true point of intersection is offset somewhat from the center (cf. Longley et al. 2001, p. 88). True to their name and

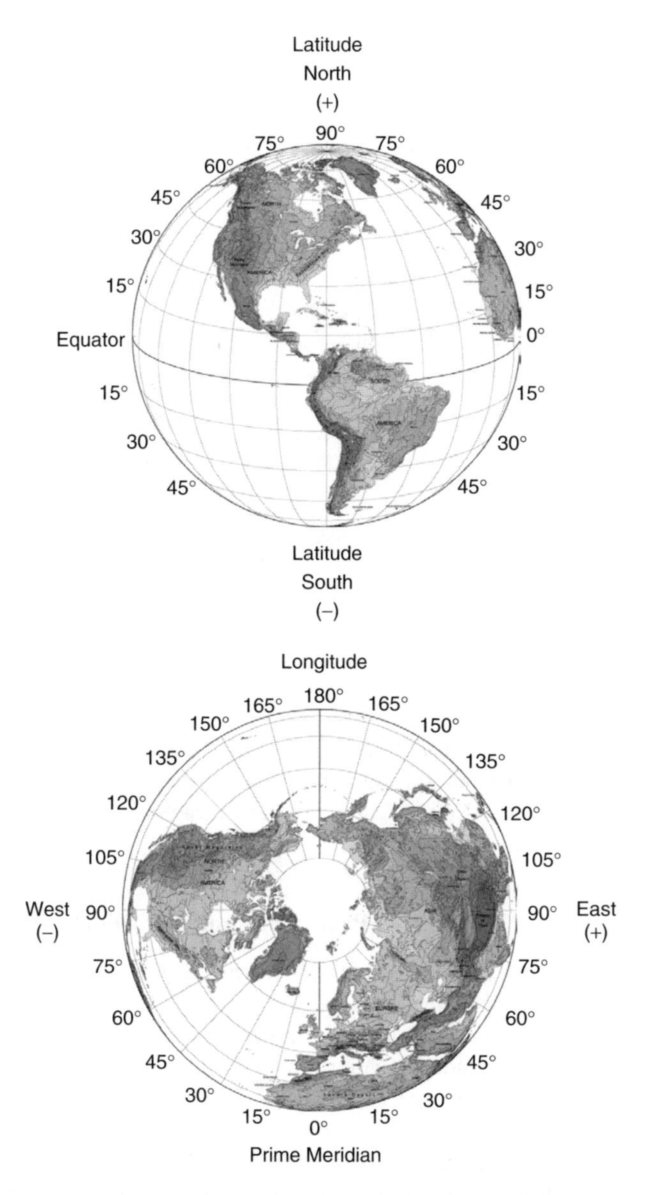

FIG. 3.1 Geometric definitions of latitude and longitude on a spherical Earth.

unlike meridians, parallels are parallel to one another, and differences in latitude are constant over Earth's surface. One degree latitude is approximately 69 miles.

Any point on Earth, s, can be georeferenced by the coordinate pair (longitude, latitude). Each coordinate can be as finely measured as we need it to be by dividing degrees into 60 minutes and each minute into 60 seconds. For example, a longitude value written as 46°22′38″W denotes a point that is located 46 degrees, 22 minutes,

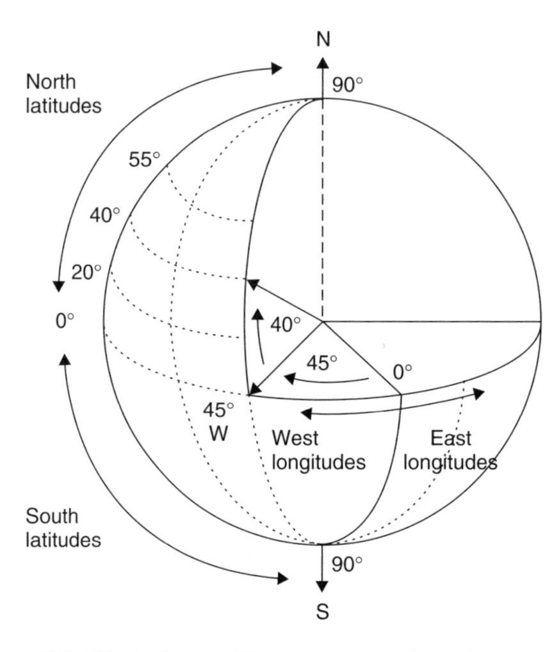

FIG. 3.2 Latitude and longitude system of coordinates.

and 38 seconds west of 0°. For calculations, this specification is often translated into *decimal degrees* in much the same way as we would translate 1 hour and 30 minutes into 1.5 hours. Also, "E" and "W" are designated by "+" and "−" so $46°22'38''$W is the same as $-46.3772°$.

3.2.2 Flattening the Globe: Map Projections and Coordinate Systems

A three-dimensional globe often is not as convenient as a two-dimensional map. A *map projection* is a mathematical transformation used to represent a spherical (or ellipsoidal) surface on a flat map. The transformation assigns each location on the spherical Earth to a unique location on the two-dimensional map. However, we cannot fit the curved surface of Earth to a plane without introducing some distortion. Map projections differ in the degree of distortion introduced into areas, shapes, distances, and directions. *Conformal* (e.g., Mercator) projections preserve local shape. Typical uses of such maps involve measuring angles (e.g., navigation charts and topographic maps), since a line drawn in a particular direction will appear straight in a conformal projection. Small areas are relatively undistorted, but conformal projections are unsuitable for large regions because areas are distorted. *Equal-area* (e.g., Albers' equal-area) *projections* preserve area, so regions will maintain their correct relative sizes after projection. Equal-area projections are useful for representing distributions of attributes (e.g., population size/density and land use) over large areas. Projected maps of these types of attributes produced using an equal-area projection will maintain the relative sizes of each region, and

Table 3.1 Distances (in Miles) between Route Locations for Various Projections

Route	Projection			
	Unprojected	Albers'	Mercator	Equidistant
Atlanta–Seattle	2185	2098	2930	2180
Atlanta–Chicago	588	617	751	601
Atlanta–New York	754	737	931	742
Atlanta–Knoxville	161	171	175	151

hence the relative extents of the associated attributes. These types of maps can be misleading when using another projection in which the areas are distorted. *Equidistance projections* preserve distance relationships in certain directions along one or a few lines between places on the map. These projections allow accurate measures of surface distances by the corresponding measured distances on the map.

Each type of projection can preserve only one property. Thus, a conformal mapping distorts areas, and an equal-area projection distorts shape. There are many compromise projections that are not conformal, equal-area, or equivalent, and each can be thought of as providing a projection providing *minimum total error* as defined by a summary of resulting distortions in area, shape, distance, and direction. Snyder (1997) provides a summary of a wide variety of map projections and discusses the strengths and weaknesses of each. Figure 3.3 shows four different maps of the continental United States. Notice how the relative sizes and shapes of the states vary among the maps. Table 3.1 shows how distances can vary as well.

The first step in a projection is the definition of the shape of the Earth we plan to project and the relationship between this shape and locations on Earth. As noted in Section 3.2.1, Earth is not a perfect sphere and is somewhat flattened at the poles. As a result, an ellipsoid (or spheroid) provides a better starting approximation, and several standard ellipsoids exist (with different ones providing different levels of accuracy). The position and orientation of the ellipsoid relative to Earth also need to be defined. When an ellipsoid is fixed at a particular orientation and position with respect to Earth, it is called a *geodetic datum*. With a *local datum*, the ellipsoid more closely approximates Earth for a particular area. For example, the NAD27 datum has the location (98°32′30″W, 39°13′30″N), corresponding to Meades Ranch, Kansas, as the reference point. At this point, the ellipsoidal model of Earth and true Earth coincide exactly. The NAD83 datum is an example of one widely used Earth-centered geodetic datum, calculated using the center of the Earth as a reference point. The WGS84 (World Geodetic System of 1984) is not referenced to a single datum, but instead, defines an ellipsoid whose placement, orientation, and dimensions best fit Earth's surface. Longley et al. (2001, p. 88) list several other standards. Different datums have different coordinate values for the same location, so two maps referenced to different datums can give locations for the same point that differ by several hundred meters.

Having chosen our standard ellipsoid, we can geometrically project locations on the ellipsoid Earth onto any of three types of surfaces, called *developable surfaces,*

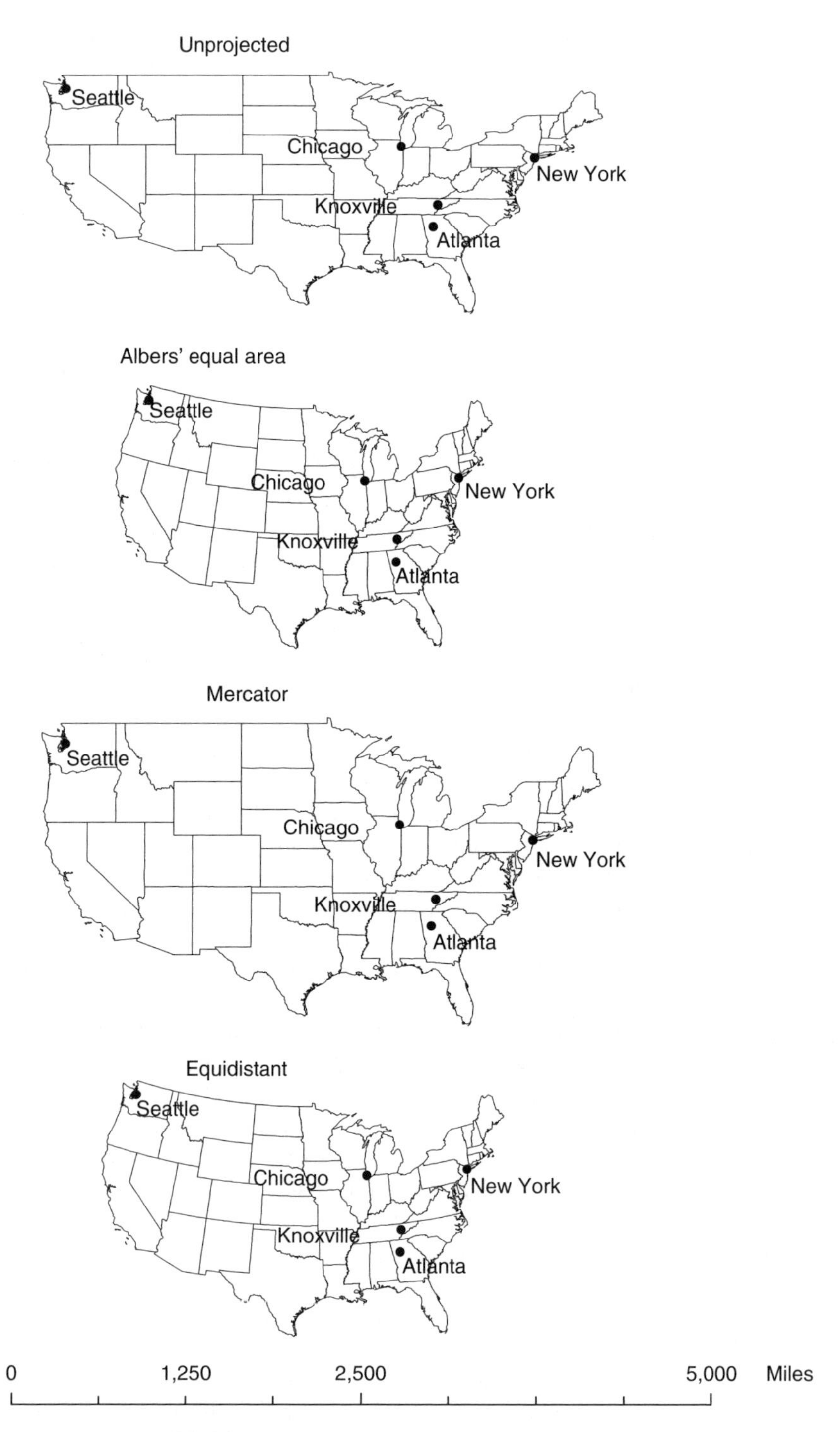

FIG. 3.3 Comparative view of different map projections.

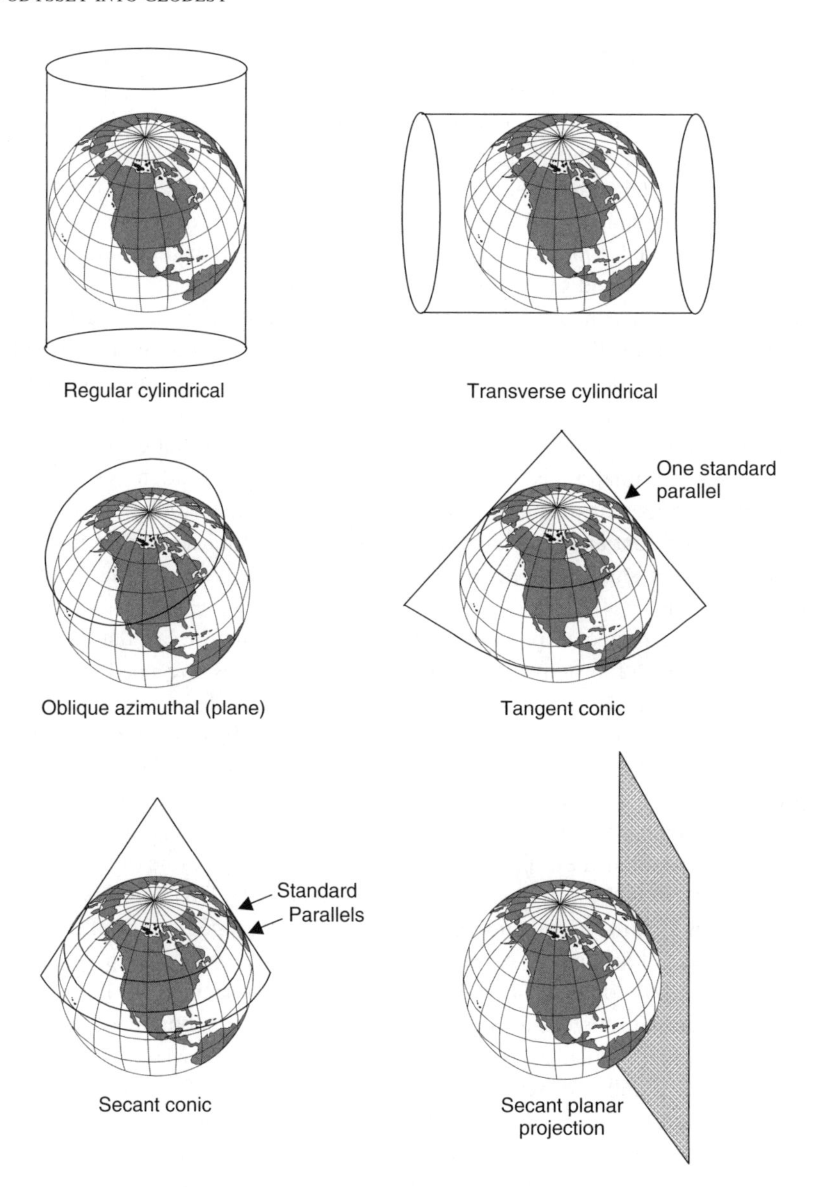

FIG. 3.4 Developable surfaces used in map projections.

that have the property that they can be flattened without distortion. Developable surfaces include planes, cones, and cylinders, resulting in *planar* or *azimuthal*, *conic*, and *cylindrical projections*, respectively (see Figure 3.4). Thus, each type of projection described above (e.g., conformal, equidistant) can also be classified by the appropriate developable surface and whether that surface is tangent to or intersects the surface of the ellipsoid. For example, for conic projections, the point of the cone falls along the axis of rotation and the cone is either tangent to the ellipsoid along a circle (one *standard parallel*) or intersects the ellipsoid at two circles (two standard parallels). One popular example is Lambert's conformal conic projection, with two standard parallels. Azimuthal projections preserve direction from one point to all other points, but preserve distance only along the standard parallel(s). As mentioned above, azimuthal projections can be combined with equal-area, conformal, and equidistant projections, creating, for example, the Lambert equal-area azimuthal and the azimuthal equidistant Projections.

A map *scale* is the relationship between a distance on the map and the corresponding distance on the ground. It is expressed as a fraction such as 1:24,000, meaning that 1 unit on the map corresponds to 24,000 units on the ground. If the units are in miles, then 1 mile on the map represents 24,000 miles on the ground. Because of the projection, the scale actually varies over the flattened map. Thus, an average approximation is usually given in the map legend to give the map interpreter some idea of distance. Small-scale maps (e.g., 1:1,000,000) show little detail but great extent and thus have low spatial resolution. Large-scale maps (e.g., 1:1000) are much smaller in extent, but show greater detail and thus have high spatial resolution.

Once we have projected points on Earth to a two-dimensional, flat surface, we need to set up a grid system to reference each point. Thus, we need to designate the center of the grid, the units, the central meridian, and the *scale factor* used in the projection. The scale factor (usually, a value ≤ 1.0) is applied to the scale of the centerline of a map projection where the developable surface intersects the ellipsoid (usually, the central meridian or a standard parallel). Scale values less than 1.0 are used to reduce the overall distortion of a projection. Most coordinate systems have already specified these parameters for us. For example, one commonly used coordinate system is the Universal Transverse Mercator (UTM) coordinate system. It results from a conformal mapping onto a cylinder wrapped around the poles of the Earth instead of around the equator as with the ordinary Mercator projection (cf. Longley et al. 2001, pp. 92–94). This projection is very accurate in narrow zones around the meridian tangent to the cylinder. The globe is subdivided into narrow longitude zones, 6° wide, each projected with a transverse Mercator projection. These zones are numbered with zone 1 between 180° and 174° west longitude and moving eastward to zone 60 between 174° and 180° east longitude. The lower 48 U.S. states are covered by zone 10 on the west coast through zone 19 on the upper east coast (Figure 3.5). In each zone we report UTM coordinates in meters north (*northings*) and east (*eastings*). To avoid negative numbers for locations south of the equator, the value 10,000,000 meters represents the equator. Each zone contains a central meridian assigned a value of 500,000 meters. Grid values to the west of this central median are less than 500,000, and to the east they are greater than 500,000. More complete descriptions of the UTM coordinate system as well as other map projections can be found in Snyder (1997) and Clarke (2001).

With all the different projections and coordinate systems, how do we know which one to use? Quantitative uses of a map (e.g., measurement of distances, areas, and angles) are more likely to reflect projection distortions than are visually

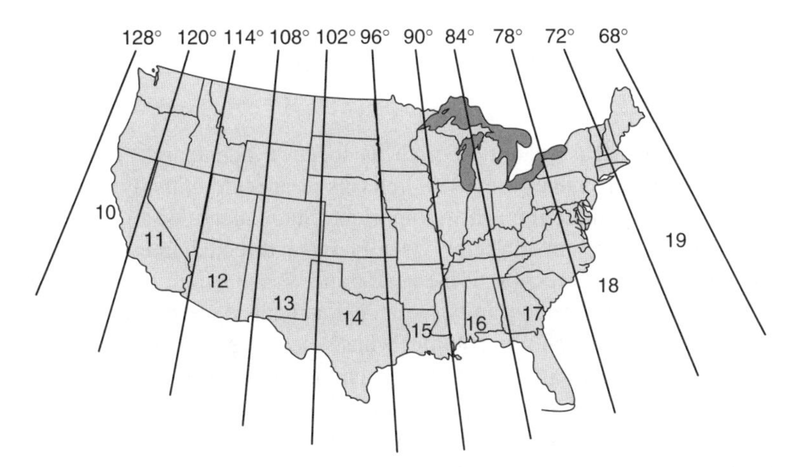

FIG. 3.5 UTM zones of the continental United States (from the U.S. Geological Survey). The upper set of numbers gives the longitude value, and the center numbers denote the UTM zones.

based subjective determinations. Thus, if we do not require a high level of accuracy for locations (e.g., we will not be performing queries based on location and distance, or we just want to make a quick map), we may not need to transform our data to a projected coordinate system; a planar display based on latitude and longitude coordinates (the default in most automated mapping software) will suffice. Scale, distance, area, and shape are all distorted, with the degree of distortion increasing with distance from the equator. If, however, we need to make precise measurements on our map, or we want to preserve one or more of these properties (area, shape, distance, or direction) for calculations or accurate visual depiction, we should choose a projected coordinate system. The system you should use depends on what you want to display. The amount of distortion resulting from a projection depends on the location, size, and shape of the region of interest. Distortion is least for small, compact regions and greatest in maps of the world. Popular projections include the Robinson projection (a compromise projection) for maps of the world, and the Albers equal-area conic and Lambert azimuthal or polyconic projections for maps of continental extent in the middle latitudes (e.g., North America). UTM coordinates (comprised of multiple local projections as outlined above) provide another common projection system for maps of the United States. Individual states (within the United States) often use the state plane coordinate system for regional mapping. This system is philosophically similar to the UTM system, but each zone may be projected differently than the others. More specific details, examples, comparisons, and mathematics that may be useful when choosing a particular coordinate system are given in Maling (1973), Snyder (1997), and Clarke (2001).

3.2.3 Mathematics of Location: Vector and Polygon Geometry

Once we have a set of locations projected onto a plane, we use vector notation and linear algebra to summarize common quantities such as distances, directions, and paths through locations. This notation provides the symbolic language for the statistical methods developed in subsequent chapters, and we provide a brief overview here.

Vectors Some physical quantities, such as location and length, are completely determined when their values are given in terms of specific units. For other quantities, such as velocity, direction is also important. Such quantities are called *vectors*. It is common to represent a vector visually by a directed line segment whose direction represents the direction of the vector and whose length represents its magnitude. Mathematically, vectors in two-dimensional space are often represented by a matrix with two rows and one column, whose elements give the u and v coordinates of the vector starting from $(0, 0)$ and ending at location (u, v) in the plane. To add two vectors, say $\mathbf{h}_1 = (u_1, v_1)'$ and $\mathbf{h}_2 = (u_2, v_2)'$, simply add the corresponding components together: $\mathbf{h}_1 + \mathbf{h}_2 = (u_1 + u_2, v_1 + v_2)'$. Subtraction can be done analogously. The *length* or *magnitude* of a vector $\mathbf{h} = (u, v)'$ is denoted by $\|\mathbf{h}\| = \sqrt{u^2 + v^2}$. This is also called the *norm* of the matrix $(u, v)'$. The *zero vector*, denoted $\mathbf{0}$, is a vector whose length is zero.

Polygons A polygon is a closed planar figure with three or more sides and angles. We are probably most familiar with rectangles, which are one of the simplest polygonal forms. We are probably also familiar with how to find the center of a rectangle and its area. However, many of the polygons in spatial analysis (e.g., the boundaries of census blocks, counties, and states) are more complex than simple rectangles. In some applications, we may even want to specify our own polygons, which describe boundaries of regions of interest to us. We may also want to specify the "location" of a polygon and determine its area.

In the plane, a polygon is specified mathematically by an ordered set of points, $\{u_i, v_i,\ i = 0, \ldots, n\}$, connected by line segments. These points define the *vertices* of the polygon. We adopt a notation for which the first and last vertex are equivalent, so that $u_0 = u_n$, $v_0 = v_n$. In some instances, we wish to define the center of a polygon in order to define some notion of distance between polygons. One definition of *center* is the *central value* of a polygon, obtained by averaging the u values and the v values to obtain location (u_m, v_m). Another definition of center is the *centroid* of a polygon defined by the center of mass (or balancing point) of the polygon. The coordinates of the centroid of a polygon, R are given by

$$c_u = (1/A) \iint_{\mathrm{R}} u \, du \, dv$$

$$c_v = (1/A) \iint_{\mathrm{R}} v \, du \, dv,$$

where A denotes the area of polygon R. Since the centroid depends on the vertices only through their definition of the perimeter of R, the centroid is less influenced than the central value by the number of vertices along any boundary of R. For example, consider a polygon with one edge defined by a curving feature such as a river. If we attempt to represent the curve through many line segments (hence many vertices), we will drive the central value toward the edge containing many vertices, while the centroid value remains relatively stable.

At first glance, the centroid seems more difficult to compute than the central value, and the area of a general polygon can be difficult to derive mathematically. However, many simple algorithms for computing the area and centroid of a polygon do exist. One that we have found useful is

$$A = \left| (1/2) \sum_{i=0}^{n-1} u_i v_{i+1} - u_{i+1} v_i \right|$$

$$c_u = [1/(6A)] \sum_{i=0}^{n-1} (u_{i+1} + u_i)(u_i v_{i+1} - u_{i+1} v_i)$$

$$c_v = [1/(6A)] \sum_{i=0}^{n-1} (v_{i+1} + v_i)(u_i v_{i+1} - u_{i+1} v_i).$$

Both central values and centroids can fall outside the polygons if the polygons have very unusual shapes (e.g., crescent, donut). In these cases, we may use known point locations to reference the polygons spatially.

For many analysis applications, we will not need the central values or the centroids of the polygons. However, many spatial analyses rely on distances (and directions) among locations to describe spatial relationships. In such cases we calculate distances between central values or centroids and use these to infer distances between polygons. For most applications, it matters little if we use the central value or the centroid to indicate the location of a polygon as long as we use the same definition consistently throughout the analysis. However, spatial analyses based on distances computed using central values may differ from those using distances computed using centroids since distances among central values probably differ from distances among centroids. Summarizing the location of a polygon by any one point in space necessarily introduces uncertainty in the analysis that we may want to adjust for when interpreting the results.

How Far? Distance Measures and Proximity As we mentioned in Chapter 1, one of the key concepts in spatial statistics is the idea that attribute values measured on features near one another tend to be more similar than those measured on features farther apart. Thus, to quantify this for use in statistical analysis, we need mathematical descriptions of *near* and *far*. We can quickly think of a very easy description: the distance between two features. However, there are many ways to measure distances, and as we saw for polygons, sometimes the idea of the location of a feature can be a bit vague. In this section we describe several different measures of distance that quantify the degree of closeness between two spatial features.

As the World Turns: Great Arc Length Suppose that we are using the longitude/latitude coordinate system to pinpoint locations on Earth's surface and we have two such locations, $s_1 = (\lambda_1, \phi_1)$ and $s_2 = (\lambda_2, \phi_2)$, where λ denotes the longitude coordinate and ϕ denotes the latitude coordinate. Then, the shortest distance between these two locations along the surface of a spherical Earth is given by

$$d(s_1, s_2) = (6378) \cdot \arccos[\sin \phi_1 \sin \phi_2 + \cos \phi_1 \cos \phi_2 \cos(\lambda_1 - \lambda_2)], \qquad (3.1)$$

where 6378 kilometers is the radius of the (spherical) Earth.

As the Crow Flies: Euclidean Distance Suppose, instead, that we are working with a projected coordinate system and we have two locations, $s_1 = (u_1, v_1)$ and $s_2 = (u_2, v_2)$, in a two-dimensional plane. Then the shortest distance between these two locations on a flat map is given by

$$d(s_1, s_2) = \sqrt{(u_2 - u_1)^2 + (v_2 - v_1)^2}. \qquad (3.2)$$

Using the notation for vectors, this distance can also be referred to as $\|s_2 - s_1\|$. This is called the *Euclidean norm*, and the distance measure in equation (3.2) is called *Euclidean distance*. We could also use the longitude and latitude coordinates, $s_1 = (\lambda_1, \phi_1)$ and $s_2 = (\lambda_2, \phi_2)$, in this formula, but the resulting distance would not take into account the curvature of the Earth. In general, the Euclidean distance measure should not be used to compute distances between sets of longitude and latitude coordinates, particularly if the distances are over a large area. Since no adjustment is made for the curvature of the Earth, distances affected by this curvature will be distorted.

As the Person Walks: City-Block Distance In some situations, measuring the shortest distance is not at all meaningful. For example, in urban areas where there are one-way streets and buildings between blocks, we cannot travel a straight line to our destination. Thus, we have to go "around the block," and to do this we drive or walk along a series of perpendicular segments. This gives rise to the idea of the "city-block" distance between two locations, $s_1 = (u_1, v_1)$ and $s_2 = (u_2, v_2)$:

$$d(s_1, s_2) = |(u_2 - u_1)| + |(v_2 - v_1)|. \qquad (3.3)$$

There are other distance measures for analogous situations [e.g., "as the fish swims" (Little et al. 1997) and "as the water flows" (Cressie and Majure 1997)]. More details on using these distance measures in spatial analysis are given in Section 8.4.6.

Across the Picket Fence: Adjacency When we have polygonal features instead of point locations, we can index the location of each polygon by its centroid and then use any of the distance measures described above to compute distances between centroids. This gives one measure of the distance between two polygons. However, sometimes a meaningful measure of the "closeness" of two polygonal features is simply whether or not they share a boundary (i.e., whether or not they are adjacent). This gives rise to a binary proximity measure

$$w_{ij} = \begin{cases} 1 & \text{if polygons } i \text{ and } j \text{ share a boundary} \\ 0 & \text{otherwise.} \end{cases}$$

We use the term *proximity* here rather than *distance* since the distance measures described above are actually topological *metrics* that must satisfy certain relationships not necessarily satisfied by proximity measures. There are many different proximity measures that can be used to define the closeness between two polygonal features, and we discuss these in more detail in Sections 4.4.1 and 7.4.2. As we shall see throughout this book, both distance measures and proximity measures have their useful place in spatial data analysis.

3.3 SOURCES OF SPATIAL DATA

The availability of spatially referenced data continues to increase at a rapid pace. Based on our experience, we focus our outline of available resources on data for the United States and Canada. However, similar data exist for other countries (or collections of countries). The following references or organizations offer access or descriptions of other geographically referenced data sets: Lawson (2001) (United Kingdom), Statistics Finland (Finland), Pan American Health Organization (Central and South America), World Health Organization, and the United Nations. Geographic scope and support (e.g., enumeration districts, counties, states, nations) of particular data sets vary widely.

In Canada and the United States, digital spatial features (i.e., spatial data that can be described by numbers) are produced by the national mapping agencies, agencies responsible for the decennial census, and other national organizations. Considerable effort has been made to coordinate and standardize the production and distribution of digital geographic data and most of these data are now readily available free on the Internet. In the following sections we describe some of the types of spatial data available that are of potential interest to public health professionals. We avoid giving actual Internet addresses, since such addresses change over time. Instead, we provide names of organizations, programs, and surveys and enough detail to enable Internet search engines to locate particular data sources. With the exception of some health data, most of the data that we describe are also available on CD-ROM for minimal processing fees.

3.3.1 Health Data

Data regarding health events vary widely in terms of purpose, ranging from specific clinical trials and localized observational studies to national (and international) disease surveillance efforts. Many spatial analyses of public health data utilize health outcome data collected and summarized by governmental agencies, often state health departments, and then released for public use.

Stroup et al. (1994) provide a thorough overview of and comprehensive bibliography to data sources relating to public health. We summarize several types of health data collected by various national and local governments, with particular attention to spatial aspects of various data sources. Many of the data sources listed below are publicly available through contact with the agency or organization responsible for the data (although we note that "publicly available" need not always equate with "easily available"). The different types of data involve a variety of collection methods and purposes, and accordingly, vary in terms of availability, spatial coverage, and spatial support.

As noted in Chapter 2, confidentiality affects the availability and spatial resolution of public health data. Reporting agencies must balance the individual's right to privacy with the public's right to know. This balance tips in different directions at different times under different governmental domains and regulations, so the spatial support available for similar types of data sources may vary between reporting units.

Vital Statistics Certification of death (issuance of death certificates) represents one of the earliest attempts to routinely gather and summarize health-related information. Parish records in western Europe dating from the fifteenth century and London's Bills of Mortality, a weekly report of deaths categorized by causes beginning in 1537, are early examples of data collection and reporting efforts relating to vital (birth and death) statistics. Stroup et al. (1994, pp. 38–44) provide a thorough overview of the history and development of the collection of vital statistics noting that vital statistics are the only health-related data available from many countries in a standard format. About 80 countries or areas currently report vital statistics to the World Health Organization, coded according to the *International Classification of Disease* (ICD) (ninth or tenth edition).

In the United States, the National Center for Health Statistics (part of the Centers for Disease Control and Prevention) collects, coordinates, and maintains vital statistics, including mortality data, some published recently in atlas form (Pickle et al. 1996; Devesa et al. 1999; Casper et al. 2000; Barnett et al. 2001). In general, spatial resolution is no finer than the county level, and for particularly rare causes of death in sparsely populated counties, numbers may be suppressed due to confidentiality concerns. The National Cancer Institute's *Atlas of Cancer Mortality in the United States, 1950–94* (Devesa et al. 1999) reports mortality for counties and for state economic areas, collections of counties within states based on demographic and economic variables as measured in 1960. The atlas does not include maps when many of the small areas (counties or state economic areas) contain sparse data, so maps are not reported for some disease/race/gender combinations. The National Center for Health Statistics' *Atlas of United States Mortality* (Pickle et al. 1996) reports for health services areas, another aggregation of counties based on a cluster analysis (classification algorithm) linking counties based on where residents aged 65 years and over obtained short-term hospital care in 1988. Unlike state economic areas, health service areas cross state boundaries.

Notifiable Diseases Due to their devastating impact and high infectivity, certain diseases often motivate surveillance by governmental public health units in order to stem outbreaks, monitor trends, and plan intervention strategies. *Notifiable diseases* are those associated with regulatory reporting requirements (i.e., by law, each incident case must be reported to a reporting agency or system upon diagnosis or laboratory verification). Stroup et al. (1994) provide a history of notifiable disease-reporting systems for the United States and internationally.

In the United States, the Centers for Disease Control and Prevention (CDC) maintains the Nationally Notifiable Disease Surveillance System to manage information on 54 reportable diseases. Some states add to the list of notifiable diseases. The National Electronic Telecommunications System for Surveillance (NETSS) provides the CDC with weekly data regarding each of the nationally reportable diseases. The data include the date of diagnosis, age, gender, race/ethnicity, and county of residence of each reported case, but no personal identifiers (e.g., name of the case). The NETSS provides information summarized in the CDC's *Morbidity and Mortality Weekly Report* (MMWR), but the CDC is currently upgrading from the NETSS to the National Electronic Disease Surveillance System (NEDSS) to address some of the reporting difficulties experienced by NETSS users.

Registries *Disease registries* differ slightly from vital statistics and notifiable disease data collection mechanisms in that registries link multiple sources of information for each case. Examples of information sources include hospital-discharge reports, death certificates, pathology reports, billing records, and in some cases the medical charts themselves. Registries attempt to consolidate information by patient so that each case appears only once in the registry.

Stroup et al. (1994) contrast *case series* and *hospital-based registries* from *population-based registries*. Case series and hospital-based registries attempt to provide information to improve patient care, and often do not provide accurate estimates of incidence rates (proportions) for the population. In comparison, population-based registries seek broader coverage in order to provide accurate estimates of overall incidence and (possibly) for local areas.

Individual registries focus on particular diseases, such as cancer and birth defects. Several cancer registries operate internationally. In the United States, the North American Association of Central Cancer Registries (NAACCR) serves to coordinate efforts and monitor quality among population-based cancer registries. NAACCR recently produced a report providing an overview and introduction to basic geographic information system (GIS) practices for cancer registries that addresses issues directly relating to spatial coverage, support, and analysis of cancer registry data in the United States (Wiggins 2002). For birth defects in the United States, the Birth Defects Monitoring Program (BDMP) links individual states, the CDC, the National Institute of Child Health and Human Development, and two nonprofit organizations (the March of Dimes and the Commission on Professional and Hospital Activities) to provide ongoing surveillance of the incidence of birth defects through registry programs (Oakley et al. 1983).

Different registries offer different spatial coverages and support. For instance, the National Cancer Institute's Surveillance, Epidemiology, and End Result (SEER) cancer registry is most likely the largest population-based cancer registry in the Western world. The SEER registry provides comprehensive incidence data since 1973, but only for the 11 SEER sites, which include state registries in Utah, New Mexico, Iowa, Hawaii, and Connecticut, and regional registries in Detroit, Seattle–Puget Sound, Los Angeles, San Francisco–Oakland, San Jose–Monterey, and Atlanta. The SEER registry also includes supplemental sites, including a Native American registry for the state of Arizona, a collection of rural Georgia counties, and the Alaska Native Tumor Registry. Planned expansion to the SEER program include registries in New Jersey, greater California, Kentucky, and Louisiana. The National Program of Cancer Registries (NPCR), established in 1992 by a U.S. congressional mandate and managed by the CDC, offers coordination and certification for registries covering non-SEER areas and states. For those seeking information on international cancer registry activities, the International Agency for Research on Cancer (IARC), part of the World Health Organization (WHO), collects information from cancer registries around the world, and provides a point of contact.

Health Surveys In contrast to registries and surveillance that seek to record all incident events within a given time period, health surveys use population-based statistical samples to draw inference regarding incidence and prevalence of health outcomes and related demographic and risk factor information. Analysts typically use design-based estimation to provide inference for the reference population, typically the aggregate population from which researchers draw the sample.

The National Health and Nutrition Examination Survey (NHANES) and the National Health Interview Survey (NHIS) are two examples of national health surveys in the United States (Korn and Graubard 1999). NHANES involved three separate data collection efforts. NHANES I collected data from civilian, noninstitutionalized individuals aged 1 to 74 years between the years 1971 and 1974 (with some follow-up in 1974 and 1975). NHANES II collected similar data from 1976–1980 (with the minimum age decreased to 6 months), and NHANES III collected data from 1988–1994 (with the minimum age decreased to 2 months and removal of an upper bound on age). The NHANES design involved primary sampling units of counties (or collections of contiguous counties). Within sampled areas, researchers collected data from household interviews and medical examinations performed in mobile examination centers (thereby providing some clinical measures linked to interview data). In comparison, the NHIS uses counties or metropolitan areas as primary sampling units, then conducts household interviews within selected units. The NHIS has been in continuous operation since 1957, with some modifications from time to time. A key difference between NHANES and NHIS data is the presence of some clinical measures (e.g., blood pressure and blood lead) in the NHANES data, collected by mobile examination centers in addition to the household interview data.

The Behavioral Risk Factor Surveillance System (BRFSS) provides an example of an annual health survey conducted by each state within the United States (Centers for Disease Control and Prevention 1998). Based on a structured telephone interview, the BRFSS collects information on health outcomes and behavioral and lifestyle factors such as exercise and diet. States collect data sufficient for obtaining statewide estimates and within any particular year, states with large numbers of counties (e.g., Texas and Georgia) will have several counties not contributing to the sample.

Surveys are designed for estimation at a particular level of aggregation (e.g., a nation for NHANES and NHIS, a state for BRFSS). As we might expect, there is often interest in obtaining sample-based estimates for local regions within the entire study area (e.g., states within a nation, or counties within a state). Cost often rules out obtaining adequate sample sizes to support design-based estimation within each local administrative unit, so researchers often use *small-area estimation* to combine data from regions statistically to stabilize estimates (Ghosh and Rao 1994, Schaible 1996, Malec et al. 1997). Only recently have small-area estimation procedures included spatial correlations, and Ghosh et al. (1998) provide an example using county-level lung cancer mortality rates in Missouri.

3.3.2 Census-Related Data

In the United States and Canada, the agencies responsible for collecting and disseminating census data provide a number of digital data sets that can be useful in public health applications. In the United States, in preparation for the 1990 census, the U.S. Bureau of the Census developed the TIGER (Topologically Integrated Geographic Encoding and Referencing) system to standardize, encode, and aid in processing of census questionnaires. TIGER/Line files cover the 50 states, the District of Columbia, Puerto Rico, the Virgin Islands, and the outlying areas of the Pacific Ocean over which the United States has jurisdiction. The spatial data contained in these files includes street networks, address ranges for street segments, railroads, political boundaries (including digital boundaries of census block groups, census tracts, counties, and states), and the boundaries of major hydrographic features, all geographically referenced by longitude and latitude coordinates. TIGER/Line files do not contain demographic attribute data, but they do contain region identifiers allowing one to link attributes from the associated census with TIGER polygons. Typical linked attribute data include feature names and codes (e.g., codes for state, county, census tract, and block) and may include population and housing unit counts, income, racial classification, and housing values. Not all attributes are available for every geographic level; for example, only the total population and housing unit counts are available at the census block level. Many local governments and software development companies have enhanced, reorganized, or simplified TIGER files for their own use. Statistics Canada produces similar spatial data sets.

3.3.3 Geocoding

Much of the public data collected in the United States is comprised of individual records, often specified by a person's address. If you have an emergency and call "911," one of the first pieces of information the operator will ask you for is your address. This address provides definitive location information for the purposes of dispatching emergency care. However, it is not definitive for automated, computer-based cartography. For this, we need geographic coordinates of the address. One way to obtain these coordinates is through *geocoding:* the process of assigning a spatial location to an address record.

Geocoding involves matching records in (at least) two databases: the database containing the address information and a reference geographic base file that contains both addresses and the geographic coordinates of those addresses. This assumes that a complete, easily available, accurate geographic base file exists, which is usually not the case except at a very local level using digital municipal data files. More commonly, the Census TIGER/Line data described in Section 3.3.2 provide the geographic base file, address ranges, and street segment records for geocoding. Some mode of interpolation then provides the actual location of the address within the street segment. Some location error remains in most geocoded addresses, and the error could be quite large for rural areas containing few street segments. Thus, the geographic base file providing address and/or street location is critical to achieving accurate locations. A variety of geographic base files are now available from both public-domain and private-sector publishers. If you provide addresses that are complete, specific (i.e., have ZIP + 4 designation), and accurate (i.e., contain no typographical errors and record address elements such as street names in a standard format), it will usually be possible to match 80–90% of your addresses to the addresses and associated geographic coordinates in the base file.

3.3.4 Digital Cartographic Data

In the United States, the U.S. Geological Survey (USGS) has long been a source of maps: topological maps, detailed quadrangle maps, geological maps, and so on. Most of these maps are now available in digital formats. The USGS's Digital Line Graph (DLG) data set includes transportation lines, hydrography, political boundaries, and elevation contours for the entire United States. The USGS land use/land cover data set delineates urban areas, agricultural lands, forests, and wetlands. The USGS has also enhanced the comprehensive digital elevation data first produced by the U.S. Defense Mapping Agency. These data sets provide an elevation value for any location in the United States and provide necessary information for many engineering and urban planning applications.

3.3.5 Environmental and Natural Resource Data

As with the health surveys (cf. Section 3.3.1), the U.S. government also conducts a number of different environmental surveys, designed to monitor the status and trends of ecological and natural resources. Many of these are national, long-term monitoring and assessment programs. Some collect data at monitoring stations (point locations), others collect information over small areal units, and some programs operate at state or regional levels. The type of attribute data collected varies widely across programs. Many use probability sampling to select the units for measurement; others select units based on judgment/convenience. Below we provide a brief overview of some of the major national environmental monitoring programs that provide public-domain data that might be useful in public health studies. Much of our information is based on the work of Olsen et al. (1999), and more detailed, statistical information about many of the surveys we describe can be found in this work.

Agriculture and Natural Resources The National Resources Inventory (NRI), part of the Natural Resources Conservation Service (NRCS) within the U.S. Department of Agriculture (USDA), collects data on land use, wetlands, soil erosion, conservation practices, and habitat diversity. The primary sampling unit is a square plot, containing approximately 160 acres. Some data are collected on these units (e.g., land use, habitat diversity), while more specific information is recorded at individual locations within each unit. NRI data provide estimates of natural resource conditions and changes in these conditions that are used to develop natural resource conservation programs.

The National Agricultural Statistics Service (NASS), also within the USDA, collects data on agricultural lands. It maintains a huge database of agricultural statistics such as crop acreage and production. Some of the information collected pertains to environmental monitoring on agricultural lands. For example, NASS maintains an agricultural chemical-use database that includes information on the type of chemical applied (e.g., specific type of fertilizer, insecticide, or herbicide), the total amount applied, the percentage of cropland treated, and so on. It is also a probability-based survey, based on a stratified, two-stage random sample of segments in land-use strata, combined with a list frame sample of individual farms. The spatial resolution depends on the information collected, most of which is at the state or county levels. NASS is one of the oldest and largest national survey organizations; the survey was mandated by Congress in 1839. Today, NASS publishes 400 national and 9000 state reports each year (Olsen et al. 1999).

Water Quality The Environmental Protection Agency (EPA)'s Environmental Monitoring and Assessment Program (EMAP) is another national probability-based survey. It was initiated to provide information on the status and trends in environmental quality and to identify emerging environmental problems by developing reliable and specific ecological indicators. It is based on a triangular grid covering the entire United States and uses systematic random sampling to determine units for measurement. EMAP Estuaries monitors all U.S. coastal waters measuring indices of ecological condition (e.g., the benthic index, based on surveying benthic invertebrates and combining measures of their abundance and diversity into a single index) and exposure indicators (e.g., dissolved oxygen). EMAP Surface Waters monitors rivers, streams, reservoirs, and lakes (except the Great Lakes). This program collects measurements on a variety of indicators that can be used to infer the "health" of the stream or river, including water quality measurements (e.g., pH), sediment toxicity, and chemical contaminants in fish. More specific information about EMAP design and component programs is provided in Stevens (1994) and Olsen et al. (1999).

The U.S. Geological Survey (USGS) implements several water quality assessment programs. One of the largest, the National Water-Quality Assessment (NAWQA) program, was initiated to collect information on the quality of the nation's ground and surface waters. The sampling design is not probability-based, but instead, study units were selected by a linear optimization algorithm, and the units now participating in the program represent 50 major hydrogeologic basins that comprise the majority of the nation's water use. The data collected on each study unit depend on the characteristics of each particular unit, but often include measurements on water pH, temperature, dissolved oxygen, and nutrient concentrations. Different programs within NAWQA focus on more specific water quality characteristics. For example, the NAWQA Pesticide National Synthesis Project aims to provide a national assessment of pesticides in surface and ground waters and supplies important information to the U.S. EPA for regulations concerning pesticide use and biodegradability requirements.

Air Quality In addition to environmental programs that focus on terrestrial and aquatic ecosystems, the U.S. government also directs many national atmospheric monitoring programs. Under the guidance of the EPA, the National Atmospheric Deposition Program (NADP) and the Clean Air Status and Trends Network (CASTNET) were developed to provide data necessary to assess the effectiveness of air pollution control efforts. Such effectiveness can be assessed by monitoring changes in atmospheric deposition, primarily acid deposition levels, high levels of which are caused by industrial and automobile emissions. The NADP collects weekly wet acid deposition samples from almost 200 sites across the United States. Each site in this network measures important components of precipitation chemistry such as sulfate, hydrogen ion, and chloride. CASTNET consists of over 70 monitoring stations across the United States that provide information on dry acid deposition, ground-level ozone, and other forms of atmospheric pollution. Sites in this network measure weekly average atmospheric concentrations of sulfate and nitrate and hourly concentrations of ozone and meteorological data used to compute acid deposition rates. The monitoring sites in both the CASTNET and NADP programs are located in rural areas and so provide information on natural background pollution concentrations. Other monitoring networks [e.g., the National Air Monitoring Stations (NAMS) network] have stations located in urban areas, and data from these networks can be combined with CASTNET information for a more comprehensive national air quality assessment.

Climate The National Climatic Data Center (NCDC), part of the National Oceanic and Atmospheric Administration (NOAA), is the world's largest archive of global climate data. It collects weather data from the National Weather Service, the Federal Aviation Administration, the U.S. military, and from several international agencies as well. NCDC data are used to provide short- and long-term national and regional climate forecasts. They also provide a complete historical record that can be used to measure global climate change. In environmental health studies, data from the NCDC are often used in modeling the effects of climate on human health and in adjusting models quantifying the effects of air pollution on human health for climatic effects.

3.3.6 Remotely Sensed Data

Remotely sensed data are data collected from a distance. The most common example of remotely sensed data is the aerial photograph. Such photographs can provide reliable spatial measurements such as elevation, soil type, and land use, but the exercise often is not as simple as snapping a photograph: The entire scientific discipline of *photogrammetry* revolves around this endeavor (Jensen 1996). Another approach to collecting remotely sensed data is through the use of satellite images. These are produced from sensors located on satellites that measure the reflected and emitted radiation from Earth's surface. This type of radiation cannot be detected by ordinary photographic film. The images are obtained directly in digital form and are comprised of cells called *pixels* (picture elements). Each pixel corresponds to an area on the ground, and the size of this area determines the *resolution* of the image. Associated with each pixel is a wave of electromagnetic energy. Different features on the ground will emit different energy waves that can then be analyzed (using our knowledge of light and electromagnetism) and interpreted to infer physical characteristics. Today, satellite imagery produces some of the most accurate and globally comprehensive information on the Earth, and many disciplines, including public health (particularly in vector-borne diseases), are finding creative and cost-effective uses for this technology (Cline 1970; Beck et al. 1994; Washino and Wood 1994; Messina and Crews-Meyer 2000; Xiang et al. 2000).

3.3.7 Digitizing

Any map available in hard copy can be scanned into a computer and digitized to produce an electronic file of digital boundaries. To tie the digitized map to a preexisting georeferenced coordinate system (e.g., longitude and latitude), the digitizer must specify the true coordinates of at least three separate locations on the map. This approach provided the initial means for transferring paper maps based on historical land surveys to the digital spatial data sets currently available.

3.3.8 Collect Your Own!

The global positioning system (GPS) is a system of 24 satellites orbiting the Earth. A GPS receiver locates the nearest satellites and receives a signal from each of them. By knowing the time differential between the signals, the positions of the satellites, and details about their orbit, it is possible to determine the exact location (longitude, latitude, and elevation) of the receiver. GPS receivers are quickly finding their way into all kinds of equipment (including automobiles), and handheld GPS receivers are now a cost-effective scientific tool. In conjunction with a laptop computer and some software, analysts can use a handheld GPS receiver to record the boundaries of the spatial features of interest. We may also measure attributes associated with these features (e.g., administer questionnaires to people; take water, soil, or blood samples and have them analyzed by a laboratory). Of course, we do not need a GPS to collect our own spatial data. All we need is a way to record the location of our features relative to other features. For example, we could designate an arbitrary point somewhere as (0,0) and then record attribute information on a regular grid extending from this origin. Agricultural scientists and ecologists have been using this approach for decades and have developed systematic sampling and mapping strategies designed to collect spatial information quickly and easily (e.g., Seber 1986; Stehman and Overton 1996; Wollenhaupt et al. 1997). Thus, public health practitioners should not rely solely on the large, existing spatial data sets described above. Much scientific discovery and understanding remains to be obtained by conducting our own studies that collect the information, both spatial and nonspatial, that we believe is important and relevant.

3.4 GEOGRAPHIC INFORMATION SYSTEMS

The term *geographic information system* (GIS) means many things to many people and has various definitions. The literature on GISs extends back at least to the mid-1960s and the development of the Canada Geographic Information System for the Canadian Land Inventory (Longley et al. 2001, pp. 10–13). From our point of view, a GIS is a complex, interactive software for the management, synthesis, and display of spatial data. As Bonham-Carter (1994) notes, the word *geographic* means that the spatial locations can be specified by geographical coordinates, latitude and longitude. The term *information* implies that the data input into a GIS can by organized in a useful way facilitating interpretation (e.g., through maps, images, charts, and tables). Finally, the word *system* indicates that a GIS is comprised of several different but interrelated components working together. As noted by Clarke (2001), a GIS allows easy visualization of geographic features comprised of points, lines, and areas and allows us easily to address questions regarding features' respective sizes, shapes, orientation, and spatial distribution, such as: Where? How far? In what direction? How big? Several such aspects of spatial features are illustrated in Figure 3.6. A GIS also allows us to link this information with various *attributes* associated with these features. Thus, we can also answer questions such as: Where are the features associated with large attribute values? How close are features with the same attribute value? These are simple but important questions, not quickly answered without GIS technology. Answers to these questions form the basic building blocks for more complex questions, including those addressed in subsequent chapters.

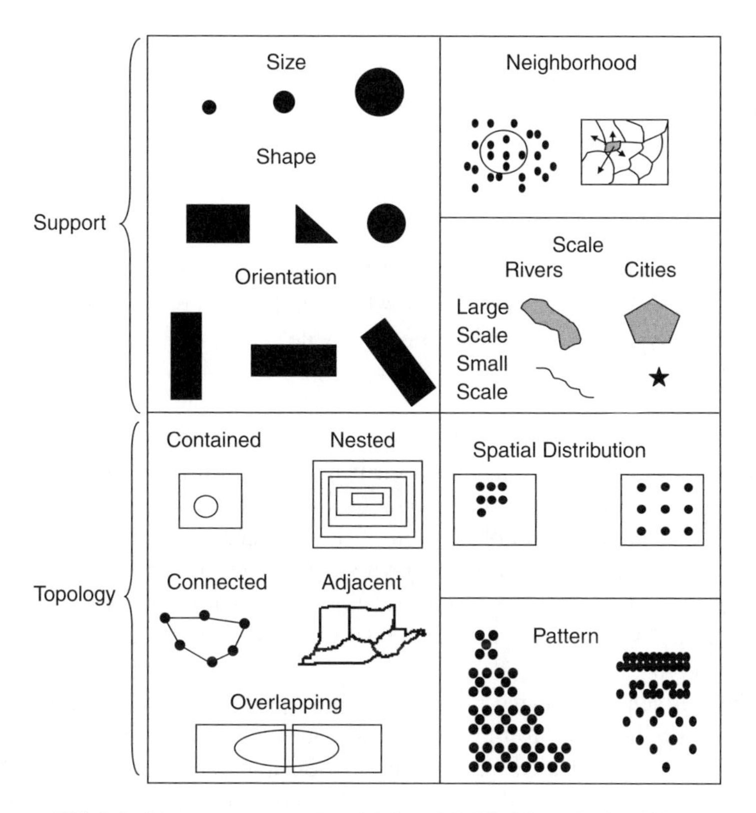

FIG. 3.6 Important aspects of spatial data. [Modified from Clarke (2001).]

3.4.1 Vector and Raster GISs

The literature distinguishes between *vector* and *raster* GISs, depending on whether locations are stored as points/lines/areas or as pixels, respectively. The underlying geographic data structures determine both the computational storage burden and the primary GIS operations of interest. Vector data often involve much less storage since we store attribute data only for points, lines, and areas rather than for every pixel, as in raster data, although various image compression systems significantly reduce the storage requirements of raster data. The speed of computational operations varies between vector and raster data. For instance, we may search through vector data by iteratively referencing each point, line, and/or area from a reference list, while a brute-force search of raster data could involve looping through the grid of pixel points (typically much larger than the vector database). Although many modern GISs manage both vector and raster data, the different storage, searching, and algorithmic strategies associated with the data types merit retention of the distinction.

Different types of data fall more naturally into the vector and raster frameworks. For instance, health or demographic data summarized to census enumeration regions fit well into the vector paradigm, due to the assignment of multiple attributes to each of a set of polygons covering the study area. In contrast, satellite imagery and aerial photography better fit into the class of raster data where each image consists of multiple pixels and their associated values.

3.4.2 Basic GIS Operations

Although particular GIS packages may differ in interface and functionality, there are certain operations central to every GIS. Although these operations do not constitute statistical analysis per se, the operations provide means for querying and linking spatial data.

Spatial Query The operation distinguishing a GIS from any other relational database is the ability to query data elements with respect to their locations as well as their attribute values. The spatial query allows us to request summaries of attribute values in the subset of locations meeting a spatial criterion (e.g., the number of pediatric asthma case residences within 500 meters of a major roadway). The spatial query underlies most GIS functionality and provides the means for sorting, subsetting, and summarizing data with respect to location and distances.

Layering Much as its name implies, the GIS operation known as *layering* consists of overlaying several different spatial data sets, linking values by location. Conceptually, think of a set of maps printed on transparencies, where each map represents a different set of data collected over the same study area (e.g., a map of population density, a map of roads, and a map of land cover). Stacking or layering the maps provides a single map consisting of the composite information from all maps.

Computationally, the GIS matches attribute values based on common locations, allowing one to query the combined attributes by a single location reference file. The term *spatial join* defines the algorithmic operation linking the layered data into a combined (joined) data set.

Layering provides a powerful visualization and data linkage tool. In public health, layering allows one to combine census data providing information on local demographics, disease registry data providing local health outcomes, and environmental monitoring data providing locations of pollution sources, each collected over the same area. As a particular example in a public health setting, Xiang et al. (2000) layered two spatial data sets: a map of maternal residences at the time of birth for infants born between 1991 and 1993 in Weld County, Colorado, and a (raster) map of crop type for 30-meter by 30-meter pixels as determined by satellite imagery. Xiang et al. (2000) next inferred pesticide use based on crop type and a survey of Colorado farmers regarding the type and application patterns of particular pesticides by crop. Through these GIS operations, Xiang et al. (2000) created a combined data set which allowed preliminary assessments of the associations between patterns of low birth weight and pesticide use.

The ability to combine several data sets collected by different agencies for different purposes is both a strength and a weakness of layering. Data merging is a strength in that it allows us to address questions we could not answer using any of the individual data sets alone. In contrast, data merging may be a weakness in that the issue of data quality becomes murky. That is, while each individual layer may meet quality levels sufficient for its intended purpose, the data may not be accurate enough to address the requirements for inference regarding the combined data. For instance, air monitoring stations installed to measure pollution levels near an industrial park may not offer accurate exposure information for subjects throughout the study area. Thus, we emphasize again that the great availability of spatial data and the ease with which such data can be combined and displayed in a GIS are still not substitutes for more focused studies designed to obtain reliable and relevant information.

Buffering *Buffering* refers to a particular type of spatial query, the definition of the area within a specified distance of a particular point, line, or area. For example, Xiang et al. (2000) define areas (*buffers*) of 300 and 500 meters, respectively, around each maternal residence in their study, then assign pesticide values within the buffer based on the remotely sensed satellite data. Other typical applications of buffering in public health studies include the definition of exposure (or *exposure potential*) zones around sources of hazard (e.g., hazardous waste sites). Buffering, too, has advantages and disadvantages. It allows us to combine spatial data collected on different features with differing supports, but in doing so, we have introduced errors and uncertainty into any analysis and the resulting conclusions.

3.4.3 Spatial Analysis within GIS

Many authors note the analytical and predictive capabilities of GISs. Some (e.g., Bailey and Gatrell 1995) distinguish between *spatial analysis*, the study of phenomena occurring in a spatial setting using the basic GIS operations outlined above, and *spatial data analysis*, the application of statistical description and modeling to spatially referenced data. The distinction provides a boundary between standard GIS operations and queries and the application of data analysis algorithms for estimation, prediction, and simulation familiar to many statisticians. Other authors use the term *spatial analysis* quite broadly as a field and include inferential statistics among the tools. For instance, Longley et al. (2001, p. 282) describe six general categories for GIS-based spatial analysis: queries (enabled by the spatial relational database underlying the GIS), measurements (e.g., length, shape, distance), transformations (e.g., spatial joins, and conversion from vector to raster, or vice versa), descriptive summaries (e.g., calculating the mean response in a particular area), optimization (e.g., searching for minima/maxima across a spatial area), and hypothesis testing. The last category specifically involves inferential statistical methods, while the other categories describe a variety of tools for quantifying trends, features, and patterns within a spatial data set. We focus on statistical methods (spatial data analysis) in this book but note that nonstatistical GIS operations often provide necessary precursory elements for the estimation, testing, and modeling approaches outlined in the following chapters.

With the exception of recent software modules implementing the geostatistical methods discussed in Chapter 8, most modern GISs allow little in the way of routine calculations for *spatial data analysis* involving statistical inference. As a result, most analyses described in subsequent chapters involve the use of separate statistical packages and are not analyzed within a GIS setting. Like any set of software packages, the capabilities of a GIS stem from the needs of the users as addressed by software developers. As more users seek spatial statistical modeling capabilities within (or in concert with) GISs, developers will seek to meet the need. *Scripts* (much like macros in SAS and functions in S-Plus or R) can greatly extend the statistical capabilities of a GIS. In addition, a growing variety of *applets* (Web-based application tools) for both statistical and GIS computing provides toolboxes for further development of software tools for spatial data analysis.

3.5 PROBLEMS WITH SPATIAL DATA AND GIS

The apparent availability of spatial databases and the ease with which these can be used and combined within a GIS make it seem easy to obtain relevant and important information for almost any study. However, as alluded to above, there are also common problems, misuses, and limitations associated with the use of spatial databases. Understanding these limitations, and anticipating them a priori, will help to ensure more productive analyses.

3.5.1 Inaccurate and Incomplete Databases

Any database can contain typographical errors and misspellings. Spatial databases are no exception, and such errors can occur in both the location values and in the attribute values. Sometimes, these errors are fairly easy to notice simply by plotting the locations on a map using a GIS. For example, when a location plots outside the domain of interest, it is often the case that the latitude and longitude coordinates were reversed, a negative sign was deleted from the longitude values, or the first digit in one of the georeferenced locations is incorrect. When two spatial databases appear to be offset by a small amount, differing datums could be the culprit.

A quality control program including simple edit checks can help to identify potential problems. For example, we could check to make sure that the date of birth and the age of the person are consistent (i.e., the person cannot be older or younger than the difference between the date of the study and their date of birth), and we can check to see that fields for city, ZIP code, county, and state are all consistent, and so on. These types of checks can be automated easily; it is just a matter of developing a comprehensive system of checks and balances.

Such quality control checks will take us only so far. If we do not know what the attribute values mean, the projection used, and the time frame over which the database was compiled, the database will have limited value. The Federal

Geographic Data Committee (FGDC) has been developing a standard for what is now called *metadata*, or "data about the data." Metadata give us important information about the database, such as who created it, when it was created, when it was last updated, the map projection used, and data quality assessments such as the accuracy of both attribute and locational information. Thus, we should always be sure to look for and understand any metadata before working with a particular spatial database.

It is very difficult if not impossible to find a complete and comprehensive spatial database ideally suited to our interests. Most databases will suffer from one of two problems: lack of extent or lack of resolution. For example, most environmental data are often of point support, but they are usually very localized, pertaining to a county or a region. Some national databases are very sparse, having but one point per state. On the other hand, it is easy to obtain comprehensive, national, state-level health data, but such data are usually not available at finer resolutions (e.g., counties). For any particular study, we will probably have to work very hard to supplement the existing spatial databases with data specific to our needs.

3.5.2 Confidentiality

Many health data sets contain sensitive information. Good ethical practice, and in many cases, federal laws, require us to protect confidential information. The FGDC is developing consistent guidelines that ensure the protection of confidential information, but many institutions have developed their own standards. For example, the U.S. Bureau of the Census will not release any individual-level information, and many U.S. government agencies have "cell suppression" rules for tables (e.g., if a count in a particular cell of a table contains five or fewer individuals, the value will not be released). While the usual patient identifiers such as name and address can obviously be used to identify patients, point locations obtained from geocoding or GPS can be used in the same way. Thus, many institutions refuse to share this type of data or have developed policies that restrict access to such data. For example, to work with some of the data collected by NCHS at the county level, screened users must conduct their research at NCHS, where their use of the data can be carefully controlled and monitored. Unfortunately, these policies and precautions also limit health research studies and the conclusions that can be obtained from them. Recently, *geographical masks* have been designed that preserve the confidentiality of individual health records but also allow analyses that require specific locational information to address important research questions of interest. Armstrong et al. (1999) provide a comprehensive review and discussion of many different types of geographical masks.

3.5.3 Use of ZIP Codes

Since geocoding is expensive or time consuming, many health studies georeference individuals to ZIP codes since patient records often contain a ZIP code field as part of the address. It is very important to remember that ZIP codes were created by the

U.S. Postal Service for delivering mail. Unlike census tracts and blocks, they were not created to be homogeneous with respect to sociodemographic variables, and in many instances, they will not manifest such homogeneity. Sociodemographic information is available by ZIP code, but it is often averaged from census block data. This averaging, over units not necessarily homogeneous, can often lead to misleading conclusions about data mapped at the ZIP-code level. For example, Krieger et al. (2001) report the results of a comprehensive study on whether or not the choice of area-based geographic units really matters when mapping data for public health surveillance. They found that when health outcomes were reported and mapped at the ZIP-code level, ZIP code measures failed to detect gradients or detected trends and patterns that were contrary to those observed with block groups or census tracts.

3.5.4 Geocoding Issues

Address matching works best for completely specified, correctly spelled addresses in urban areas. In many cities, a designation such as "East" or "North" is very important. For example, in Atlanta, North Peachtree Street is in a very different location than Peachtree Street. It is also important to provide all the aliases for a given street (e.g., Peachtree is often abbreviated as "P'tree"). Address matching does not work well in rural areas, and it cannot be used for P.O. boxes or rural route designations.

Achieving a 100% match rate occurs only when we geocode error-free addresses using an error-free base map. Of course, a high match rate does not ensure correct spatial coordinates for each address. Cromley and McLafferty (2002, p. 87) note that it is not uncommon for 7% of locations assigned to addresses within a base map to be incorrect. In addition, Krieger et al. (2001) report variable accuracy in a comparison of four independent geocoding vendors, each assigned the same original set of addresses. Thus, we stress that although many automated geocoders may match most addresses within seconds, geocoding is an iterative process that requires substantial checking and verification to ensure accurate spatial information.

3.5.5 Location Uncertainty

Even a foolproof geocoding approach will not obviate all locational issues. In human health applications, we traditionally assign the residence location to each case. Although we will use residential location for the examples below, such locational assignment may not be entirely satisfactory for some applications. For instance, assigning residence location to each case ignores human mobility and may assign cases to locations far from areas where relevant (e.g., occupational or school-based) exposures occur. Also, people move from place to place during the course of the day and may receive significant environmental exposures at their workplace, in their car, or in other locations. Finally, in studies of chronic diseases (such as various cancers) where disease onset may occur years after the suspected relevant exposure(s), appropriate locational assignment may involve collection of historical housing and occupational data for each case and any relevant noncases collected as a comparison group.

Lilienfeld and Stolley (1984, pp. 138–139) and Cromley and McLafferty (2002, pp. 214–215) both provide an example of location issues based on a study of endemic typhus fever in Montgomery, Alabama, originally published by Maxcy (1926). Maxcy mapped residences of cases revealing little spatial pattern. Maxcy then mapped occupational sites for cases showing a concentration of cases in the city's central business district. Closer examination of additional data associated with type of occupation showed higher incidence for employees of food depots, groceries, feed stores, and restaurants, suggesting a rodent reservoir of the disease with transmission via fleas, mites, or lice. This study illustrates two important points: (1) residence may not be the primary location of interest (e.g., location of the relevant exposure), and (2) additional, nonspatial data (here, type of business) often refine theories linking cases, and eventually, provide more detailed etiologic hypotheses than location alone.

These are some of the problems that we may encounter when working with spatial data. There are undoubtedly more that we can expect with particular applications. It is important to be aware of them, but we should not let them deter us from spatial analysis. We hold spatial data to very high standards: We do not seem to expect other types of data to be so widely and publicly available, nor do we have entire committees ensuring their accuracy and mandating their documentation!

In this chapter we have provided an overview of spatial public health data, from attributes and features, through geocoding, geodesy, and GIS, to sources, surveys, and use of ZIP codes. We turn now to spatial data analysis, and as we will see in the next chapter, this begins with the principles of cartography and the art and science of visualization.

CHAPTER 4

Visualizing Spatial Data

map: *Unlike photographs, maps are selective and may be prepared to show various quantitative and qualitative facts, including boundaries, physical features, patterns, and distribution.*

The Columbia Encyclopedia, 6th ed., 2001

A plague upon it! I have forgot the map.

William Shakespeare (1564–1616), Henry IV,
Part 1, act 3, scene 1, lines 5–6

Maps provide a powerful means to communicate data to others. Unlike information displayed in graphs, tables, and charts, maps also provide bookmarks for memories. They remind us of places we visit, a childhood home, and locations of historical events. In this way, maps are not passive mechanisms for presenting information. The *mapmaker* filters the data and its summaries to emphasize what he or she thinks is important. The *map reader* filters the map through his or her previous knowledge. Thus, the reader may not see what the mapmaker intended, and different readers may see different things in the same map. Consequently, maps inevitably include many avenues for misunderstanding.

More specifically, maps differ from statistical graphics because the geographic setting portrayed in the map almost always triggers memories, opinions, and conclusions wholly separate from (but perhaps related to) the intent of the mapmaker. As an example, in viewing a national weather map we almost instinctively examine our home city first rather than the perhaps more meteorologically interesting storm brewing across the country. In contrast, in a scatterplot of height versus weight, many readers note the overall pattern of points first, then try to identify their own coordinates in reference to the trends depicted in the plot. In studies of health and potential environmental effects, the "where's my house?" syndrome affecting map readers makes maps a very dynamic communication device, as people familiar with a particular location often bring additional local information into the discussion. For example, long-term residents of a neighborhood may add relevant information regarding the precise location of a closed and demolished gas station in a study

Applied Spatial Statistics for Public Health Data, by Lance A. Waller and Carol A. Gotway
ISBN 0-471-38771-1

of spatial patterns of leukemia incidence. In this setting, although the mapmakers may not have been aware of and did not include the potential exposure, some map viewers interpret the map in light of this additional information. It is often difficult (and sometimes impossible) to incorporate such information within a formal statistical analysis of a particular data set (e.g., such recollections may not occur in other areas containing similar exposures but no putative increase in health risk, thereby biasing any estimate of association between exposure and outcome), but the additions can provide important insight into the potential strengths and limitations of study conclusions.

In addition to these considerations, map readers often relate the accuracy of the display of the geographic setting of a data set to the accuracy of the data displayed. For example, if a map shows particular local geographic features (e.g., roads or rivers) accurately, map readers often suppose that the same level of accuracy applies to the local disease rates displayed in the same map. In short, a good map of bad data often seems much more believable than a bad map of good data, so it is in the spatial analyst's best interest to create good maps of the best data available.

This chapter reviews the role of mapmaking in spatial data analysis for public health through an overview of the field of cartography. We provide a review of the typical types of maps used in public health studies, notes regarding cartographic symbolization (i.e., choices regarding point, line, and area symbols, including color choices), and an introduction to statistical methods for stabilizing local rate estimates based on small numbers of people at risk. We conclude with a description of geographic, epidemiologic, and statistical issues arising in the analysis of data aggregated to and mapped in small areas. These topics provide the tools necessary for constructing accurate and effective maps of data and output for the statistical models described in subsequent chapters.

4.1 CARTOGRAPHY: THE ART AND SCIENCE OF MAPMAKING

The science of geodesy defines, through geometrical models of the Earth and map projections, the planar system within which we display our data. *Cartography* involves our decisions of which data to display and how we will display them; it is simply the art and science of mapmaking. The science provides the canvas and the frame, and the art provides the pens, brushes, and palette for creating the map. The art analogy is not too farfetched since we often cannot display all data items simultaneously in a single map, so we select certain features to highlight, and use the map and the symbols contained therein to aid in making and communicating the conclusions of our spatial analyses. As noted in the introduction to this chapter, the map serves as a point of communication between the mapmaker (in our case, the spatial analyst) and the map reader (e.g., a research collaborator, a journal reader or referee, or the general public). This communication has been the focus of much of the research literature in cartography since World War II. Monmonier (1996) provides a readable introduction to issues relating to making and reading a map; Slocum (1999) gives a comprehensive introduction into the principles of cartography illustrated with many examples; while MacEachren (1994, 1995) provide a more detailed typology of cartographic elements, their purposes, and their uses.

MacEachren (1995, pp. 2–6) cites two developments since World War II driving much of modern cartography: the publication of Arthur H. Robinson's dissertation in 1952 (Robinson 1952), followed by the developing view of cartography as a communication science in the 1970s. Robinson (1952) recognized that a solely artistic consideration of map design could often lead to increased map misinterpretation and proposed the detailed study of map perception in order to develop objective rules for map design. This view, coupled with an increasing appreciation of the communicative nature of maps, provides a rich array of methods for the cartographic display of spatially referenced data.

The rise of modern computing also dramatically affected the field of cartography (National Research Council 1997, p. 57). This impact is evident not only in the development of GISs to store, manage, and link spatial data but also in the evolution of new visualization techniques, including dynamic animated maps (Slocum 1999, Chapter 14) and interactive and multimedia maps linking geographic information with videos, sounds, pictures, and text. In the public health field, one of the earliest animated maps for desktop computers involved visualization of the spread of AIDS at the county level for Pennsylvania (Gould 1989; National Research Council 1997, p. 58). The capability to link additional information and to allow users to explore maps and related data personally led to the growth and expansion of electronic atlases. The development and design of Internet-based mapping tools remains an active area of cartographic development.

4.2 TYPES OF STATISTICAL MAPS

There are many different ways to classify map types in order to discuss and illustrate general mapping approaches and cartographic principles. Such approaches and principles necessarily vary with the purpose of the map. For example, the information we need from a map to be used for urban planning and zoning will be quite different from the information we need to hike the Grand Canyon. Thus (this being a statistics book and not a hiking guide), we focus our attention on some of the general types of maps that can be useful for displaying the spatial variation of quantitative data (e.g., disease rates, exposure levels, and population densities). We use data from the following map study for illustration and discussion.

MAP STUDY: Very Low Birth Weights in Georgia Health Care District 9 Rogers et al. (2000) presented the results of a case–control study of the risk of having a very low birth weight (VLBW) baby, defined as weighing less than 1500 grams at birth. The study area comprises 25 contiguous counties in southeastern Georgia, collectively referred to as Georgia Health Care District 9 (GHCD9) (Figure 4.1). Cases were identified from all live-born, singleton infants born between April 1, 1986 and March 30, 1988. Controls were selected for this study by drawing a 3% random sample of all live-born infants weighing more than 2499

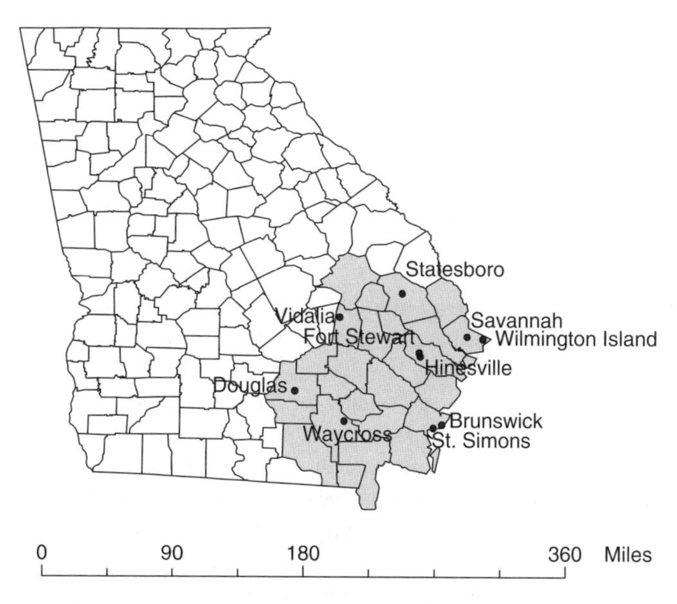

FIG. 4.1 Counties comprising Georgia Health Care District 9.

grams at birth. This sampling was constrained so that the controls met the same residency and time-frame requirements as the case subjects.

The addresses of the birth mothers were geocoded to produce georeferenced point location data. The maps presented in this chapter are based on a total of 230 cases and 550 controls. The number of live births per county was also recorded, enabling calculation of a VLBW rate for each county.

Emissions data for 1986–1988 on 32 industrial facilities within GHCD9 were obtained from the Georgia Environmental Protection Division (GAEPD) of the Georgia Department of Natural Resources. These industries produce chemicals, plastics, fertilizers, asphalt, wood, paper, and gypsum, and according to the GAEPD, account for almost 95% of the approximately 45,000 tons of total suspended particulate (TSP) emissions in the area per year. An atmospheric transport model was used to predict TSP exposure at the case and control residence locations. Further details of this study are described in Rogers et al. (2000).

For purposes of illustration in this chapter, we investigate the spatial distribution of several different variables: (1) the locations of the 230 cases and 550 controls; (2) the number of live births per county; (3) the VLBW rate per county; (4) 32 original TSP emissions values [in tons per year/1000 located by universal transmercator (UTM) coordinates]; and (5) the predicted TSP exposure at each of the 780 point residence locations (in $\mu g/m^3$). In the following subsections we use these variables to illustrate several different types of statistical maps and discuss some of the cartographic principles and issues associated with each one. Unfortunately, we are limited to black-and-white figures; more informative maps may be made by creative use of color (cf. Brewer 1994, 1999; Brewer et al. 1997).

4.2.1 Maps for Point Features

Many types of data used in public health studies are point features in that they can be associated with specific geographic point locations. Examples include residential addresses, locations of hospitals, locations of hazardous waste facilities, and locations of air pollution monitoring stations. There are several different ways to display this type of spatial data, depending on the type of attribute data associated with the point features.

Point Maps A point map uses symbols to delineate the locations in a point feature class. The main goal of a point map is visualization of the spatial distribution of the point features. Thus, if there is no attribute information associated with the locations, or we just want to see where the point locations are relative to one another and to other features of interest, a point map can be useful. Often, the symbols are simply filled dots, and in such situations, point maps are often called *dot maps*. A dot map of the VLBW case locations in GHCD9 appears in Figure 4.2.

Dot maps of health data are frequently used to monitor the spread of infectious diseases and can be useful in identifying potential point sources of disease outbreaks. John Snow's map depicting the clustering of cholera cases around the Broad Street pump is a famous example (Snow 1855; Frerichs 2000). However, such maps must be interpreted with caution since the underlying population also varies spatially. Disease occurs where people are, and any apparent clusters could simply be due to a large concentration of residents in a given area. This could be

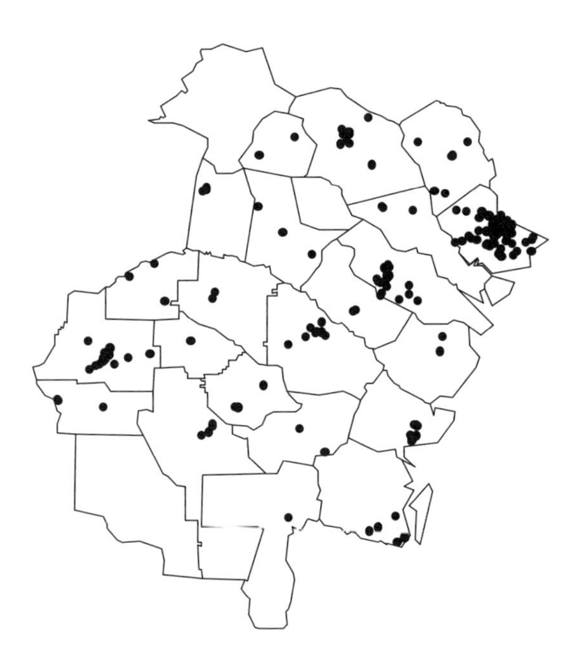

FIG. 4.2 Point map of cases of very low birth weight in Georgia Health Care District 9.

the situation conveyed by Figure 4.2, where the largest concentrations of VLBW cases correspond to the large cites shown in Figure 4.1. Note that dot maps of data that are not based on population (e.g., dot maps delineating the locations of landfills or monitoring stations) do not have this interpretive problem.

Another type of point map, called a *graduated color map*, can be used to address this difficulty (Figure 4.3). Here, the locations of both cases and controls are plotted on the same map with the same symbol, but two different colors are used to differentiate cases from controls. The assumption here is that the controls are a representative sample of the underlying population at risk and thus their spatial distribution is similar to that of the underlying population at risk. With this type of map, the spatial distribution of cases is compared to that of controls rather than to the distribution of the underlying population that is inferred by the reference map of the counties in GHCD9.

We can also plot point features with continuous attribute information (e.g., pH or air pollution concentration). With a continuous attribute, we divide values into several different classes and use different colors and/or symbols to delineate each class. Such a map is sometimes referred to as a *postplot*. The goal here is to allow the map viewer to see the spatial distribution of all locations as well as judge relative differences in attribute values without the smoothing that results from contouring. As an example, we use such a map to look at the spatial distribution of predicted TSP concentration values associated with each residence (Figure 4.4). Here, we are not interested in the relative arrangement of locations but in the spatial variation in TSP concentrations.

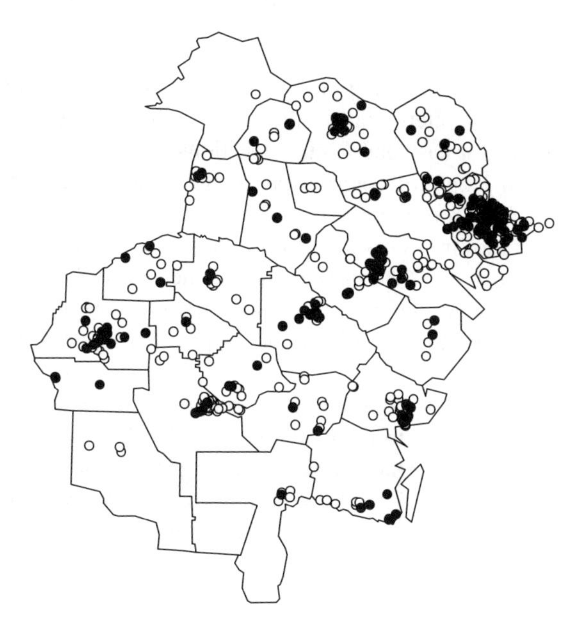

FIG. 4.3 Graduated color map of cases of very low birth weight and controls in Georgia Health Care District 9. Case locations are indicted with filled circles; control locations are designated by the open circles.

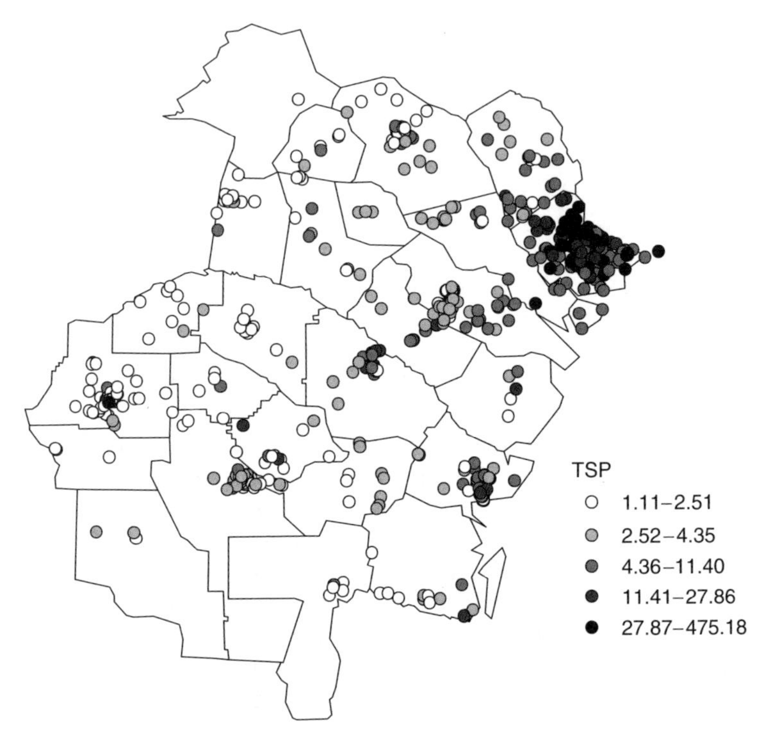

FIG. 4.4 Graduated color postplot of predicted TSP concentrations (in tons per year) in GHCD9.

Many other options for symbology in point maps also exist. With a *point symbol map,* different events of interest are indicated by different symbols (e.g., using filled and open circles for case and control locations as in the example above). We can also use pictorial icons to represent particular locations (e.g., red crosses for hospitals, airplanes for airports, flags for schools).

There is no reason to limit ourselves to the two-dimensional map view. We can also use the usual statistical *scatterplot* in three dimensions. With this type of plot, we plot attribute values on the z-axis and plot locations in the (u, v) plane. An example based on the original 32 TSP values appears in Figure 4.5.

Contour Maps For spatially continuous attribute variables with point support, point maps may be inadequate to really allow us to visualize the spatial distribution of the attribute values. For example, referring to Figures 4.4 and 4.5, we can easily see where the high and low TSP concentrations are, and we can obtain an overall indication of broad geographic trends. However, we really cannot assess more complicated trends and spatial patterns in the values. Also, point maps may not be very informative if we have a large number of points or if some of the spatial locations are very close together.

Another approach to visualizing spatially continuous attribute values is to use a *contour map.* Contour maps represent values of an attribute variable in two

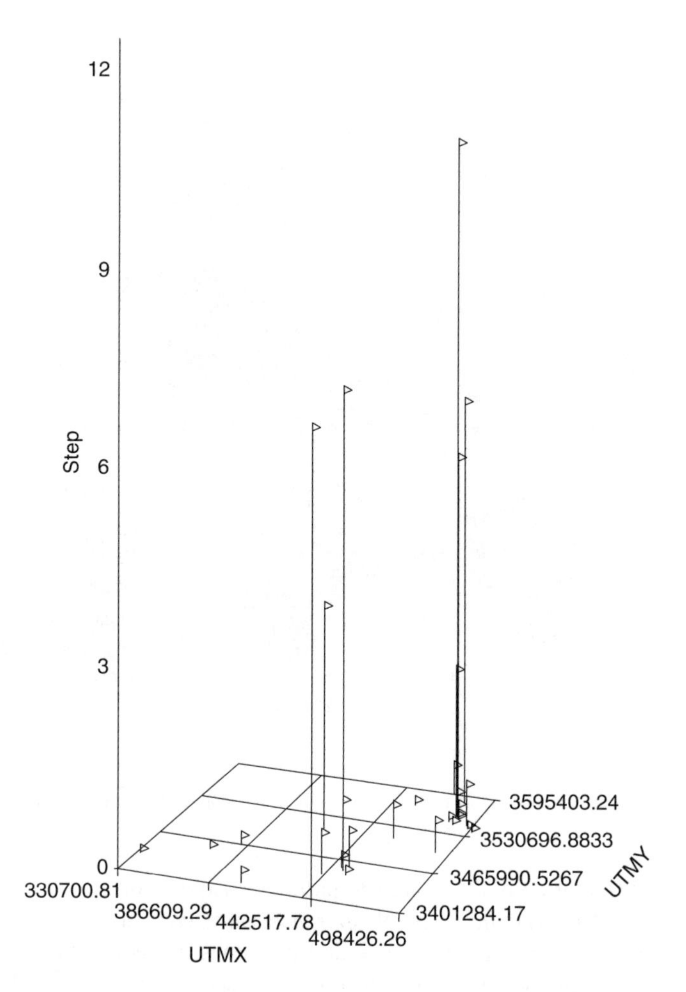

FIG. 4.5 Three-dimensional scatterplot of the original 32 TSP concentrations (in tons per year/1000) in GHCD9. UTMX denotes the u-axis and UTMY the v-axis (measured in UTM coordinates).

dimensions using lines of equal values, called *isolines,* across the extent of the map. To construct a contour map, we must first "fill in the holes" between the data locations. This is done with a process called *gridding,* the systematic interpolation of attribute values onto a regular arrangement (or grid) of spatial locations with our domain of interest. We discuss statistical methods for gridding in Section 8.3. For now, we simply focus on the visualization aspect of the maps and not their methods of construction.

We can display a contour map in several ways. First, we must decide how many isolines to use. Certainly, if we use just one isoline, our map will be too vague, and if we use too many isolines, our map will be too busy. Typically, between 5 and 10 isolines are used. We can draw the isolines and label them numerically on the

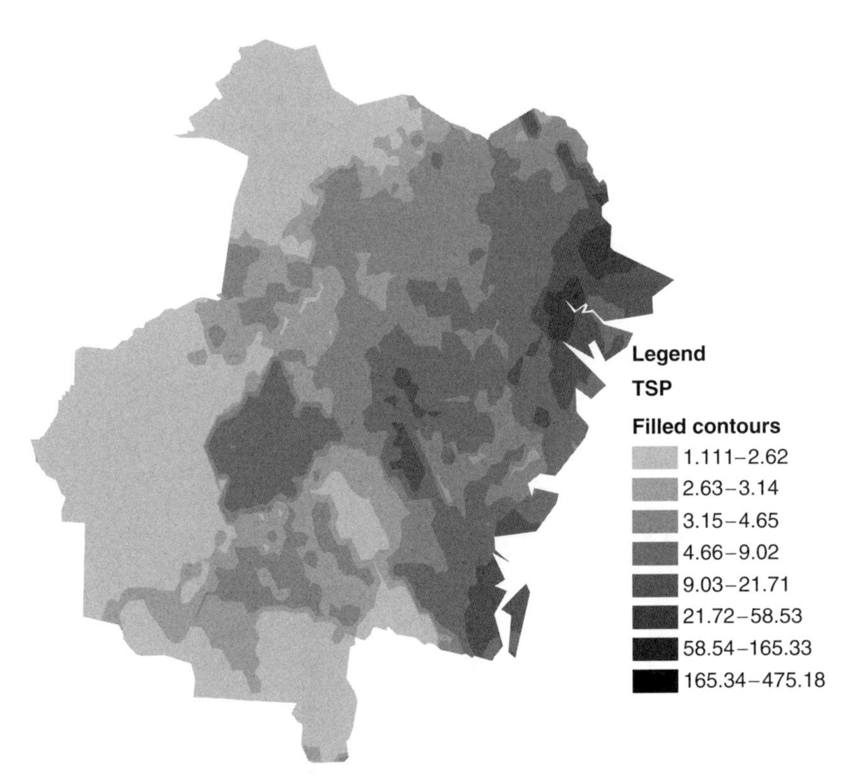

FIG. 4.6 Filled contour map of predicted TSP concentrations (in tons per year) in GHCD9.

map, or use different colors to designate particular isolines or sets of isolines. For example, if the data contain a central reference value (e.g., a mean concentration or regulatory limit), one can used thick and thin lines to mark isolines associated with values above and below the reference value, respectively. One popular contour map, called a *filled contour map*, uses color and patterns between the contour lines. Figure 4.6 illustrates this type of map for the TSP concentrations predicted. This map is a smooth version of the postplot in Figure 4.4. It is much easier to see the spatial distribution in the TSP concentrations in this map than it is in the postplot.

Again, we are not limited to two-dimensional display. A *surface map* is a three-dimensional representation of gridded attribute data. Instead of shading the attribute values like we do when constructing a contour map, we simply plot the interpolated attribute values on the z-axis as a function of the spatial locations in the x, y plane. A surface map of the predicted TSP concentrations is shown in Figure 4.7. This map is a smooth version of the three-dimensional scatter diagram in Figure 4.5.

Image Maps Image Maps show the values of a spatially continuous attribute variable as variation in colors assigned to a regular array of pixels. The most common examples of image maps are satellite images and aerial photographs. An example of an aerial photograph is shown in Figure 4.8.

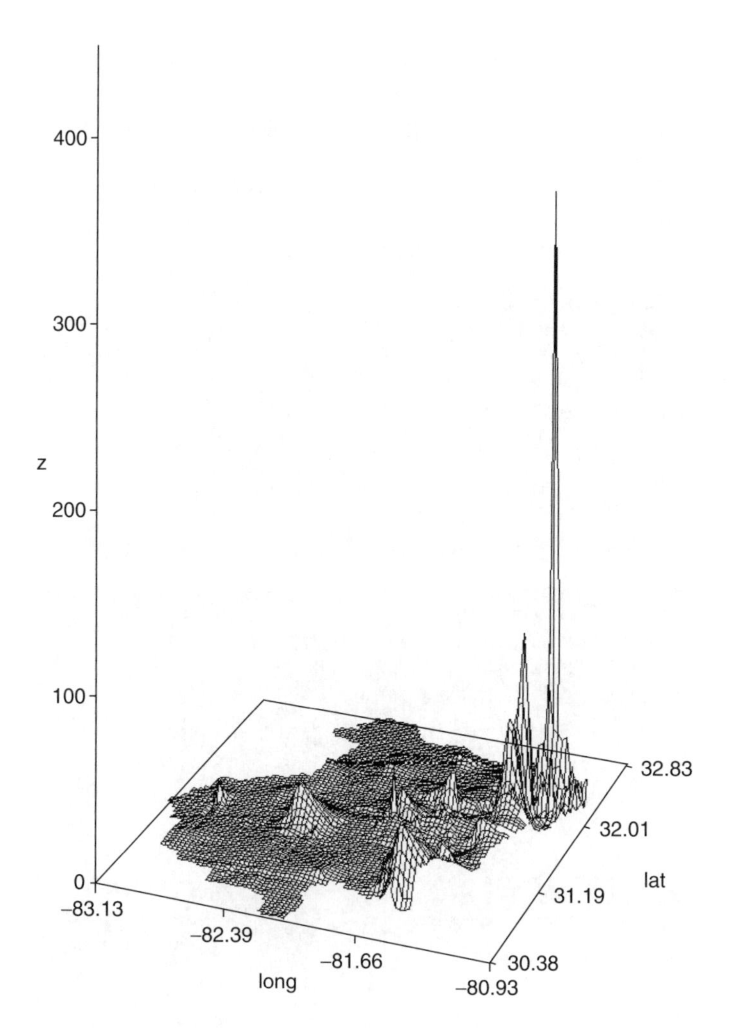

FIG. 4.7 Surface map of predicted TSP concentrations (in tons per year) in GHCD9.

4.2.2 Maps for Areal Features

Often, attribute values are associated with an area as opposed to a specific point on the map, for example, the number of births per county in GHCD9. Information associated with an area on a map is called *areal* or *regional data*. There are several approaches for visualizing areal data.

Classed Symbol Maps With these maps, a symbol is located at the center of each region and the attribute value associated with each feature is indicated by the choice of symbol. With a *graduated symbol map* the symbol size (often, a filled circle) varies with the attribute value or class of values. Figure 4.9 displays the number of very low birth weight babies per county in using a graduated symbol map.

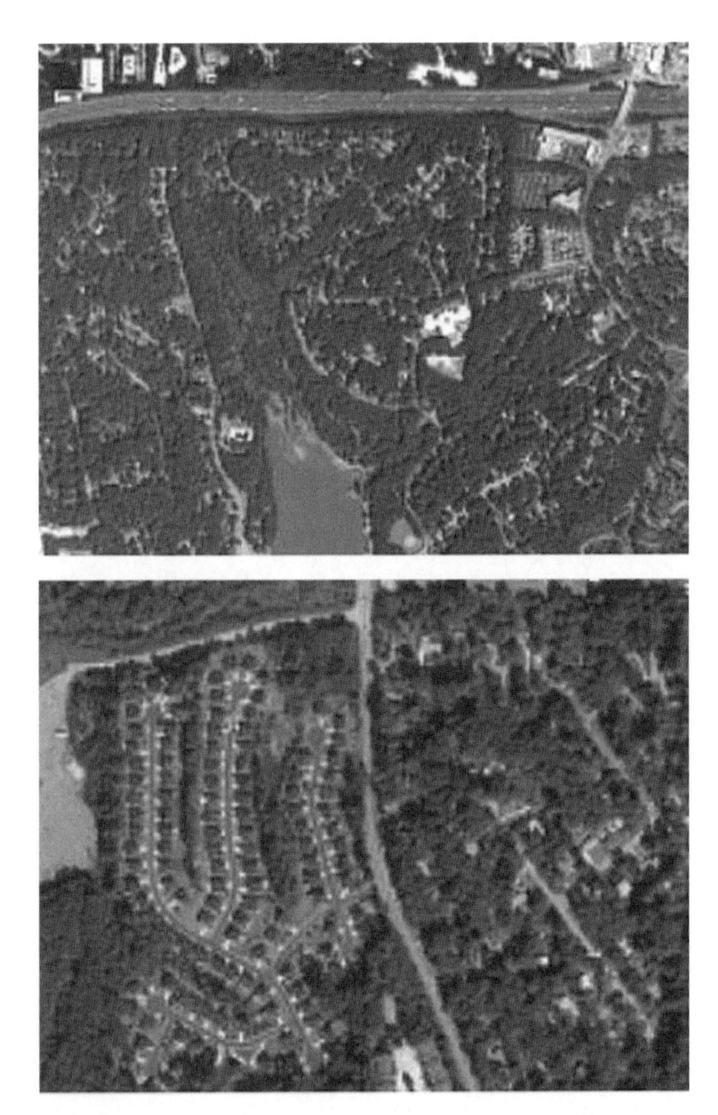

FIG. 4.8 Aerial photographs. The top photograph is Carol Gotway's neighborhood and the bottom photograph is Lance Waller's neighborhood. Both neighborhoods are in Atlanta, Georgia.

With a *proportional symbol map* the symbol size is proportional to the magnitude of the attribute values in each class. Figure 4.10 is an example of a proportional symbol map where the size of each stork indicates the relative number of live births per county.

Choropleth Maps Choropleth maps are probably the most common type of map for the display of areal data. These maps use different color and pattern combinations to depict different values of the attribute variable associated with each

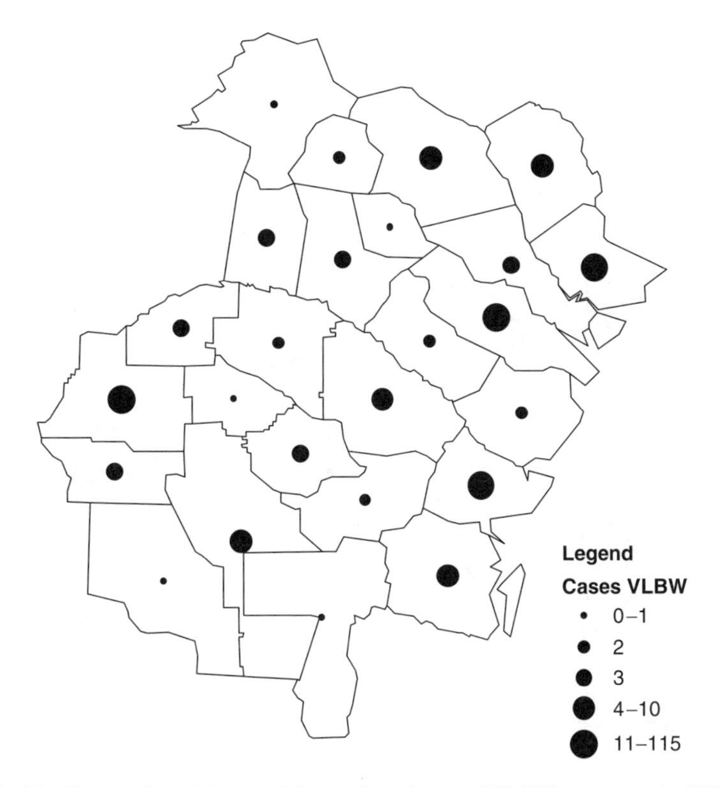

FIG. 4.9 Graduated symbol map of the number of cases of VLBW per county in GHCD9.

area. Each area is colored according to the category into which its corresponding attribute value falls. Figure 4.11 is a choropleth map of very low birth weight rates per county in Georgia Health Care District 9. Here, counties with the darkest shading have the highest rates of very low birth weight births; counties with the lightest shading have the lowest rates. The legend provides us indication of the overall magnitude of the rates and the magnitude of the relative differences in attribute values that correspond to the range of colors used in the map.

Many cartographers find the choropleth map a relatively crude method of displaying data, particularly data such as disease rates or exposure values, which vary continuously in space. Several statisticians share this view; for instance, Tukey (1988, p. 116) offers the following advice to users of choropleth ("patch") maps: "Pray." A primary reason for these concerns is that a choropleth map of continuous values presents the true (unknown) surface, often assumed to be smoothly varying, as a piecewise set of constant regional levels. However, many demographic data (e.g., age, race, and gender) utilized in studies of public health are only available in aggregate for enumeration units associated with the decennial census and projections from these data for intercensus years. As a result, choropleth maps often figure predominately in public health studies.

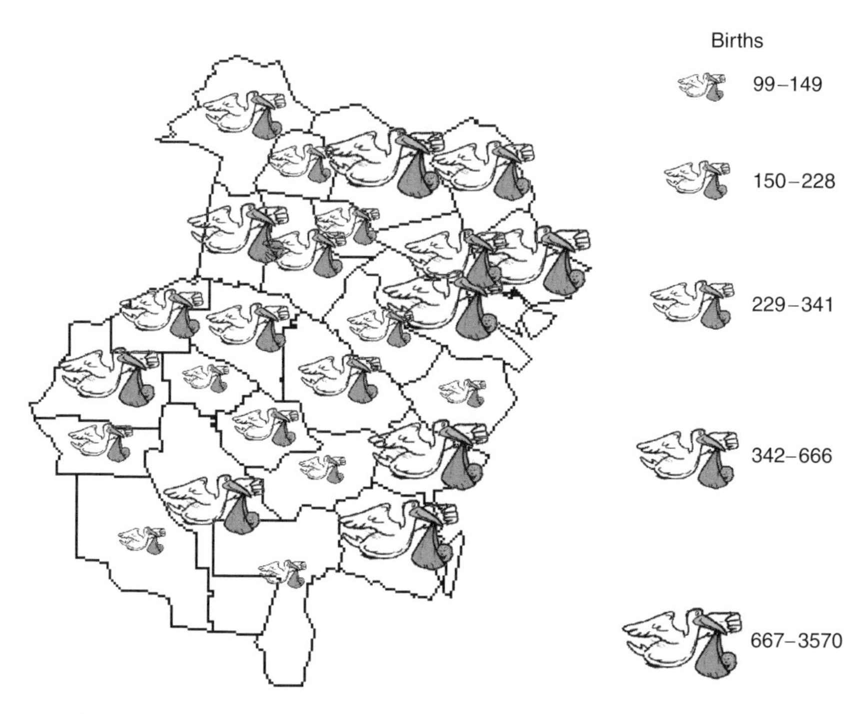

FIG. 4.10 Proportional symbol map of the number of live births per county in GHCD9.

A variety of cartographic possibilities exists, even within the family of choropleth maps. *Classed choropleth maps* (e.g., Figure 4.11) assign to each region a color, gray scale, or pattern associated with one of a set of nonoverlapping intervals covering the full range of data values. Intervals may be of equal length, or defined by data quantiles, "natural breaks" in the observed data, or standard deviation units, or based on substantive considerations (e.g., pollutant levels associated with particular levels of regulatory action). Some classification schemes optimize particular criteria, but all should be considered in light of the application at hand. Quantiles provide (roughly) equal numbers of regions in each class, while equal intervals provide interpretable ranges and can better indicate skewness in the outcome distribution. Slocum (1999, Chapter 4) provides a valuable summary of options for data classification for choropleth maps and illustrations of the differences between them.

Unclassed choropleth maps assign color, gray scale, or pattern according to a continuous range (e.g., saturation of a single hue going from light to dark red) where the value associated with each region corresponds to a unique assignment along this continuum and no two regions share precisely the same color, gray scale, or pattern unless they have the same attribute value. Debates regarding the relative merits of classed and unclassed maps peppered the cartographic literature from the 1970s into the 1990s, and Slocum (1999, Section 4.2) provides an overview of the issue and many examples of both types of maps, illustrating the advantages and disadvantages of each.

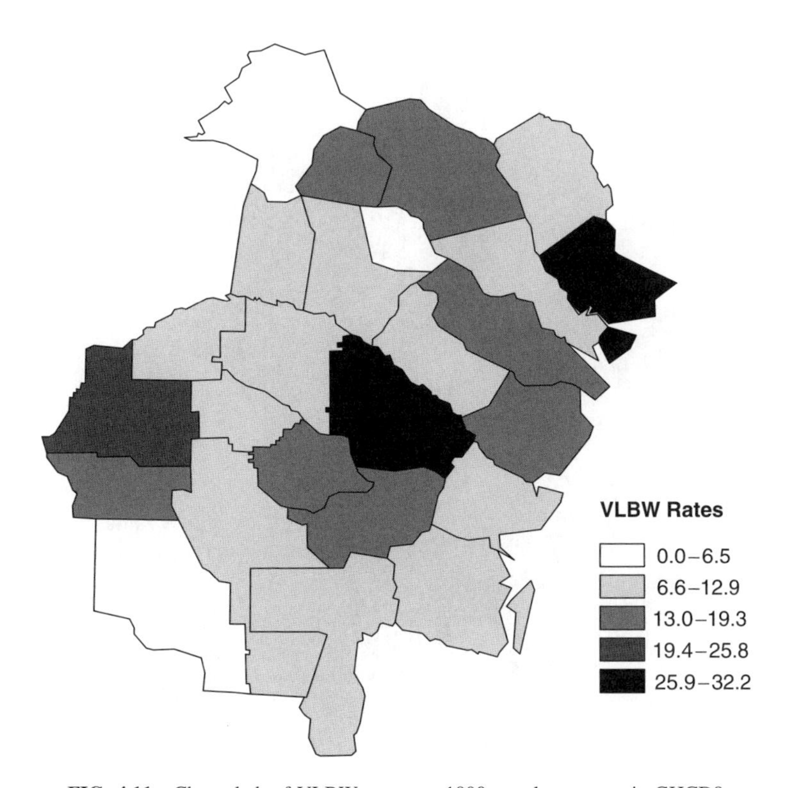

FIG. 4.11 Choropleth of VLBW rates per 1000 people per year in GHCD9.

The appropriate selection of a map type depends on the experience and familiarity of the map *readers* as well as the map creators. With particular reference to maps of disease rates, Pickle et al. (1994) report that the epidemiologists they interviewed preferred classed choropleth maps and used them more accurately than competing types of maps. As a result, we expect classed choropleth maps to remain in fairly wide use within public health for some time to come.

Three-Dimensional Display The three-dimensional depiction of a choropleth map is called a *prism map* or a *stepped statistical surface* (see Figure 4.12). It uses raised polygons, or prisms, of different heights, patterns, or colors to indicate the values or classes of values of the attribute variable. *Block maps* are similar but use blocks (narrow rectangular prisms within each region) instead of area-shaped prisms to indicate the relative values of the attribute variable. These types of maps make it easier to see connected regions with the same class of values. However, it can be difficult to choose a good angle (*tilt*) and perspective (*rotation*) for viewing, particularly if there are many regions.

Dot Density Maps Not to be confused with dot maps described in Section 4.2.1, dot density maps derive from aggregated data. Each region has an associated

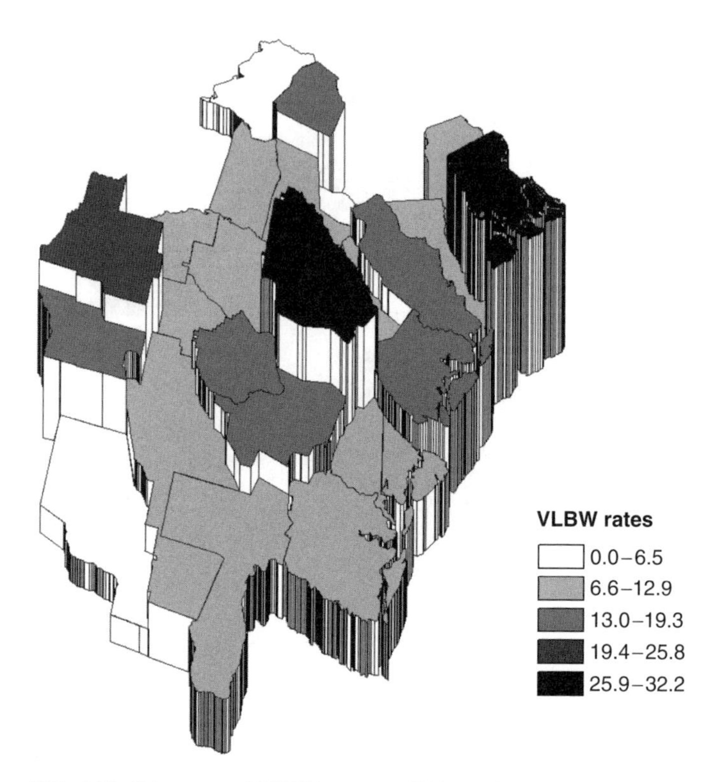

FIG. 4.12 Prism map of VLBW rates per 1000 people per year in GHCD9.

attribute value (e.g., the number of live births in a given time period). Instead of representing each regional value through shading or a proportional symbol, we add a number of dots to each region, representing that region's attribute value. For instance, we could assign a dot for each 100 live births in a county over the study period. We place dots randomly within each region. Visually, the density of dots in each region represents the value in a given area. The more points in a given area, the higher the attribute value in that area.

Dot density maps can be very misleading in public health applications since it is easy for map readers to assume that each dot on the map represents the actual location of an event. For example, consider the number of cases of very low birth weight for each county obtained by adding the total number of cases of VLBW in each county. Figure 4.13 shows a dot density map constructed from these aggregated data. Since there are very few cases of VLBW per county, we use one dot for each case. In this instance, the number of dots per county represents the number of cases, but the locations of the dots within each county are randomly generated and do not represent the location of case residences. Recall that case locations appear in Figure 4.2. We find it far too easy for map readers to assume that the map in Figure 4.13 represents the same spatial information as the map in Figure 4.2, when, in fact, the accuracy of event locations is actually very different

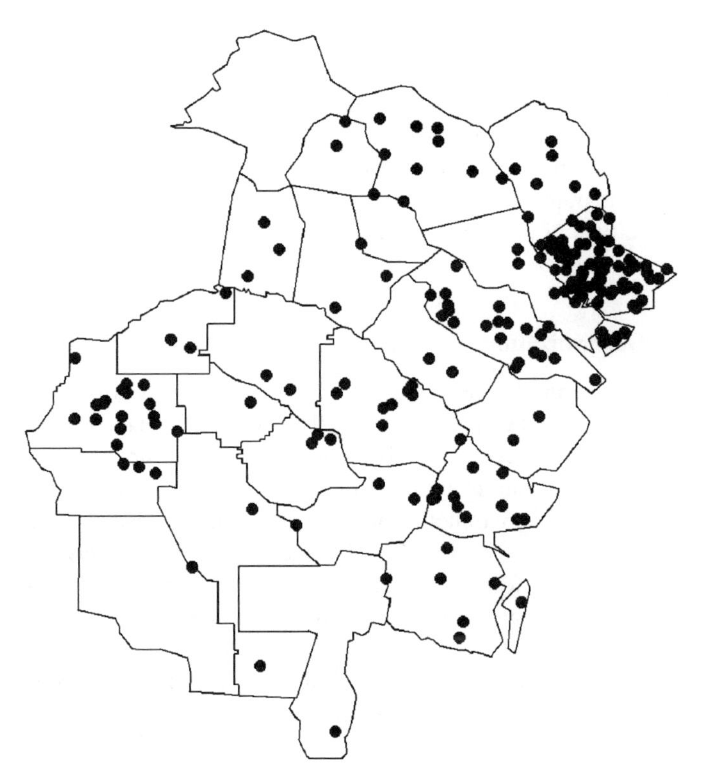

FIG. 4.13 Dot density map derived from the number of cases of VLBW aggregated by county. One dot corresponds to one case of VLBW.

between the two maps (accurate to the county level or accurate to the individual level, respectively). While dot density maps most often assign multiple events to each dot (e.g., a single dot represents 100 cases), we find the visual temptation to interpret mapped dots as actual case locations to be far too strong to recommend use of dot density maps for public health applications.

Other Maps Although we review and illustrate several basic types of maps used to visualize spatial data in this section, there are many others (some of which we mention briefly in Section 4.6). Which type of map we use and our selection of particular visualization options (e.g., classes and colors in a choropleth map) depend on the type of spatial features, the nature of the attribute values, and the message we want to convey. Often, the best approach is to try different maps with different visualization options and then compare results. For example, with the very low birth weight births, the nature of the spatial variation and our color limitations (to shades of gray only) lead us to prefer a choropleth map over a prism map. The tilting and rotation used to obtain a decent viewpoint seems to distort the prism map somewhat, and even then, some of the higher prisms hide lower prisms, making this map visually unappealing and difficult to read.

4.3 SYMBOLIZATION

Once we choose a map type (or perhaps types) to display our data, we must also consider the *symbolization* used to display the data within the map. Computer-based mapping routines with GISs offer a wide variety of point, line, and area symbols to consider. Cartographic principles offer guidance on symbolization, which again depends on the type of data, the message to be delivered, and the medium used to deliver it.

4.3.1 Map Generalization

The first consideration is that of *map generalization*, which governs the level of detail represented in geographic features displayed on a map. For instance, we display most linear features such as rivers or roads as collections of connected line segments. The generalization question involves how many segments we should use to approximate the continuous nature of our "linear" feature. Generalization affects issues in GIS map layering. For instance, if we use two layers containing boundaries of the same feature (e.g., a census tract) stored at different levels of generalization, we may have difficulty resolving the borders. Generalization issues are often internal to many GISs, but can affect the construction of maps with layers from a variety of data sources. McMaster and Shea (1992) provide an overview of map generalization and its basic components.

4.3.2 Visual Variables

Next we consider the choice of symbols to represent particular geographic features (Monmonier 1996, Chapter 10). Bertin (1983) defines the basic typology of visual variables pertaining to the symbolization of maps. These variables include location in the plane, size, shape, orientation, texture, gray-scale value, and color. Slocum (1999, p. 23 and Section 2.3) presents these in some detail, and both Monmonier (1996, p. 20) and MacEachren (1994, p. 16) provide tables illustrating these variables for points, lines, and areas.

The first two variables are fairly straightforward. *Location* in the plane provides the spatial structure and support of our geographic data. Size of point features indicates actual or relative value, or identifies subgroups of points. Size of line features typically corresponds to width, where, for example, wider lines correspond to interstate highways and narrower lines correspond to local streets. Using size symbolization for area-based data typically involves the use of graduated symbols within each area (e.g., Figures 4.9 and 4.10).

Shape corresponds to icons associated with each geographic feature. Point features may be displayed using pictorial representations providing the map reader with widely differing visual impressions. As a quick example of the impact of symbolization, if we replace the largest storks in Figure 4.10 by skulls and crossbones, our first impression is likely one of distress for areas associated with this symbol.

Orientation provides another mode of visual distinction. One example is the use of wind direction symbols in meteorologic maps, but the idea is quite general. We could indicate local positive and negative deviations from an overall mean by slanting lines to the right or the left at points, along lines, or within areas.

Texture, *gray-scale value*, and *color* refer to the graphical patterns or colors assigned to points, lines, and areas. The primary consideration in the assignment of textures, gray-scales, and colors should be the message the mapmaker wishes to convey. In the next section we present recommendations drawing primarily from research involving color (Brewer 1994, 1999; Brewer et al. 1997), but many of the same principles apply to texture and gray-scale values.

4.3.3 Color

Monmonier (1996, Chapter 11) provides an introduction to the "attraction and distraction" of the use of color in maps, and Brewer (1994) and Slocum (1999, Chapter 6) provide thorough reviews of the role of color in modern cartography. Color is a three-dimensional concept consisting of *hue* (e.g. red, green, or blue), *lightness* or *value* (e.g., light versus dark), and *saturation* or *chroma* (e.g., dull versus vivid). Varying one or more of these dimensions results in different colors. Brewer (1994) notes that viewers tend to perceive *differences* between colors most readily when changing hue, and perceive *ordering* most readily when changing lightness (with darker colors perceived as "higher"). That is, a map viewer can quickly tell that a green region is somehow different from a red region, but can more readily report that the light green region is somehow "lower" than the dark green region. While chromatic (rainbow) colors have an optical ordering (red < orange < yellow < green < blue < violet), ordering, say, orange relative to green often requires more thought than ordering light green and dark green (Monmonier 1996, p. 168).

Brewer (1999) suggests dichotomies helpful in determining the appropriate use of color for maps, based on the underlying message that a mapmaker wishes to convey. The first is the distinction between *sequential* and *diverging patterns* in mapped values. With sequential patterns, we want our map readers to readily identify which values are higher or lower than other values. As noted above, lightness is the color dimension best suited for sequential perception. For diverging patterns, we want our map readers to easily identify ordering in two directions. For instance, if we assign blue to counties having lower than average rates and red to counties having higher than average rates, the reader can quickly separate the blue from the red counties. Brewer (1999) notes that map readers identify differences in hue more readily than differences in lightness or saturation for diverging patterns. By varying lightness within each hue (e.g., light to dark blue for intervals moving farther below the mean, and light to dark red for intervals moving farther above the mean) we allow readers to quickly identify counties with rates above or below the state rate and to order counties within each of these two classes. The *Atlas of United States Mortality* (Pickle et al. 1996; Brewer et al. 1997) uses this sort of scheme for precisely these reasons.

Brewer (1999) also considers *qualitative* and *binary* mapping goals where we want our map viewer to be able to distinguish between several or two categories, respectively. In these cases, differences in hue provide the preferred color scheme, but some thought should go into the particular hues. For instance, three categories colored bright yellow, dark green, and dark blue do not provide equal visual distinction between all categories.

Finally, color choices also involve considerations of color choices for colorblind readers, color choices for display on computer terminals, color choices for color printing, and color choices for various projection options. Cynthia Brewer synthesizes much of her research (referenced above) in the "ColorBrewer" Web site, which provides automated assessments of particular color schemes with respect to these particular presentation issues.

4.4 MAPPING SMOOTHED RATES AND PROBABILITIES

We now turn from choices governing the type and structure of a map, to considerations of what values to map. The typical goal of mapping public health data is to provide insight into geographic variations in disease risk. *Risk* is simply the probability that an unfortunate event occurs. In public health, the unfortunate event is usually the contraction of or death from a specific disease. When we make a map of disease counts, proportions, or rates, we are ultimately intending to convey inferences about disease risk. However, a map of raw counts is not the best tool for inference about disease risk, since we expect regions with larger populations to have higher disease counts. We can account for population differences by using rates (disease incidence per person per time) as measures of risk. Higher disease rates reflect greater chances for contracting the disease, and thus, viewed this way, rates reflect a person's risk for disease. However, a map of rates may still obscure the spatial pattern in disease risk, particularly if the rates are based on populations of very different sizes. Since the variability in the estimated local rates depends on population size, some rates may be better estimated than others, and this may obscure spatial patterns in disease risk. Rates based on small populations or on small numbers of disease cases are likely to be elevated artificially, reflecting lack of data rather than true elevated risk. As a simple example, consider a large metropolitan area with 2 million residents and 2 observed cases of a disease. Suppose that the study area consists of subregions each containing 100 persons at risk. For the entire study area the crude incidence rate is 1/1,000,000, while two of the small areas contain crude rate estimates of 1/100. This is often referred to as the *small number problem*.

There are several solutions to this problem. First, we could calculate rates over larger areas (e.g., use states instead of counties), although this comes at the expense of giving up some of the geographic information we wish to convey. Second, we could make a comparative map, one that compares each rate to a common measure and, in doing so, adjusts for different population sizes. One such map is a *probability map* (described in Section 4.4.4). Another approach is *spatial smoothing*, one method for reducing the noise in rates associated with geographic regions. Spatial smoothers are analogous to scatterplot smoothers in regression analysis and to moving-averaging methods in time series, adapted to two dimensions. The basic idea is to "borrow" information from neighboring regions to produce a better (i.e., more stable and less noisy) estimate of the rate associated with each region and thus separate out the "signal" (i.e., spatial pattern) from the noise. There are many different approaches to spatial smoothing. We tend to favor those with theoretical statistical foundations and those that lead to statistical models. Thus, we have limited our discussion to commonly used approaches that satisfy these criteria and do not rely on a lot of assumptions, tedious derivations, or complex computations procedures. Other methods are described in Section 4.6.4 or are given in the references.

4.4.1 Locally Weighted Averages

We can obtain a smoothed value for each region by simply averaging the values associated with neighboring regions. With *disk smoothing*, a circular or disk smoothing window of specified radius is centered at the centroid of each region. The smoothed value for each region is then taken to be the average of all the values associated with centroids that lie within the disk. Thus, if $r_1, r_2, \ldots, r_N$ are the observed rates, smoothed rates can be calculated as

$$\tilde{r}_i = \frac{\sum_{j=1}^{N} w_{ij} r_j}{\sum_{j=1}^{N} w_{ij}}, \tag{4.1}$$

where the weights are given by

$$w_{ij} = \begin{cases} 1 & \text{if } d_{ij} < \delta \\ 0 & \text{otherwise.} \end{cases} \tag{4.2}$$

Here d_{ij} is the distance (Euclidean, city-block, or any other distance metric) between the centroids of regions i and j and δ is the disk radius. Casper et al. (2000) utilize disk smoothing in their atlas of heart disease in women for the United States.

We may also want simultaneously to weight by population, so that more stable rates (i.e., those based on larger populations) receive more weight than those based on smaller populations. Thus, we may want to use

$$w_{ij} = \begin{cases} n_j & \text{if } d_{ij} < \delta \\ 0 & \text{otherwise.} \end{cases} \tag{4.3}$$

Instead of using circular disks of constant radius defined by geographic proximity, Talbot et al. (2000) recommend the use of moving windows defined in terms of constant population size. More generally, we may want to define a *smoothing neighborhood* that identifies, for each region, the set of regions whose values are to be used in the local average. A common approach to defining smoothing neighborhoods is through a *spatial proximity measure* (discussed in more detail in Section 7.4.2) that specifies the neighborhood structure and provides suitable weights for the values being averaged. Different smoothers result from different choices for the weights. One example, described in Section 3.2.3, is to use adjacency to define neighbors. Thus, we could use

$$w_{ij} = \begin{cases} 1 & \text{if regions } i \text{ and } j \text{ share a boundary} \\ 0 & \text{otherwise.} \end{cases}$$

Sometimes, it is advantageous to separate the ideas of neighborhood structure and distance, population, or other types of weighting approaches. Thus, we define $\mathcal{N}_i = \{j : \text{region } j \text{ is a neighbor of region } i\}$, as the *neighborhood set* of the ith region, where $j \in \mathcal{N}_i$, implies that region j is a *neighbor* of region i. Thus, we can write the locally weighted mean as

$$\tilde{r}_i = \frac{\sum_{j=1}^{N} w_{ij}^* r_j I[j \in \mathcal{N}_i]}{\sum_{j=1}^{N} w_{ij}^* I[j \in \mathcal{N}_i]}, \tag{4.4}$$

where

$$I[j \in \mathcal{N}_i] = \begin{cases} 1 & \text{if regions } i \text{ and } j \text{ are neighbors} \\ 0 & \text{otherwise} \end{cases} \tag{4.5}$$

and w_{ij}^* can be any weights of our choosing. For example, choosing $w_{ij}^* = n_j$ and $\mathcal{N}_i = \{j : d_{ij} < \delta\}$, will give us the same overall weighting as using the weights in equation (4.3) with the smoother in equation (4.1).

Regardless of the weighting function chosen, all means (weighted or not) are sensitive to extreme observations and skewed distributions. More resistant smoothers can be constructed by using medians rather than means. With median-based disk smoothing, smoothed values are obtained as the median of all values in each disk. This idea can be extended to incorporate weighted medians and other robust measures of central tendency.

4.4.2 Nonparametric Regression

Suppose that we have data $Y_1, Y_2, \ldots, Y_N$ from a probability distribution $f(y|\xi)$, where ξ is an unknown parameter that we wish to estimate. The locally weighted mean described in Section 4.4.1 is a special case of a more general class of local estimators that are derived by maximizing the weighted log-likelihood of the data given by (Brillinger 1990)

$$\sum_{j=1}^{N} w_{ij} \log f(y_j|\xi).$$

Different estimators can be obtained for different distributions and for different problems. For example, if the data are Gaussian with means ξ_i and common variance σ^2, we can estimate ξ by maximizing the weighted log-likelihood with respect to ξ. Thus,

$$\hat{\xi}_i = \frac{\sum_{j=1}^{N} w_{ij} Y_j}{\sum_{j=1}^{N} w_{ij}},$$

which is the locally weighted mean given in equation (4.1) based on the Y_j, suggesting that equation (4.1) makes theoretical sense if we assume that local rates follow a normal distribution. We note that the variance, σ^2, affects any estimate of standard errors, but not the point estimates $\hat{\xi}_i$.

More often, we consider rates, $r_i = Y_i/n_i$, where Y_i is assumed to follow a Poisson distribution with mean (and variance) $n_i\xi$. Here ξ represents the probability of any person contracting a disease (i.e., the risk of disease), and we wish to map locally smoothed estimates of ξ to investigate whether the individual risk (rate) or disease appears to vary across the study area. In this setting, the approach of Brillinger (1990) yields a locally weighted estimate of ξ for the ith region, the locally smoothed rate $\tilde{r}_i$ given by

$$\tilde{r}_i = \frac{\sum_{j=1}^{N} w_{ij} Y_j}{\sum_{j=1}^{N} w_{ij} n_j}. \tag{4.6}$$

This estimate differs from the locally weighted mean given in equation (4.1) and represents a ratio of two smoothers, one applied to the Y_i and one applied to the n_i (cf. Kafadar 1996). Such a smoother might be advantageous if we also want to explicitly consider, and smooth out, variations in population data that might arise from sampling or counting errors.

As before, different estimators result from different choices of weights. We can use a very general notion of weights through the use of *kernel functions*, by defining

$$w_{ij} = \text{kern}\left(\frac{\boldsymbol{s}_i - \boldsymbol{s}_j}{b}\right),$$

where $\boldsymbol{s}_i$ and $\boldsymbol{s}_j$ denote the spatial locations of the centroids of regions i and j. The kernel function, kern$(\cdot)$, is a bivariate probability density function that is symmetric about the origin and integrates to 1 over the domain. The parameter b, called the *bandwidth*, controls the amount of smoothing. Here we assign decreasing weight to observations Y_j as the distance between locations $\boldsymbol{s}_j$ and $\boldsymbol{s}_i$ increases. Larger values of b result in including more areas in the smoothing neighborhood and lead to maps with less geographic variation (i.e., "smoother" maps). With kernel smoothing, smoothed rates are computed as

$$\tilde{r}_i = \frac{\sum_{j=1}^{N} \text{kern}\left(\frac{\boldsymbol{s}_i - \boldsymbol{s}_j}{b}\right) Y_j}{\sum_{j=1}^{N} \text{kern}\left(\frac{\boldsymbol{s}_i - \boldsymbol{s}_j}{b}\right) n_j}.$$

We provide a much more detailed description of kernel smoothing and examples of kernel functions in Section 5.2.5.

We can also consider local polynomial regression estimators. Instead of a locally weighted mean, a weighted regression estimate is obtained in each neighborhood. This approach was first proposed by Cleveland (1979) for scatterplot smoothing and is now known as a class of smoothers referred to as *loess smoothers*. It was then adapted to multivariate smoothing by Cleveland and Devlin (1988). Let $\boldsymbol{s}_i = (u_i, v_i)$ be the centroid of region i and let Y_i denote the corresponding outcome variable of interest. In loess smoothing, we regress Y_i or r_i on functions of u_i and v_i using just the values at the locations closest to (u_i, v_i). The number of neighboring values used in each local regression is specified as a fraction of the values, called the *span*. The regression is weighted using a user-specified function of the distance between $\boldsymbol{s}_i$ and the centroids of its neighboring regions. The smoothed value at each $\boldsymbol{s}_i$ is then the predicted value from the locally weighted regression surface.

4.4.3 Empirical Bayes Smoothing

The smoothing approaches outlined earlier "borrow" information from nearby regions to stabilize local estimates through the use of various weighting schemes. One set of smoothed rates results from a set of weighted average of neighboring rates, the other from a weighted average of incidence counts divided by a weighted average of population sizes. Another, somewhat more formal approach uses probability models to obtain smoothed estimates consisting of a compromise between the observed rate for each region and an estimate from a larger collection of cases and persons at risk (e.g., the rate observed over the entire study area or over a collection of neighboring regions). The compromise combines the rate from each region, which can be statistically unstable due to the rarity of the disease and the relatively small number of people at risk, with an estimated rate from a larger collection of people which is more statistically stable but has less geographic resolution.

Clayton and Kaldor (1987) propose a Bayesian approach to this problem which defines the analytic form of the compromise estimator. Bayesian statistics in general treats all unknown model parameters as random variables, and the goal of inference is to define the distributions of these variables, thereby providing point and interval estimates, predictions, and probability calculations. Analysts derive these distributions based on a combination of prior information or beliefs regarding the variables and the observed likelihood of parameter values in light of the data. Analysts summarize *prior* beliefs regarding the possible values through specification of a *prior distribution* assigning a probability distribution without regard or reference to the data. Data inform on the variables of interest through the *likelihood function* (the same likelihood function used in maximum likelihood analysis). The likelihood function summarizes the conditional probability distribution of the data, given the value of the unknown parameters. The *posterior distribution* reflects the conditional distribution of model parameters, given the data, and represents a compromise between the prior distribution and the likelihood function, thereby summarizing the distribution of the random variable(s) of interest, taking into account both prior beliefs and the information observed in the data. To be more specific, if we have a vector of data values $\mathbf{Y} = (Y_1, \ldots, Y_N)'$, and a corresponding vector of model parameters $\boldsymbol{\xi} = (\xi_1, \ldots, \xi_N)'$, and if we allow $f(\cdot)$ to denote a general probability density function, we have

$$\begin{aligned}
\text{prior} &= f(\boldsymbol{\xi}) \\
\text{likelihood} &= f(\mathbf{Y}|\boldsymbol{\xi}) \\
\text{posterior} &= f(\boldsymbol{\xi}|\mathbf{Y}) = f(\mathbf{Y}|\boldsymbol{\xi})f(\boldsymbol{\xi})/\text{const},
\end{aligned}$$

where "const" denotes a normalizing constant [equal to $\int f(\mathbf{Y}|\boldsymbol{\xi})f(\boldsymbol{\xi})d\boldsymbol{\xi}$, ensuring the posterior density $f(\boldsymbol{\xi}|\mathbf{Y})$ integrates to 1]. Bayes' theorem provides a connection that allows the reversal of conditioning between the likelihood function and the posterior distribution, leading to the term *Bayesian statistics*. In a Bayesian setting, all inference regarding the model parameter $\boldsymbol{\xi}$ stems from the conditional distribution of $\boldsymbol{\xi}$ given the data $\mathbf{Y}$ (i.e., the posterior distribution). Carlin and Louis (2000) and Gelman et al. (2004) provide thorough introductions to Bayesian inference and its application in a wide variety of data analysis settings.

Bayesian inference depends on the prior distribution. The use of a "non-informative" prior distribution results in a posterior distribution very similar to the likelihood function, while an overly "informative" prior may result in a posterior far removed from the likelihood function. The central role of the prior distribution is a point of contention for many regarding the utility and applicability of the Bayesian paradigm. An in-depth discussion of the philosophical issues involved in this debate is beyond the scope of this book. Instead, we illustrate how incorporation of particular prior distributions achieves our goal to borrow information (often termed *borrowing strength* in the statistical literature) from other areas to stabilize local rates while maintaining a very sensible probabilistic structure to the problem.

To begin, we build a probability model describing our data. Assume that the disease counts Y_i represent random variables, each following a Poisson distribution with mean equal to $n_i\xi_i$, where ξ_i denotes the risk of a person residing in region i contracting the disease during the study period. Given this local probability of disease, we have

$$Y_i|\xi_i \overset{\text{ind}}{\sim} \text{Poisson}(n_i\xi_i). \tag{4.7}$$

Under this model, we are assuming that the Y_i are conditionally independent given the ξ_i. This does not mean that the Y_i are mutually independent; rather, this implies that any spatial correlation observed in the Y_i is a function of spatial trends in either the population sizes n_i (considered to be fixed, known quantities) or in the local individual risks ξ_i for $i = 1, \ldots, N$.

In a Bayesian analysis, the likelihood function is defined by the conditional distributions defined in equation (4.7) (recall that the likelihood represents the distribution of the data given the model parameters). Since the Y_i are conditionally independent given the ξ_i parameters, the likelihood takes a particularly simple form and is defined as the product, across all regions $i = 1, \ldots, N$, of the conditional distributions given in equation (4.7).

A Bayesian analysis treats the ξ_i as random variables, and we next define a prior distribution for each ξ_i. To begin, we follow Marshall (1991) and denote the prior mean by $E_\xi(\xi_i) = m_{\xi_i}$ and the prior variance by $\text{Var}_\xi(\xi_i) = v_{\xi_i}$. Equation (4.7) gives the mean and variance of the observed local count, Y_i, conditional on the value of ξ_i, as $n_i\xi_i$. Therefore, the conditional mean and variance of the local rate observed, r_i, of disease are

$$E(r_i|\xi_i) = E[(Y_i/n_i)|\xi_i] = \xi_i$$

and

$$\text{Var}(r_i|\xi_i) = \text{Var}[(Y_i/n_i)|\xi_i] = \xi_i/n_i,$$

respectively.

To find the unconditional mean of the rate observed in region i, r_i, we need to take the expectation over ξ_i of the conditional expectation:

$$E_r(r_i) = E_\xi E(r_i|\xi_i) = E_\xi(\xi_i) = m_{\xi_i},$$

where E_r and E_ξ denote expectation with respect to the marginal distributions of r and ξ, respectively. The unconditional variance of r_i equals the sum of the variance of the conditional mean with respect to ξ_i and the expectation of the conditional variance:

$$\text{Var}_r(r_i) = \text{Var}_\xi(\xi_i) + E_\xi(\xi_i/n_i) = v_{\xi_i} + m_{\xi_i}/n_i.$$

Deriving the best linear Bayes estimator of ξ_i by minimizing the expected total squared-error loss yields (Marshall 1991)

$$\begin{aligned} \hat{\xi}_i &= m_{\xi_i} + C_i(r_i - m_{\xi_i}) \\ &= C_i r_i + (1 - C_i) m_{\xi_i}, \end{aligned} \tag{4.8}$$

where $C_i = v_{\xi_i}/(v_{\xi_i} + m_{\xi_i}/n_i)$ is the ratio of the prior variance to the data variance. This ratio is called the *shrinkage factor* since it defines how much the crude rate, $r_i = Y_i/n_i$, "shrinks" toward the prior mean. Note that the estimator defined in equation (4.8) corresponds to a weighted average of the crude estimate and the prior mean. When the population size, n_i, is small, $C_i \to 0$, and the Bayes estimator is close to the prior mean, m_{ξ_i}. However, when the expected count is large, $C_i \to 1$, and the Bayes estimator approaches the rate observed. In short, the Bayes estimator provides an approach that *borrows strength* from the prior mean, where the amount of strength borrowed depends on the stability of the crude local estimate as measured by the prior variance.

To compute the estimates, we require values for m_{ξ_i} and v_{ξ_i}. In a fully Bayesian approach, these parameters are also considered to be random variables and given prior distributions called *hyperpriors*. The hyperpriors may depend on random variables that are also assigned prior distributions. This hierarchical specification can continue through many levels, but at the last stage of the hierarchy, values must be given for any unknown parameters. In *empirical Bayes estimation*, the unknown parameters are estimated from the data. In the case described above, Marshall (1991) assumed that $m_{\xi_i} \equiv m_\xi$, and $v_{\xi_i} \equiv v_\xi$ (i.e., the same prior mean and variance for all regions) since the model is otherwise overspecified (i.e., there are more unknown parameters than there are data values). With this assumption, Marshall (1991) uses the method of moments to estimate m_ξ, v_ξ, and C_i. The method-of-moments estimator of the overall mean, m_ξ, is just the weighted sample mean,

$$\tilde{m}_\xi = \frac{\sum_{i=1}^N r_i n_i}{\sum_{i=1}^N n_i}. \tag{4.9}$$

The weighted sample variance is

$$s^2 = \frac{\sum_{i=1}^N n_i (r_i - \tilde{m}_\xi)^2}{\sum_{i=1}^N n_i}$$

and has expected value (ignoring estimation of m_ξ) $v_\xi + m/\overline{n}$, where $\overline{n} = \sum_{i=1}^{N} n_i/N$. Thus, the method-of-moments estimator of v_ξ is

$$\tilde{v}_\xi = s^2 - \frac{\tilde{m}_\xi}{\overline{n}}. \tag{4.10}$$

If this quantity is negative, we will use zero as our estimate of v_ξ, to avoid negative variance estimates. Substituting $\tilde{m}_\xi$ and $\tilde{v}_\xi$ from equations (4.9) and (4.10), respectively, into the expression for C_i gives the method-of-moments estimator of the Bayes shrinkage factor as

$$\tilde{C}_i = \begin{cases} \dfrac{s^2 - \tilde{m}_\xi/\overline{n}}{s^2 - \tilde{m}_\xi/\overline{n} + \tilde{m}_\xi/n_i} & \text{if } s^2 \geq \tilde{m}_\xi/\overline{n} \\ 0 & \text{otherwise.} \end{cases}$$

Substituting these values into equation (4.8) yields the empirical Bayes estimator

$$\hat{\xi}_i = \tilde{m}_\xi + \tilde{C}_i(r_i - \tilde{m}_\xi). \tag{4.11}$$

This estimator, based on method-of-moments estimates of the prior mean and variance, provides the most straightforward empirical Bayes estimates of local disease rates. We can derive other Bayes estimators by assuming different prior information about the ξ_i or by using different methods to estimate the prior parameters (cf. Clayton and Kaldor 1987; Marshall 1991; Bailey and Gatrell 1995, pp. 303–308). However, all empirical Bayes estimators have the general form given in equation (4.8), namely, a weighted sum of the prior mean and the crude local rate. Devine et al. (1994) provide a thorough discussion and illustration of the use of different empirical Bayes estimators in epidemiology.

We note that the Bayes estimators described above are global in that they "shrink" each observed rate toward the prior mean, m_ξ. We could obtain local empirical Bayes estimators by considering locally defined prior means (e.g., define a prior distribution for ξ_i that results in shrinkage to the mean of rates observed from regions neighboring region i). In this case, the estimates shrink each r_i to its neighborhood mean rather than the global mean. We illustrate such an approach in the data break following Section 4.4.5.

Compared to the smoothing methods defined in Sections 4.4.1 and 4.4.2, empirical Bayes smoothers may seem more complicated in definition and implementation. The additional structure comprising the Bayesian framework offers a richer framework for modeling covariate effects and spatial correlation structures, somewhat offsetting the initial effort in model specification and estimation.

For instance, suppose that we wish to consider age-standardized rates to adjust for differing age distributions among persons at risk within each region. The weighted averages presented in Sections 4.4.1 and 4.4.2 do not accommodate differing age structures easily. However, Clayton and Kaldor (1987) illustrate a fairly simple adjustment to the empirical Bayes estimates above, adjusting regional disease risks (rates) for differences in age or other risk factors. First, suppose that our data involve not only the disease counts $Y_1, Y_2, \ldots, Y_N$ observed from each of N regions, but also include a set of counts $E_1, E_2, \ldots, E_N$ *expected* for the same regions. Second, suppose that the counts expected represent standardized counts based on the age structure of the population at risk (see Section 2.3). Recall from Section 2.3.2 that the ratio of observed to expected counts, Y_i/E_i, corresponds to the local observed *standardized mortality ratio* (SMR_i). SMR_i represents the maximum likelihood estimate of the *relative risk* experienced by persons residing in region i [i.e., the multiplicative increase or decrease in disease risk compared to the risk (or risks) defining the expected count E_i]. Since we treat the expected counts as fixed and known (not random) quantities, local SMRs suffer the same statistical instability as local rates (Y_i/n_i) for areas with few persons at risk, particularly for areas with few cases expected during the study period. Therefore, we need to borrow information from the other regions to stabilize our local SMRs.

Clayton and Kaldor (1987) propose an empirical Bayes solution based on a reparameterization of the basic probability model defined in equation (4.7). We assume that each Y_i (the random variables representing the disease count in region i) follows a Poisson distribution with mean (and variance) $E_i\zeta_i$, where ζ_i represents the relative risk associated with people residing in region i. Specifically, we assume that

$$Y_i|\zeta_i \overset{\text{ind}}{\sim} \text{Poisson}(E_i\zeta_i). \tag{4.12}$$

The primary difference between equations (4.7) and (4.12) involves the unknown parameter. In the former setting we seek a smoothed estimate of an unknown local risk of disease ξ_i; here we seek a smoothed estimate of an unknown local relative risk ζ_i. Otherwise, the probability models are identical: The conditional mean of Y_i is the product of a known constant [n_i in equation (4.7) and E_i in equation (4.12)] and an unknown parameter (ξ_i or ζ_i). Therefore, we may define a method-of-moments empirical Bayes estimate of the SMR_i by replacing n_i with E_i in the preceding development.

The full advantage of the approach of Clayton and Kaldor (1987) arises when we wish to include additional covariates and/or consider various spatial correlation structures to the relative risk parameters ζ_i. Besag et al. (1991) provide a widely applied expansion of the basic structure above, allowing very general application of Poisson regression with correlated errors. These extended models allow us to assess covariate effects and incorporate spatial correlation. To avoid a (lengthy) digression into statistical modeling at this point, we defer discussion of such models to Chapter 9, and limit our consideration here to the smoothing and visualization properties of empirical Bayes estimators simulations in the examples in this chapter.

4.4.4 Probability Mapping

Noting the problems with rate maps based on small populations, Choynowski (1959) suggested the use of a probability map as an alternative. If we assume that the disease counts, $Y_1, Y_2, \ldots, Y_N$ are independent Poisson random variables, we can calculate the probability of any observed disease count, Y_i, for each region using the Poisson distribution. We simply need an estimate of the expected count, E_i, for each region. We can use an overall mean risk estimate over the entire domain as $\hat{\xi} = \sum_{i=1}^{N} Y_i / \sum_{i=1}^{N} n_i$, or perhaps an age-adjusted estimate, as in the preceding section. Using the overall mean risk for simplicity, we calculate the expected count in each region as $\hat{E}_i = n_i \hat{\xi}$. This implies that the risk is the same in all areas, and we refer to this as the *constant risk hypothesis* in later chapters. Next, we calculate the probability of being more extreme than our observed count in each region, denoted p_i, via

$$p_i = \begin{cases} \Pr[Y_i \geq y_i | E(Y_i) = \hat{E}_i] & \text{if } y_i > \hat{E}_i \\ \Pr[Y_i \leq y_i | E(Y_i) = \hat{E}_i] & \text{if } y_i < \hat{E}_i. \end{cases}$$

The p_i values are based on cumulative probabilities from a Poisson distribution and provide an index of deviation from the hypothesis of equal risk. For visualization, we post the probabilities on a choropleth map and consider regions with probabilities less than 0.05 to have rates significantly different from the average. Cressie and Read (1989) illustrate this approach using sudden infant deaths in North Carolina. As demonstrated in both Choynowski (1959) and Cressie and Read (1989), these maps may be much more informative than maps of raw rates. However, as Cressie (1993) points out, if the n_i are very different, it may not be possible to distinguish deviations from the constant risk assumption from lack of fit of the Poisson distribution. Moreover, users of probability maps will usually infer significance for regions with relatively high population sizes since there is intuitively more statistical power for detecting differences from a background risk in these regions. Nevertheless, probability maps offer one approach to assessing the significance of high rates as opposed to visual inference from a choropleth map or ranking of the rates themselves in which at least one rate must appear to be the highest.

4.4.5 Practical Notes and Recommendations

In this section we draw on the discussion in this chapter, our experience, and additional literature to offer some practical recommendations pertaining to the advantages and disadvantages of smoothing, when to smooth, and which smoother to use.

Advantages and Disadvantages of Smoothing There are two main advantages to smoothing rates. The first is that smoothing allows us to stabilize rates based on small numbers by combining available data at the resolution of interest. We do not have to aggregate to larger regions to achieve stable rates for mapping. The second advantage to smoothing is that it reduces noise in the rates caused by different population sizes, thus increasing our ability to discern systematic patterns in the spatial variation of the underlying risk.

Smoothing also has some disadvantages. Smoothed maps are maps of values other than the raw data values. Many people are leary of statistically adjusted numbers, particularly if money or power is to be allocated based on them. In fact, Walter and Birnie (1991) reports that very few official disease atlases include any sort of smoothing, although two recent U.S. atlases do include smoothed rates (Pickle et al. 1996; Casper et al. 2000). Another disadvantage of smoothing is that it can introduce artifacts and autocorrelation into the rate map (see, e.g., Gelman and Price 1999; Gelman et al. 2004). Thus, smoothing may replace one set of artifacts (e.g., unstable estimates) in mapped rates with another set of artifacts (e.g., correlated estimates) in altered rates. Still, we believe that the visual inferences obtained from maps of raw rates can often be so misleading that smoothing is a better choice.

When to Smooth We want to avoid hard-and-fast rules concerning smoothing, since it is important for people familiar with an actual application or study to use their knowledge and their instincts in the smoothing decision. Nevertheless, here are some general guidelines that indicate when rates may be unstable and for which smoothing should be *considered:*

1. If the addition of one event (e.g., disease case) or one more person at risk results in a large difference in one or more of the rates.
2. If a rate changes by 25% or more (although what constitutes such a large difference should be judged on a case-by-case basis).
3. If the number of events that forms the numerator of one or more of the rates is less then 3.
4. If the number of persons at risk per region is small (e.g., less than 500 or 100 people) and the numbers change by an order of magnitude or more across the regions. For example, rates based on 10 people are not easily comparable to rates based on 100 people.

On the other hand, if we are not looking for individual regions (e.g., counties, tracts) with elevated rates, but instead want to get a general assessment of broad trends and patterns, smoothing will help reduce the noise and make the trends and patterns more clear. Smoothing can reduce our attention to large rates that may be outliers by focusing it on the overall picture.

What Smoother to Use The most important property of a smoother is its accuracy: It should correctly identify regions of high and low rates and smooth over rates that are artificially elevated due to instability. It should not indicate trends or patterns when no such trends or patterns exist. Using these criteria, Kafadar (1994) put several smoothers to the test (e.g., locally weighted average, empirical Bayes, loess, and a technique known as *headbanging* (cf. Section 4.6.4), applying them to carefully simulated data where the true spatial variation in the data was known. Kafadar (1994) found that the locally weighted average smoothers with weights inversely proportional to distance were the most accurate. Loess and local empirical

Bayes did not perform as well, particularly in what Kafadar (1994) called high-noise situations, where there was a lot of variability in the data. However, in such cases, all smoothers were better than no smoothing.

In addition to the overall accuracy criterion considered by Kafadar (1994), we suggest that two additional criteria are also important. The first of these is simplicity or ease of use. Since these smoothers are meant to be exploratory tools for descriptive statistics, a smoother that can be calculated quickly without complex estimation rules, difficult or tedious programming, and specification of extra parameters is preferred. Thus, these criteria argue against the use of empirical Bayes or loess approaches. However, when we want to go beyond exploratory methods to inferential statistics in which we can adjust for confounders and perform hypothesis tests, Bayesian and empirical Bayes methods offer several advantages. Another important criterion in selecting a smoother is whether or not we can obtain standard errors for the smoothed estimates. The ability to quantify uncertainty is perhaps the distinguishing characteristic of the field of statistics. For the linear smoothers (e.g., locally weighted averages, kernel smoothing, empirical Bayes with C_i known), deriving standard errors for the smoothed rates is straightforward. For nonlinear smoothers such as headbanging or empirical Bayes with C_i estimated, developing such a measure of uncertainty is much more difficult.

CASE STUDY: Smoothing New York Leukemia Data To illustrate some of the ideas and methods presented in this section, we consider leukemia data reported and analyzed by Waller et al. (1992, 1994). The data here are the number of incident leukemia cases from 1978–1982 per census tract in an eight-county region of upstate New York (Figure 4.14). This figure is enlarged in Figure 4.15, so we can see the tracts more clearly. Note that the census tracts are smaller in urban than in rural areas.

The data include 592 leukemia cases among 1,057,673 people at risk. As described in Waller et al. (1994), most of the leukemia cases were originally georeferenced to census block groups, but some of the cases could not be georeferenced to this resolution. These cases were then allocated proportionally among the block groups, so that some of the resulting disease counts are not necessarily integers. For our purposes here, we aggregate the number of cases per block group to census tracts. The number of cases per tract ranged from 0.00 to 9.29 cases. Leukemia

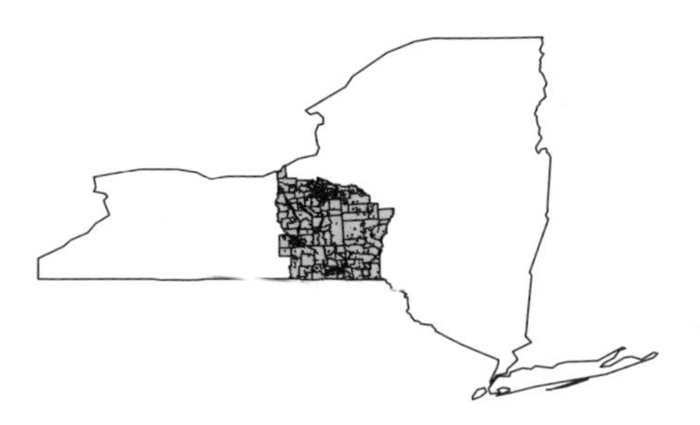

FIG. 4.14 Eight-county study area in New York.

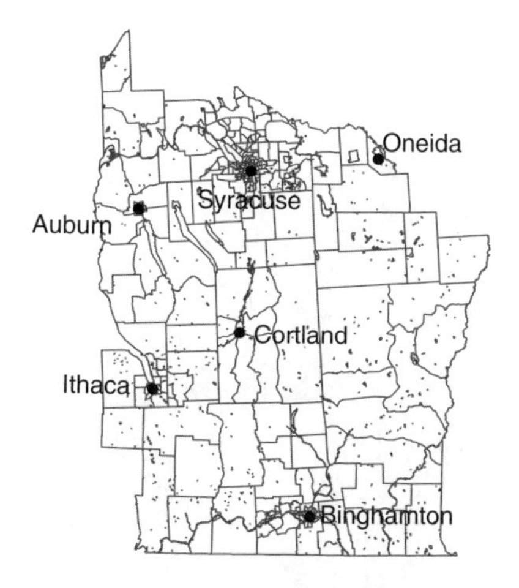

FIG. 4.15 Major cities in the eight-county region.

rates per tract were computed by dividing the number of leukemia cases per tract by the 1980 population per tract and then again by 5 to obtain rates per 100,000 people per year. Figure 4.16 displays the census tract leukemia rates.

Regions with high observed leukemia rates are of particular interest, so we will have a closer look at these areas. The tract with the highest rate per 100,000 people, 139.86, is located in Syracuse (it is difficult to see this on the map since the census tract is very small), but it is based on only 1 case of leukemia and 143 people at risk. The average population size per tract is 3764 people. Of the highest 10% of the rates, 15% (5) of these have leukemia counts ≤ 2.1 and these five tracts are located within the Syracuse area. There does not seem to be a trend in the rates (i.e., no apparent tendency to increase or decrease systematically in any direction), but high rates do seem to occur near the larger cities. Some of these cities are also the locations of hazardous waste sites, and the relationship between the locations of these sites and the occurrence of the leukemia cases is explored further following Section 7.6.5. The map shows a great deal of variability, some of which may be due to the small number of cases used to compute the rates, or to the variation in population sizes, rather than trends or patterns in the underlying leukemia risk.

To illustrate the effects of smoothing, we first smoothed each rate using the global empirical Bayes smoother given in equation (4.11) (see Figure 4.17). The effects of smoothing are obvious: Tracts with low rates have been smoothed upward toward the mean, and tracts with high rates have been smoothed downward toward the mean. The spatial variation in the rates has been reduced drastically. The smoothed rates range in value from 5.46 to 24.27, much different than the same extrema for the original rates (ranging from 0.0 to 139.86). Even so, a few of the tracts with high original rates (e.g., those near Cortland and Syracuse) still appear relatively high.

Next we used a local empirical Bayes smoother. The smoothed rates are again computed using equation (4.11), but in local neighborhoods. We defined

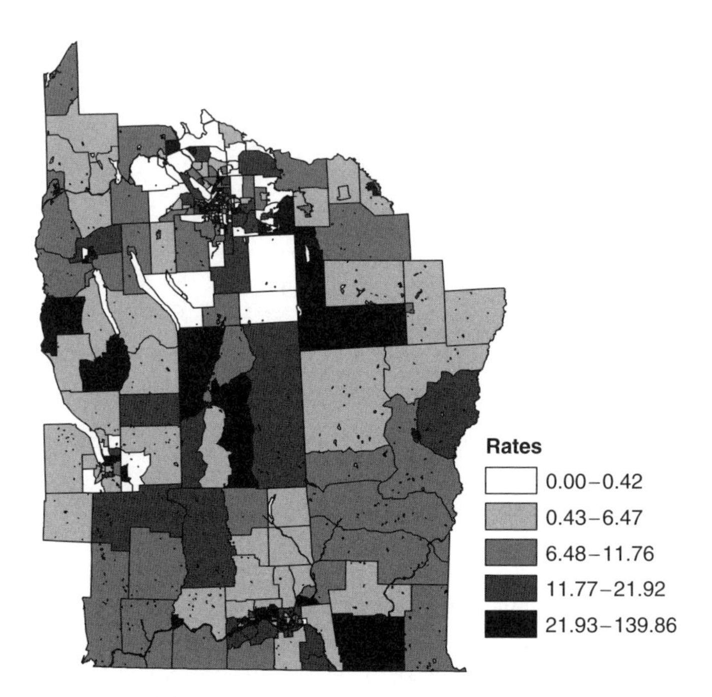

FIG. 4.16 Original leukemia rates per 100,000 people per year.

neighborhoods by adjacency:

$$\mathcal{N}_j = \{j : \text{tract } j \text{ shares a boundary with tract } i\}.$$

The resulting map appears in Figure 4.18. There is more variability in these smoothed rates, with values ranging from 0.29 to 26.81. Comparing this map to the map of the original rates and to the map from global empirical Bayes smoothing, we can see the effects of the local smoothing: Local smoothing allows more variability in areas where adjacent tracts have moderately different rates. If the differences between rates in adjacent tracts are large, the highest rates will be smoothed down and the lowest rates will be smoothed up to the local mean.

Finally, we computed a locally weighted-average smoother using the same adjacency-based neighborhood as with the local empirical Bayes smoother. We used weights equal to the population size in each tract in order to compare the results more directly with those obtained using empirical Bayes. This smoother is the same as that of equation (4.11) but without the shrinkage factor and implemented locally. The resulting map is given in Figure 4.19. This map is very similar to that produced using local empirical Bayes.

Even after smoothing, a few tracts appear to have relatively high rates. This will always be the case in this type of analysis: by definition, 5% of the rates will exceed the 95th percentile of the distribution of the rate values. On a choropleth map, the largest values will necessarily be shaded in the same color, often the

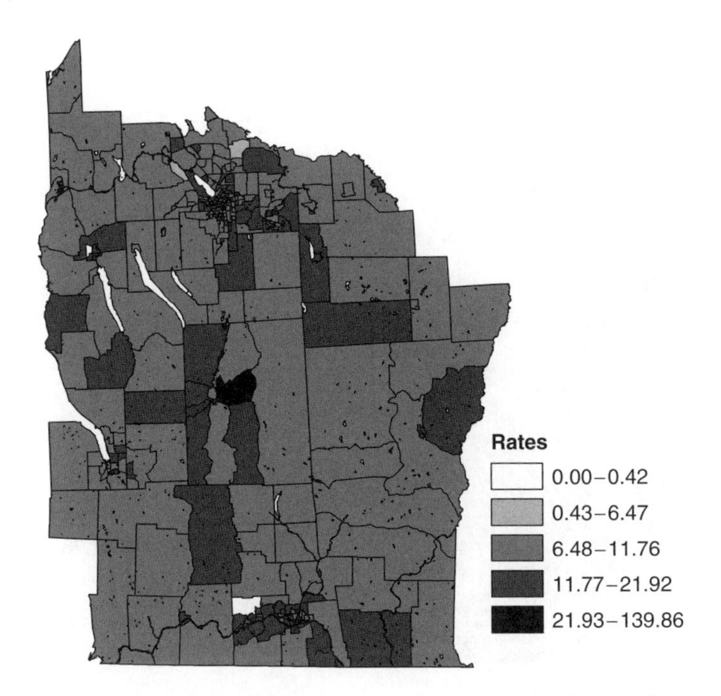

FIG. 4.17 Smoothed leukemia rates using the global empirical Bayes estimator.

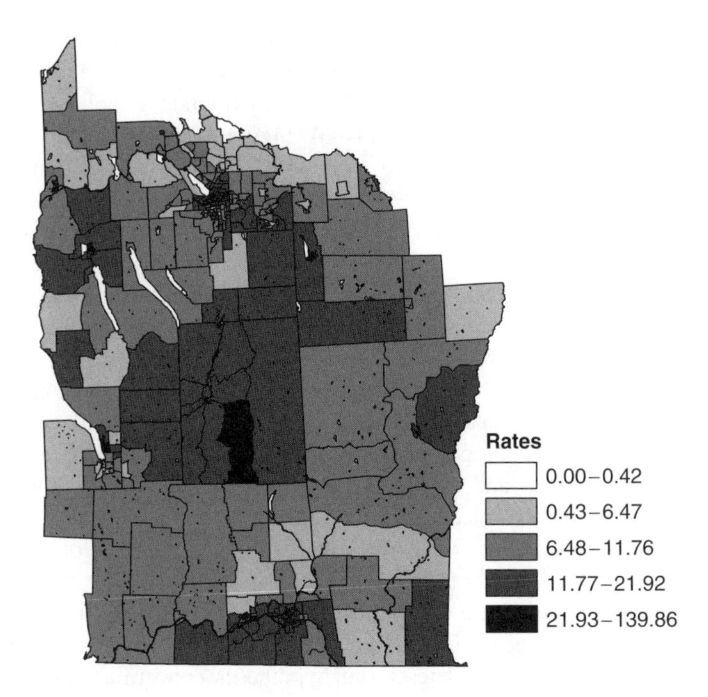

FIG. 4.18 Smoothed leukemia rates using a local empirical Bayes estimator.

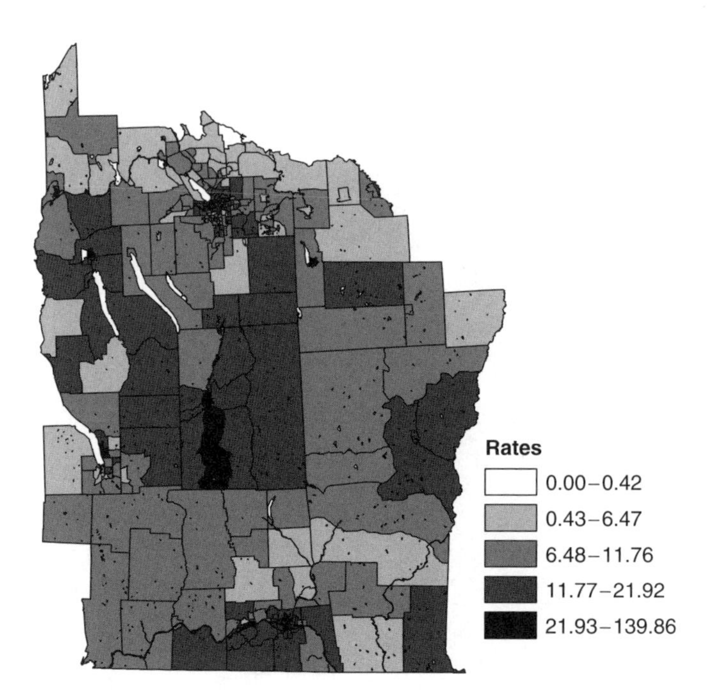

FIG. 4.19 Smoothed leukemia rates using a locally weighted-average estimator.

darkest. Yet we have to wonder if these rates are unusually high in some sense (e.g., when compared to an overall background rate). We investigate this hypothesis more precisely in Chapter 7, but as an additional exploratory tool, we construct a probability map as described in Section 4.4.4 (Figure 4.20). This map depicts, for each tract, the probability of observing a rate as extreme or more extreme than our original rate, under the null hypothesis that all rates are equal to a mean rate. If a probability is small, there is some evidence against this null hypothesis and we conclude that the corresponding tract has an unusually high or low rate.

We might be more interested in the rates that are significantly high. Thus, in Figure 4.21 we have indicated the tracts for which the probability of a higher rate under the null hypothesis of a constant mean rate is < 0.05. Most of these tracts are located in large cities, where we would expect the power of detecting elevated rates to be much higher than in other tracts, due to the large populations in these tracks. However, many of these tracts were also identified as tracts of concern using the local empirical Bayes and weighted-average smoothers. Notice, however, that some of the tracts initially of concern (as indicated on the map of original rates in Figure 4.16)—those in the westernmost part of the state, south of Auburn, and those in the northeast region, southwest of Oneida—are not significant on this map.

Although these methods are exploratory, some areas are consistently indicated as areas of concern, all near cities: Binghamton, Cortland, Ithaca, Syracuse, and Auburn. We consider additional tests and hypotheses concerning these leukemia rates in Chapter 7.

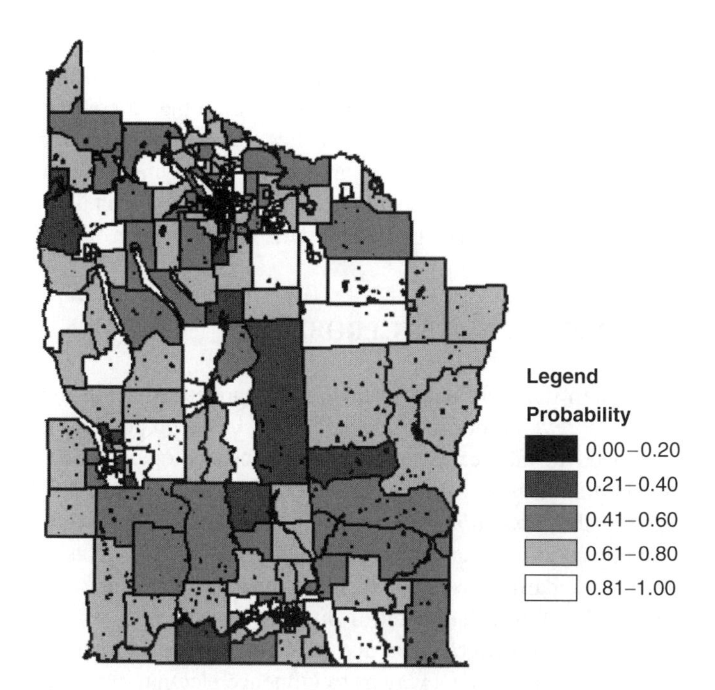

FIG. 4.20 Probability map based on the unadjusted leukemia rates in the eight-county study area.

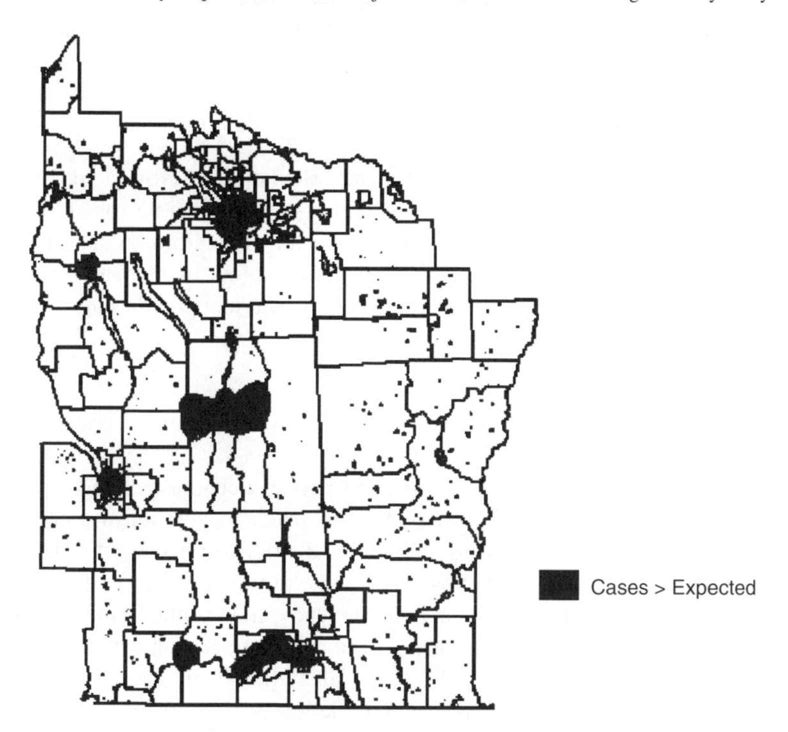

FIG. 4.21 Tracts with significantly higher-than-average leukemia rates, based on Figure 4.20.

In summary, smoothing methods offer statistical approaches for stabilizing rate (or proportion) estimates from small areas. Both smoothing and probability maps offer a first step toward clarifying the signal by attempting to control (or at least model) the noise inherent in the summary statistics and to pool values having similar expectations. Although such approaches aid us in displaying and understanding summary values from small areas, they do not address a fundamental issue involved in the analysis of geographically aggregated data, as outlined in the next section.

4.5 MODIFIABLE AREAL UNIT PROBLEM

Once we map health data, we need to take great care in inferring individual risk from local area rates, even if our rates are stable and based on populations of similar size. First, we need to take care not to commit the ecological fallacy (inferring individual-level relationships from group-level data; see Section 2.7.4). Second, we need to avoid the *modifiable areal unit problem* (MAUP). This problem is a geographic manifestation of the ecological fallacy in which conclusions based on data aggregated to a particular set of districts may change if one aggregates the same underlying data to a different set of districts.

The MAUP forms the geographical and mathematical basis for gerrymandering (defining voting districts in such a way as to influence election outcomes), a subject of intense interest each census cycle in the United States and other countries where politicians use the census results to define "representative" districts. The problem becomes even more perplexing because, in many instances, spatial aggregation is necessary to create meaningful units for analysis. An early description of the latter aspect appears in Yule and Kendall (1950, p. 312), where they state:

> [G]eographical areas chosen for the calculation of crop yields are modifiable units and necessarily so. Since it is impossible (or at any rate agriculturally impractical) to grow wheat and potatoes on the same piece of ground simultaneously we must, to give our investigation any meaning, consider an area containing both wheat and potatoes and this area is modifiable at choice.

Geographers have long appreciated the problems associated with the use of modifiable units, leading Openshaw and Taylor (1979) to first coin the term *modifiable areal unit problem*.

Gehlke and Biehl (1934) were among the first to document changes in statistical inference due to the scale of aggregation when they found a tendency for the magnitude of the correlations to increase as districts formed from census tracts increased in size. Working with 252 census tracts in the Cleveland area, they considered the correlation of male juvenile delinquency, in absolute numbers, with the median equivalent monthly rental costs for the census tracts. They then considered this same correlation based on the 200, 175, 150, 124, 100, 50, and 25 areas formed by joining contiguous census tracts. The correlation became increasingly negative, being −0.502 for the 252 individual tracts and decreasing to −0.763 for the 25 areas. However, when they repeated the exercise using a random grouping for 252 tracts and 25 and 150 areas, the correlations showed no relationship to size.

To better understand the nature of the problem and to suggest efficient groupings for geographical data, Openshaw and Taylor (1979) constructed all possible groupings of the 99 counties in Iowa into larger districts. Their results are somewhat startling. When considering the correlation between the percentage of Republican voters and the percentage of elderly voters in the 1976 election, they were able to construct sets of 12 districts producing correlations ranging from -0.97 to $+0.99$. Moreover, Openshaw and Taylor (1979) found no obvious relationship between the spatial characteristics of the districts and the variation in the resulting correlation coefficients.

More closely related to health data, Monmonier (1996, p. 158) illustrates the MAUP with an application to John Snow's 1854 cholera data. Monmonier (1996, p. 158) aggregates the cholera deaths to three different sets of districts. In two of these, the effects of the Broad Street cluster are diluted or obliterated completely. Monmonier's example is particular fitting for our discussion, as it takes a classic disease map based on point locations and illustrates the effect of aggregating these locations into each of three sets of districts. Thus, as noted by Yule and Kendall (1950, p. 312), maps are only able to "measure the relationship between the variates for the specified units chosen for the work. They have no absolute validity independently of those units, but are relative to them."

What causes the MAUP? Theoretical reasons for the increase in correlations that occurs as the level of aggregation increases have been provided by several authors, including the early work of Robinson (1950), who suggested areal weighting to alleviate the effects of the MAUP on statistical inference. However, areal weighting offers an effective solution to this problem only in very specialized situations (Thomas and Anderson 1965). A simple example [modified from those considered in Robinson (1956), Thomas and Anderson (1965), and Jelinski and Wu (1996)] illustrates some of the key ideas. Comparing configurations A–C in Figure 4.22, the effects of aggregation are clearly visible. The means (top number) do not change between configurations B and C, but the variances decrease and the correlations increase with increasing aggregation. Area weighting has no effect because the units within each of these configurations are all the same size and shape. In configurations D–F, we aggregate the basic units in various ways to produce larger units. Note that configurations B and D have the same number of aggregated units, but we aggregate horizontally in B and vertically in D. Configurations C and E are comparable in a similar way. Comparing these configurations shows the change in variance that can result when the orientation of the aggregation is altered but the number of aggregated units remains the same. Finally, by comparing configurations C, E and F, we see that even when the number of aggregated units is held constant (here at $n = 4$ units), the means, variances, and correlation coefficient all change with the spatial configuration of the aggregated units, even when areal weighting is used to adjust these statistics.

This example serves to illustrate that the MAUP is not one, but two interrelated problems. The first concerns the different results and inferences obtained when

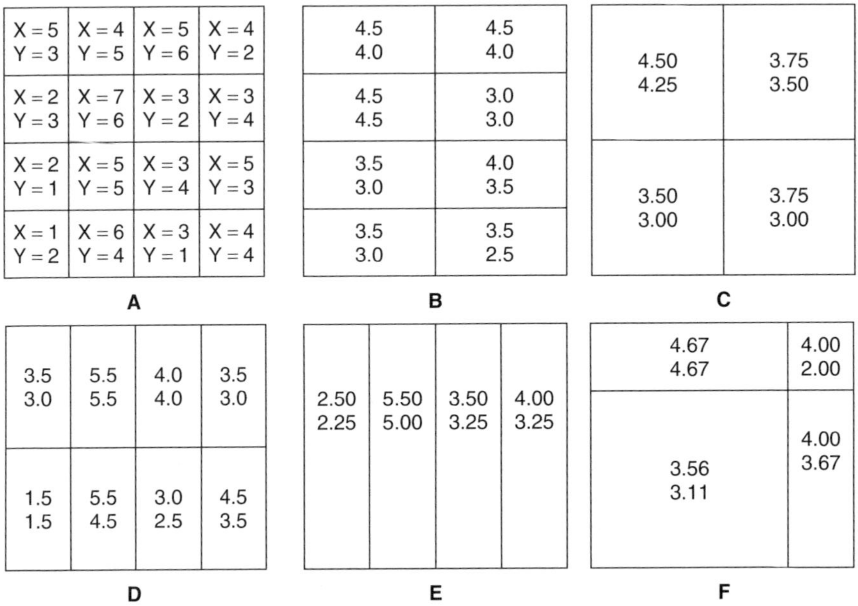

X = 5 Y = 3	X = 4 Y = 5	X = 5 Y = 6	X = 4 Y = 2
X = 2 Y = 3	X = 7 Y = 6	X = 3 Y = 2	X = 3 Y = 4
X = 2 Y = 1	X = 5 Y = 5	X = 3 Y = 4	X = 5 Y = 3
X = 1 Y = 2	X = 6 Y = 4	X = 3 Y = 1	X = 4 Y = 4

A

4.5 4.0	4.5 4.0
4.5 4.5	3.0 3.0
3.5 3.0	4.0 3.5
3.5 3.0	3.5 2.5

B

4.50 4.25	3.75 3.50
3.50 3.00	3.75 3.00

C

3.5 3.0	5.5 5.5	4.0 4.0	3.5 3.0
1.5 1.5	5.5 4.5	3.0 2.5	4.5 3.5

D

2.50 2.25	5.50 5.00	3.50 3.25	4.00 3.25

E

4.67 4.67	4.00 2.00
3.56 3.11	4.00 3.67

F

	Unweighted					Weighted				
	$\bar{X}$	$\bar{Y}$	s_X^2	s_Y^2	r_{XY}	$\bar{X}$	$\bar{Y}$	s_X^2	s_Y^2	r_{XY}
A	3.88	3.44	2.36	2.37	0.66	3.88	3.44	2.36	2.37	0.66
B	3.88	3.44	0.30	0.40	0.88	3.88	3.44	0.30	0.40	0.88
C	3.88	3.44	0.14	0.26	0.94	3.88	3.44	0.14	0.26	0.94
D	3.88	3.44	1.55	1.34	0.95	3.88	3.44	1.55	1.34	0.95
E	3.88	3.44	1.17	0.98	0.98	3.88	3.44	1.17	0.98	0.98
F	4.06	3.36	0.16	0.93	0.64	3.88	3.44	0.18	0.48	0.80

FIG. 4.22 Impact of aggregation of spatial data. The top number in each cell of configurations B–F is the aggregated value of X obtained by averaging the original values comprising the larger cell; the lower number is the corresponding aggregated value of Y. Areal weighting follows formulas in Robinson (1956).

the same set of data is grouped into increasingly larger areal units. This is often referred to as the *scale effect* or *aggregation effect*. The second, often termed the *grouping effect* or *zoning effect*, considers the variability in results due to alternative formations of the areal units, leading to differences in unit shape at the same or similar scales (Openshaw and Taylor 1979; Openshaw 1984; Wong 1996). Figure 4.23 illustrates both aggregation and zoning effects.

The effects of the MAUP go beyond simple statistics such as the variance and the correlation coefficient discussed here. Inferential problems also occur in multivariate regression analysis, Poisson regression, hierarchical models, spatial

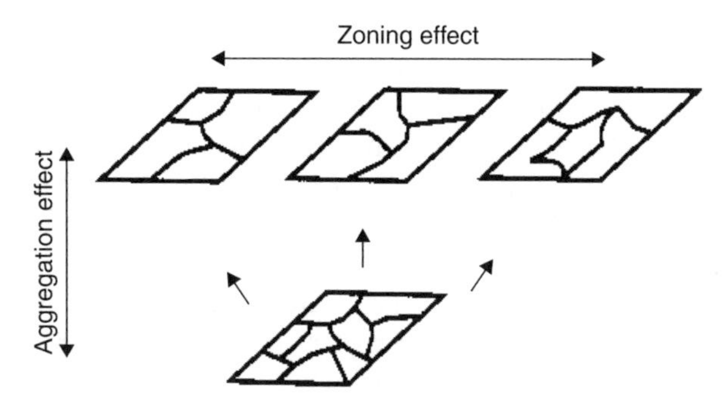

FIG. 4.23 Aggregation and zoning issues in the modifiable areal unit problem. [Adapted from Wong (1996).]

autocorrelation statistics, and probably most other statistical modeling and estimation procedures as well.

In the field of geostatistics (cf. Chapter 8), both the MAUP and the ecological inference problem can be considered special cases of what is called the *change of support problem* (COSP). Recall from Chapter 3 that the support of a spatial feature is the size, shape, and orientation of the feature. Thus, the COSP arises when features (points, lines, or areas) are altered to produce other features. Changing the support of a variable (typically by averaging or aggregation) creates a new variable. This new variable is related to the original one but has different statistical and spatial properties. The problem of how the spatial variation in one variable relates to that of the other variable is called the *change of support problem.*

Is there a solution to the MAUP or the COSP? This rather straightforward question does not have a straightforward answer. The most obvious answer is "no," since there is no way to completely recover information lost in aggregation, and how the aggregation is done will definitely affect the resulting inference. However, this answer would be misleading since there are things that we can do to ameliorate the effects of the MAUP and, under certain assumptions for certain problems, provide a solution to the MAUP (e.g., the solutions to the ecological inference problem described in Section 2.7.4).

First, just being aware of the problem may lead to two very simple solutions: (1) we can refrain from making individual-level inference from aggregate data (e.g., we frame our conclusions in terms of rates not risk and in terms of the specific set of districts used); or (2) we collect/use data only on features about which we want to make inferences. If we want to make inferences about people, we need to have data on people. Of course, this may be difficult and expensive, but if we *really* want to make inferences about people, this is the best approach.

Second, we should think more about the statistics used to make inferences and use scale-independent statistics when possible. As King (1997, p. 250) noted:

> Despite the clarity with which MAUP seems to be stated, most statements have propagated a fundamental confusion between the definition of theoretical quantities of interest and the estimates that result

> in practice. Geographers and statisticians have studied the MAUP by computing a statistic on areal data aggregated to different levels, or in different ways, and watching the results vary wildly in sign and magnitude. ... Unfortunately, the statistics used to study these issues have not been aggregation-invariant (or "scale-invariant"). If a researcher wishes to have statistics that are invariant to the areal units chosen, then there is no reason to choose correlation coefficients, which depend heavily on the definition of available areal units. Solving the MAUP only requires developing statistics that are invariant to the level of aggregation.

In fact, even the slope coefficient from simple linear regression would be a better choice for inference than the correlation coefficient, and there are rules under which this coefficient is invariant to changes in scale (Prais and Aitchison 1954; Cramer 1964; Firebaugh 1978). In the spatial setting, Richardson (1992) elaborated on these rules in the context of geographical correlation studies, and Cressie (1996) showed that a similar result holds in aggregated spatial linear regression models by properly including geography as a latent variable. Tobler (1989) took this idea further by suggesting that methods of spatial analysis should be independent of the spatial coordinates used; the problem is not in the choice of units, but with the choice of models and methods used in the analysis. Cressie (1996), Fotheringham (1989), and Tobler (1989) further suggested choosing models whose parameters change in a predictable manner at various levels of aggregation. Thus, although the variance (and any p-values) will be affected by changes in scale or zoning, at least we will infer the correct magnitude and sign (positive/negative) of the effect.

Finally, several solutions to particular COSPs have been proposed. These solutions differ inherently with respect to the assumptions made, the validity of these assumptions, and the nature of any "extra" information used to reconstruct the missing individual-level statistics. Most of these solutions have a common strategy: They all build a model from point support data (even if no observations were taken at this level of support) and then develop methods to optimally estimate important parameters. A few of these solutions are examined in more detail in Sections 4.6.4 and 8.3.2. A more complete review can be found in Gotway and Young (2002).

4.6 ADDITIONAL TOPICS AND FURTHER READING

Addressing the question: "How do we map data effectively to explore patterns and communicate results?" covers a wide variety of geographic, cartographic, epidemiologic, and statistical issues. In seeking to provide broad coverage of relevant issues, we necessarily omit some details. Interested readers may wish to explore the references cited below for more information regarding any of the areas covered.

4.6.1 Visualization

Few (if any) will view or create maps in the same way after reading *How to Lie with Maps* (Monmonier 1996), which should be required reading for anyone interested in making maps. For readers interested in more detailed discussion of cartographic visualization, the texts by MacEachren (1994, 1995) and Slocum (1999) provide an excellent introduction to the field of cartography and access to the cartographic literature.

A wide variety of types of maps have been used to display health-related data, and the literature contains several historical reviews. Walter and Birnie (1991) reviewed the statistical and cartographic techniques used in disease atlases from several countries (and noted the relative lack of truly international health mapping activities). Howe (1989) and Walter (2000) provide concise overviews of the history of health mapping, including several historical examples. Finally, in the course of preparing the *Atlas of United States Mortality* (Pickle et al. 1996), its authors collaborated with cartographers, statisticians, and epidemiologists, generating several reports on particular aspects of the mapping process [cf. Pickle (2000) for a review of the process and issues considered]. The publications resulting from this effort (e.g., Lewandowsky et al. 1993; Pickle and Herrmann 1995; Hastie et al. 1996; Herrmann and Pickle 1996; Brewer et al. 1997) provide a valuable contribution to the medical geography literature.

4.6.2 Additional Types of Maps

Cartography is far from a stagnant field and contains many new developments in mapping (particularly for computer mapping). With respect to health maps, Carr et al. (2000) describe two new map templates with application to public health data: *linked micromap plots* and *conditioned choropleth maps*. We describe each template in turn below. Although such maps have not yet seen wide application in public health, we note that the U.S. National Cancer Institute recently implemented linked micromap plots as a means for users to explore cancer mortality data on its Internet sites. As the software becomes more widely available [see the appendix of Carr et al. (2000) for addresses and Internet access to the software], we expect greater use of these types of maps in the public health (and other) settings.

Linked micromap (LM) plots are a collection of related plots presenting many statistical summaries (e.g., rates for each county and their associated confidence intervals) from spatially referenced data in one graphical setting. Figure 4.24 illustrates an LM plot for low birth weight (LBW) rates by county in Georgia Health Care District 9. The template for LM plots involves four key components (Carr et al. 2000, p. 2527). As the first component, LM plots include at least three parallel panels containing items linked by location. The first panel consists of a vertical series of small maps (micromaps) that provide geographic setting of the data. Rather than create a single map displaying the rate of LBW births for all counties at once, the LM plot displays only a small number of counties in each of several maps. The second panel provides a legend identifying the name and symbology (e.g., color)

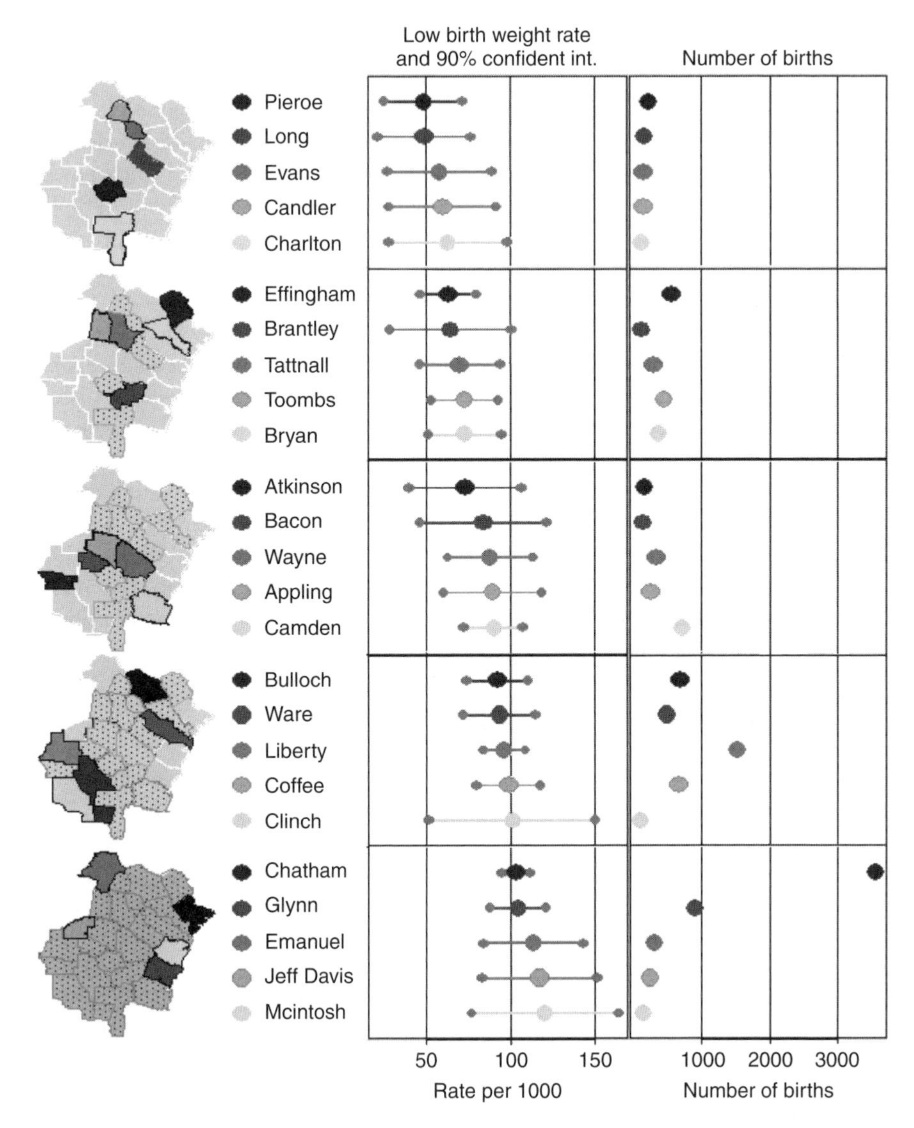

FIG. 4.24 LM plot for LBW rates in GHCD9. (Plot courtesy of Dan Carr, George Mason University.)

used to identify spatial areas within each micromap. The third panel provides some sort of statistical graphics, such as confidence intervals or histograms. The second component of a LM plot is the sorting of geographic units by the summary statistic of interest (e.g., sorting counties in Georgia Health Care District 9 by LBW rate). The third component partitions the regions into groups to focus attention on a few regions at a time. The fourth component links study units across the three panels.

Referring to Figure 4.24, on the left we see a repeated, relatively low-resolution map of the set of counties under consideration. Each map displays rates for five counties. The next column contains the county names and the gray scale used to denote that county in the adjacent micromap. Note that we use shading to distinguish counties within a particular micromap, not necessarily to identify numerical values. In particular, the same gray scale does not indicate the same numerical value of a rate between micromaps (e.g., light gray denotes the county with the lowest observed rate of the five displayed in a particular micromap). The third vertical panel contains the point estimate of the LBW rate for each county and a 95% confidence interval for this rate. Note that we order counties from top to bottom by increasing observed rates. Finally, Figure 4.24 contains a fourth vertical display reporting the observed number of births in each county (the denominator of the LBW rate). Note that those counties with the most unstable rates (those with the widest confidence intervals) correspond to those counties with small numbers of births. Any spatial patterns in the data appear in the series of micromaps. As we move from low to high LBW rates, those counties appearing in previous micromaps are outlined so that the reader may scan and follow how the pattern of high-rate counties emerges. In the case of increasing LBW rates, there is some slight suggestion that lower rates tend to occur in counties near the center of Georgia Health Care District 9 and then increase as we move toward the coast and northwestern edge of the district. However, the confidence intervals overlap quite a bit and the statistical suggestion of a changing pattern is not particularly strong.

Conditioned choropleth (CC) maps represent the second type of map proposed by Carr et al. (2000). This format provides a collection of mapped outcomes partitioned by categories of potential categorical variables. For instance, consider a single map of county-specific LBW rates in Georgia Health Care District 9, where we shade counties one of three colors based on whether the county falls into the lowest, middle, or highest third (tertile) of rates reported. Such a map indicates patterns in outcome but does not reveal whether the patterns observed correspond to any particular potential explanatory variables. Suppose that we wish to see if the pattern observed in rates corresponds well to the pattern of exposure to total suspended particulates (TSP) across counties. Further suppose that we divide county-specific TSP exposures into thirds (tertiles) also. Conditioned choropleth maps provide a separate choropleth map for each category of the explanatory variable (here, tertiles of TSP). We use the same color categories (different shades for rate tertiles), but a particular map displays values only for those counties falling into the TSP tertile associated with that map. In other words, we obtain three maps, a choropleth map of rate tertiles for counties in the lowest TSP tertile, a choropleth map of rate tertiles for counties in the middle TSP tertile, and a choropleth map of rate tertiles for counties in the highest TSP tertile. Carr et al. (2000) also illustrate the use of CC maps with two potentially interacting covariates. For example, if we wish to assess spatial patterns of LBW in Georgia Health District 9 with respect to tertiles of TSP and tertiles of maternal age, we could create a 3×3 grid of maps where each column represents a tertile of TSP and each row represents a tertile of maternal age. We examine patterns observed to see whether high rates of LBW tend to occur for particular combinations of TSP and maternal age (e.g., for high TSP and low maternal age).

Other examples of applications of LM plots and CC maps appear in Carr et al. (1998, 2000), and Carr (2001) and the references therein.

4.6.3 Exploratory Spatial Data Analysis

The famous statistician Oscar Kempthorne used to preach in lectures on experimental design: "Look at your data!" Tukey (1977) provided the first set of tools for data exploration, now known comprehensively by the term *exploratory data analysis* (EDA). EDA is a set of statistical techniques, many of them graphical and implemented interactively, that allow us to look at our data in various ways. The goals of EDA include extracting important variables; identifying outliers, anomalies, and unusual observations; detecting patterns and trends; and refining scientific hypotheses. The emphasis is on descriptive rather than inferential statistical methods. Many EDA techniques are probably familiar: five-number summaries, stem-and-leaf diagrams, boxplots, scatterplots, smoothing, and the more visual and interactive ideas of brushing, rotating, and spinning (Cleveland 1985). Other ideas, such as "polishing" two-way tables to detect factor effects (similar to analysis of variance) or using robust statistics, may be less familiar. Two excellent references for comprehensive EDA are Tukey (1977) and Velleman and Hoaglin (1981).

When working with spatial data, we need to put an "S" in EDA: *exploratory spatial data analysis* (ESDA). The goals and techniques of ESDA are similar to those of traditional EDA, but adapted for spatial data. All of the EDA techniques may be used "as is" with spatial attribute data, but we need additional techniques that explicitly use the spatial arrangement of the observations. For example, Haining (1990, Chapter 6, pp. 214–215) provides ESDA techniques that can be used to detect spatial outliers, observations that may not be unusual overall but that are unusual with respect to neighboring values. Cressie (1993, pp. 42–44) illustrates the use of a "pocket plot" for detecting localized atypical areas. Cressie (1984) extended the median polish technique of Tukey (1977), providing a robust method for detecting trends in spatial data. This technique is another type of spatial smoother, one that Kafadar (1994) included in her evaluation of spatial smoothers. Median polish and many other ESDA methods are described and illustrated in Cressie and Read (1989), Haining (1990), and Cressie (1993).

Much recent attention has been focused on software development for ESDA, including work by Brunsdon and Charlton (1996) and Dykes (1996) and the development of ESDA software for use within a GIS (e.g., Haining et al. 1996, 1998). Wise et al. (1999) provide a more recent overview of scientific visualization and ESDA. XGobi is a system for visualizing multivariate data that has been adapted to ESDA through a link to ArcView GIS (Cook et al. 1996; Symanzik et al. 1998). GeoVISTA *Studio*, a JAVA-based toolkit for ESDA developed at Pennsylvania State University and described in Takatsuka and Gahegan (2002), integrates both complex computations and visualization with the laudable goal of a codeless visual programming environment for ESDA and spatial data analysis.

4.6.4 Other Smoothing Approaches

Headbanging One median-based smoothing procedure, known as *headbanging* (Tukey and Tukey 1981; Hansen 1991), emphasizes local directional trends. Recent applications include smoothed national mortality maps, where analysts preferred headbanging's ability to preserve steep transitions between regions that can often be "oversmoothed" by other methods, particularly mean-based or linear smoothers (Mungiole et al. 1999).

The headbanging algorithm consists of two basic steps. The first step is identification of the values to be used in a median smoother. For each value to be smoothed, r_i, we first identify its k nearest neighbors. We then select pairs of these nearest neighbors so that the angle formed by the two segments with r_i in the center, say η, exceeds a specified value, η^*. Ideally, we want each *triple*, a pair plus r_i, to be roughly collinear. If there are many triples that satisfy this condition, we use only NTRIP of them whose angles are closest to 180° (NTRIP is a parameter of the smoothing algorithm that can be specified by the user). For edge or corner points that have few pairs satisfying this condition, the algorithm creates artificial triples by linear extrapolation from pairs of neighboring points. Once the triples have been identified, the second step is an iterative smoothing algorithm that proceeds as follows. For each pair associated with the ith value to be smoothed, let (l_j, u_j) be the lower and higher of the two values in the jth pair. Let $L = \text{median}\{l_j\}$ and $U = \text{median}\{u_j\}$. Then the smoothed value of r_i is $\tilde{r}_i = \text{median}\{L, r_i, U\}$. The smoothed value is used in place of the original value and the procedure is repeated until there is no change in the smoothed values. Greater smoothing results from using larger values of k, NTRIP, and η^*. Hansen (1991) suggests setting $\eta^* = 135°$; this default seems to give good results in most applications. To account for differing variances among the rates, Mungiole et al. (1999) developed a weighted headbanging algorithm that replaces the use of medians in the foregoing algorithm with weighted medians. Mungiole et al. (1999) used reciprocals of the standard errors associated with the rates as weights, but any specified weighting function could be used.

Splines and Generalized Additive Models Other smoothing approaches build on the nonparametric regression smoothers were introduced in Section 4.4.2. Suppose that we have spatial data $Y_1, Y_2, \ldots, Y_N$, associated with spatial locations $\mathbf{s}_i = (u_i, v_i)$. With spline smoothing our goal is to find a function, $f(u, v)$, that minimizes the trade-off between goodness of fit to the data and the smoothness (or equivalently, the roughness) of the resulting surface. There are many ways to measure surface smoothness, but one way is to use partial derivatives to measure the change in f; for example (Wahba 1990),

$$J_2(f) = \iint \left[\left(\frac{\partial^2 f}{\partial u^2} \right)^2 + 2 \left(\frac{\partial^2 f}{\partial u \partial v} \right)^2 + \left(\frac{\partial^2 f}{\partial v^2} \right)^2 \right] du\, dv.$$

Then our function f, called a *thin-plate smoothing spline*, minimizes

$$1/N \sum_{i=1}^{N} [Y_i - f(u_i, v_i)]^2 + m J_2(f).$$

The first term is a measure of goodness of fit to the data, the second term is a measure of surface smoothness, and the parameter m controls the trade-off between the two. If $m = 0$, there is no penalty for rapid changes in f, and thus the best-fitting surface will be the one that passes though all the data points. This function is then called an *interpolating* spline. Different choices of m lead to very different surfaces, some perhaps too smooth and others perhaps not smooth enough. One objective approach is to let the data determine m though a technique called generalized *cross validation* (see Wahba 1990). Wahba (1983) derives confidence intervals for the smoothing spline estimator.

Alternatively, we could use regression to fit a surface to the data. In this case, $E(Y) = \beta_0 + \beta_1 u + \beta_2 v$, and we could estimate the parameters using least squares. An alternative is to use an *additive model*, which assumes that $E(Y) = f_0 + f_1(u) + f_2(v)$, where the f_i are smooth functions. Splines and loess smooths are common choices for the f_i. Instead of a linear model, we could assume a generalized linear model (cf. Section 2.6.1) $g(E(Y)) = f_0 + f_1(u) + f_2(v)$, where g is a *link function* such as the log or the logit. This model is called a *generalized additive model* (GAM). Details on fitting GAMs can be found in Hastie and Tibshirani (1990), and a particular application to spatial epidemiology appears in Kelsall and Diggle (1998). Because of their flexibility in modeling nonlinear surfaces, splines and GAMs are very popular. However, other than cross-validation, which many find can produce surfaces that seem to be too smooth, there are few objective criteria governing the choice of the number of terms to include in the model, the nature of these terms, and the choice of m with smoothing splines and the span in loess. Thus, depending on the choices we make, we can essentially get any surface from least squares to an interpolating spline. GAMs are great exploratory tools, but it is very easy to overfit the data. We question their use with semiparametric models that include covariates of potential interest for which hypothesis testing is desired.

Centroid-Free Smoothing A third alternative smoothing approach seeks to eliminate the dependence on centroids for determining distances and neighborhoods. The use of centroids in determining the distance between areal features ignores the support of the spatial features. It also introduces an extra source of uncertainty into the results of smoothing since these results will depend on whether we base our distance calculations on centroids, centers, capitals, or some other point in each region. Tobler (1979) suggests one of the earliest centroid-free smoothers of aggregated data. He assumes the existence of an underlying intensity function, $\lambda(u, v)$, which is nonnegative and has a value for every location $s = (u, v) \in D$. (We define and use intensity functions beginning in Chapter 5.) Thus, we assume the underlying population to be distributed according to a spatial density function proportional to $\lambda(s)$, and the number of people in any region A is $Z(A) = \int_A \lambda(s)ds$. Tobler suggested that such an intensity function should be smooth and that adjacent regions should influence each other in the estimation process. Thus, given aggregated data (counts or totals), $Z(A_1), \ldots, Z(A_N)$ observed in regions A_i within a domain $D \subset \Re^2$, he suggested choosing $\lambda(u, v)$ to minimize

$$\iint \left[\left(\frac{\partial^2 \lambda}{\partial u^2} \right)^2 + \left(\frac{\partial^2 \lambda}{\partial v^2} \right)^2 \right] du\, dv, \qquad (4.13)$$

subject to the constraints $\lambda(\boldsymbol{s}) \geq 0$ and

$$\int_{A_i} \lambda(\boldsymbol{s})\, d\boldsymbol{s} = Z(A_i) \quad \text{for } i = 1, \ldots, N. \qquad (4.14)$$

When applied to point data, the intensity surface that minimizes equation (4.13) is the same as the spline surface described above. In the case of areal data, with the additional constraint of equation (4.14), the surface is constrained to preserve volume: The intensity process integrates to the data observed for each region. Tobler (1979) called this constraint the *pycnophylactic property* (or volume-preserving property). Tobler used finite difference methods to solve this constrained minimization. His approach is a very elegant solution to a complex problem, although standard errors for the smoothed values are difficult to obtain.

Finally, Brillinger (1990, 1994) consider a different optimization criterion based on a locally weighted analysis. Brillinger used the estimator given in equation (4.6) to estimate the value of $\lambda(u, v)$ based on a linear combination of aggregate data values [i.e., $\hat{\lambda}(\boldsymbol{s}) = \sum_{i=1}^{N} w_i Z(A_i)$]. Each weight, $w_i(u, v)$, determines the effect of region A_i on location (u, v). Brillinger (1990, 1994) suggested using weights that were integrals of the usual kernel functions, accounting for the support of the regions and avoiding the use of centroids. Müller et al. (1997) adapted Brillinger's ideas to estimation of the intensity function of disease incidence, where the total number of disease cases and the total population at risk are available for each region. They developed a modified version of locally weighted least squares where the squared differences between observations and local fits are integrated over the regions. Unlike Tobler's method, both of these estimators have standard errors and allow adjustment for covariates. However, they are much more computationally involved than the solution proposed by Tobler (1979).

These approaches explicitly recognize the different supports of the regions and do not reduce spatial analysis to simple computations involving point locations. Thus, they provide solutions to COSPs. Since we can use them to infer the intensity at any point location from aggregate data, they also provide one solution to the ecological inference problem. Integrating the intensity estimates over different regions is a solution to the MAUP.

4.6.5 Edge Effects

Observations near the edges of the study area have fewer local neighbors than observations in the interior. As a result, smoothed values near the edges often average over or borrow less neighboring information than their interior counterparts. For this reason, the behavior of spatial smoothing algorithms can be suspect near the edges of the study area. Accurate assessment of the impact of edge effects and development of flexible adjustments remain open areas for further research, for which Gelman and Price (1999), Lawson et al. (1999), and Gelman et al. (2000) provide recent developments.

4.7 EXERCISES

4.1 Derive the locally weighted estimator in equation (4.6).

4.2 Assuming that $Y_i \sim$ Poisson $(n_i \xi)$ and $r_i = Y_i/n_i$, find the expected value and variance of the locally weighted-average smoother in equation (4.1).

4.3 Derive the method-of-moments estimators of α and β from the Poisson–gamma model discussed in Section 4.4.3. Then give the resulting empirical Bayes smoother.

4.4 Table 4.1 gives the number of low birth weight babies born in 1999, the number of live births in 1999, and the number of very low birth weight babies born in 1999 for each county in Georgia Health Care District 9. The numbers of very low birth weight babies presented here are masks of the true values, obtained by adding random noise to the original counts. For confidentiality reasons, we could not release the true values. The table also gives the centroids of each county in UTM coordinates (in meters).

(a) Compute the rate of very low birth weight for each county. Make a choropleth map of the rates.

(b) Make a probability map using the very low birth weight rates you computed in part (a). Which counties have significantly high rates?

(c) Use the global empirical Bayes estimator given in equation (4.11) to smooth the rates.

(d) Implement this estimator locally using neighborhoods based on distance between centroids and defined by the weights in equation (4.2).

(e) Implement the empirical Bayes estimator locally using neighborhoods defined by adjacency weights given in equation (4.5). Lee and Wong (2001) have a nice collection of scripts that can be used to determine the neighbors of each county using a GIS.

(f) Repeat these exercises using the number of low birth weight babies.

(g) What are your conclusions about smoothing? Do the VLBW rates need to be smoothed? Do the LBW rates need to be smoothed? Which neighborhood structure did you prefer, and why? Which smoother did you prefer, and why? Which counties may have unusually high VLBW rates?

Table 4.1 Georgia Health Care District 9 Data[a]

County	No. Live Births	No. Low Birth Weight	No. Very Low Birth Weight	Easting	Northing
Emanuel	308	35	0	380775.664	3606798.382
Bulloch	693	64	9	429643.221	3587905.874
Effingham	570	36	8	467554.861	3581547.440
Candler	151	9	3	398199.760	3581861.311
Toombs	454	33	2	375444.918	3558825.264
Tattnall	300	21	5	400212.232	3549337.656
Evans	155	9	0	415835.404	3560344.423
Bryan	370	27	2	454305.848	3544080.578
Liberty	1525	147	19	446806.707	3524848.421
Long	164	8	1	434104.476	3505692.396
Jeff Davis	238	28	2	344402.500	3524049.993
Appling	257	23	1	374321.622	3513589.072
Chatham	3570	369	100	493865.557	3539584.049
Wayne	341	30	10	412989.631	3497227.698
Coffee	666	66	18	325675.232	3487194.532
Bacon	143	12	2	364082.121	3494227.776
McIntosh	149	18	3	463548.477	3486352.845
Pierce	228	11	2	383019.454	3473351.819
Ware	492	46	3	366888.053	3438399.181
Glynn	908	95	12	454245.142	3456655.732
Atkinson	164	12	5	321340.050	3464443.158
Brantley	124	8	1	408546.111	3453357.994
Clinch	99	10	2	334630.866	3423796.886
Camden	722	65	7	440181.095	3425482.335
Charlton	127	8	0	388725.451	3424758.917

[a]To protect data confidentiality, the counts of very low birth weight cases have been masked, so their true values are not presented here.

CHAPTER 5

Analysis of Spatial Point Patterns

Woes cluster. Rare are solitary woes;
They love a train, they tread each other's heel.
Edward Young, *Night Thoughts*, Night iii, Line 63

A primary goal in the analysis of mapped point data is to detect patterns (i.e., to draw inference regarding the distribution of an observed set of locations). In particular, we wish to detect whether the set of locations observed contains clusters of events reflecting areas with associated increases in the likelihood of occurrence (e.g., unusual aggregations of cases of a particular disease).

In this chapter we introduce mathematical models for random patterns of events and outline basic related analytic methods for spatial point processes. We pay particular attention to data restrictions, common assumptions, and interpretation of results. The models and methods introduced in this chapter provide the basis for the analytic approaches in Chapters 6 and 7 specifically assessing spatial patterns observed in public health data.

5.1 TYPES OF PATTERNS

It is human nature to assign order to our observations and to seek patterns in collections of seemingly random events. Here, we use mathematical definitions to identify patterns in the spatial distribution of a set of locations. In public health data, one pattern of particular interest is the presence of a tendency of locations to *cluster* together (i.e., occur more frequently in close proximity to one another) than one would expect from a set of cases with no common causative factor (e.g., environmental exposure). We explore such applications more thoroughly in Chapter 6, but the notion of clustering offers a starting point for discussions of spatial pattern.

To define spatial *clustering*, we begin by defining its absence. We define an *event* as an occurrence of interest (e.g., an incident case of a disease) and associate

Applied Spatial Statistics for Public Health Data, by Lance A. Waller and Carol A. Gotway
ISBN 0-471-38771-1

an *event location* with each event. We follow terminology in Diggle (1983) and distinguish between an event and a point. A *point* is any location in the study area where an event could occur; an *event location* is a particular location in the study area where an event did occur. A data set consists of a collection of observed event locations and a spatial domain of interest. The spatial domain is a very important aspect of the data set. It may be defined by data availability (e.g., a state or county boundary), but in many problems the analyst must define the boundary with thoughtful consideration. Examples in this chapter illustrate how different choices for the domain can result in different inferences about the spatial data under study.

Next, we consider what is meant by a "random" pattern. Technically speaking, all of the models in this chapter generate random patterns since each is based on a particular probability structure. However, in general usage, the phrases *random pattern*, *at random*, or *by chance* typically refer to a distribution of events that is not influenced by various factors under investigation (e.g., the local level of a toxic substance).

As our first model of a random pattern, *complete spatial randomness* (CSR) defines a situation where an event is equally likely to occur at any location within the study area, regardless of the locations of other events. That is, events follow a *uniform distribution* across the study area, and are *independent* of one another. We use the term *uniform* in the sense of following a uniform probability distribution across the study area, not in the sense of "evenly" dispersed across the study area. Figure 5.1 illustrates six realizations (sets of events) arising from a CSR model. We present several realizations (data sets) based on the same model to illustrate a range of patterns possible under CSR. Note that each of these spatially random patterns of events contains collections of nearby events (apparent clusters), and large gaps between events. The apparent clusters illustrate that a certain degree of clustering occurs by chance, making visual assessment of particular clusters or overall patterns of clustering difficult.

Complete spatial randomness serves as a boundary condition between spatial processes that are more clustered than random and processes that are more regular than random. Figure 5.2 illustrates three examples of patterns more clustered than CSR (top row), and three examples of patterns more regular than CSR (bottom row). It might be easy to distinguish the three different types of patterns in Figures 5.1 and 5.2, but it is difficult to do so in practice, and an "eyeball" comparison can often be misleading. Moreover, observed patterns do not always fall neatly into one of the three classes: clustered, random, or regular. Figure 5.3 illustrates realizations from a process consisting of regular patterns of clusters (clusters are centered at points arranged like the "five" on a die) and from a process consisting of clusters of regular patterns (each regular pattern consists of five points in a similar relative arrangement). Although admittedly contrived, these patterns of 100 events each illustrate the critical role played by *spatial scale* in describing observed patterns (i.e., clustering exists at one level of spatial scale, regularity at another). Issues of spatial scale are often discussed in the ecology literature. Indeed, an extensive literature exists regarding the determination of the spatial scale of species, behaviors,

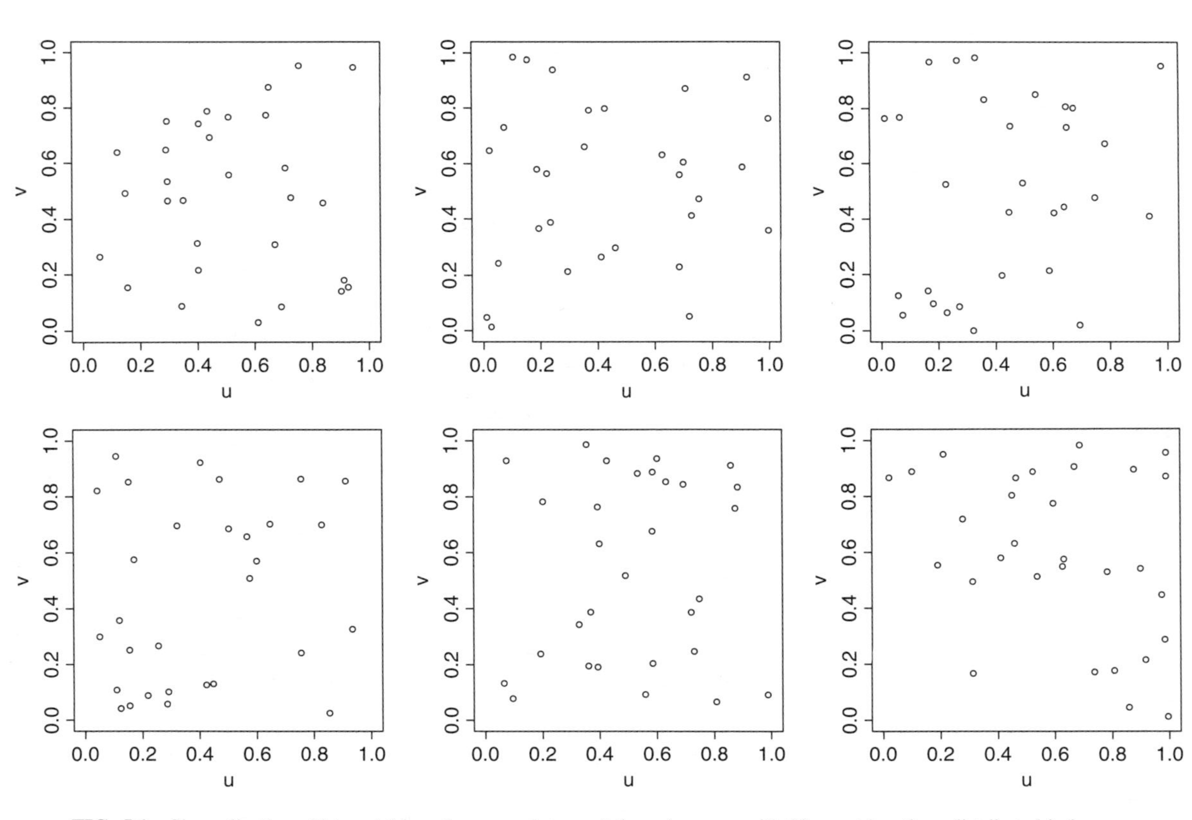

FIG. 5.1 Six realizations (data sets) based on *complete spatial randomness*, with 30 event locations distributed independently (no interactions between events) and uniformly (events equally likely at any locations) across the unit square.

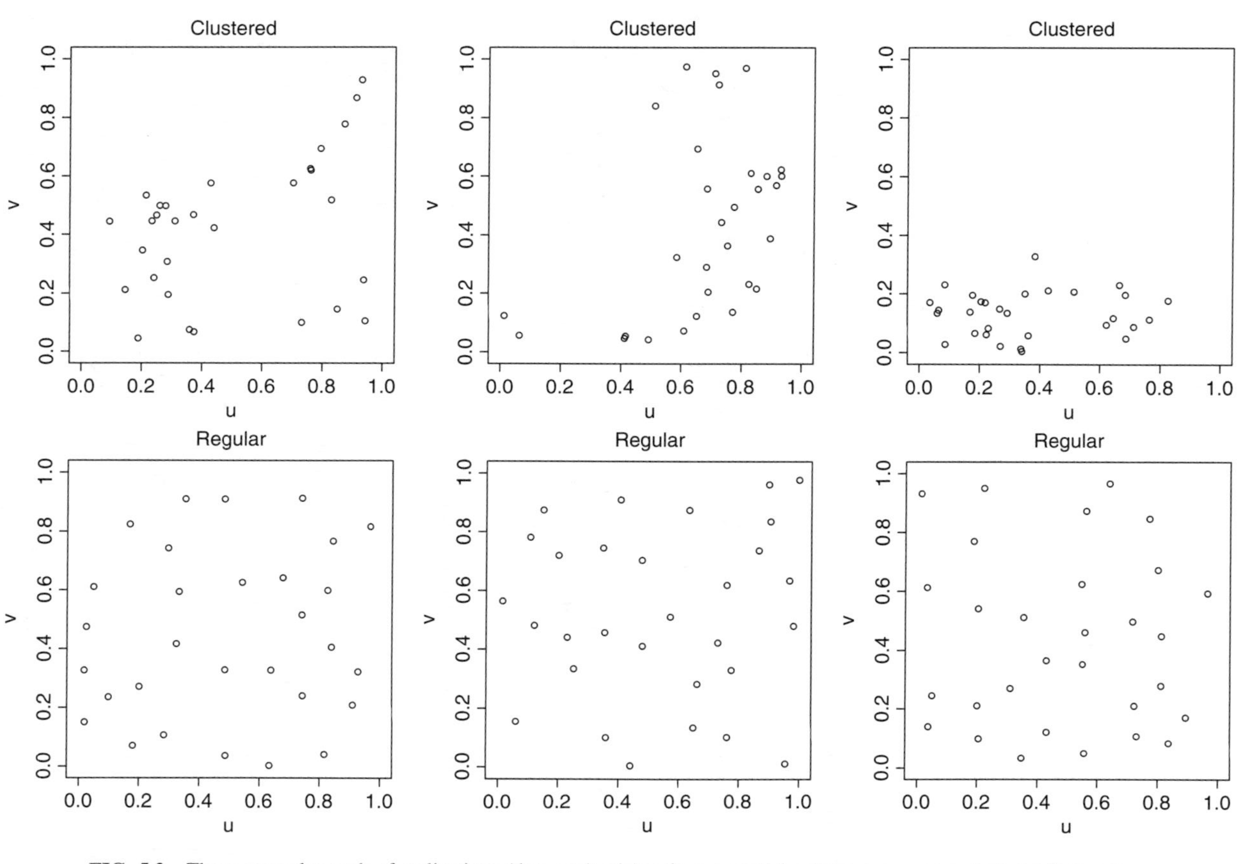

FIG. 5.2 Three examples each of realizations (data sets) arising from a spatial point process more clustered that complete spatial randomness (top row), and a spatial point process more regular than complete spatial randomness (bottom row). Each data set contains 30 event locations within the unit square.

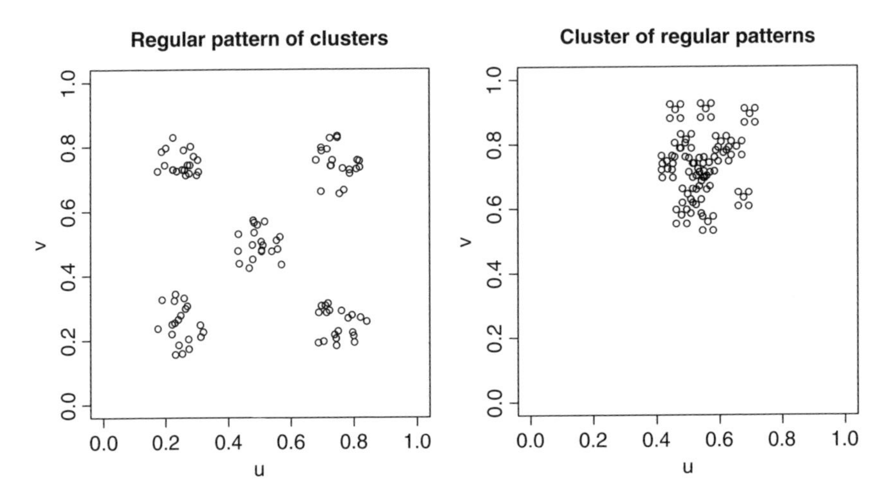

FIG. 5.3 Realizations of two hypothetical spatial point processes containing both clustering and regularity at different spatial scales.

and diseases in plants and animals (see, e.g., Turner et al. 1989; Levin 1992), but little appears to date in the epidemiologic literature [but see Prince et al. (2001) for an example].

With a general notion of clustered, random, and regular patterns (and an appreciation to the limitations of the simple categorization illustrated in Figure 5.3) we next seek to define probabilistic models of spatial patterns in order to motivate methods for detecting clustering among health events.

5.2 SPATIAL POINT PROCESSES

A *stochastic process* is a probabilistic model defined by a collection of random variables, say $\{X_1, X_2, \ldots, X_N\}$. In most cases each X_i is a similar measurement occurring at a different time or place (e.g., the number of persons in a post office queue at the ith time period, or the amount of rainfall at the ith location). A *spatial point process* describes a stochastic process where each random variable represents the location of an event in space. A *realization* of the process is a collection of locations generated under the spatial point process model; that is, a realization represents a data set resulting from a particular model (either observed or simulated). The patterns illustrated in Figures 5.1–5.3 display realizations from various spatial point process models. In some instances, a data set may consist of a sample from a realization of a particular pattern (e.g., we may map a simple random sample of residential locations of disease cases in a registry), and in such cases we must take care to consider the spatial impact (if any) of the sampling procedure (cf. Diggle 1983, Chapter 3).

Ripley (1981, Chapter 8), Diggle (1983), and Cressie (1993, Chapter 8) provide details regarding theory and applications of spatial point processes from many diverse fields (e.g., forestry, astronomy, cellular biology). We focus primarily on basic structures in spatial point process models and their application to assessments of pattern in public health data.

5.2.1 Stationarity and Isotropy

Two underlying concepts provide a starting place for modeling spatial point processes. Mathematically, a process is *stationary* when it is invariant to translation within d-dimensional space, and *isotropic* when it is invariant to rotation about the origin. In other words, relationships between two events in a stationary process depend only on their relative positions, not on the event locations themselves. Starting with a stationary process, adding an assumption of isotropy involves a further restriction that relationships between two events depend only on the distance separating their locations and not on their orientation to each other (i.e., relationships depend only on distance, not direction). However, neither property (isotropy nor stationarity) implies the other.

These two properties offer a notion of replication within a data set. For example, two pairs of events in the realization of a stationary process that are separated by the same distance and relative direction should be subject to the same relatedness. Similarly, two pairs of events from a realization of a stationary and isotropic process separated by the same distance (regardless of relative direction) should be subject to similar properties. These two assumptions offer a starting point for most of the estimation and testing procedures outlined in this chapter. In some cases we move beyond assumptions of stationarity and isotropy, and we take care to note these instances.

5.2.2 Spatial Poisson Processes and CSR

We next outline a particular set of spatial point processes and illustrate its equivalence with CSR. Specifically, we consider the family of stationary *homogeneous spatial Poisson point processes* defined by the following criteria (Diggle 1983, p. 50; Stoyan et al. 1995, p. 33):

1. The number of events occurring within a finite region A is a random variable following a Poisson distribution with mean $\lambda|A|$ for some positive constant λ and $|A|$ denoting the area of A.
2. Given the total number of events N occurring within an area A, the locations of the N events represent an independent random sample of N locations, where each point (location where an event could occur) is equally likely to be chosen as an event.

Criterion 2 represents the general concept of CSR (events uniformly distributed across the study area), and criterion 1 introduces the idea of an *intensity* λ representing the number of events expected per unit area. The Poisson distribution allows the total number of events observed to vary from realization to realization while maintaining a fixed (but unknown) expected number of events per unit area. Dividing the total number of events observed by the total area provides a straightforward estimate of λ (i.e., $\widehat{\lambda} = N/|A|$). This estimate serves well for most of the examples in this book; however, we note that other estimators can provide better performance in certain situations, particularly those involving estimates based on sparse samples of the set of events observed (Byth 1982; Diggle and Cox 1983).

For further insight into the properties of homogeneous Poisson processes, consider an equivalent definition listed in Cressie (1993, p. 634):

(a) The numbers of events in nonoverlapping regions are statistically independent.

(b) For any region $A \subseteq D$,

$$\lim_{|A| \to 0} \frac{\Pr[\text{exactly one event in } A]}{|A|} = \lambda > 0$$

where $|A|$ is the area of region A, D is the domain of interest (study area), and

(c)

$$\lim_{|A| \to 0} \frac{\Pr[\text{two or more events in } A]}{|A|} = 0.$$

Component (a) is particularly important to the analysis of regional counts (e.g., the number of incident disease cases observed in a partition of the study area into enumeration districts). Diggle (1983, p. 50) formally establishes the link between criteria 1 and 2 and component (a). Component (b) implies that the probability of a single event in an increasingly small area A (adjusted for the area of A) is a constant (λ) independent of the location of region A within the study area of interest. Component (c) implies that the probability of two or more events occurring in precisely the same location is zero. As above, the quantity λ is the Poisson parameter, or the intensity of the process, and is equal to the mean number of points per unit area. Since the intensity of events is constant at all locations in the study area, we say that the process is *homogeneous*. Mathematically, stationarity and homogeneity are related but separate concepts (e.g., a process defined within a finite study area cannot be stationary). However, the differences are largely technical and have relevance beyond the scope of this book, and we use the terms fairly interchangeably in the examples that follow.

The definition of a homogeneous Poisson process given by criteria 1 and 2 not only describes the mathematical model underlying CSR, but also a straightforward two-stage approach for simulating realizations from CSR in a study area D. Such simulations prove extremely useful in the analysis of spatial point process data, and we outline the simulation procedure here. First, we generate the total number of points, $N(D)$, from a Poisson distribution with mean $\lambda|D|$ (where $|D|$ denotes the area of D). Next, we place events within D according to a uniform distribution. If D is rectangular, we may generate u and v coordinates using uniform random number generators on the intervals corresponding to the width and height of D, respectively. It is worth noting that many pseudorandom number generators used in computer simulation contain deterministic (nonrandom) patterns for some pattern length. As a result, a single string of such pseudorandom numbers may appear sufficiently random, but the sets of k values exhibit a pattern, typically resulting in the pseudorandom values falling along sets of parallel lines in k-dimensional space [see Ripley (1987, pp. 22–26) for details]. For our purposes in two or three dimensions, the uniform random number generators in most statistical packages will function well, but some experimentation in the form of plotting pairs or triplets of consecutive values is often a good idea. For simulating CSR within a nonrectangular study area D, one option is to embed D within a larger rectangle R, and generate event locations within R until $N(D)$ events occur within D, and use these $N(D)$ events as the realization. For more details and other approaches for nonrectangular areas, see Stoyan et al. (1995, pp. 28–30, 44–46).

5.2.3 Hypothesis Tests of CSR via Monte Carlo Methods

To detect clustering (or regularity) statistically, we need to ascertain departures from CSR. Even with the same underlying CSR process, Figure 5.1 indicates a fair amount of variability between realizations. In many applications we observe a single realization from the underlying (but unknown) point process. We need a method to describe how much variation we expect under CSR and to tell us when an observed pattern of event locations appears to differ *significantly* from CSR. Hypothesis tests and Monte Carlo simulation techniques provide versatile tools for such assessments.

A statistical hypothesis test typically compares the observed value of a quantitative summary of the data observed (the test statistic) to the probability distribution of that summary under the assumptions of the null hypothesis. For example, we might want to compare the average interevent distance observed for a set of event locations to the distribution of average interevent distances occurring from repeated independent realizations from CSR. For many test statistics, one may rely on asymptotic arguments to derive their associated null distributions theoretically under CSR [Table 8.6 on page 604 of Cressie (1993) provides an outline of many of these tests and their associated distributions]. However, these arguments often require certain assumptions about the shape of the study area (either rectangular or square), and base asymptotics on the number of observed events going to infinity. In many health applications, the study area is shaped irregularly and the number of events depends more on an underlying disease incidence rate than on sampling considerations (i.e., sample size increases only by observing cases over a longer period of time, leading to a loss of temporal resolution in the data). In such cases, the usual asymptotic distributions may be inappropriate and inaccurate.

In contrast, the general frequentist notion of comparing the observed value of a test statistic to its distribution under the null hypothesis combined with the ease of simulating data from CSR (even subject to the constraints of a fixed or reduced sample size and/or an irregularly shaped boundary) suggest the use of *Monte Carlo* (simulation-based) methods of inference. In Monte Carlo testing, we first calculate the test statistic value based on the data observed and then calculate the same statistic for a large number (say, N_{sim}) of data sets simulated independently under the null hypothesis of interest (e.g., simulated under CSR as described above). A histogram of the statistic values associated with the simulated data sets provides an estimate of the distribution of the test statistic under the null hypothesis. The proportion of test statistic values based on simulated data exceeding the value of the test statistic observed for the actual data set provides a Monte Carlo estimate of the upper-tail p-value for a one-sided hypothesis test. Specifically, suppose that T_{obs} denotes the test statistic for the data observed and $T_{(1)} \geq T_{(2)} \geq \cdots \geq T_{(N_{\text{sim}})}$ denote the test statistic values (ordered from largest to smallest) for the simulated data set. If $T_{(1)} \geq \cdots \geq T_{(\ell)} \geq T_{\text{obs}} > T_{(\ell+1)}$ (i.e., only the ℓ largest test statistic values based on simulated data exceed T_{obs}), the estimated p-value is

$$\widehat{\Pr}[T \geq T_{\text{obs}} | H_0 \text{ is true}] = \frac{\ell}{N_{\text{sim}} + 1}$$

where we add one to the denominator since our estimate is based on $N_{\text{sim}} + 1$ values ($\{T_{(1)}, \ldots, T_{(N_{\text{sim}})}, T_{\text{obs}}\}$). One calculates lower-tail p-values in an analogous manner. Besag and Diggle (1977), Ripley (1981, pp. 16–18), Cressie (1993, pp. 635–636), and Stoyan et al. (1995, pp. 142–142) provide further details regarding the application of Monte Carlo tests to the analysis of spatial point patterns.

Due to their reliance on simulated data sets, Monte Carlo methods are not precisely replicable. That is, an independent set of N_{sim} realizations will result in a slightly different estimated p-value than the first set of simulations. However, the larger the value of N_{sim}, the more stable the resulting estimates, and one can calculate the variability (Monte Carlo error) as a function of N_{sim} (Ripley 1987). Note the difference between the asymptotics associated with N_{sim} (a sample size we define, irrespective of the data) and the asymptotics associated with the number of events (a feature of the data not often under our control). The former define the accuracy of our estimate of the correct null distribution; the latter define a distribution that is only known to be correct for large numbers of events.

Finally, we note that CSR is only one example of a null hypothesis of interest, but the Monte Carlo testing procedure is quite general. We illustrate Monte Carlo testing in a variety of contexts relevant to health data below and in Chapters 6 and 7.

5.2.4 Heterogeneous Poisson Processes

As mentioned in Section 5.2.2, the Poisson process is homogeneous when the intensity, λ, is constant across the study area. In the analysis of health events, we may find a homogeneous model too restrictive. In particular, CSR may not be an appropriate model for the lack of clustering, since the population at risk is not distributed uniformly across space; rather, people tend to live in towns and cities. Instead, we often consider the *constant risk hypothesis* as a model of "no clustering." Under the constant risk model, each person has the same risk of disease during the observation period, regardless of location, and we expect more cases in

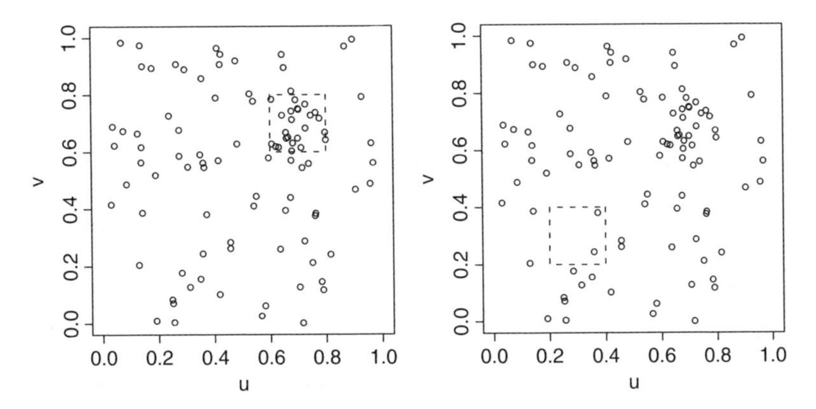

FIG. 5.4 Example of a process that appears clustered with respect to CSR but not clustered with respect to a hypothesis of constant risk. The box represents an area of high population density. The set of event locations is the same in both plots. In the plot on the left, we observe a higher intensity of events in the high-population area, consistent with a constant risk hypothesis but inconsistent with CSR. In the plot on the right, the cluster occurs outside the area of high population density, reflecting an area of increased local risk and a clustered process with respect to both CSR and constant risk.

areas with more people at risk. Clusters of cases in high population areas could violate CSR but not the constant risk hypothesis. Typically, for noninfectious diseases we are most interested in clustering above and beyond that due to geographic variations in the density of the population at risk (i.e., clustering of disease events after accounting for known variations in population density). We wish to interpret the observed pattern of cases with respect to the observed pattern of people at risk. Figure 5.4 provides a simplified example. Both plots show the same set of event locations. Suppose that the dashed square represents the boundary of a small area of high population density within the study area. In the left-hand plot, a cluster of events occurs within the high-population-density area, consistent with a hypothesis of constant risk, but inconsistent with CSR. In the right-hand plot, the cluster now occurs outside the high-population-density area, inconsistent with both a constant risk hypothesis and CSR.

The constant risk hypothesis requires a generalization of CSR where we define the intensity as a spatially varying function defined over our study area D [i.e., the intensity is a function $\lambda(s)$ of the spatial location $s \in D$]. Specifically, one defines a *heterogeneous Poisson process* by the following criteria:

1*. The number of events occurring within a finite region A is a random variable following a Poisson distribution with mean $\int_A \lambda(s)\, ds$.

2*. Given the total number of events N occurring within an area A, the N events represent an independent random sample of N locations, with the probability of sampling a particular point s proportional to $\lambda(s)$.

The number of events observed in disjoint regions still follow independent Poisson distributions, but the expectation of the event count in a region A becomes $\int_A \lambda(s)\, ds$, and events are distributed according to a spatial density function proportional to $\lambda(s)$.

That is, we expect more events in areas corresponding to higher values of $\lambda(\boldsymbol{s})$ and fewer events in areas corresponding to lower values of $\lambda(\boldsymbol{s})$. Note that heterogeneity (as defined by a spatially varying intensity function) necessarily implies nonstationarity as the point process is no longer translation invariant (stationarity). Since we define isotropy with respect to rotation invariance around a single point (typically referred to as the *origin*), heterogeneity in the intensity function results in an anisotropic process only if $\lambda(\boldsymbol{s})$ itself is anisotropic (i.e., not symmetrical around the origin).

The intensity function $\lambda(\boldsymbol{s})$ is a first-order (mean) property of the random process, describing the expected density of events in any location of the region. Events remain independent of one another, but clusters appear in areas of high intensity. Under a heterogeneous Poisson process clusters occur solely due to heterogeneities in the intensity function and individual event locations remain independent of one another.

To illustrate, consider a scenario of five cases of acute lymphocytic leukemia observed in a census region. Since under the constant risk hypothesis, our concept of whether this constitutes a cluster or not depends on the size of the population at risk, our model of no clustering should depend on the observed population density across our study area. As population sizes increase, so should our expected number of cases under a model of constant individual-level risk of disease at all locations. The heterogeneous Poisson process offers a convenient null model (model of no clustering) for our tests of disease clustering that allows for geographic variations in population size.

As an example of a heterogeneous Poisson process, the spatially varying intensity function in Figure 5.5 exhibits two modes (areas of high intensity) at $\boldsymbol{s} = (u, v) = (3, 3)$ and $(16, 14)$, respectively. The intensity is more peaked around the former and more broad around the latter. Figure 5.6 illustrates six realizations of 100 events

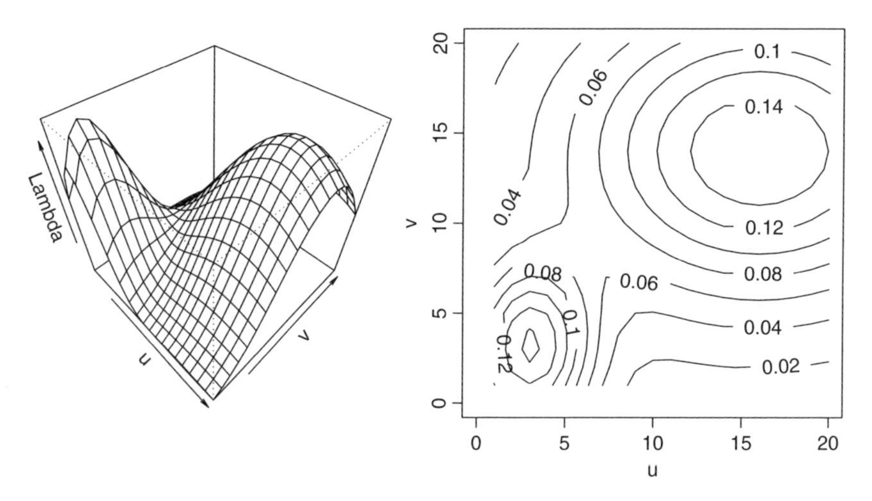

FIG. 5.5 Example intensity function, $\lambda(s)$, for a heterogeneous Poisson point process defined for $s = (u, v)$ and $u, v \in (0, 20)$.

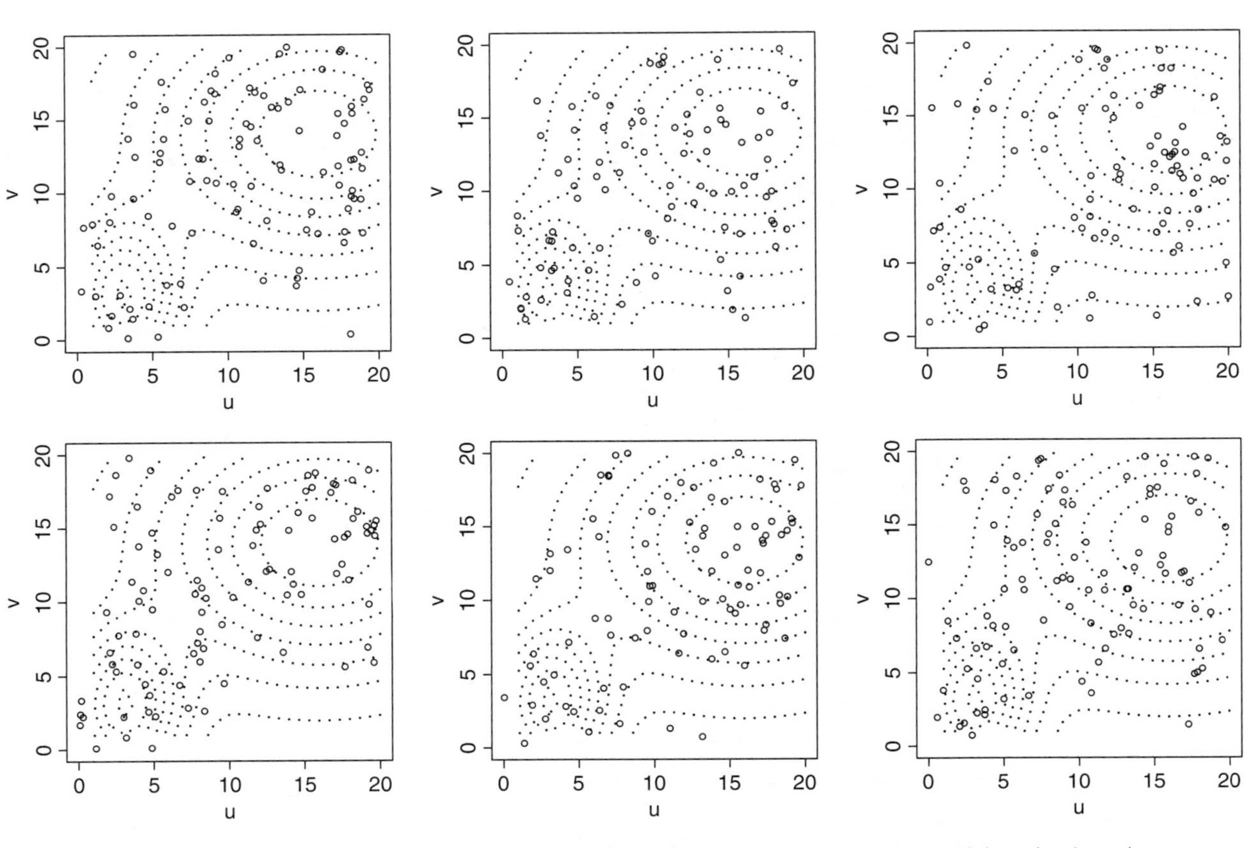

FIG. 5.6 Six simulated realizations of 100 events each from an inhomogeneous Poisson process with intensity shown in Figure 5.5.

each from a heterogeneous Poisson process with intensity $\lambda(s)$ shown in Figure 5.5. The examples reveal a relative lack of events in the area between the modes, and proportionally more events in the broader rise in $\lambda(s)$ surrounding the mode at (16, 14) than in the smaller, peaked area around (3, 3). Note that collections of events generally suggest areas of higher intensity, although the specific locations of the modes can be difficult to spot from a single realization. The problems at the end of this chapter outline an algorithm for simulating realizations from a heterogeneous Poisson process with known intensity function, offering further exploration of this issue.

5.2.5 Estimating Intensity Functions

A contour or surface plot of the intensity function for a heterogeneous Poisson process indicates areas with higher and lower probabilities of an event occurring. As an exploratory measure, we may compare peaks and valleys in the intensity function with maps of covariates and look for similarities between the observed spatial patterns of events and covariates, respectively. We may also compare the estimated intensities of event locations associated with incident cases of a disease and that of a sample of nondiseased subjects (controls) over the same study area.

First we need to define a way to estimate the intensity function from a set of observed event locations. Suppose that we have a data set consisting of N locations, $s_1, \ldots, s_N$, and we wish to estimate $\lambda(s)$ from these locations. A common method involves *kernel density estimation* (Silverman 1986; Scott 1992; Wand and Jones 1995). Conceptually, think of mapping events on a tabletop and then placing an identical mound of modeling clay over each event. The mounds of clay will overlap for groups of events occurring close together, resulting in a higher pile of clay in such areas. When considered together, the clay represents a surface reflecting a nonparametric estimate of the intensity function.

To illustrate, consider the one-dimensional example in Figure 5.7. Our data set consists of the event locations marked $\times$ along the s-axis within the unit interval. We center our mound of clay, represented by a symmetric "kernel," at each observed data location. Intensity functions must be positive at all locations and integrate to a finite number, so often, known parametric density functions provide convenient kernels. In Figure 5.7 we use kernels proportional to a Gaussian density function with different standard deviations illustrating differing amounts of overlap between kernels. To estimate the shape of the intensity function $\lambda(s)$ underlying the distribution of events, we plot the curve defined by summing the heights of all kernels at any point along the s-axis. Here, the kernel variance reflects the square of the *bandwidth* (standard deviation) or extent of influence of each data point and governs the overall smoothness of the intensity estimate.

Kernel estimation methods originally focused on estimating a probability *density function* $f(s)$ rather than an *intensity function* $\lambda(s)$. With respect to a spatial point process, a density function defines the probability of observing an event at a location s, while the intensity function defines the number of events expected per unit area at location s. (Note that for a continuous intensity function, this "expected number

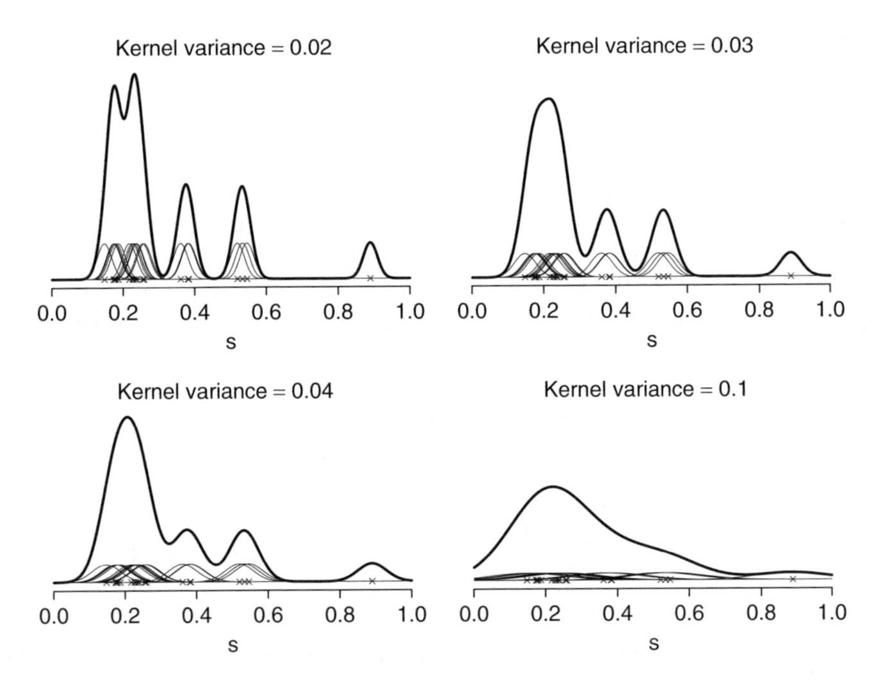

FIG. 5.7 Kernel intensity estimates based on the same set of 20 event locations and four different kernel bandwidths [kernel variances reflect the square of the bandwidth (standard deviation)].

of events per unit area" varies smoothly from location to location.) By definition, a density integrates to one across a study area D. In contrast, an intensity estimate integrates to the overall mean number of events per unit area (i.e., the total number of events observed divided by $|D|$, the area of D) (Diggle 2000). Dividing the intensity $\lambda(\boldsymbol{s})$ by its integral over D yields the density $f(\boldsymbol{s})$. As a result, the density function and the intensity function differ by a constant of proportionality, which can result in visual stretching or shrinking of the modes (peaks) in perspective or contour plots of the intensity compared to similar plots of the densities. However, the relative spatial pattern (e.g., locations of peaks and valleys) in densities and intensities will be the same. Most kernel estimation software estimates densities rather than intensities, and it is fairly common to use a kernel density estimate, denoted $\tilde{f}(\boldsymbol{s})$, as an estimate of $\lambda(\boldsymbol{s})$ without rescaling. Authors sometimes use the terms *density* and *intensity* interchangeably when the spatial variation in the functions rather than their precise values is of primary interest, but some care is required for describing, reporting, and interpreting actual numerical values.

Mathematically, the definition of a kernel density estimate in one dimension based on observations $u_1, u_2, \ldots, u_N$ is

$$\tilde{f}(u) = \frac{1}{Nb} \sum_{i=1}^{N} \text{kern}\left(\frac{u - u_i}{b}\right) \tag{5.1}$$

where u is a location in one-dimensional space, kern$(\cdot)$ is a kernel function satisfying

$$\int_D \text{kern}(s)\, ds = 1$$

and b denotes a smoothing parameter (bandwidth). Again, the bandwidth corresponds to the width of the kernel function. To obtain a kernel estimate of the density function, replace N^{-1} by $|D|^{-1}$ in equation (5.1).

The one-dimensional kernel estimate in equation (5.1) extends to multiple dimensions. For our two-dimensional spatial point process data, we consider two-dimensional *product kernels* based on the product of two one-dimensional kernels. Product kernels are a natural extension when we do not assume any interaction or dependence between the u and v coordinates of the observed event locations in our data set. The two-dimensional kernel estimate of the density function at location $s = (u_0, v_0)$ is defined by

$$\tilde{f}(u_0, v_0) = \frac{1}{N b_u b_v} \sum_{i=1}^{N} \left\{ \text{kern}\left(\frac{u_0 - u_i}{b_u}\right) \text{kern}\left(\frac{v_0 - v_i}{b_v}\right) \right\} \quad (5.2)$$

where b_u and b_v are the bandwidths in the u and v directions, respectively. In practice, we evaluate equation (5.2) at a grid of locations $s = (u_0, v_0)$ covering the study area, then create a surface or contour plot of these values, representing our estimate of the overall intensity surface. Note that in the product kernel formulation, we apply one-dimensional kernels in the u and v directions separately, then multiply the two kernels together. In addition to product kernels, other bivariate kernel formulations are available [see Scott (1992) and Wand and Jones (1995) for further discussion and examples].

In applying kernel estimation, we must specify two items: the kernel function and the bandwidth. We may use any positive function integrating to 1 as a kernel function; however, several particular functions appear regularly in the literature and have well-studied theoretical properties. Table 5.1 lists the one-dimensional form of many commonly used kernels, using u^* to denote the distance between the general location u and the ith observation u_i, divided by the bandwidth:

$$u^* = ((u - u_i)/b),$$

in the ith summand of equation (5.1). While some kernel functions have better mathematical or computational properties than others, the differences between estimates based on different kernel functions are often small. Hence, for most purposes any symmetric kernel is adequate. Computational efficiency typically dictates simplicity in the kernel's functional form, so in practice we often use computationally simpler functions than the Gaussian kernel used in Figure 5.7 (see Silverman 1986, pp. 76–77).

In the examples below we use one of two bivariate kernel functions. First, we consider a product kernel based on univariate Gaussian kernels in the u and

Table 5.1 Common One-Dimensional Kernel Functions Centered at the ith Observation u_i[a]

Kernel	Kern(u^*)
Uniform	$\frac{1}{2b} I\left(\lvert u^*\rvert \le 1\right)$
Triangle	$\frac{1}{b(2-b)}\left(1-\lvert u^*\rvert\right) I(\lvert u^*\rvert \le 1)$
Quartic (biweight)	$\frac{15}{16b}\left[1-(u^*)^2\right]^2 I(\lvert u^*\rvert \le 1)$
Triweight	$\frac{35}{32b}\left[1-(u^*)^2\right]^3 I(\lvert u^*\rvert \le 1)$
Gaussian	$\frac{1}{\sqrt{2\pi}b}\exp\left[-\frac{1}{2}(u^*)^2\right]$

[a] u^* represents the difference between location u and u_i divided by the bandwidth b [*i.e.*, $(u-u_i)/b$] (see text). The function I(expression) is the indicator function taking the value 1 if the expression is true and 0 otherwise.

v directions. The second kernel is the computationally simpler two-dimensional analog of the *quartic kernel* defined in Table 5.1. Bailey and Gatrell (1995, p. 85) define the two-dimensional quartic kernel as

$$\text{kern}(\boldsymbol{s}) = \begin{cases} \frac{3}{\pi}(1-\boldsymbol{s}'\boldsymbol{s})^2 & \boldsymbol{s}'\boldsymbol{s} \le 1 \\ 0 & \text{otherwise,} \end{cases}$$

where $\boldsymbol{s}'$ denotes the transpose of the vector $\boldsymbol{s}$. The corresponding estimated intensity

$$\tilde{\lambda}(\boldsymbol{s}) = \sum_{\|\boldsymbol{s}-\boldsymbol{s}_i\| \le b} \frac{3}{\pi b^2}\left(1 - \frac{\|\boldsymbol{s}-\boldsymbol{s}_i\|^2}{b^2}\right)^2$$

is easy to compute and interpret (only events within distance b of point $\boldsymbol{s}$ contribute to the estimated intensity at $\boldsymbol{s}$).

Although the precise form of the kernel weakly influences intensity estimates, the bandwidth can have a profound impact. Figure 5.7 illustrates the intensity estimates based on a variety of bandwidths. Technically, the optimal bandwidth (i.e., the bandwidth minimizing the mean integrated square error between the estimate and the true intensity) depends on the unknown underlying function $\lambda(\boldsymbol{s})$, an unfortunately circular relationship. However, Silverman (1986, pp. 43–61) describes several approaches for determining bandwidth, each based on different criteria, noting that the appropriate choice of bandwidth always depends on the purpose intended for the smoothed estimate. Large bandwidths result in more smoothing; small bandwidths retain more local features but exhibit spikes at isolated event locations. Exploratory analyses may consider several bandwidths to determine general patterns, and the analyst may determine somewhat subjectively the sensitivity of the intensity estimate to the choice of bandwidth.

A more formal criterion for bandwidth selection involves the *asymptotic mean integrated squared error* (AMISE) of the estimate, defined as the limit of the expected value of

$$\int \left[\tilde{\lambda}(s) - \lambda(s)\right]^2 ds$$

as the sample size (number of events) goes to infinity. Wand and Jones (1995) offer a detailed description of bandwidth selection methods based on AMISE. For our purposes, Scott (1992, p. 152) offers an easy-to-remember data-based bandwidth selection rule for Gaussian product kernels in dimensional space, based on the components of an expansion of the AMISE. The estimated bandwidth for the component of the product kernel associated with the u-coordinate is

$$\widehat{b}_u = \widehat{\sigma}_u N^{-1/(\text{dim}+4)} \tag{5.3}$$

where $\widehat{\sigma}_u$ is the sample standard deviation of the u-coordinates, N represents the number of events in the data set (the sample size), and "dim" denotes the dimension of the study area. We define $\widehat{b}_v$ (the bandwidth for the v-coordinate component of the product kernel) in a similar manner, replacing $\widehat{\sigma}_u$ with $\widehat{\sigma}_v$.

We illustrate the kernel estimation approach in the following example.

DATA BREAK: Early Medieval Grave Sites Alt and Vach (1991) describe an archaeological investigation of an early medieval burial ground in Neresheim, Baden-Württemberg, Germany. The anthropologists and archaeologists involved wonder if this particular culture tended to place grave sites according to family units. To investigate this hypothesis, the archaeologists consider 152 grave sites and use inherited features in the teeth of excavated skeletons (namely, missing or reduced wisdom teeth) to mark a subset of 31 grave sites. For illustrative purposes, we consider a subset of 143 of these 152 grave sites, which includes 30 of the original 31 affected sites. The research question is whether the spatial pattern of the 30 graves with affected teeth (graves of "affected individuals") differs from the pattern of the 113 nonaffected graves. How could estimates of the intensity functions for the affected and nonaffected grave sites, respectively, help answer this question?

Figure 5.8 illustrates the locations of affected and nonaffected grave sites, revealing several interesting features. First, we note that the locations occur in an irregularly shaped region within the figure, perhaps because of local topographic features. Second, we suspect heterogeneity in the intensity, as some areas seem to have a higher concentration of events than others (regardless of their affected/nonaffected status).

For an initial exploration of the data, we assume that the collections of affected and nonaffected grave site locations follow heterogeneous Poisson processes with unknown intensity functions $\lambda_1(s)$ and $\lambda_0(s)$, respectively (e.g., the early medieval

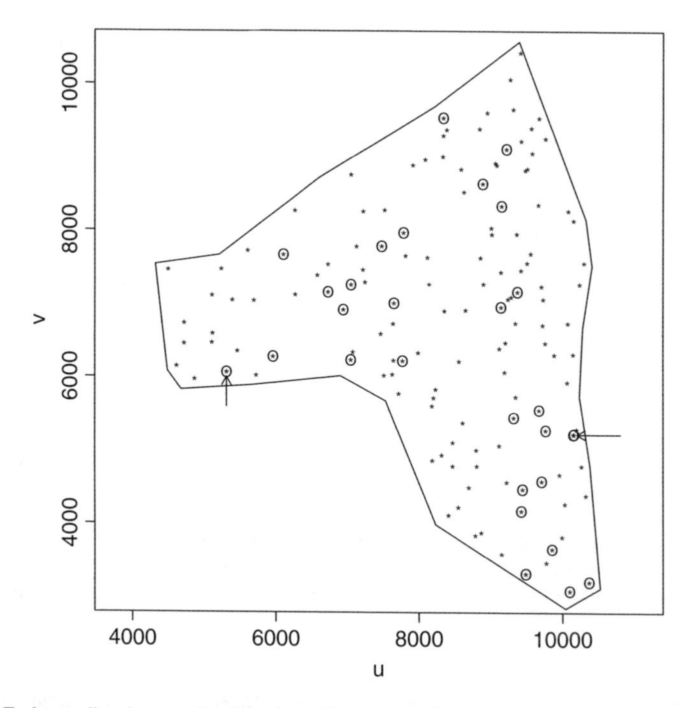

FIG. 5.8 Early medieval grave site locations. Circled locations denote those grave sites where the person shows evidence of a particular tooth defect ("affected individuals"). The polygon surrounding the points represents the edge of the study area. Arrows indicate two locations, each containing two grave sites occurring at such small distances that visual distinction of event locations is difficult at the scale of the figure. The question of interest: Do the burial sites of affected individuals tend to cluster?

culture chose grave sites at random in this general area, with the likelihood of choosing any particular location dependent on smoothly varying spatial features such as soil type and vegetation). At this stage, for simplicity, we assume independence between the two processes. Figures 5.9 and 5.10 illustrate kernel density estimates (proportional to the intensity functions) for affected and nonaffected sites, respectively, using Gaussian product kernels. Recall that *density functions* differ from *intensity functions* only by a multiplicative constant, so the two functions exhibit the same spatial pattern, but the numerical value (height) of the functions depend on a multiplicative constant corresponding to the integral of the intensity function over the study area.

Scott's rule suggests bandwidths $\widehat{b_u} = 872.24$ in the u direction and $\widehat{b_v} = 997.45$ in the v direction for the affected sites, and bandwidths $\widehat{b_u} = 695.35$ and $\widehat{b_v} = 734.82$ for the nonaffected sites. The bandwidths are fairly comparable between the two point patterns, with slightly smaller bandwidths for the nonaffected sites, due primarily to the slightly larger sample size. The resulting intensity function estimates suggest some local differences in the two spatial patterns. Both patterns imply two modes (areas of highest intensity of grave sites), but the modes appear in slightly different places. As an exploratory tool, our density estimates lend some

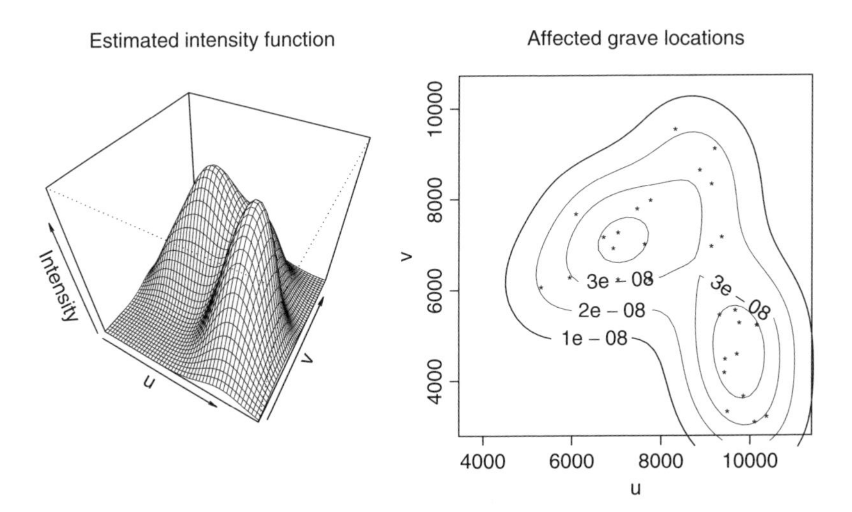

FIG. 5.9 Kernel smoothed density estimate (proportional to the intensity function) for affected locations (grave sites with tooth defect) in an early medieval grave site data set. Bandwidth set to 872.24 in the u direction and 997.45 in the v direction based on Scott's rule [equation (5.3)] for Gaussian kernels (see text).

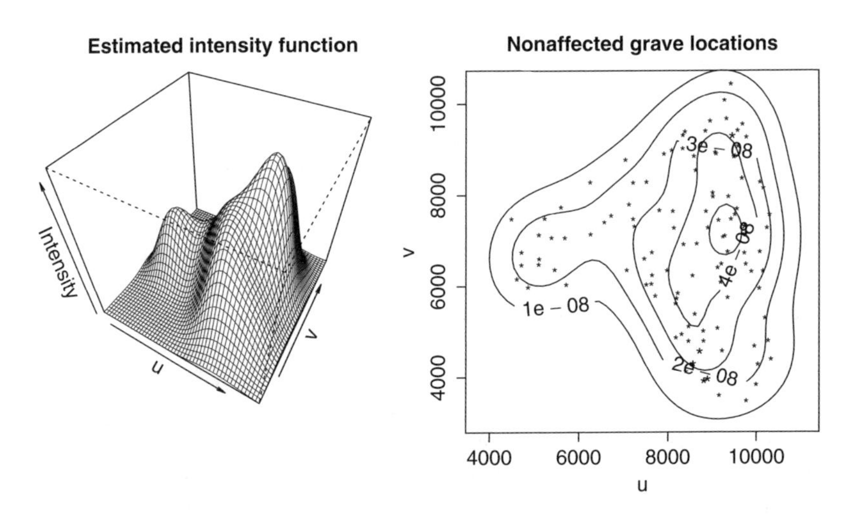

FIG. 5.10 Kernel smoothed spatial density estimate (proportional to the intensity function) for nonaffected locations (grave sites without tooth defect) in early medieval grave site data set. Bandwidth set to 695.35 in the u direction and 734.82 in the v direction based on Scott's rule [equation (5.3)] for Gaussian kernels (see text).

credence to the suspected different burial patterns; however, the estimates do not yet provide any notion of the "statistical significance" of any observed differences between the patterns. We outline more formal comparisons between these patterns in Section 5.3.3.

5.3 *K* FUNCTION

In addition to the intensity function's description of the spatial pattern of the expected number of events per unit area, we may also be interested in how often events occur within a given distance of other events. Where an intensity function informs on the mean, or *first-order, properties* of a point process, the relative position of events informs on the interrelationship between events, or *second-order properties* (similar to variance and covariance) of the process. Bartlett (1964) introduced the notion of second-order properties of spatial point processes, while Ripley (1976, 1977), expanded on these ideas and provided estimation techniques and examples for applying second-order analyses to observed data sets. We base much of our development on Diggle (1983, pp. 47–48), which provides a readable introduction to first- and second-order properties of spatial point processes.

Second-order properties of spatial point processes allow the analyst to summarize spatial dependence between events over a wide range of possible spatial scales. The most common form of second-order analysis for spatial point process is termed the *K function* or *reduced second moment measure* (Ripley 1977; Diggle 1983), defined as

$$K(h) = \frac{E[\text{number of events within } h \text{ of a } \textit{randomly} \text{ chosen event}]}{\lambda} \tag{5.4}$$

for any positive distance (or *spatial lag*) h. One does not include the randomly chosen event in the number of events within distance h, so some definitions specify "the number of additional events." Equation (5.4) assumes stationarity and isotropy through the constant intensity λ and by taking the expectation across all events in the study area (which assumes a process operating identically at all locations). Analogs of the K function exist for nonstationary (Baddeley et al. 1999) or anisotropic (Stoyan et al. 1995, pp. 125–132, 134–135) processes, but we focus our attention on the isotropic and stationary version. Even for a nonhomogeneous Poisson process, the stationary K function defined in equation (5.4) can provide valuable information as outlined below.

Ripley (1977) shows that specifying $K(h)$ for all h is equivalent to specifying $\text{Var}(N(A))$ (the variance of the number of events occurring in subregion A), for any subregion A of the study region. In this sense, $K(\cdot)$ is associated with the second moment of the process and is indeed a second-order property of the underlying spatial point process. The popularity of the K function lies primarily in its ease of estimation compared to other second-order measures.

Intuitively, the definition of the K function (the average number of events within distance h of a randomly chosen event divided by the average number of events per unit area) implies that under CSR, the value of $K(h)$ is πh^2 (the area of a circle of radius h). For processes more regular than CSR, we would expect fewer events within distance h of a randomly chosen event than under CSR, so $K(h)$ would tend to be less than πh^2. Conversely, for processes more clustered than CSR, we would expect more events within a given distance than under CSR, or $K(h) > \pi h^2$.

5.3.1 Estimating the K Function

Estimation of the K function proceeds by replacing the expectation in its definition [equation (5.4)] with a sample average. Initially, this suggests that

$$\widehat{K}(h) = \widehat{\lambda}^{-1} \frac{1}{N} \sum_{i=1}^{N} \sum_{\substack{j=1 \\ j \neq i}}^{N} \delta(d(i, j) < h) \tag{5.5}$$

for a realization of N events, where $d(i, j)$ denotes the Euclidean distance between events i and j, and $\delta(d(i, j) < h)$ equals 1 if $d(i, j) < h$ and 0 otherwise. Note that the assumed stationarity and homogeneity of the process allows us to replace λ in equation (5.4) with the estimate $\widehat{\lambda} =$ (number of events in $A/|A|$), where A is the study area and $|A|$ denotes the area of A.

The estimator in equation (5.5) is not entirely satisfactory when one considers events near the boundaries of the study area. For h larger than the distance of a particular event to the nearest boundary, the count of events within distance h of other events provided by $\sum_i \sum_{j \neq i}^{N} \delta(d(i, j) < h)$ would not include events occurring just outside the boundary but nevertheless within distance h of an event in the data set. The potential undercount becomes more of an issue as the distance h increases. One solution for closed study areas (i.e., ones having no "holes" where events could occur but are not observed) is to collect event locations from the entire study area plus an additional "guard area" of width h^* around the boundary and only calculate $\widehat{K}(h)$ for $h \leq h^*$. Another approach, proposed by Ripley (1976), uses a weighted version of equation (5.5), namely

$$\widehat{K}_{\text{ec}}(h) = \widehat{\lambda}^{-1} \sum_{i=1}^{N} \sum_{\substack{j=1 \\ j \neq i}}^{N} w_{ij} \delta(d(i, j) < h) \tag{5.6}$$

where "ec" denotes "edge corrected" and w_{ij} is a weight defined as the proportion of the circumference of the circle centered at event i with radius $d(i, j)$ which lies within the study area. Note that $w_{ij} = 1$ if the distance between events i and j is less than the distance between event i and the boundary of the study area. Also note that w_{ij} need not equal w_{ji} and that equation (5.6) is applicable even if the study area is not closed (i.e., has "holes"). Conceptually, w_{ij} denotes the conditional probability of an event occurring a distance $d(i, j)$ from event i falling within the study area, given the location of event i (and again assuming a homogeneous process). Most software packages providing estimates of the K function use equation (5.6) or some variant thereof. Since the edge correction in equation (5.6) depends on the definition of the study area's borders, w_{ij} is most easily calculated for rectangular or circular study areas. Other edge correction strategies appear in Ripley (1988) and Stoyan et al. (1995).

5.3.2 Diagnostic Plots Based on the K Function

Under CSR, $K(h) = \pi h^2$, a parabola. Plotting an estimate of $K(h)$ versus h requires one to visually assess deviation from a curve. Besag (1977) suggested a transformation allowing comparison of an estimated K function to a straight line, an easier visual task. Specifically, since $K(h) = \pi h^2$ implies that

$$\left(\frac{K(h)}{\pi}\right)^{1/2} = h,$$

plotting

$$h \text{ versus } \left[\frac{\widehat{K}_{ec}(h)}{\pi}\right]^{1/2} - h$$

provides a useful diagnostic plot. If we define $\widehat{L}(h) = [\widehat{K}_{ec}(h)/\pi]^{1/2}$, then (under CSR) the expected value of $\widehat{L}(h) - h$ is zero. Hence, deviations from the horizontal line $\widehat{L}(h) - h = 0$ provide evidence of departures from CSR. Deviations above the zero line suggest clustering (more events within distance h than expected), while deviations below zero suggest regularity (fewer events within distance h than expected). We refer to such a plot as an $\widehat{L}$ *plot*. To add to the diagnostic ability of the $\widehat{L}$ plot we need a method to illustrate the random error associated with estimating the K function from a finite realization of the underlying spatial process. Although some asymptotic properties of estimates of the K function exist, most depend on circular study areas or hold only for a fixed, predefined distance (Cressie 1993, p. 642; Stoyan et al. 1995, pp. 50–51). Thus, for general inference regarding K functions we again turn to Monte Carlo methods as introduced in Section 5.2.3.

5.3.3 Monte Carlo Assessments of CSR Based on the *K* Function

We begin (as with any Monte Carlo test of CSR) by generating many simulations of CSR and estimating the K function for each realization. Since we are interested in the behavior of the estimated K function across a range of distances, and since each simulation provides an estimated *function* (rather than a single test statistic value), we construct *envelopes* or *bands* around the value expected under the null hypothesis. Many applications plot the upper and lower envelopes based on the lines connecting the minimum and maximum $\widehat{L}(h) - h$ values obtained at a collection of distances h for many simulations. If one can afford a large number of simulations, it may be more interesting to compute envelopes defining certain percentiles (e.g., the 5th and 95th percentiles) in addition to those defining the minima and maxima. Such percentiles offer diagnostic suggestions of spatial scales (distances) at which observed patterns appear to differ from the null hypothesis (see the data break below for an example) but do not provide formal statistical inference in the form of a test statistic.

If we are interested in hypothesis tests, we may conduct a Monte Carlo test (as described in Section 5.2.3) with test statistic $T = \widehat{L}(h) - h$ for a value of h specified prior to analysis, or consider a test for deviations of $\widehat{L}(h) - h$ from its null value over a range $0 \leq h \leq h_{\max}$, where one specifies $h_{\max}$ a priori (e.g., $h_{\max} =$

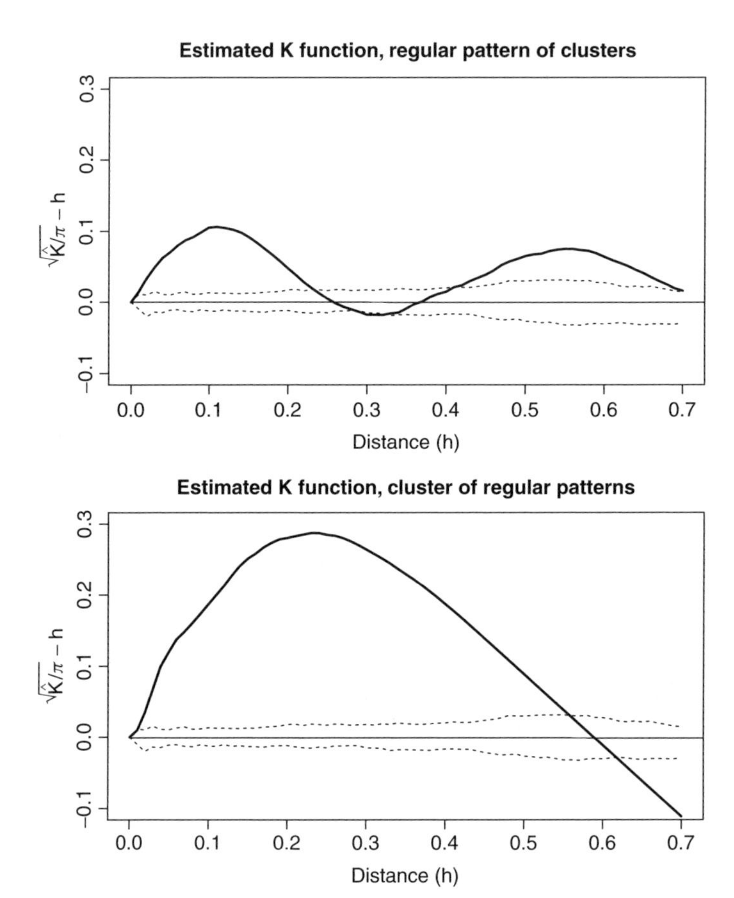

FIG. 5.11 $\widehat{L}$ plots for the regular pattern of clusters (top) and the cluster of regular patterns (bottom) from Figure 5.3. Dashed lines represent the maxima and minima of $\widehat{L}(h) - h$ at each distance h, based on 500 simulations of complete spatial randomness.

one-half the maximum observed interevent distance). Stoyan et al. (1995, p. 51) describe an example of the latter with test statistic

$$T = \max_{0 \le h \le h_{\max}} \left| \widehat{L}(h) - h \right|.$$

(Again, see the data break below for an example.) One could conduct similar tests for any predefined interval of interest.

Since second-order properties offer a way to distinguish among CSR, clustered, and regular processes at different distances, the $\widehat{L}$ plots described above offer insight into the question of different tendencies at different spatial scales raised by the example given in Figure 5.3. The top figure in Figure 5.11 shows $\widehat{L}$ plots for the example of a regular pattern of clusters, while the bottom figure shows the same plot for the example of a cluster of regular patterns.

Figure 5.11 also shows minimum–maximum Monte Carlo envelopes based on 500 simulations for each point process. For this example, each simulation consists of the same number of events (100) as shown in Figure 5.3, but distributed uniformly across the unit square. For the regular pattern of clusters we see the plotted values above the K functions based on the simulated patterns (indicating clustering) for distances below $h = 0.2$ and again for $h \in (0.4, 0.7)$. The "bumps" indicate more pairs of events observed at these distances than one would expect under CSR. The first bump corresponds to pairs of events within a single cluster; the second (slightly wider) bump corresponds to pairs of events from different clusters. The second bump is slightly wider than the first, corresponding to the variation in distance between pairs of clusters. In this case, the $\widehat{L}$ function provides some insight into the spatial scale of clustering for the process. Overall, the $\widehat{L}$ plot suggests a pattern with several tight, distinct clusters, with regularity between clusters.

The $\widehat{L}$ plot for the cluster of regular patterns (bottom plot in Figure 5.11) captures the cluster clearly but does not clearly identify the regular pattern. The regular pattern occurs only at the very smallest observed distances, and our regular patterns overlap, thereby generating pairs of points (from different regular patterns) at distances smaller than the interevent distance in a single regular pattern. Hence, the regularity is not captured in the $\widehat{L}$ function.

DATA BREAK: Early Medieval Grave Sites (*cont.*) Recall the medieval grave site data illustrated in Figure 5.8. Previously, we considered first-order summaries of the patterns observed. Here we continue our analysis by considering second-order properties of the set of all locations, the set of affected locations, and the set of nonaffected locations. Figure 5.12 illustrates the $\widehat{L}$ plots (based on $\widehat{K}_{ec}$) for each of the collections of events. The dashed lines represent the simulation envelopes (minimum and maximum values at each distance) based on 500 simulations of CSR in the region defined by a rectangle bounding the minimum and maximum u and v values. All three show clear departures from CSR, suggesting clustering for most distance values, first departing the tolerance envelopes at distances near 400 units. Unlike the intensity estimates in Figures 5.9 and 5.10, the K functions do not suggest *where* clusters occur, but rather, at what distances events tend to occur from other events with respect to distances expected under CSR.

Closer examination reveals several features of Monte Carlo analysis, allowing more specific inference. First, in our simulations of CSR, the total number of events varies according to Poisson distributions with means defined by the numbers of grave sites observed, grave sites affected, and grave sites nonaffected, respectively. Does it make sense to allow the total number of events to vary in our application? Assuming a thorough archaeological survey, we should not expect any more grave sites within the study area. Perhaps we should restrict our inference to the observed number of grave sites within each category. In that case, we seek an answer to more specific questions, moving from "Do the grave sites follow CSR?" to "Do the observed 143 (or 30 or 113) grave sites appear to be uniformly distributed in space?" That is, we are investigating patterns of a fixed number of grave sites to see if their locations appear to be distributed randomly.

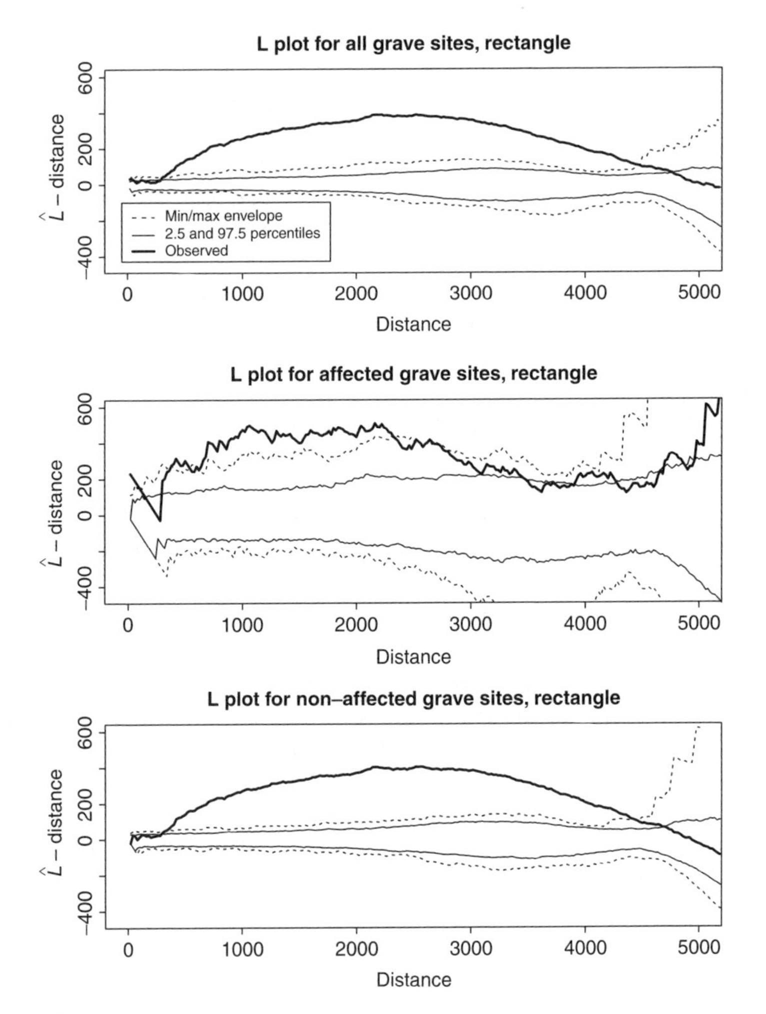

FIG. 5.12 $\widehat{L}$ plots for the early medieval grave site data shown in Figure 5.8. The dashed lines represent the upper and lower simulation envelopes based on 500 simulations of CSR. The thin solid lines represent the upper 97.5th and lower 2.5th percentiles of simulated $\widehat{L}(h)$ values at each distance h. Here simulations place events throughout the rectangular area defined by the minimum and maximum coordinates observed for both the u and v directions.

Second, does CSR on a rectangle offer a sensible null hypothesis? The event locations clearly occur within an irregularly shaped, nonconvex polygon contained within the rectangular boundary of Figure 5.8, while CSR over a rectangle can (and does) assign grave sites uniformly throughout the rectangle (including locations outside the irregular polygon). The clustering suggested by Figure 5.12 may be due entirely to the occurrence of events *within the enclosing polygon.*

Some refinement of our simulations addresses both concerns. Suppose that we fix the number of events in each simulation to the number observed and then simulate

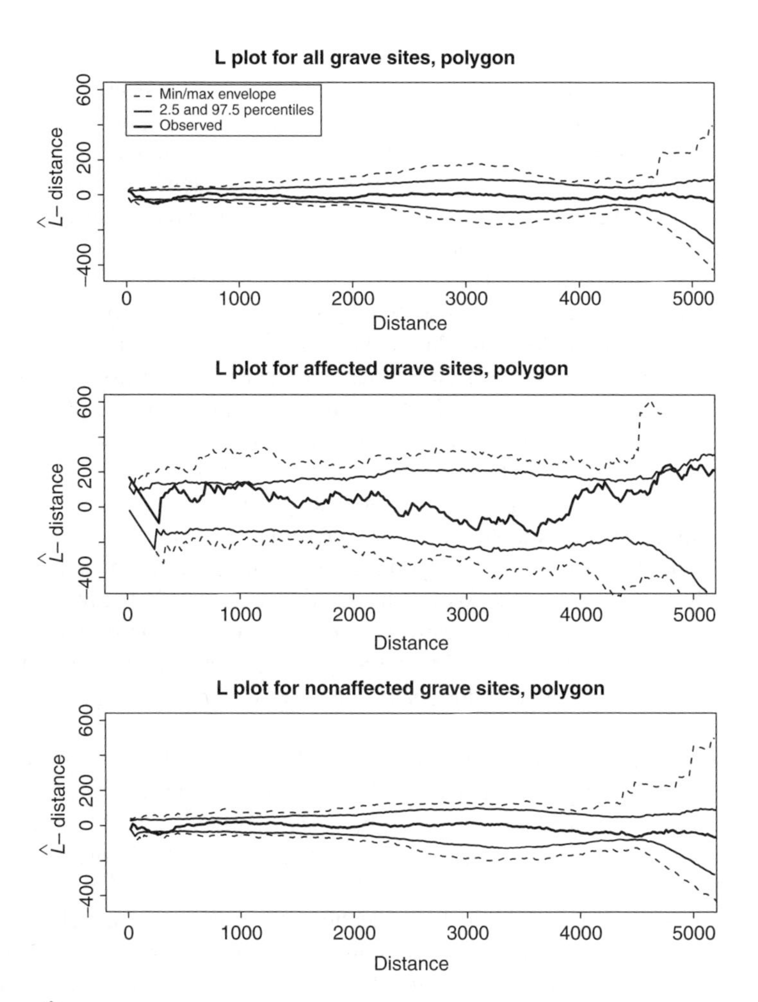

FIG. 5.13 $\widehat{L}$ plots for the early medieval grave site data shown in Figure 5.8 based on edge-corrected estimates of the K function. The dashed lines represent the upper and lower simulation envelopes based on 500 simulations of CSR *within the bounding polygon* shown in Figure 5.8. The thin solid lines represent the upper 97.5th and lower 2.5th percentiles of simulated $\widehat{L}(h)$ values at each distance h. Compare to Figure 5.12.

CSR *within a polygon* containing the locations observed. Figure 5.13 illustrates the $\widehat{L}$ plots when we limit inference to the polygon surrounding the collection of all grave site locations. Note the "noisier" point estimate of $\widehat{L} - h$ and associated wider simulation envelopes for the set of affected sites, due to the much smaller sample size (31) compared to the other two plots (sample sizes of 143 and 113, respectively). Fixing the number of events within each simulation serves to narrow the simulation envelopes over what would be observed with a Poisson number of grave sites in each simulation. Limiting comparisons to events within the polygon serves to remove the suggestion of clustering observed in Figure 5.12. The revised

$\widehat{L}$ plots exceed the 95% simulation envelopes only for the shortest distances in the affected sites, probably due to the two locations indicated in Figure 5.8 with two affected graves occurring very close together. By refining our simulations we refined the question under investigation from "Are grave sites clustered within a square?" to the more appropriate "Are grave sites clustered within the study area?".

Figures 5.8, 5.9, and 5.13 provide comparisons of the spatial patterns (summarized through estimated intensities and K functions) between the set of affected sites and CSR, and between the set of nonaffected sites and CSR. Such comparisons allow us to compare patterns in the affected and nonaffected sites only through their respective comparisons to CSR. We next consider using K functions to compare directly the patterns of affected and nonaffected sites (i.e., to assess whether the spatial pattern of affected sites is similar to the spatial pattern of nonaffected sites).

Suppose we assume that the set of all grave sites is fixed and we are interested in the patterns of the 30 affected graves *among these 143 sites*. A non-CSR but equally valid model of "no pattern" is that each grave site is equally likely to be an affected grave. This is known as the *random labeling hypothesis*, which differs slightly from the constant risk hypothesis of Section 5.2.4. The random labeling hypothesis always conditions on the set of locations of all events observed, whereas the constant risk hypothesis may or may not condition on the total number, depending in part whether the overall risk of disease is estimated from the data or known with some certainty based on other information (e.g., the scientific literature), respectively.

The random labeling hypothesis, introduced by Diggle (1983, p. 93), offers one approach for assessing the pattern of affected graves within the set of all graves. Failure to reject the random labeling hypothesis suggests similarity in the underlying processes, but rejection of the random labeling hypothesis suggests that the set of affected graves appear to be selected from the set of all graves via some mechanism other than simple random selection. As noted by Diggle (1983, p. 93), random labeling neither implies nor is implied by the stricter notion of statistical independence between the pattern of affected sites and that of nonaffected sites. Independence and random labeling are only equivalent when both point patterns follow homogeneous Poisson processes. Further discussion contrasting independence and random labeling and associated tests appears in Diggle (1983, Sections 6.2, 6.3, 7.2.2, and 7.2.3).

In our example, the random labeling hypothesis offers a reasonable formulation of our question of interest: Do the affected graves appear to follow the same K function as the nonaffected? To test the random labeling hypothesis, we condition on the set of all grave site locations, using the same 143 locations in all simulations, with the Monte Carlo step drawing a sample of 30 locations from the set of 143 observed locations (randomly without replacement), and calculating the corresponding K function for the 30 sampled locations. Under the random labeling hypothesis, the 30 sampled locations reflect a random "thinning" of the set of all locations. The theoretical K function of the thinned process is identical to that of the process generating the entire set of 143 locations, but (naturally) we observe some variability in $\widehat{K}_{ec}(h)$ between random samples, due to estimation based on finite samples.

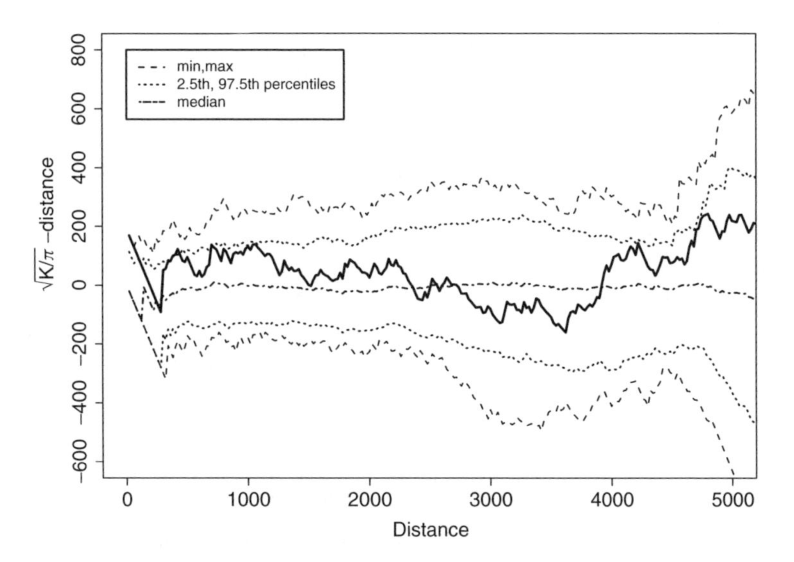

FIG. 5.14 $\widehat{L}$ plot for the early medieval grave site data shown in Figure 5.8, compared to a random labeling hypothesis (see text). The solid line illustrates $\widehat{L}(h) - h$ for the case data (comparable to the middle plot of Figure 5.13). The dashed, dotted, and dash-dotted "envelopes" represent the minimum, maximum, 2.5th percentile, 97.5th percentile, and median values, respectively, based on 499 random samples of 30 sites each from the set of 143 sites.

Figure 5.14 shows the $\widehat{L}$ plot for the observed data (dark solid line), the minima/maxima-based envelopes (dashed lines), the 2.5th and 97.5th percentile-based envelopes (dotted lines), and the median value (dot-dashed line) based on 499 random labelings. The observed values lie mostly within the envelopes, wandering beyond only for the very smallest distances (as in the $\widehat{L}$ plot for the affected sites in Figure 5.13), reflecting the two pairs of grave sites at very small distances of one another (possibly multiple graves), and for one other very short interval.

To determine statistical significance of any clustering, we consider the Monte Carlo test defined above using the test statistic

$$T = \max_{0 \leq h \leq h_{\max}} \left(\widehat{L}(h) - h \right).$$

This test is attractive since it investigates deviations over a range of distances from zero to $h_{\max}$, a distance we define. Technically, we must define $h_{\max}$ a priori, prior to our analysis of the data. Specifically, for our hypothesis-testing assumptions to hold, we must define $h_{\max}$ based on it being a distance of interest for the problem at hand rather than as the most suggestive distance shown in Figure 5.14. If we select $h_{\max} = 2000$, then based on 499 simulations, we obtain a Monte Carlo p-value of 0.453, suggesting little statistical evidence for clustering beyond that expected under a random labeling hypothesis for distances between 0 and 2000.

Reviewing our analysis of the grave site data, the $\widehat{L}$ plots suggest that the pattern of 113 nonaffected grave sites observed does not differ appreciably from a random allocation of locations within our study polygon. The pattern of affected sites observed is also fairly consistent with a random selection of sites within the polygon except for a suggestion of clustering at the smallest distances. Comparison of the estimated second-order properties with those arising under the random labeling hypothesis also gives little reason to suspect a more clustered site selection process for the affected sites than for the nonaffected sites, where again the only suggestion of clustering occurs at very short distances. If we rerun the analyses generating Figures 5.13 and 5.14 omitting one of each pair of the locations circled in Figure 5.8, all suggestion of clustering (at any distance) disappears. In summary, our second-order analysis of the grave site data suggests a largely homogeneous site selection process across the study area for the culture under study, with the exception of two locations containing pairs of graves in very close proximity, both of which are affected grave sites.

5.3.4 Roles of First- and Second-Order Properties

First-order (intensity function) and second-order (K function) analysis provide different but complementary insight into the analysis of spatial point patterns. In our medieval grave site example, our second-order (K function) analysis of the medieval grave site data provides insight into *global* aspects of the point pattern (are there general patterns of clustering and/or regularity with respect to CSR or another pattern?), whereas first-order properties (intensity functions) provide *local* insight (where do the patterns appear to differ?). Although we did not make explicit inferential comparisons here of the intensity functions we explore this issue (and the distinction between local and global properties of spatial point patterns) with special emphasis in Chapters 6 and 7.

The examples in this chapter show that the estimated intensity (first-order property) and K function (second-order property) provide insight into the process underlying observed point patterns. We next consider whether the first- and second-order properties *uniquely* define a spatial point process. Baddeley and Silverman (1984) indicate that this is not the case and provide an interesting counterexample illustrating two very different spatial point processes defined on the unit square with identical intensity and K functions. The two processes are a homogeneous Poisson process (CSR) with intensity function $\lambda = 1$ and the point process defined by the following:

1. Divide the plane into unit squares by random placement of a square grid.
2. In each unit square, place N_s events uniformly and independently, where N_s comes from the distribution

$$\Pr[N_s = 0] = \frac{1}{10}$$

$$\Pr[N_s = 1] = \frac{8}{9}$$

$$\Pr[N_s = 10] = \frac{1}{90}.$$

3. A realization consists of only the set of events (i.e., the grid cell boundaries are not observed).

In the second process, most cells have exactly one event. Some cells are empty. Very rarely (1/90 of the time) we observe a cluster of 10 events. For a study area A with $|A|$ close to 1 square unit, we generally observe very few events per realization, with rare exceptions. For study areas closer to 100 square units in size, we tend to observe one cluster of 10 events, while the other events tend to be more regularly distributed than we would expect under CSR. The equality of intensities is readily apparent, since for the second process,

$$\lambda|A| = [0(1/10) + 1(8/9) + 10(1/90)]|A| = |A| = \lambda_{\text{CSR}}|A|.$$

Baddeley and Silverman (1984) provide proof of equality of the associated theoretical K functions, based on equality of $\text{Var}(N(A))$ between the two processes for any area A (recall that this is equivalent to showing equality between the processes' respective K functions).

In summary, just as first and second moments provide some information about possible probability distributions driving observations of a univariate random variable but do not identify the particular distribution uniquely, the estimated first- and second-order properties of an observed spatial point pattern provide valuable but only partial insight into possible underlying probabilistic mechanisms.

5.4 OTHER SPATIAL POINT PROCESSES

The homogeneous and heterogeneous Poisson processes introduced in Section 5.2 play a key role in the development of statistical methods for the analysis of chronic disease data and form the basis for many of the methods outlined in Chapters 6 and 7. However, such models allow clustering only through inhomogeneities in the intensity function. Clusters could also arise through processes such as randomly located cluster centers, each emitting mutually independent but still clustered events, or through interactions between events (e.g., through some sort of contagion process), although applications of such models to the analysis of public health data are currently rare. A variety of other spatial point process models exist and provide alternative approaches for the analysis of observed spatial point patterns. An appreciation of the underlying structure of each set of models, and determination of the appropriateness of a given model for a particular application, drives the choice of the appropriate family of models. We provide brief overviews of three general model classes here and defer the reader to Diggle (1983), Cressie (1993), and Stoyan et al. (1995) for more complete definitions, examples, and relevant references.

5.4.1 Poisson Cluster Processes

The *Poisson cluster process* defines a spatial point process wherein each event belongs to a particular cluster. Specifically, the process consists of a set of *parent locations* each of which generates a set of *child locations*. The parent locations are not observed and the realization of the Poisson cluster process consists of the locations of the children only. Typically, the parent locations follow a Poisson spatial point process (either homogeneous or heterogeneous), the number of children per parent follows a discrete probability distribution (typically Poisson), and the child locations follow a spatial probability density function, generally peaked at the associated parent location, and decaying with distance from the parent (e.g., a bivariate Gaussian density centered at the parent location) (Cressie 1993, p. 662). Conceptually, think of a set of trees in a forest where seeds are most likely to fall near the parent tree but (less often) may be carried some distance away by wind or animals. Again, a realization of a Poisson cluster process consists only of the children's locations, and does not include the parents.

The family of Poisson cluster processes grew from models described in Neyman (1939) and Neyman and Scott (1958), with the latter defining a particular class of Poisson cluster processes where (1) the parent locations follow a homogeneous or heterogeneous Poisson process, (2) the numbers of children per parent are independent and identically distributed according to the same probability distribution for each parent, and (3) the locations of children around their respective parent are independent and identically distributed according to the same bivariate probability density for each parent. The restriction to identical distributions for both the number and the location of child events with respect to their parent event provides enough replication to yield some underlying theoretical properties, and the literature refers to such processes as *Neyman–Scott processes*. Briefly, a Neyman–Scott process is stationary and isotropic if the parent process is stationary and the child-dispersal distribution is isotropic. Diggle (1983, p. 55) and Cressie (1993, pp. 664–666) illustrate that the theoretical K function for stationary and isotropic Neyman–Scott processes is equal to the K function for CSR plus a strictly positive term based on the distribution of the number of children per parent and the spatial distribution of children around parents (i.e., the K function for the Poisson cluster process exceeds that for CSR, indicating clustering).

The definition of a Poisson cluster process above provides an algorithmic recipe for simulating realizations. Edge effects can play a key role in such simulations, particularly regarding observations of children for parents located outside the study area. One pragmatic solution involves either generation of parents and children in a much larger area encompassing the study area and observing children only within the study area. Another, applicable only to rectangular study areas, involves a *toroidal correction* wherein one assigns child locations generated, say, d units outside the study area to occur d units inside the opposite side of the study area (where the top and bottom of the rectangle are "opposite" sides, as are the right and left sides of the rectangle). This approach effectively simulates locations on a torus where the top of the study area connects to the bottom, and the right edge connects to the left edge.

Finally, one could extend the notion of a Poisson cluster process to multiple generations (children generating children). Although conceptually easy to implement via simulation, such processes quickly become mathematically intractable and do not appear extensively in the literature.

5.4.2 Contagion/Inhibition Processes

Other spatial point processes focus on the direct modeling of interevent interactions such as contagion or inhibition wherein the occurrence of an event raises or lowers (respectively) the probability of observing subsequent events nearby. Contagion models are particularly appropriate for modeling the spread of infectious diseases, while inhibition models address applications wherein each event precludes the occurrence of other events in a nearby area (e.g., the territory of an animal or the volume of a cell).

Inhibition and contagion provide a wide realm of possibilities for spatial modeling. Inhibition may be absolute (i.e., there may be a "hard core" radius around each event within which no other events may occur) or may simply result from a reduced (but still positive) probability of nearby events. A wide variety of models for inhibition and/or contagion exist (e.g., Markov point processes and Gibbs processes), where we define *contagion* rather loosely to refer to the increased likelihood of events near other events. Many such models involve specification of the local interaction between events via some functional relationship, such as a pair-potential function (Stoyan et al. 1995, p. 169). In addition, one may specify such functions in a manner resulting in regularity at some spatial scales and clustering at others, thereby addressing the issue raised in Figure 5.3 in a more substantial manner. The definition and estimation of spatial interaction functions, and the simulation of such processes, are beyond the scope of this book and we refer the interested reader to Diggle (1983, pp. 63–66), Cressie (1993, Sections 8.5.4 and 8.5.5), Stoyan et al. (1995, Chapter 5), van Lieshout (2000), and the references therein for details.

5.4.3 Cox Processes

We next contrast the specific models of spatial clusters in Sections 5.4.1 and 5.4.2 with the clustering observed among independent events generated by a spatially varying intensity function of the heterogeneous Poisson processes of Section 5.2.4. In our public health applications to chronic disease data, we typically think of events as independent of one another, but we consider the intensity function $\lambda(\boldsymbol{s})$ to reflect some sort of environmental heterogeneity in disease occurrence (e.g., due to a heterogeneous population at risk or a heterogeneous risk of disease based on some environmental factors). In some applications we may wish to consider this heterogeneity a random factor that changes from year to year (e.g., due to population mobility or to variation in environmental exposures). In such a case we could consider the intensity function $\lambda(\boldsymbol{s})$ as a random quantity drawn from some probability distribution of possible intensity functions over our study area. Such processes are referred to as *Cox processes* based on their development in one dimension by Cox (1955) and are said to be *doubly stochastic* (i.e., the random location of events depends on a random process itself).

Perhaps the simplest example of a Cox process is an extension of CSR where we assume the intensity λ (a constant) follows some probability distribution. Such a model would be appropriate if we assume a uniform distribution of events in the study area but allow the expected total number of events ($E[N(D)]$) to vary from realization to realization. One could generalize such a model to a heterogeneous Poisson process where the allowable intensity surfaces are proportional to one another (hence each is proportional to the same probability density in space) but again, the expected total number of observed events can vary between realizations.

Lawson (2001, Chapter 11) considers a general class of heterogeneous Poisson process models for infectious disease modeling. The intensity function consists of a product of spatial clustering functions (as in the Poisson cluster processes above) and temporal clustering functions. Such functions typically involve parameters that may be assigned by the analyst (yielding a heterogeneous Poisson process) or estimated from the data (resulting in a Cox process approach).

The Cox process offers a very broad class of models. Recently, Møller et al. (1998) defined the subclass of *log Gaussian Cox processes* as a parameterization allowing fairly complex spatial modeling of the intensity function based on covariates and spatial correlation, in a manner utilizing many of the structures considered in this book in Chapters 7 and 8. Computational implementation is still rather intricate [see Møller et al. (1998) and Brix and Diggle (2001) for examples], but the very general modeling structure in such models offers much promise for more advanced applications.

5.4.4 Distinguishing Processes

Distinguishing between possible underlying processes based on observed data can be problematic. For instance, based on a single realization, there is no mathematical way to distinguish between a process of independent events generated under a heterogeneous intensity and a process of dependent events generated under a homogeneous intensity. With replicate realizations, one may be able to distinguish the patterns since realizations with a heterogeneous (but fixed) intensity will tend to have concentrations of events in the same locations in each realization (see Figure 5.6), while realizations of dependent observations would tend to have concentrations of events in different locations in each realization.

If we allow the heterogeneity itself to be random (moving from a heterogeneous Poisson process to a Cox process), the mathematical boundaries between processes become murkier and in some cases vanish entirely. Bartlett (1964) formally established the mathematical equivalence between Neyman–Scott processes with Poisson numbers of children per parent and Cox processes. That is, for any Neyman–Scott process with a Poisson number of children, one can derive an equivalent Cox process. To gain intuition for Bartlett's equivalence, consider any fixed set of parent locations and define a heterogeneous intensity function consistent with the child dispersal process (i.e., with a mode over each parent and a distance decay matching the probability of observing a child event around that parent). Next, assign an appropriate probability to each intensity, corresponding to a possible set of parent locations. This defines a Cox process equivalent to the Neyman–Scott process under consideration [see Cressie (1993, pp. 663–664) for a more formal argument]. We note that the results establish an equivalent Cox process for any Neyman–Scott process (with Poisson numbers of children), but the reverse does not hold, as the class of Cox processes is much larger than those equivalent to Neyman–Scott processes. For example, consider the simple Cox process based on CSR with a variable intensity λ. No realization of this process involves clustering consistent with a Neyman–Scott process (unless one considers a degenerate uniform child-dispersal distribution). Finally, although the conceptual description of Bartlett's equivalence above might suggest that any Poisson cluster process yields an equivalent Cox processes, formalizing the argument mathematically requires precise definitions of valid probability structures, and Cressie (1993, p. 664) points out that the general result remains unproven.

5.5 ADDITIONAL TOPICS AND FURTHER READING

In this chapter we provide only a brief introduction to spatial point processes and their first- and second-order properties. The methods outlined above provide the probabilistic tools to develop the analytic methods in Chapters 6 and 7 for investigating spatial patterns of disease. Many of the applications in Chapters 6 and 7 build from heterogeneous Poisson processes, and our discussion here tends to focus accordingly, resulting in limited treatment of some concepts covered in more detail in more general texts on spatial statistics. In particular, we only provide the barest details regarding tests of CSR. Cressie (1993, Chapter 8) provides a more thorough presentation of such methods.

Due to our focus on heterogeneous Poisson processes, we ignore the sizable literature regarding nearest-neighbor distance distributions. The literature refers to the *F function* and the *G function* to represent cumulative distribution functions of the distances between either a randomly chosen point in the study area or a randomly chosen event to the nearest-neighboring event, respectively. See Diggle (1983, Section 2.3) and Cressie (1993, Sections 8.2.6 and 8.4.2) for further details. In addition, van Lieshout and Baddeley (1996) consider the ratio of the F and G functions (termed the *J function*) as a measure of spatial interaction in a spatial point processes. Van Lieshout and Baddeley (1999) provide an analog to the J function for multivariate point processes (e.g., point processes with more than one type of event, as in the grave site example).

Finally, there are also a wide variety of point process models in addition to the Poisson processes outlined above. We refer the reader to Diggle (1983), Ripley (1988), Chapter 8 of Cressie (1993), Stoyan et al. (1995), and Lawson (2001) for further details and examples.

5.6 EXERCISES

5.1 Suppose that we have a realization of a spatial point process consisting of N event locations $\{s_1, \dots, s_N\}$. Let W_i denote the distance between the ith event and its nearest-neighboring event. The literature refers to the cumulative distribution function of W (the nearest event–event distance) as the *G function*. What is the G function under complete spatial randomness; that is, what is $\Pr[W \le w]$? (*Hint:* Consider the probability of observing no events within a circle of radius w.)

5.2 Simulate 100 realizations of complete spatial randomness in the unit square with 30 events in each realization. For each realization, calculate the distance between each event and its nearest-neighboring event, denoted W_i for the ith event in the realization. Calculate $2\pi\lambda\sum_{i=1}^{30} W_i^2$ (Skellam 1952) for each realization and compare the distribution of values to a χ^2_{2N} distribution where $N = 30$ denotes the number of events, λ the intensity function (30 for this application), and π is the familiar mathematical constant.

5.3 Repeat Exercise 5.2, letting the number of events in each realization follow a Poisson distribution with mean 30. What changes in the two settings? Under what assumptions is Skellam's chi-square distribution appropriate?

5.4 Simulate 100 realizations of a Poisson cluster process and calculate Skellam's statistic for each realization. Compare the histogram of values to that obtained in Exercise 5.2. How does the distribution of the statistic change compared to its distribution under complete spatial randomness?

5.5 For each of $\lambda = 10$, 20, and 100, generate six realizations of CSR on the unit square. For each realization, construct a kernel estimate of $\lambda(\mathbf{s})$ (supposing you did not know that the data represented realizations of CSR). How does each set of six estimates of $\lambda(\mathbf{s})$ compare to the known constant values of λ? What precautions does this exercise suggest with regard to interpreting estimates of intensity from a single realization (data set)?

5.6 The following algorithm outlines a straightforward acceptance–rejection approach to simulating realizations of N events from a heterogeneous Poisson process with intensity $\lambda(\mathbf{s})$. First, suppose that we can calculate $\lambda(\mathbf{s})$ for any point $\mathbf{s}$ in the study area A, and that we know (or can calculate) a bounding value λ^* such that $\lambda(\mathbf{s}) \le \lambda^*$ for all $\mathbf{s} \in A$.

Step 1. Generate a "candidate" event at location $\mathbf{s}_0$ under CSR in area A.

Step 2. Generate a uniform random number, say w, in the interval [0, 1].

Step 3. If $w \le \left(\lambda(\mathbf{s})/\lambda^*\right)$ [i.e., with probability $\left(\lambda(\mathbf{s})/\lambda^*\right)$], keep the candidate event as part of the simulated realization; otherwise, "reject" the candidate and omit it from the realization.

Step 4. Return to step 1 until the collection of accepted events numbers N.

In this algorithm, events have a higher probability of being retained in the realization in locations where the ratio $\left(\lambda(\mathbf{s})/\lambda^*\right)$ is higher. The closer the value λ^* is to $\max_{s \in A} \lambda(s)$, the more efficient the algorithm will be (as fewer candidates will be rejected overall). [See Lewis and Shedler (1979), Ogata (1981), and Stoyan et al. (1995, Section 2.6.2) for more detailed discussions of this and similar algorithms.]

For a heterogeneous intensity $\lambda(s)$ and study area A of your choice, generate six realizations with 30 events each from the same underlying heterogeneous Poisson process. For each realization, estimate $\lambda(s)$ via kernel estimation. Plot the realizations with respect to your known intensity $\lambda(s)$. Provide separate plots of each kernel density estimate and compare to the true intensity function $\lambda(s)$.

On a separate plot, indicate the location of the mode (maximal value) of each kernel estimate of $\lambda(s)$. How do these six values compare to the true mode of $\lambda(s)$? What (if any) implications do your results suggest with respect to identifying modes of disease incidence based on intensity estimated from a single data realization (e.g., a set of incident cases for a single year)?

5.7 The medieval grave site data set introduced in Section 5.2.5 appear in Table 5.2. Estimate the intensity functions for affected and nonaffected sites for a variety of bandwidths. For what bandwidths do the two intensities appear similar? For what bandwidths do they appear different?

Table 5.2 Medieval Grave Site Data[a]

u	v	Aff	u	v	Aff	u	v	Aff
8072	8970	0	9004	7953	0	8614	8528	0
9139	8337	1	8876	8641	1	8996	8039	0
7898	8892	0	8320	9010	0	9052	8923	0
9130	7438	0	9194	6474	0	9338	5737	0
8102	7636	0	9334	6740	0	9183	6073	0
8889	7272	0	8639	6916	0	9110	6393	0
8167	5609	0	9272	7095	0	8341	6903	0
8546	6218	0	9419	4177	1	9215	4570	0
8400	4117	0	9110	5067	0	9310	5450	1
9361	7166	1	8303	4935	0	8536	4226	0
9435	4473	1	8189	5720	0	8797	4787	0
8326	9300	0	8457	4785	0	8326	9541	1
5100	6466	0	8373	9379	0	7042	8761	0
4714	6455	0	4492	7463	0	7212	8262	0
7209	7467	0	7468	7789	1	7768	7972	1
7796	7657	0	7639	7009	1	7237	7299	0
7620	6039	0	6934	6918	1	9149	3588	0
7708	5776	0	7119	7784	0	7042	7264	1
7039	6234	1	8778	3844	0	9485	3319	1
5305	6065	1	5306	6065	1	5456	6353	0
5717	6023	0	5597	7725	0	5231	7472	0
6092	7671	1	4862	5969	0	6252	8271	0

(continued overleaf)

Table 5.2 (*continued*)

u	v	Aff	u	v	Aff	u	v	Aff
6720	7164	1	6569	7391	0	6258	7127	0
9558	9403	0	9208	9114	1	9352	7957	0
9473	8826	0	7505	6024	0	7974	6332	0
7634	6229	0	8126	7269	0	9756	9257	0
9752	6468	0	10073	8273	0	9405	10431	0
10147	8141	0	10100	3085	1	9262	10068	0
9990	3824	0	9305	9661	0	8831	9393	0
9570	9059	0	9656	8356	0	9547	7690	0
9416	9223	0	9502	8846	0	8937	9611	0
10263	4790	0	10324	4389	0	10232	7271	0
9497	7564	0	9412	7463	0	9722	7065	0
9757	5276	1	9879	6309	0	10061	5937	0
9716	6713	0	9699	7240	0	9665	5554	1
10156	5225	1	10143	6317	0	10373	3208	1
8575	8840	0	9072	8894	0	8846	7633	0
9131	6958	1	9230	7068	0	8217	5835	0
8458	5106	0	8685	4497	0	8175	4862	0
8598	5377	0	8789	5006	0	5101	7115	0
4716	6733	0	5109	6590	0	7507	8280	0
7459	6591	0	8861	3882	0	7068	6341	0
5683	7046	0	4612	6147	0	5385	7052	0
6720	7541	0	5952	6278	1	7759	6222	1
7628	6730	0	10070	6739	0	9770	3469	0
9850	3656	1	9667	9541	0	9702	4581	1
10030	4274	0	10292	7562	0	9953	4673	0
10192	5291	0	10148	5222	1			

[a] u and v denote the coordinates of each location and "Aff" indicates whether the grave site included missing or reduced wisdom teeth (Aff = 1) or did not (Aff = 0). See text for details.

5.8 Simulate 10 realizations from the Baddeley and Silverman (1984) process defined in Section 5.3.4 on a 100×100 unit grid. Plot the K function for each realization and plot the average of the 10 K functions at each distance value. Does the average of the K-function estimates appear consistent with the K function for complete spatial randomness? Does each of the 10 estimated K functions appear consistent with the K function from complete spatial randomness?

CHAPTER 6

Spatial Clusters of Health Events: Point Data for Cases and Controls

It is no great wonder if in long process of time, while fortune takes her course hither and thither, numerous coincidences should spontaneously occur.

Plutarch, *Life of Sertorius*

The methods outlined in Chapter 5 provide a basis for addressing a very common question related to mapped health data: Are there clusters of disease? As we saw in Chapter 5, this question in deceptively simple to ask and considerably more difficult to answer. In this chapter and the next, we review basic issues affecting our assessment of clustering related to data types, answerable questions, assumptions, and interpretation of results.

The typical data structure for assessments of spatial health patterns involves a collection of locations of incident events over a particular period for a given study area. For example, one might record the locations of residences for children diagnosed with acute lymphocytic leukemia in a given year. Common questions relating to the clustering of health events include:

- Do cases tend to occur near other cases (perhaps suggesting an infectious agent)?
- Does a particular area within the study region seem to contain a significant excess of observed cases (perhaps suggesting an environmental risk factor)?
- Where are the most unusual collections of cases (the most likely clusters)?

To address such questions, we need to determine whether an observed collection of cases is somehow unusual (i.e., different than we expect under a hypothesis of chance allocation of cases among the population at risk).

The question "Are disease cases clustered?" appears to imply existence of a simple "Yes" or "No" answer, and suggests a hypothesis-testing approach based

Applied Spatial Statistics for Public Health Data, by Lance A. Waller and Carol A. Gotway
ISBN 0-471-38771-1

on a conceptual null hypothesis of

$$H_0: \text{There are no clusters of cases.} \tag{6.1}$$

However, as we will see, there are many ways to operationalize this simple idea, each differing in underlying assumptions, goals, and ways of assessing departures from this null hypothesis. The statistical literature contains a variety of hypothesis tests addressing disease clustering [see Marshall (1991), Elliott et al. (1995), Alexander and Boyle (1996), Lawson and Waller (1996), Kulldorff (1997), Diggle (2000), Wakefield et al. (2000b), Lawson (2001), and Kulldorff (2002) for reviews]. We do not attempt an exhaustive review here; rather, we focus on a variety of strategies for addressing the conceptual null hypothesis above, listing a sample of methods following each strategy.

6.1 WHAT DO WE HAVE? DATA TYPES AND RELATED ISSUES

Disease cluster investigations generally involve case data in one of two broad categories: case–control point data or regional count data. *Case–control point data* involve point locations for each of a set of cases reported (e.g., those cases reported to a disease registry or other reporting system within a given time period), and a collection of noncases, termed *controls*. *Regional count data* generally provide reported counts of incident (newly diagnosed) or prevalent (existing) cases residing in particular regions partitioning the study area (e.g., census enumeration districts). We focus on methods for case–control point data in this chapter, and on methods for regional count data in Chapter 7.

With case–control point data, the control locations provide background information on spatial patterns of the population at risk. Often, we assume that controls represent an independent random sample from subjects free of the disease of interest, and compare patterns of the cases to the pattern of people without the disease. In some cases, we select controls "matched" to the set of cases, reflecting similar proportions of demographic features such as age, gender, or race/ethnicity. Such matching of controls is common practice in epidemiology, but analysts need to be aware that matching affects the standard error of statistical estimates and often requires adjustments in calculations [see Chapter 10 of Rothman and Greenland (1998) for a general discussion of matching and Diggle et al. (2000) for issues specific to spatial point pattern analysis]. In some cases we may have complete (or very nearly complete) enumeration of cases and noncases (e.g., a complete registry of birth defects combined with a birth certificate database). In other cases we may consider sampling controls from the population at risk. For very rare diseases, we may consider the set of all persons at risk (diseased and nondiseased) as a set of controls with the bias associated with the inclusion of the cases in the set of controls diminishing with increasing rarity of disease.

Limited availability of point data for nondiseased persons often necessitates other definitions of controls. One approach uses cases of a second disease (or set of diseases) different from the disease under investigation (cf. Diggle 1989, 1990; Lawson 1989; Lawson and Williams 1993). In this case the analyst specifically assumes differences in etiology between the case and control diseases relating particularly to any exposures of interest (environmental or otherwise). As a specific example, English et al. (1999) investigate associations between pediatric asthma and traffic flow using pediatric asthma cases among children using California's Medicaid program and controls sampled from the nonrespiratory visits recorded in the same system. This choice of cases and controls explores differences between the spatial distribution of residences of children using the low-income health system for asthma-related outcomes and that of children using the same system for reasons other than respiratory ailments. Note that this is a different comparison than that between all cases of pediatric asthma and nonasthmatic children. The particular choice of controls refines the hypotheses under investigation and specifies the answerable questions in the available data.

The case and control point locations provide realizations from the underlying case and control spatial point processes. In the methods outlined below, we use ideas from Chapter 5 to find similarities or differences between these two processes.

6.2 WHAT DO WE WANT? NULL AND ALTERNATIVE HYPOTHESES

To define hypothesis tests, we first need to operationalize H_0 as defined verbally in equation (6.1). The particular implementation of a hypothesis test involves several assumptions, each determining whether observed patterns provide evidence for or against a conclusion of clustering. As discussed in Section 5.2.4, complete spatial randomness (CSR), a mathematical definition of the absence of clustering in spatial point processes, is not a satisfactory null hypothesis if the population at risk is distributed heterogeneously across the study area. As a result, many traditional tests of CSR based on nearest-neighbor distances [e.g., those outlined in Table 8.6 of Cressie (1993, p. 604)] are not appropriate tests of clustering of disease cases in heterogeneously distributed populations. One way around this problem involves defining mathematical transformations of the study area such that the population at risk is homogeneously distributed in the transformed space, allowing application of distance-based tests of CSR in the transformed data (Selvin 1991, pp. 117–124). These transformations generate *cartograms* or *density equalized map projections*. Public health applications of cartograms appear in the literature (e.g., Levison and Haddon 1965; Selvin et al. 1987, 1988; Schulman et al. 1988). However, defining a unique transformation that maintains regional adjacencies (shared borders) can be nontrivial. Since the heterogeneous Poisson process provides a flexible means for analyzing the untransformed data, we limit discussion to such approaches below.

To begin, we consider spatially varying functions defining the spatial pattern of disease and consider the relationship between these quantities and the spatial intensity function for a heterogeneous Poisson process defined in Chapter 5. Such functions allow us to assess whether the data observed appear consistent with the conceptual null hypothesis expressed in equation (6.1). Three concepts from

Chapter 2 provide a starting point: spatial variations in disease *risk*, disease *rates*, and *relative risk*. As noted in Chapter 2, the term *rate* often refers to incidence proportion rather than to a true rate (number of incident cases per time interval). Expanding the definitions of Chapter 2 to the spatial domain implies a spatially varying function risk(s), denoting the probability of a person at location s contracting the disease of interest within a specified interval, a function rate(s) denoting the proportion of people at location s contracting the disease within the interval, and a function relative risk(s) denoting the multiplicative increase in disease risk occurring at location s compared to the overall disease risk observed (i.e., the total number of cases divided by the total number of persons at risk). As noted in Chapter 2, risks are unknown and unobserved quantities specific to individuals, often estimated by rates (proportions) observed over groups of people.

If we assume that case and control locations follow heterogeneous Poisson point processes, we may consider each of the spatially varying intensity, risk (rate), and relative risk functions as ratios comparing the expected number of cases (numerator) at a location s to different reference quantities (denominators). Conditional on the total number of cases in the study area, the intensity function at location s is proportional to the spatial probability density function at location s describing the proportion of all cases observed expected to occur at location s. The risk (rate) at location s describes the proportion of at-risk persons at location s expected to contract the disease. Hence the comparison (denominator) groups for intensity and rate (risk) functions are all cases, and all at-risk persons, respectively.

Ratios of case and control intensities and ratios of spatially varying risk functions both provide insight into the spatial relative risk function. Informally, consider the *rate ratio* resulting from replacing the ratio of risks (unknown probabilities to be estimated) with proportions. The typical interpretation of the spatially varying rate ratio is

$$\frac{(\text{number of incident cases at } s)/(\text{number at risk at } s)}{(\text{total number of cases})/(\text{total number at risk})}. \tag{6.2}$$

We note that algebraic manipulation of equation (6.2) yields

$$\frac{(\text{number of incident cases at } s)/(\text{total number of cases})}{(\text{number at risk at } s)/(\text{total number at risk})}. \tag{6.3}$$

As a result, the rate ratio at location s describes the ratio of intensities in equation (6.3) (the ratio between the proportion of all cases occurring at location s and the proportion of all noncases occurring at location s) and the ratio of incidence proportions in equation (6.2) (the ratio of the incidence proportion at s to the incidence proportion for the entire study area) equally well. More formal development of the spatial relative risk with respect to intensity and density functions appears below and in Diggle (2000, pp. 89–91) and Wakefield et al. (2000b, pp. 140–141).

With estimates or summaries of spatially varying risks, rates, or relative risks, attention turns to quantifying how a particular estimate varies from what would be expected under the conceptual null hypothesis. As outlined below, different statistical methods approach this issue in different ways.

Two common methods for operationalizing the null hypothesis defined in equation (6.1) based on an assumed underlying heterogeneous Poisson process are the random labeling hypothesis for point case–control data (defined in the application of the K function to the medieval grave site data in Section 5.3.3), and the constant risk hypothesis (defined in Section 5.2.4) for regional count data. Recall that the former assumes that case and control event locations arise from the same underlying spatial point process, while the latter assumes cases reflect a random sample of the at-risk population where the probability of selection is the same everywhere (perhaps varying by risk strata, e.g., age, but with spatially constant stratum-specific risks). Accordingly, many statistical approaches for point case–control data rely on estimates of intensity or K functions, while those for regional data involve comparisons of regional summaries to those expected from independent Poisson random variables with expectations defined as the product of the assumed constant risk and the population size perhaps adjusted for demographic structure. As a result, many tests for regional count data resemble traditional goodness-of-fit tests wherein one compares the number (or proportion) of cases observed to that expected under the null hypothesis, as detailed in Chapter 7.

The two approaches to defining null hypotheses are similar but not identical. In particular, the constant risk hypothesis assumes a known (or estimated) background risk, while the random labeling hypothesis only assumes an equal probability of case–control assignment at all locations. We will refer to the constant risk hypothesis even though technically we replace risk with an estimate based on proportions (rates). The assumptions defining random labeling and constant risk can differ in the situation where we use a reference disease risk estimated from data external to the study area (e.g., applying a national rate to a local area). To illustrate, consider a situation where the external rate (risk estimate) differs appreciably from the rate observed within the data set but that this difference occurs uniformly across the study area. In this setting, tests comparing the case counts observed to those expected under the external rate would tend to find evidence against the null hypothesis, due to comparison with a discrepant overall rate rather than to local variations in disease risk within the study area. In short, when using an externally estimated reference rate, the constant risk hypothesis may be rejected by any of the following: local deviations in the disease rate within the study area (i.e., localized clustering or a nonstationary disease intensity), a uniform increase or decrease in the rate across the study area (i.e., a mismatch between the disease rate for the entire area and that of the external reference population), or some combination of both. This feature argues for careful interpretation of any rejection of the constant risk hypothesis, particularly when using reference rates based on external data. In contrast, the random labeling hypothesis assigns the case–control label using the frequency of cases and controls observed in the data. Related tests are conditional on the frequency observed, and random labeling is not sensitive to the estimated/assumed background risk in the same manner as is the constant risk hypothesis.

We may also distinguish subtle differences between different implementations of the null hypothesis by considering how we might simulate data realizations under each implementation. This approach is particularly enlightening since Monte Carlo (simulation) methods provide inference for many of the tests described below. First, consider simulating realizations under the random labeling hypothesis for case–control point data. Here, we consider the set of event (say, N_1 case and N_0 control) locations fixed and generate data sets under the null hypothesis by randomly assigning N_1 of the set of $N = N_0 + N_1$ locations as "cases." In defining our null process in this manner, we address the question: "Is there evidence of clusters or clustering in our data?" more explicitly as "Are the N_1 case locations observed consistent with a random assignment of N_1 among the N event locations observed?" Table 6.1 extends this exercise to a variety of settings, each operationalizing the conceptual null hypothesis in slightly different ways for both case–control point and regional count data.

Table 6.1 also distinguishes between null hypotheses based on fixed and variable total numbers of cases. For example, contrast the questions "Is there evidence of

Table 6.1 Specification of Questions Addressed by Different Approaches for Operationalizing the Null Hypothesis of the Absence of Clustering[a]

Null Hypothesis	Question Addressed
Random labeling Case–control point data	Are the N_1 case locations observed consistent with a random assignment of N_1 cases among the N event locations observed?
Constant risk Case–control point data (fixed total)	Are the N_1 case locations observed consistent with a random assignment of N_1 cases among the N event locations observed?
Constant risk Case–control point data (variable total)	Are the case locations observed consistent with each of the N locations observed having probability N_1/N of being a case?
Constant risk Regional count data (fixed total, risk known)	Are the regional counts observed consistent with a random assignment of N_1 cases among the population at risk?
Constant risk Regional count data (variable total, risk known)	Are the regional counts observed consistent with a random assignment of cases among the population at risk, where each person is subject to the same, known risk of disease?
Constant risk Regional count data (variable total, risk estimated)	Are the regional counts observed consistent with a random assignment of cases among the population at risk, where each person is subject to the same constant, but unknown, risk of disease?

[a] As in the text, N_0 denotes the number of controls observed, N_1 the number of cases observed, and $N = N_0 + N_1$ the total number of cases and controls. For the purposes of this table, we assume that the population at risk remains constant for the study period.

clustering of 592 cases of leukemia among 1,057,673 persons at risk?" and "Is there evidence of clustering of cases of leukemia among 1,057,673 persons at risk where each person has a risk of 592/1,057,673 of contracting leukemia in the time interval under study?" In the former we seek evidence of clusters among 592 observed cases, and each simulated data set would include 592 cases of leukemia in a Monte Carlo study. In the latter we seek evidence among a fixed population of 1,057,673 persons at risk but allow the total number of cases to vary (both conceptually and in Monte Carlo simulations) even though each person experiences a constant risk of disease. Another example involves the difference between "Do we observe evidence of clustering among the 592 cases observed this year?" and "Do we observe evidence of clustering among cases observed at this year's rate?" Bithell (1995) outlines theoretical reasons for conditioning on the total number of cases (an ancillary statistic), whereas we focus on the conceptual change in the question of interest.

In addition to differences in the null hypothesis, most tests assess deviations from the conceptual null hypothesis in equation (6.1) with respect to particular mathematical definitions of "cluster" within alternative hypotheses. Hence, different tests identify different patterns as evidence of deviations from this null hypothesis. Several possibilities exist for relevant alternative hypotheses, and Besag and Newell (1991) provide valuable terminology for distinguishing between them. First, consider the distinction between *clusters* and *clustering*. Detecting a *cluster* involves the identification of a collection of cases inconsistent with our null hypothesis of no clustering, whereas detecting *clustering* involves assessment of the overall propensity of cases to cluster together (i.e., detecting the *tendency* of cases to cluster rather than identifying a particular collection or collections of cases). A single cluster represents an anomaly in the data (i.e., a collection inconsistent with the broader pattern); clustering represents a pattern among all or most cases. Typically, a test of clustering provides a single assessment of the statistical significance of the pattern for the entire area (e.g., a single p-value), whereas tests to detect clusters often utilize multiple tests (multiple p-values) to determine which collection of cases represents the most significant cluster. We note that the distinction between detecting clusters and detecting clustering is not always clear (e.g., some cases may occur in clusters whereas others do not, there may be more than one cluster, or only a subset of cases actually exhibit a clustering tendency). Nonetheless, the categories focus our attention on different aspects of the observed spatial distribution of cases and different answers to the question "Is there evidence of clusters in my data?"

Besag and Newell (1991) further distinguish between general tests and focused tests (of clustering or to detect clusters). *General tests* test for clusters/clustering anywhere in the study area; *focused tests* test for clusters or clustering around predefined foci of suspected increased risk of disease (e.g., a contaminated well). Statistically, the difference lies again in the null hypotheses; contrast H_0 for a general test (absence of clustering) with that for a focused test:

H_0: There are no clusters of cases *around the foci*.

In a focused study, one attempts to increase statistical attention (e.g., power) on a particular set of possible clusters (those around the foci) rather than trying to find any sort of cluster in any location.

6.3 CATEGORIZATION OF METHODS

With the ideas outlined in Sections 6.1 and 6.2 in mind, we review several specific statistical approaches for case–control point data in the following sections. We note that different tests may provide differing conclusions regarding clusters/clustering present in the same set of data (Waller and Jacquez 1995). By better understanding the types of clustering/clusters associated with particular tests, we may better understand the types of patterns present in any particular data set.

In the sections below we present tests of disease clusters/clustering categorized by the type of data and the statistical strategy for detecting clusters and/or clustering:

- Methods for case–control point data using first- and second-order summaries of spatial point processes (e.g., intensity and K function estimates)
- Methods for case–control point data based on scanning local rate estimates

We believe that this classification aids in identifying differences among methods and the assumptions and goals underlying each. We present a representative (but not exhaustive) sample of case–control point approaches appearing in the statistical and epidemiologic literature, and provide references to reviews and other approaches in Section 6.7. We take care to indicate assumptions inherent in the methods and highlight the particular manner in which each method operationalizes the conceptual null hypothesis stated in equation (6.1).

6.4 COMPARING POINT PROCESS SUMMARIES

In Chapter 5 we introduced two-dimensional heterogeneous Poisson processes and defined their first- and second-order properties as summarized by the intensity function $\lambda(s)$ and K function $K(h)$, respectively. We also provided methods for estimating the intensity and K functions from an observed realization of event locations. We illustrated these methods using the medieval grave site data (listed at the end of Chapter 5), drawing only qualitative conclusions comparing the point patterns of affected and nonaffected grave sites. We now formalize inferential methods comparing intensity functions for a pair of patterns observed over the same study area. When considering the set of affected and nonaffected sites, the medieval grave site data again provide an example of case–control point data and we continue to use the data to motivate the various statistical approaches.

6.4.1 Goals

The primary goal for comparisons of intensity functions is to detect local differences between the spatial pattern in disease incidence observed in the cases from the spatial pattern observed in the controls, and to assign statistical significance to any differences observed. Most often, we wish to detect significant peaks (and/or valleys) of case incidence above and beyond the baseline pattern of individuals at risk, illustrated by the controls. As a result, the approaches below most often serve as tests to detect *clusters*, although the approaches sometimes use summary values to provide a means to assess overall *clustering* as well. Such tests of clustering assess the frequency and strength of local differences occurring anywhere in the study area rather than directly assessing a tendency of cases to occur near other cases (i.e., the presence of many individual clusters can provide evidence for clustering rather than a general tendency for cases to be near other cases). The goal of detecting local differences between the case and control patterns observed indicates that the approaches most often offer *general* inference, although we could define *focused* approaches either as special cases of a general method or as derived from the same underlying principles.

In contrast, comparison of second-order properties focuses on assessing *clustering* rather than *clusters*. Recall that the K function is a summary of the tendency for observed events to occur within a distance h for values of h ranging from zero to (typically) half the largest interevent distance observed. As such, the K function summarizes clustering tendency across all events rather than identifying particular collections of events as clusters.

6.4.2 Assumptions and Typical Output

For comparing intensities or K functions, we assume that the case locations represent a realization of a heterogeneous Poisson point process and that the control locations represent a realization of a second heterogeneous Poisson process observed over the same area. As such, we assume that each case and control event location occurs independently of other events in the same process, with spatial variation in incidence summarized by the intensity function for the appropriate process.

As mentioned in Section 6.2, methods for case–control point data often build inference based on the random labeling hypothesis, conditional on the point locations observed. All methods described in this section assume that the set of case–control locations are fixed. That is, all simulations involve random assignment of the case–control label to the existing set of locations rather than randomly assigning locations to cases. As a result, the tests seek an answer to the question: Is the labeling of event locations observed as cases and controls consistent with a random assignment of labels to this set of locations observed? Recall that random labeling does not necessarily imply independence between the case and control processes. For methods based on estimated intensity functions, we are less concerned with describing the overall pattern of events than with identifying those locations in the study area where the observed probability of an observed event being a case (versus a control) appears high. Hence, the output of our general tests to detect clusters below will typically consist of a map indicating areas where events appear more or less likely to be cases than controls, as compared to the case–control ratio observed in data aggregated over the entire study area.

Naturally, methods based on estimated first- and second-order properties of spatial point processes inherit the assumptions allowing the particular estimation methods in the first place. As a starting point, the approaches below assume independence between events within a realization (e.g., events within the case process) and therefore do not apply readily to infectious outcomes. Second, the usual implementations of kernel estimation of intensities and edge-corrected estimation of the K function employ some form of isotropy. Kernel estimation typically uses isotropic kernels, which may work well with a sufficiently large sample size (number of locations), even for an anisotropic intensity function. K-function estimation assumes isotropy of the underlying process. Both intensity estimation and K-function estimation may be extended to incorporate various anisotropies, provided that we have a priori reasons for such an adjustment. Finally, K-function estimation typically assumes stationarity of the underlying process in addition to isotropy. Diggle and Chetwynd (1991) note that one may assume stationarity for a heterogeneous Poisson process as long as one assumes that the (heterogeneous) intensity function is itself a realization of a stationary random process defining intensities (i.e., a Cox process as defined briefly in Section 5.4.3). As in the data break ending Section 5.3.3, a random labeling hypothesis based on K functions seeks to determine if the case and control processes exhibit the same sort of deviation from a homogeneous Poisson point process.

6.4.3 Method: Ratio of Kernel Intensity Estimates

Suppose that our data include the locations of N_1 case events and N_0 control events distributed throughout the same study area. The medieval grave site data from Alt and Vach (1991) introduced in Section 5.2.5 provide an example of such data. We define $\lambda_1(\boldsymbol{s})$ and $\lambda_0(\boldsymbol{s})$ as the intensities associated with the point process of cases and controls, respectively. Each intensity function is proportional to the underlying spatial probability density functions associated with the probability of observing an event of the associated type (case or control) at any particular location in the study area. Comparisons of the two intensity functions form the basis of several approaches for assessing spatial clustering in public health data (Bithell 1990; Lawson and Williams 1993; Kelsall and Diggle 1995a,b, 1998). Bithell (1990) and Lawson and Williams (1993) suggest exploratory analyses based on the ratio of these two intensities, with Bithell (1990) proposing a logistic transformation to symmetrize variances. Kelsall and Diggle (1995a,b) formalize such comparisons of intensity functions and we outline their approach here.

By assuming an underlying Poisson process, Kelsall and Diggle (1995a,b) note that conditional on the number of cases and controls, the data are equivalent to two independent random samples from (spatial) probability distributions over the study area (denoted D) with density function

$$f(\boldsymbol{s}) = \lambda_1(\boldsymbol{s}) \Big/ \int_D \lambda_1(\boldsymbol{u})\, d\boldsymbol{u}$$

for cases and

$$g(s) = \lambda_0(s) \Big/ \int_D \lambda_0(u)\, du$$

for controls. Kelsall and Diggle (1995a,b) suggest inference (conditional on N_1 and N_0) based on the natural logarithm of the ratio of the two spatial densities, i.e., inference based on

$$r(s) = \log\{f(s)/g(s)\},$$

a quantity related to the logarithm of the *relative risk* of observing a case rather than a control at location s in D. Note that algebraic manipulation of the definition of $r(s)$ yields

$$r(s) = \log\{\lambda_1(s)/\lambda_0(s)\} - \log\left\{\int_D \lambda_1(u)\, du \Big/ \int_D \lambda_0(u)\, du\right\}. \tag{6.4}$$

The second term on the right-hand side of equation (6.4) does not depend on the spatial location s, so $r(s)$ and the natural logarithm of the ratio of intensity functions contain identical information regarding spatial variation in risk. That is, a surface plot of the log ratio of the spatial density functions [$f(s)$ and $g(s)$] will be identical to that of the log ratio of the spatial intensity functions [$\lambda_1(s)$ and $\lambda_0(s)$] offset by a constant defined by the log ratio of the integrated intensities. This constant corresponds to the log overall disease rate if we observe all case and noncase locations (the complete realization of the two point processes), or may be estimated by $\log(N_1/N_0) - \log(q_1/q_0)$ if we sample proportions q_1 of N_1 cases and proportion q_0 of N_0 noncases, given values for N_0, N_1, q_0, and q_1 (Kelsall and Diggle 1995b).

Statistical analysis proceeds via estimation of $r(s)$ and inference regarding either clustering or detection of particular clusters. An advantage of analysis based on $r(s)$ is that one obtains an estimate of the (log) relative risk surface at all locations s within the study area D. Local assessment of the null hypothesis defined by equation (6.5) (i.e., assessment at particular locations $s \in D$) allows identification of those areas appearing least consistent with $r(s) = 0$ (i.e., a way to detect the locations s defining the most suspicious clusters within the study area).

To implement this approach, we require an estimate of the function $r(s)$. Kelsall and Diggle (1995a) propose a ratio of kernel estimates for $f(s)$ and $g(s)$, denoted $\tilde{f}_b(s)$ and $\tilde{g}_b(s)$, respectively, where b denotes the bandwidth. The usual considerations in kernel estimation apply, including edge-effect adjustments, kernel selection, and bandwidth selection. As noted in Section 5.2.5, the particular functional form of the kernel is not as important as the choice of bandwidth (but the numerical values of bandwidth may not be directly comparable between kernel types, as illustrated in the data break below). On the practical side, we note that the assumption of $r(s)$ as a continuous function of location s assumes that people at any location experience some nonzero risk of the disease. For small sample sizes of cases or controls, kernel estimation of the intensity function using finite-tail kernels (e.g., quartic kernels) can result in zero estimates for either $f(s)$ or $g(s)$

in locations containing few cases and/or controls. Zero estimates for $g(s)$ lead to local instabilities (division by zero) in resultant estimates of $r(s)$. Even kernels with infinite tails (e.g., Gaussian kernels) may result in numerically instable estimates if the data include wide gaps between event locations yielding very small estimates of $g(s)$. The existence and extent of such instabilities vary with the choice of the bandwidth, suggesting careful examination of plots of the estimated surfaces $f(s)$, $g(s)$, and $r(s)$ for odd behavior. An advantage to choosing a kernel with infinite tails such as a bivariate Gaussian density is that the estimate of the control density, $g(s)$, is nonzero for all locations and bandwidths, thereby avoiding division by zero in the estimate of $r(s)$. Kelsall and Diggle (1995a) note that bandwidths sensible for individual densities $\tilde{f}_b(s)$ and $\tilde{g}_b(s)$ may not be sensible for estimating $r(s)$, and suggest a common b for both when $r(s) \approx 0$.

While an optimal bandwidth based on mean integrated squared error (MISE) cannot be defined (see Section 5.2.5), an approach known as *least squares cross-validation* provides an approximation to minimizing the MISE (Silverman 1986, pp. 48–53; Wand and Jones 1995, pp. 63–66). In one dimension, least squares cross-validation approximates the MISE by the difference between the squared kernel estimate integrated over the study area and twice the averaged estimates based on kernel estimates from the data set omitting each observation in turn. Although least squares cross-validation is not perfect and can have poor performance in some situations (Wand and Jones 1995, pp. 65–66), it does provide a general strategy for bandwidth selection. We defer details of particular bandwidth selection algorithms to Wand and Jones (1995), Kelsall and Diggle (1995a,b), and Lawson (2001, pp. 66–67).

Suppose that we denote the selected bandwidth value (or values, in the case of product kernels) by b^*. At a descriptive level, a contour plot of $\tilde{r}_{b^*}(s)$ provides a map of areas where cases are more or less likely than controls [s such that $\tilde{r}_{b^*}(s) > 0$ and $\tilde{r}_{b^*}(s) < 0$, respectively]. Assessment of the significance of these deviations from zero proceeds via Monte Carlo analysis. Although a null hypothesis based on the constant risk hypothesis (actually, a constant *relative* risk hypothesis) makes intuitive sense, Monte Carlo tests are easier under the random labeling hypothesis (as is typically the case for case–control point data). We condition on the observed locations of cases and controls, and randomly assign N_1 of the $N_1 + N_0$ total locations as cases for each simulated data set. We then calculate $\tilde{r}_{b^*}(s)$ for each simulated split of locations into cases and controls (typically using the bandwidth calculated for the data both for computational ease and to remove variability associated with bandwidth estimation from our inference). If we repeat the process N_{sim} times over the same grid of locations in the study area, we can construct histograms and Monte Carlo p-values [the number of simulated values of $\tilde{r}_{b^*}(s_k)$ exceeding the value based on the observed data divided by $N_{\text{sim}} + 1$] associated with each grid point.

In addition to assessment of local *clusters*, the $\tilde{r}(s)$ surface also allows investigation of overall *clustering* via assessment of the global null hypothesis

$$H_0 : r(s) = 0 \qquad \text{for all } s \text{ in } D, \tag{6.5}$$

reflecting a situation where the spatial densities (and intensities) of cases and controls may vary across the study area but are always in the same relative proportion. That is, any heterogeneities in the spatial intensity of cases directly mirror those in the spatial intensity of controls. As written, equation (6.5) is a constant relative risk hypothesis, but as above, Monte Carlo implementation is more straightforward under the random labeling hypothesis. Note that the null hypothesis defined in equation (6.5) holds for *all* locations $\boldsymbol{s}$ within the study area, so a test of this null hypothesis provides summary inference (e.g., a single p-value) for the entire study area. For a test of overall clustering, Kelsall and Diggle (1995b, p. 2339) suggest one based on the statistic

$$\int_D \{\tilde{r}(\boldsymbol{u})\}^2 \, d\boldsymbol{u}, \tag{6.6}$$

calculated for the observed and simulated data, with inference based on Monte Carlo testing under the random labeling hypothesis. The integration summarizes all deviations between the case and control intensities across the study area, thereby providing a single statistic for the entire study area. Hence, unlike other tests of clustering proposed below, the log ratio of intensity functions provides a test of clustering using a direct mathematical summary of individual clusters.

DATA BREAK: Early Medieval Grave Sites (*cont.*) Let us reconsider the medieval grave site data of Chapter 5. In the data break in Section 5.2.5 we calculated and visually compared kernel estimates of the intensity functions for cases (grave sites with affected teeth) and controls (grave sites without affected teeth). We now apply the method of Kelsall and Diggle (1995b) to assess the statistical significance of any observed deviations between the two intensity functions.

We begin with circular symmetric Gaussian kernels for cases and controls with a common bandwidth of 700 units in all directions, where our choice represents a compromise among Scott's rule (Section 5.2.5) for bandwidths in the u and v directions for cases and controls [(872.24,997.45) for cases, and (695.35,734.82) for controls, respectively]. Recall that bandwidths meeting selection criteria for the individual case and control processes do not necessarily correspond to sensible bandwidths for the ratio of density (intensity) estimates, and we consider a variety of kernels and bandwidths below.

Figure 6.1 illustrates contour plots for the two density functions (normalized intensities) for a bandwidth of 700 units. The densities are somewhat less smooth than those presented in Figures 5.9 and 5.10, due to the slightly smaller bandwidth.

Figure 6.2 reveals the resulting log relative risk surface. No areas exceed the upper or lower pointwise 90% tolerance intervals for this choice of bandwidth based on 999 random labeling simulations, suggesting no locally significant departures from the random labeling hypothesis. This implies that the visual differences observed between the two estimated density (intensity) functions in Figures 6.1 and 5.10 do not correspond to statistically significant deviations from the random labeling hypothesis (i.e., clusters).

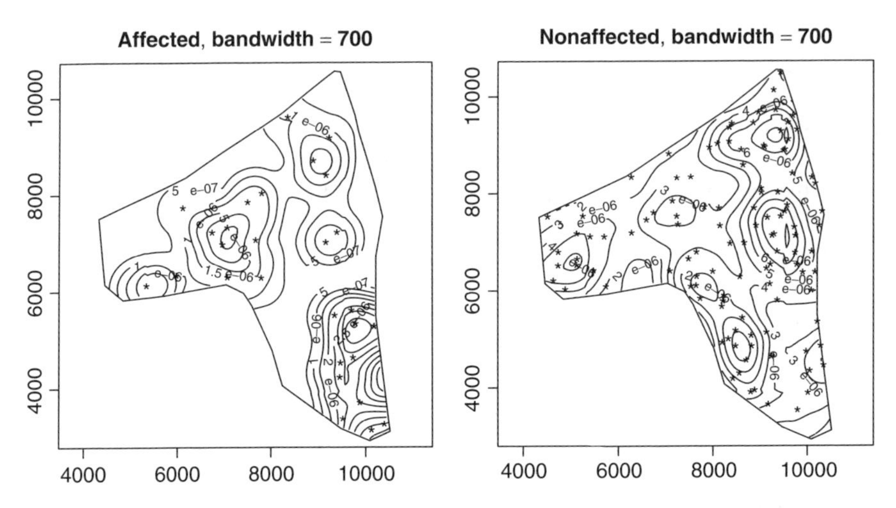

FIG. 6.1 Estimated densities (normalized intensities) using Gaussian kernels and a bandwidth of 700 units (see text). Compare with Figures 5.9 and 5.10.

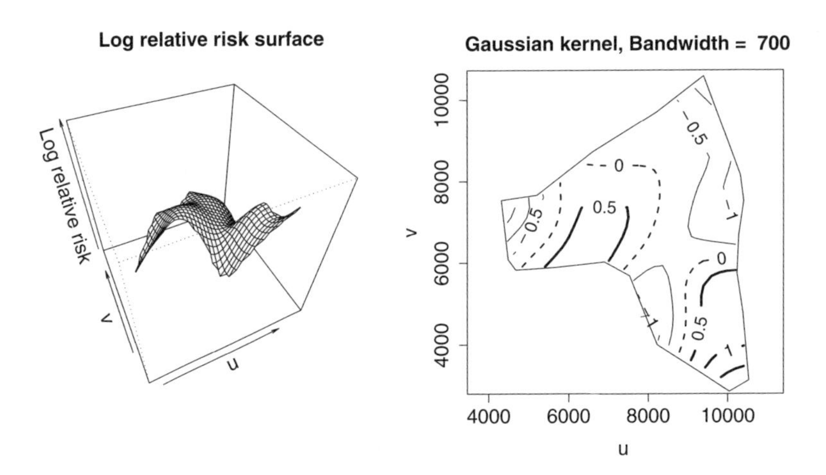

FIG. 6.2 Log ratio of density functions (proportional to the log ratio of intensity functions) for the medieval grave site data, using Gaussian kernels with a bandwidth of 700 distance units. Thin lines represent contours for log ratio values below zero, dashed contours represent log ratios of zero, and thick contours represent log ratio values above zero.

Using the same 999 random labeling assignments, the global test based on the statistic defined in equation (6.6) with Gaussian kernels and a bandwidth of 700 units yields a p-value of 0.18, suggesting that the overall difference between intensities does not suggest a global pattern of clustering.

In order to investigate the sensitivity of our inference to the selection of the bandwidth, Figure 6.3 illustrates the log relative risk surface based on radially symmetric

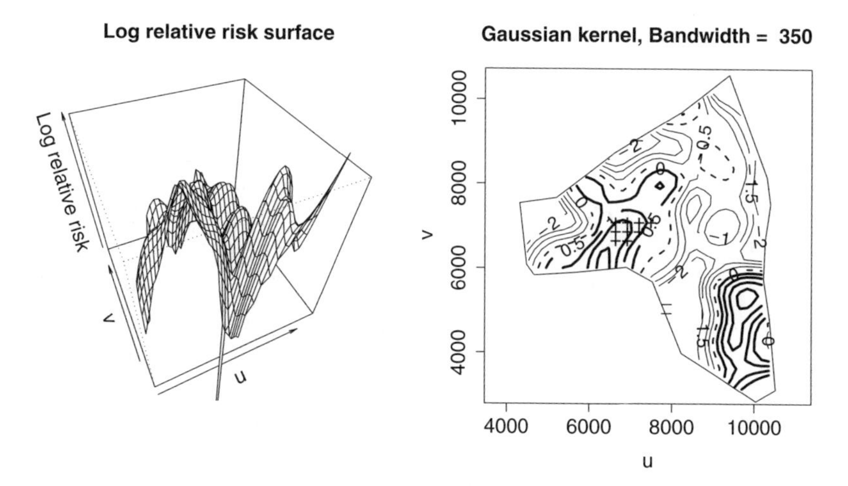

FIG. 6.3 Log ratio of density functions (proportional to the log ratio of intensity functions) for the medieval grave site data, using Gaussian kernels with a bandwidth of 350 distance units. Any collections of "+" symbols indicate areas where the observed log ratio exceeds the upper 90% tolerance region obtained by 999 simulations under the random labeling hypothesis (see text). Similarly, any collections of "−" symbols indicate areas where the observed log ratio of intensities is below the lower 90% tolerance limit. Thin lines represent contours for log ratio values below zero, dashed contours represent log ratios of zero, and thick contours represent log ratio values above zero.

Gaussian kernels with a bandwidth of 350 distance units for both cases and controls. For comparability, we use the same vertical scale, (−3,3), and contour levels in Figures 6.2 and 6.3. As expected, the smaller bandwidth results in a bumpier surface, and certain areas now exceed the upper or lower pointwise tolerance limits. In Figure 6.3 we label areas exceeding the upper pointwise 90% tolerance intervals with collections of "+" symbols, and areas of significantly reduced (log) relative risk appear as a collection of "−" symbols. These areas suggest a cluster of cases near (6500, 6500), and a deficit of cases along the southern border near (8000, 5000). The area indicated by these symbols indicate areas within the study area which are the most inconsistent with a random labeling assignment of grave sites, suggesting the most unusual clusters of affected grave sites. The area exceeding the lower tolerance limits corresponds to the sharp lower "spike" observed in the perspective (left-hand) plot in Figure 6.3. Such a deviation is due to the local deficit of cases near this edge of the study area (see Figure 6.1). The reduced bandwidth places this location out of the range of appreciable kernel weight of any of the case locations.

Again based on 999 random labeling assignments, the global test based on the statistic in equation (6.6) using Gaussian kernels and a bandwidth of 350 units yields a p-value of 0.13, suggesting that the overall difference between intensities still does not suggest a global pattern of clustering. However, we note that this does not mean that the individual deviations seen in Figure 6.3 are "insignificant," as the global test is a test for *clustering* rather than a test of the existence of any *clusters*.

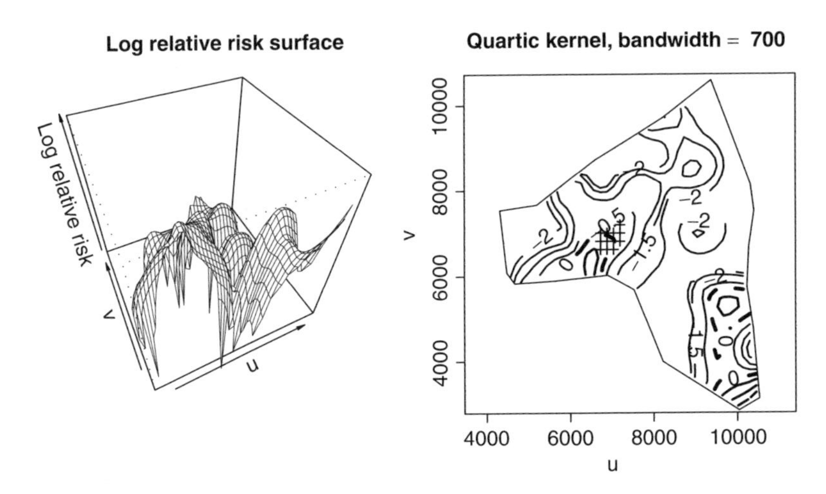

FIG. 6.4 Log ratio of density functions (proportional to the log ratio of intensity functions) for the medieval grave site data, using quartic kernels with a bandwidth of 700 distance units. Thin lines represent contours for log ratio values below zero, dashed contours represent log ratios of zero, and thick contours represent log ratio values above zero. Any collections of "+" symbols indicate areas where the observed log ratio exceeds the upper 90% tolerance region obtained by 999 simulations under the random labeling hypothesis (see text).

Next we consider kernel estimates based on radially symmetric quartic kernels rather than Gaussian kernels. Figure 6.4 shows the log relative risk function using quartic kernels and a bandwidth of 700 units, illustrating an important point regarding kernels and bandwidth selection. The log relative risk function based on a quartic kernel with bandwidth set to 700 units is very similar to the log relative risk surface based on a Gaussian kernel with bandwidth set to 350 units (Figure 6.3). Even though we note in Section 5.2.5 that kernel estimates are more sensitive to bandwidth than the particular kernel used, the bandwidth must always be interpreted in the context of a particular kernel.

To see why the log relative risk surface based on quartic kernels with bandwidth set to 700 units is similar to that based on Gaussian kernels with bandwidth set to 350 units, consider Figure 6.5, where we overlay the one-dimensional Gaussian and quartic kernels, each with bandwidth set to 700. For the Gaussian kernel, the bandwidth corresponds to the standard deviation of a Gaussian distribution; for the quartic kernel, the bandwidth corresponds to the distance beyond which locations do not contribute to the kernel estimate for the location of interest ($u = 0$ in Figure 6.5). Note the quartic kernel assigns zero weight beyond its bandwidth of 700 units, while the Gaussian kernel assigns appreciable weight to the distance beyond 700 units, resulting in a smoother kernel estimate for Gaussian kernels than for quartic kernels with the same bandwidth. The Gaussian kernel with bandwidth 350 units provides a set of kernel weights similar to those provided by the quartic kernel with bandwidth 700 units, hence a similar intensity (density) estimate.

Based on the different results for different kernels and bandwidths, which do we choose? First, we find no clear general pattern of clustering among the grave sites

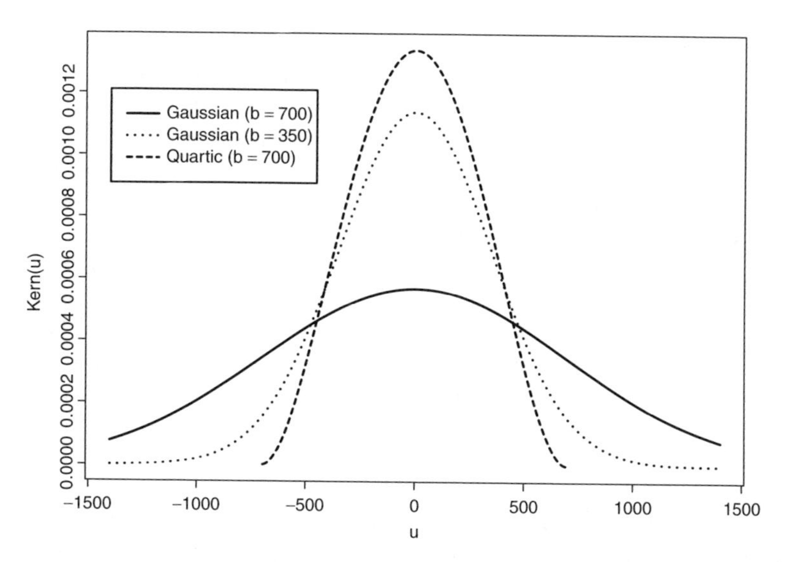

FIG. 6.5 Comparison of the one-dimensional Gaussian and quartic kernels (defined in Table 5.1) with bandwidth set to b distance units, centered at $u = 0$.

for Gaussian kernels with the bandwidth set to either 350 or 700 units. However, we do find an area with a suspicious aggregation of affected sites for Gaussian kernels with bandwidth 350 units (similarly for quartic kernels with bandwidth set to 700 units). The aggregations only appear inconsistent with the random labeling hypothesis for smaller bandwidths, suggesting fairly local impact of neighboring locations, if any.

The results are clearly dependent on the bandwidth selection. Recalling our original intent, we wish to recover a log relative risk surface accurately portraying differences in burial site selection patterns for affected and nonaffected sites. Smaller bandwidths may correspond to more local burial site selection criteria more closely than do larger bandwidths. Linking the statistical methods with the original application requires development of a reasonable bandwidth reflecting a likely "area of influence" of a familial-based burial strategy, a decision based on both statistical and archaeological input.

In summary, although the log relative risk approach alone does not prove burial by family unit, the local tests suggest areas where archaeologists may wish to seek additional evidence for familial ties through artifacts, or further laboratory testing of the remains.

6.4.4 Method: Difference between K Functions

In contrast to comparisons of estimated first-order properties, Diggle and Chetwynd (1991) consider inference based on estimated second-order properties of the case and control processes, namely the difference

$$KD(h) = K_{\text{cases}}(h) - K_{\text{controls}}(h)$$

between the K function based on cases and that based on controls for distance h. We estimate $KD(h)$ by $\widehat{KD}(h)$ replacing the K functions with their edge-corrected estimates defined in Section 5.3.1. As mentioned above, edge-corrected estimates of the K function typically assume stationarity (homogeneity) of the underlying point processes; however, Diggle and Chetwynd (1991) provide justification of their use here based on an assumption that the heterogeneous case and control intensity functions themselves arise from underlying stationarity random processes.

Under the random labeling hypothesis the expected value of $KD(h)$ is zero for any distance h. Positive values of $KD(h)$ suggest spatial clustering of cases over and above any clustering observed in the controls. Hence, distances for which $KD(h)$ exceeds zero provide insight into the spatial scale of any clustering observed. Note $KD(h)$ provides a summary of clustering within the entire data set, or at a particular distance (h), but does not pinpoint the location of specific clusters.

Diggle and Chetwynd (1991) and Chetwynd and Diggle (1998) provide derivations of the variance–covariance structure of the estimated K functions, providing pointwise interval estimates under random labeling for each value of h under consideration. However, as above, Monte Carlo interval estimates and hypothesis tests are straightforward, and we concentrate on these here. With N_1 cases and N_0 controls, conditional on the set of $(N_1 + N_0)$ locations, we repeatedly randomly select N_1 cases and define the remaining locations as controls for each of N_{sim} simulations. For each simulation, we calculate $\widehat{KD}(h)$, then calculate envelopes based on percentiles of the simulated values (or the minima and maxima values), providing Monte Carlo pointwise interval estimates of $KD(h)$ under the random labeling hypothesis.

If we wish to summarize clustering behavior over a range of distances, Diggle and Chetwynd (1991) suggest

$$KD_+ = \sum_{k=1}^{m} \widehat{KD}(h_k) / \sqrt{\text{Var}\left[\widehat{KD}(h_k)\right]}$$

as a sensible test statistic summarizing clustering over a set of m distances. Under random labeling, KD_+ approximately follows a Gaussian distribution with mean zero and variance equal to

$$m + 2 \sum_{j=2}^{m} \sum_{i=1}^{j-1} \text{corr}\left[\widehat{KD}(h_j), \widehat{KD}(h_i)\right],$$

with

$$\text{Var}\left[\widehat{KD}(h_k)\right] \quad \text{and} \quad \text{corr}\left[\widehat{KD}(h_j), \widehat{KD}(h_i)\right]$$

defined in Diggle and Chetwynd (1991). Alternatively, we may use a Monte Carlo test where we calculate KD_+ for each of our N_{sim} random labelings, rank the estimates, and define our p-value as the number of KD_+ values from simulated data exceeding the value observed in the data divided by $(N_{\text{sim}} + 1)$.

The medical literature contains applications of the difference between the K-function approach in assessments of clustering of anophthalmia and microphthalmia (Mariman 1998; Dolk et al. 1998; Cuzick 1998), primary biliary cirrhosis (Prince et al. 2001), and granulocytic ehrlichiosis in dogs (Foley et al. 2001), as well as a comparison of the geographic distributions of cancers in dogs and humans (O'Brien et al. 2000).

DATA BREAK: Early Medieval Grave Sites (*cont.*) By applying the difference of K functions (a second-order approach) to the medieval grave site data, we address a different question than we did with methods based on first-order intensity (density) functions. In this case we are not interested in determining where affected grave sites cluster; rather, we explore at what distances any observed clustering tends to occur, averaged over the entire study area. Figure 6.6 illustrates the difference between the K functions for cases and that for controls, compared to the 5th and 95th percentiles (calculated at each distance) of the difference based on 499 random labelings of cases and controls. These values offer pointwise 90% tolerance regions for the estimate of $KD(h)$ for a particular distance h.

We see the function $\widehat{KD}(h)$ stray beyond the tolerance envelopes for the smallest distances, and briefly for distances slightly less than 500 units. This suggests relatively weak evidence for an overall pattern of *clustering* at small distances, a conclusion fairly consistent with the type of *clusters* observed in comparing the

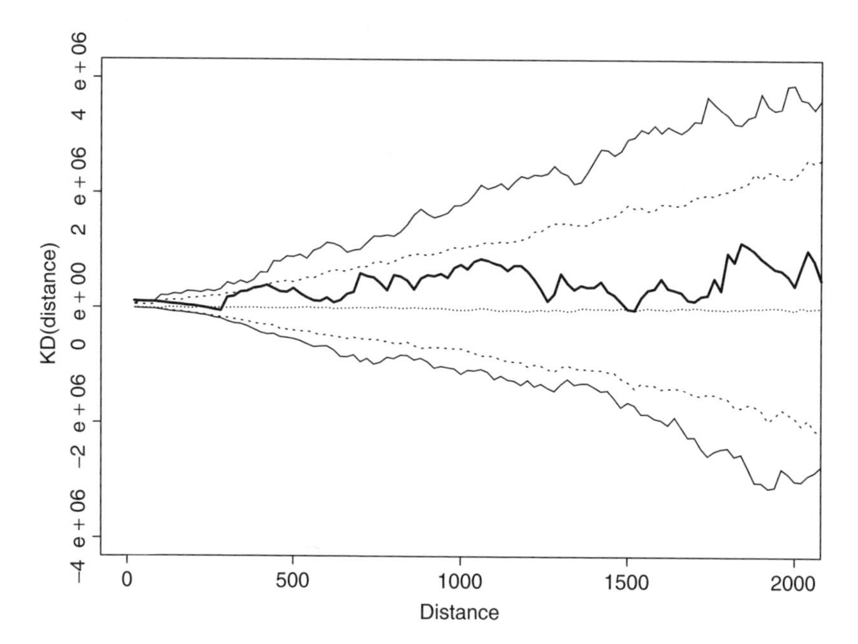

FIG. 6.6 Difference between K function for cases and that for controls for the medieval grave site data. Dashed lines represent the upper and lower bounds of pointwise Monte Carlo 90% tolerance limits calculated from 499 random labelings of cases and controls. The dotted line connects the median difference from the 499 random labelings.

intensity functions above. There we only observed a few, tight-knit regions with elevated relative risk of being a case (affected) versus being a control (nonaffected) for small bandwidths. The results in Figure 6.6 reflect this assessment by suggesting a slightly increased probability of cases near other cases, but only for small distances.

We contrast the global test of clustering based on the integrated log relative risk function defined in equation (6.6) and that based on KD_+. The former addresses the question "Do cases and controls tend to occur in the same locations?" and the latter addresses the question "Do cases tend to occur near other cases in the same manner that controls tend to occur near other controls?" For instance, it would be possible for $KD(h)$ to be near zero for all distances h but still have different intensity functions, since second-order summaries do provide inference regarding the locations of any local modes in the intensity functions.

6.5 SCANNING LOCAL RATES

While the point process summaries outlined in Sections 6.4.3 and 6.4.4 most closely follow methods for the analysis of spatial point processes introduced in Chapter 5, calculation of intensity and K-function estimates typically remain outside the standard set of tools in most statistical and geographic information system software packages. As a result, the literature includes a variety of other tests for assessing clusters and clustering, many based on particular properties of the heterogeneous point process (e.g., the number of events in an area follows a Poisson distribution), but constructed from statistics more readily available in standard software tools.

To explore such approaches, we next focus on a collection of methods for case–control point data based on comparisons of local rate estimates (e.g., methods assessing whether the ratio of cases to controls appears "significantly" elevated in certain areas). Although such methods are similar in spirit to the comparisons of intensity functions outlined above, recall intensity ratios compare the expected number of cases per unit area to the expected number of controls per unit area, whereas the methods below either compare rates (cases per persons at risk) or case/control ratios (number of cases compared to the number of controls) between different areas.

6.5.1 Goals

The primary goal of comparisons of local rates (or case/control ratios) is to determine areas where the observed rate (or ratio) appears inconsistent with the rate (or ratio) observed over the rest of the study area. As such, the approaches focus primarily on tests to detect *clusters* rather than tests of *clustering*.

6.5.2 Assumptions and Typical Output

As mentioned above, scans of local rates or case/control ratios typically seek to find the most unusual aggregation(s) of cases (i.e., the most likely clusters). The methods listed below build from basic geographic information system (GIS) operations such as calculating distances from a point, and counting case and control events occurring within a specified polygon or circle. Usually, the approach considers a set of potential clusters and ranks them by the unusualness of each. The use of statistical significance (e.g., a p-value for each potential cluster) as a measure of "unusualness" complicates statistical inference of individual clusters due to multiple testing issues, especially when potential clusters overlap and share individual cases.

Tests based on scans of local rates or case/control ratios often condition on the set of all locations and operationalize the conceptual null hypothesis of no clustering through a random labeling or a constant risk hypothesis where the effective difference hinges on whether or not the total number of cases remains fixed across simulations, respectively. By conditioning on the total number of locations, the operational difference between the random labeling and the constant risk hypotheses reduces to the difference between conducting simulations conditional or not conditional on the total number of cases (N_1), respectively.

The typical output of these methods includes a map containing an indication of the location(s) of the most likely cluster(s), often accompanied by some measure of the statistical significance of these cluster(s).

6.5.3 Method: Geographical Analysis Machine

The geographical analysis machine (GAM) of Openshaw et al. (1988) provides the prototype for the methods below. The GAM involves an algorithm for a systematic search of potential clusters and mapping of the most unusual collections of cases. At each of a fine grid of locations covering the study area, the user centers a circle of a prespecified radius (typically larger than the grid spacing in order for circles to overlap), counts the number of cases occurring within the circle, and draws the circle on the map if the count observed within the circle exceeds some tolerance level. Openshaw et al. (1988) define their tolerance level via random labeling; in particular, they draw the circle if its observed count exceeds all of the counts associated with that circle under 499 random labeling simulations. The GAM also considers a variety of circle radii in order to capture a variety of geographic sizes of potential clusters. All operations involve basic GIS functions allowing automation of the process. Subsequent modifications of the GAM replace case counts with rates or case/control ratios within each circle to account for spatial heterogeneity in the population at risk.

Openshaw et al. (1988) suggest the use of a very fine grid and a relatively large radius for each circle, resulting in a large overlap between neighboring circles and a high degree of correlation between rates estimated in adjacent circles (since they share most of the same cases). That is, if one circle meets the plotting criterion, many neighboring circles will also resulting in a map containing "blobs" of circles. The circles of the GAM are conceptually similar to circular uniform kernels; in fact, one can construct kernel estimates in a GAM-like fashion, as we will see in Section 6.5.4. However, the computational implementation differs. In the GAM, we center circles on grid locations, and in kernel estimation we center kernels around data locations. The GAM approach utilizes standard GIS operations (i.e., buffering and point-in-polygon routines), offering some advantage over the kernel approach for GIS implementation, although an increasing number of GIS packages (or add-on modules) include some sort of kernel estimation routines.

Early critics of the GAM faulted its somewhat ad hoc statistical basis and the large number of blobs drawn, leading to many false positive clusters due to the large degree of overlap between circles. However, Openshaw (1990) stresses that the goal of the GAM was not to provide a statistical test to detect clusters per se, but rather, an automated spatial surveillance tool to identify areas of potential concern.

The GAM influenced development of several related methods, including a "thinned" GAM (Fotheringham and Zhan 1996) where the user only plots a simple random sample of circles meeting the plotting criterion, thereby reducing some of the spurious blobs, consisting of only one or two circles, and focusing attention on blobs consisting of greater numbers of individual circles. Other approaches take the basic structure of GAM operations and consider a variety of techniques for providing associated statistical inference. We present several methods rooted in GAM ideas in the sections below.

6.5.4 Method: Overlapping Local Case Proportions

Rushton and Lolonis (1996) propose an exploratory method for assessing spatial variation in disease risk in case–control point data that bears similarity to both the GAM and the ratio of intensity estimators. We first define a grid of points covering the study area and, as with the GAM, consider a set of overlapping circles centered at each grid point. Unlike the GAM, Rushton and Lolonis (1996) propose using radii slightly smaller than the grid spacing, considerably reducing the number of circles sharing any particular event.

Next, we determine the number of case events and control events occurring within each circle and calculate the ratio of the number of cases to the number of cases and controls. The result is a local *case proportion*, the proportion of cases among events near each grid point. Since the circles overlap and share neighboring cases and controls, these ratios exhibit (positive) spatial correlation. The strength of this autocorrelation will vary based on the relationship between the circle radii and the grid spacing, both defined by the user. To avoid local estimated case proportions based on very few event locations, Rushton and Lolonis (1996) suggest only mapping values for circles containing a user-defined minimum number of events (cases or controls).

Rushton and Lolonis (1996) consider a Monte Carlo assessment of statistical significance conditional on the set of all locations. Within each simulation, we assign a case–control label to each location independently with probability $N_1/(N_0 + N_1)$ (i.e., the number of cases divided by the total number of locations). Although this involves random labeling of case and control locations, note the subtle difference from the random labeling hypothesis as applied previously. In the examples above, each random labeling simulation resulted in N_1 cases, and here the total number of cases varies from simulation to simulation (with an expected value of N_1). As a result, the Monte Carlo approach of Rushton and Lolonis (1996) also reflects a sort of constant risk hypothesis, where *risk* corresponds to the probability that any event location receives a "case" assignment. The simulation approach yields a Monte Carlo significance value for each grid location.

Rushton and Lolonis (1996) consider an application based on the spatial distribution of low birth weight among the population of registered live births in Des Moines, Iowa for 1983–1990. Since they have event locations for all persons under study (i.e., the set of controls represents all noncases in the study area), their local rate estimates correspond to incidence rates (incidence proportions), and their approach assesses spatial variations in local rates compared to a constant risk hypothesis. In more general application where we have a set of controls (most likely sampled from all noncases), direct application of the approach of Rushton and Lolonis (1996) results in assessment of spatial variations in the local proportion of cases within the set of cases and controls compared to a hybrid constant proportion/random labeling null hypothesis.

We note that the local Monte Carlo significance values (associated with each grid point) will also be positively spatially autocorrelated, again due to the overlapping circles, and just as was the case in consideration of the ratio of intensity estimates in Section 6.4.3, the local assessment of significance provides pointwise local inference rather than a global test of clustering. The number of pointwise significance values and their inherent correlation makes proper adjustment for multiple testing difficult, so we limit conclusions to suggestion of clusters rather than definitive identification of significant clusters.

DATA BREAK: Early Medieval Grave Sites (*cont.*) To illustrate the approach, we apply the method of Rushton and Lolonis (1996) to the medieval grave site data. We define a grid with points approximately 325 units apart in both the u and v directions and a radius of approximately 300 units. DMAP (Disease Mapping and Analysis Program), the software package implementing the approach of Rushton and Lolonis (1996), references locations in latitude and longitude, so precise distances in two dimensions depend on map projections and geodesy as outlined in Chapter 3.

Figure 6.7 illustrates contour plots of the estimated local case proportions (left) and a plot of the associated local Monte Carlo p-values (right). The "$\times$" symbols in the case proportion plot indicate grid points meeting a user-defined criterion of containing at least two (case or control) events, thereby omitting estimation and inference outside the study area and for areas within the study area with sparse collections of controls. The p-value plot (on the right) only reports p-values for the subset of these locations with at least one case in the circle (i.e., a nonzero estimate of the local case proportion). We note that (in general) the contour plot of the local case proportion displays a spatial pattern similar to that seen in the log ratio of intensity (density) functions shown in Figures 6.2–6.4 using the log ratio of intensity functions, particularly for small bandwidths.

In fact, the method of Rushton and Lolonis (1996) is very similar to the ratio of intensity estimators using circular uniform kernels. The methods are equivalent

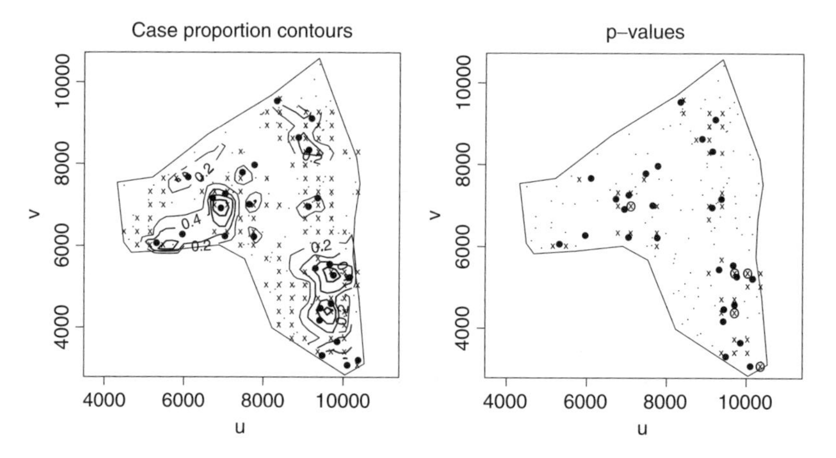

FIG. 6.7 Contour maps of local case proportions (left) and associated pointwise Monte Carlo p-values (right) based on 499 simulations under a constant case proportion (see text). Large black dots represent affected sites. The small "×" symbols in the case proportion plot represent grid points with a circle of radius of 300 units containing at least two controls (i.e., grid points with calculated local ratios). Small "×" symbols in the p-value plot represent locations with nonzero estimated local case proportions. Circled "×" symbols in the p-value plot represent locations with Monte Carlo local p-values less than 0.05.

if we replace local case proportions with local case/control ratios (the ratio of the number of cases to the number of controls in each circle), and if we only exclude circles containing no controls (where the case/control ratio is undefined). Prince et al. (2001) do precisely this, applying the method of Kelsall and Diggle (1995b) with circular uniform kernels to assess spatial variations in the incidence of primary biliary cirrhosis in a set of cases and controls in northeast England. To see the relationship between the ratio of intensities and the method of Rushton and Lolonis (1996) applied to case/control ratios, suppose that we wish to estimate the case/control ratio at each of a set of grid points (thereby allowing a contour or surface plot). As noted above in Section 6.5.3, counting cases and controls within circles centered at grid points more readily utilizes standard GIS operations than does counting the number of kernels (centered at case or control locations) overlapping each grid point.

Figure 6.8 illustrates the equivalence between the two approaches and the different types of calculation involved. In the left-hand plot, the circle around the central grid point contains two cases and two controls leading to a (local) case/control ratio of 1. In the right-hand plot, the central grid point falls within two control and two case kernel boundaries. Since this point receives zero kernel weight from any other case or control, the ratio of intensity functions is also 1. Finally, Figure 6.9 contrasts the one-dimensional uniform kernel (bandwidth 300 units) to the quartic and Gaussian kernels used in Figures 6.2–6.4. As with the quartic kernel, the uniform kernel assigns no weight to observations beyond the bandwidth.

The equivalence between the local case/control ratios and the ratio of intensity (density) estimates raises two issues regarding selection of the grid points and the

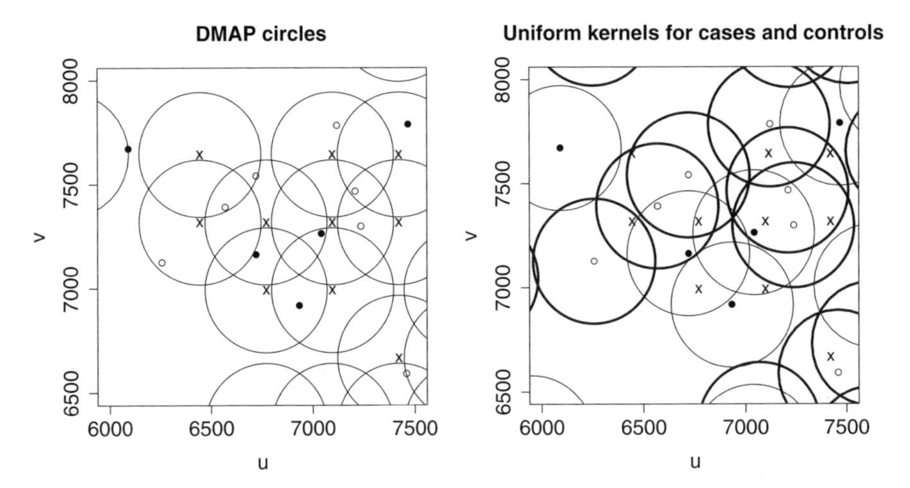

FIG. 6.8 Equivalence between the case/control ratio within circles surrounding grid points (left-hand plot) and the ratio of intensity (density) functions based on circular uniform kernels (right-hand plot). Case locations appear as filled small circles, control locations as open small circles, and grid points as "×" symbols. In the left-hand plot, large circles represent radii of 300 units around each grid point. In the right-hand plot, dark circles represent control kernel radii, and lighter circles represent control kernel radii (both 300 units).

circle radii. First, Rushton and Lolonis (1996) describe the choice of circle radii as a compromise between the overall smoothness of the surface and the ability to discern local peaks and valleys, precisely equivalent to the role of bandwidth selection. Although Rushton and Lolonis (1996) do not specifically require that the circle radius be less than the distance between grid points, their examples do suggest that such a restriction and the current version of the DMAP package will not accept radii larger than the grid spacing. Such a restriction constrains our analysis of the grave site data, since we would like fairly small grid spacing (to provide estimates for much of the study area), but small bandwidths allow inclusion of only a few events in each circle. Viewing the circle diameters as kernel bandwidths indicates that no such limit is needed, and Prince et al. (2001) utilize a cross-validation approach to choose bandwidths (circle radii), unconstrained by grid spacing. Second, for relatively sparse data (such as the grave site data), perhaps nonuniform kernels provide better performance as kernel weights decrease more gradually than the uniform kernel, allowing additional events to have diminishing (but nonzero) impact as distance increases.

A few features of our application merit attention. First, the output of the method of Rushton and Lolonis (1996) is limited to circles meeting our (user-defined) criterion of a minimum of two events (case or control). The low-birth-weight data considered by Rushton and Lolonis (1996) contain 2406 case locations and a large number of controls (8506 non-low-birth-weight births in Des Moines, Iowa, over a period of eight years), and similarly, the analysis of Prince et al. (2001) includes over 3000 controls. However, the grave site data contain only 143 event locations,

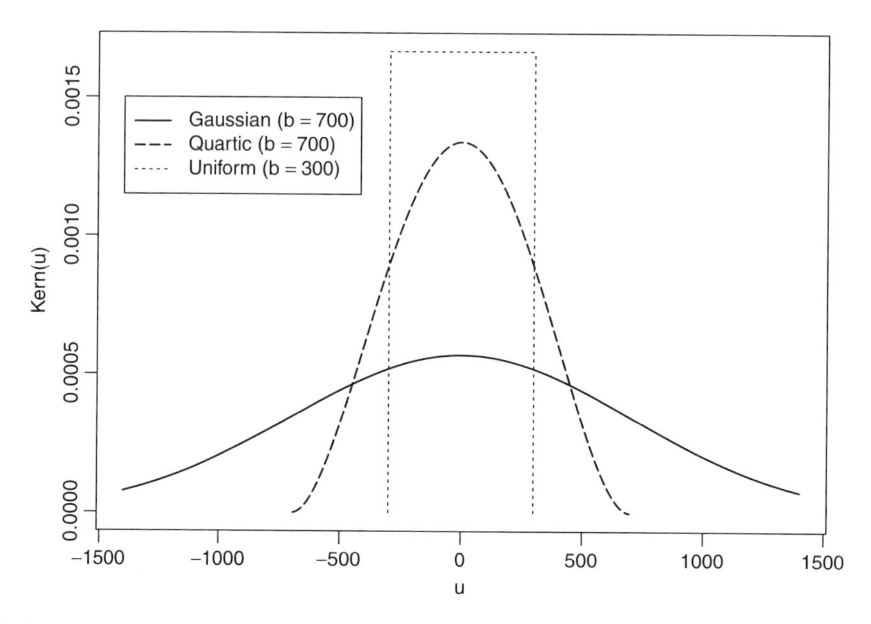

FIG. 6.9 Comparison of the one-dimensional Gaussian, quartic, and uniform kernels for bandwidths 700, 700, and 300, respectively.

limiting estimation to those grid points indicated by a "×" symbol in Figure 6.7. In addition, the overall case proportion (30/143) is much higher than the typical disease rates considered in public health applications of tests of clusters and clustering. Together, the relatively small number of controls, the relatively large overall case proportion, and a fairly tight grid result in circles with very small numbers of cases and controls.

Our choice of a minimum number of events is a compromise between maintaining coverage of a large proportion of the study area with a tight enough grid to provide local variations in the case proportions. However, the choice is not particularly satisfactory, since it results in many circles containing zero cases, providing a local case proportion of zero for many of the circles meeting the "greater than two cases or controls" criterion. In addition, the circles contain between two and six controls and between zero and three cases, so the possible observed values of the case/control ratio are severely limited. For example, circles containing two events can only experience case proportions of 0.0, 0.5, or 1.0 in each simulation (resulting in the relative high number of 0.5 values observed in the left-hand plot in Figure 6.10). The highly discrete distribution of the case proportions also limits the observable pointwise p-values, as illustrated in Figure 6.10, a feature not immediately obvious from the contours displayed in Figure 6.7. (Recall that under the null hypothesis, p-values will follow a uniform distribution for test statistics with continuous distributions; see, e.g., Sackrowitz and Samuel-Cahn 1999.)

This example illustrates both the type of output of the method of Rushton and Lolonis (1996) and the sort of care that one should take in interpreting the output

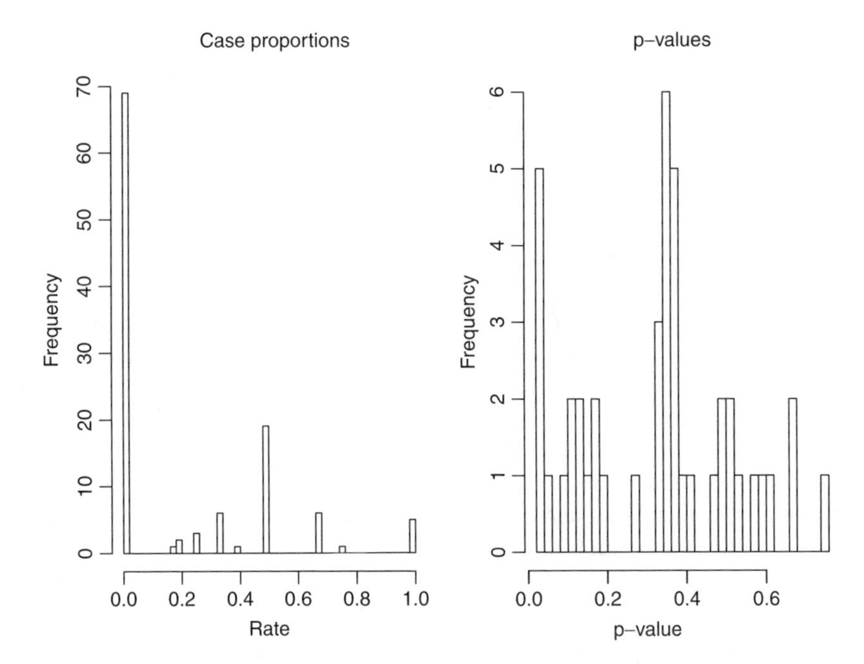

FIG. 6.10 Histograms of estimated local case proportions (left) and local p-values (right), across all grid points containing at least two event locations. Note the highly discrete distribution of the local case proportions, due to the fairly small number of controls expected within 300 units of each grid point.

maps, especially for modest numbers of events. In addition, the example highlights the interpretation of the output as case proportions, which approximate disease rates for a rare disease (where the ratio of cases to cases and controls approximates the ratio of cases to the number at risk), but do not when controls represent a sample of noncases.

6.5.5 Method: Spatial Scan Statistics

Scan statistics provide another approach similar to the local case/control ratios of Rushton and Lolonis (1996). A scan statistic involves definition of a moving "window" and a statistical comparison of a measurement (e.g., a count or a rate) within the window to the same sort of measurement outside the window. A large literature exists on the theoretical aspects of scan statistics in one dimension (cf. Glaz et al. 2001) and their application to the detection of temporal clusters of disease (Wallenstein 1980; Sahu et al. 1993; Wallenstein et al. 1993).

Kulldorff (1997) defines a spatial scan statistic very similar to the GAM and the method of Rushton and Lolonis (1996), but with a slightly different inferential framework. As with the two preceding methods, the primary goal of a scan statistic is to find the collection(s) of cases least consistent with the null hypothesis [i.e., the most likely cluster(s)]. Kulldorff (1997) goes a bit further and seeks to provide a significance value representing the detected cluster's "unusualness," with an adjustment for multiple testing.

Like Openshaw et al. (1988) and Rushton and Lolonis (1996), Kulldorff (1997) considers circular windows with variable radii ranging from the smallest observed distance between a pair of cases to a user-defined upper bound (e.g., one-half the width of the study area). The spatial scan statistic may be applied to circles centered at either grid locations (like the previous two methods) or the set of observed case–control locations, but note that these two options define different sets of potential clusters, and therefore may not provide exactly the same answers, particularly for very spatially heterogeneous patterns.

Kulldorff (1997) builds an inferential structure based on earlier work where Loader (1991) and Nagarwalla (1996) note that variable-width one-dimensional scan statistics represent collections of local likelihood ratio tests comparing a null hypothesis of the constant risk hypothesis compared to alternatives where the disease rate within the scanning window is greater than that outside the window. Let $N_{1,\text{in}}$ and $N_{\text{in}} = N_{0,\text{in}} + N_{1,\text{in}}$ denote the number of case locations and persons at risk (number of case *and* control locations) inside a particular window, respectively, and similarly, define $N_{1,\text{out}}$ and $N_{\text{out}} = N_{1,\text{out}} + N_{0,\text{out}}$ for outside the window. The overall test statistic is proportional to

$$T_{\text{scan}} = \max_{\text{all windows}} \left(\frac{N_{1,\text{in}}}{N_{\text{in}}}\right)^{N_{1,\text{in}}} \left(\frac{N_{1,\text{out}}}{N_{\text{out}}}\right)^{N_{1,\text{out}}} I\left(\frac{N_{1,\text{in}}}{N_{\text{in}}} > \frac{N_{1,\text{out}}}{N_{\text{out}}}\right), \tag{6.7}$$

where $I(\cdot)$ denotes the indicator function (i.e., we only maximize over windows where the observed rate inside the window exceeds that outside the window). Although developed for circular windows, the general structure of T_{scan} allows application for other shapes of clusters (e.g., within 0.5 mile of a particular stream, or a highway).

The maximum observed likelihood ratio statistic provides a test of overall general clustering and an indication of the most likely cluster(s), with significance determined by Monte Carlo testing of the constant risk hypothesis. The Monte Carlo method differs somewhat from those proposed above and merits a detailed description. The GAM and the method of Rushton and Lolonis (1996) raise multiple testing issues by assessing the unusualness of each possible cluster. However, the spatial scan statistic focuses attention on the single potential cluster generating the maximum likelihood ratio statistic [equation (6.7)]. As mentioned above, all methods in this section, including the spatial scan statistic, provide results conditional on the set of all case–control locations. As a result, the infinite number of potential clusters defined by the infinite possible radii considered generates only a finite number of test statistic values since the test statistic defined in equation (6.7) only changes for radii where an additional case or control location joins the potential clusters. However, the number of potential clusters remains large. Following a Monte Carlo approach proposed by Turnbull et al. (1990) (outlined in Section 7.3.4), Kulldorff (1997) randomly assigns cases to the set of all locations (a random labeling assignment), calculates and stores the test statistic [equation (6.7)], and repeats several times, thereby obtaining a Monte Carlo estimate of the distribution of the test statistic under a random labeling null hypothesis.

As a result, the spatial scan statistic provides a single p-value for the study area, suggesting that it is a test of clustering. However, the test statistic observed is generated by a well-defined set of cases, and we can map the potential cluster generating the test statistic value observed, thereby identifying the most likely cluster. So, in a sense, the spatial scan statistic provides both a test of clustering and a test to detect the most likely cluster. We tend to favor the latter categorization, as the term *clustering* as described in Section 6.2 tends to refer to a pattern of clustering over the entire study area rather than the presence of a single cluster, as suggested by the spatial scan statistic.

The literature contains a considerable number of applications of the spatial scan statistic and space–time extensions (cf. Kulldorff et al. 1998; Hjalmars et al. 1999; Viel et al. 2000; Gregorio et al. 2001; Sankoh et al. 2001) due in part to the availability of SaTScan, a free software package developed and distributed by the U.S. National Cancer Institute.

DATA BREAK: Early Medieval Grave Sites (*cont.*) We utilize the SaTScan package to apply the spatial scan statistic to the medieval grave site data. We consider potential clusters centered around all case and control locations, with radii varying from the minimum interevent distance (between cases, controls, or case–control pairs) up to half of the maximum interevent distance. Figure 6.11 indicates the most likely cluster occurs in and covers much of the lower right section of the map, very similar to the areas with high log relative risk (based on the ratio of intensities) (Figures 6.2–6.4) and the smoothed case/control ratios (Figure 6.7). The most likely cluster has a p-value of 0.067 based on 999 simulations, again suggesting relatively weak statistical evidence for any clustering (or clusters) in the data.

6.6 NEAREST-NEIGHBOR STATISTICS

6.6.1 Goals

We next turn to a class of methods based on characteristics of the nearest neighbors of case–control point event locations. Rather than examine point process summaries or estimated local rates or case/control ratios, these methods examine local patterns of cases in the vicinity of other cases. Evidence for clustering involves observing more cases among the nearest neighbors of cases than one would expect under the random labeling hypothesis. Simply put, the method seeks an answer to the question: Are there more cases than we would expect under random labeling in the q locations nearest each case?

6.6.2 Assumptions and Typical Output

By the nature of the question of interest, nearest-neighbor statistics summarize clustering behavior across the study area and therefore provide tests of clustering rather than tests to detect clusters. Such tests typically derive inference under a random labeling hypothesis and as a result, are conditional on the set of all case–control

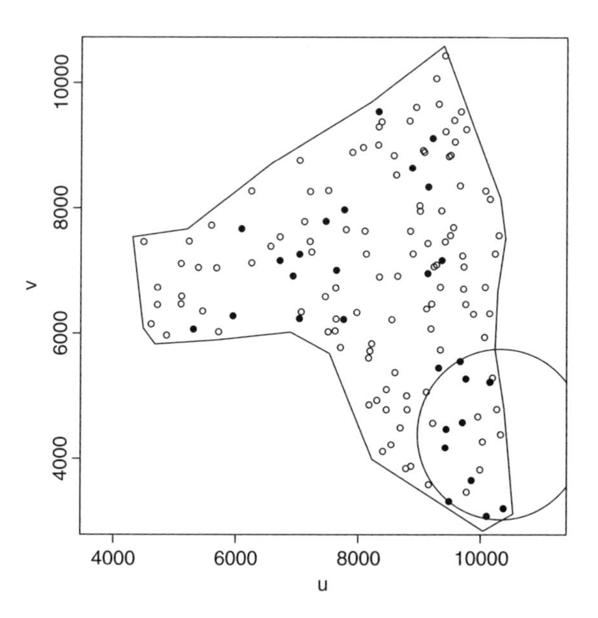

FIG. 6.11 The spatial scan statistic's most likely cluster for the medieval grave site data with Monte Carlo p-value 0.067 based on 999 simulations (see text). Filled circles represent affected sites (cases) and empty circles represent nonaffected sites (controls). The method selects from among circular clusters centered at each case or control location and radii varying from the minimum distance between any pair of case or control locations up to half the extent of the study area.

locations. The output involves an overall p-value summarizing the significance of the clustering observed compared to patterns expected under random labeling.

6.6.3 Method: q Nearest Neighbors of Cases

Independent of one another, Cuzick and Edwards (1990) and Alt and Vach (1991) developed identical random labeling approaches based on the nearest-neighbor properties observed in case–control point data. Specifically, for N_1 case and N_0 control locations ($N = N_0 + N_1$ locations in all), the test statistic represents the number of the q nearest neighbors of cases that are also cases. The user defined q then calculates the nearest-neighbor adjacency matrix $\boldsymbol{W} = \{w_{i,j}\}$, where

$$w_{i,j} = \begin{cases} 1 & \text{if location } j \text{ is among } q \text{ nearest neighbors of location } i \\ 0 & \text{otherwise.} \end{cases} \tag{6.8}$$

Both Cuzick and Edwards (1990) and Alt and Vach (1991) consider the test statistic

$$\begin{aligned} T_q &= \sum_{i=1}^{N} \sum_{j=1}^{N} w_{i,j} \delta_i \delta_j \qquad (6.9) \\ &= \boldsymbol{\delta}' \boldsymbol{W} \boldsymbol{\delta}, \end{aligned}$$

where $\delta_i = 1$ if the ith location represents a case, $\delta_i = 0$ if the ith location represents a control, and $\boldsymbol{\delta} = (\delta_1, \delta_2, \ldots, \delta_N)'$ is the vector of case indicators for all (case and control) locations. Note that equation (6.9) simply accumulates the number of times $\delta_i = \delta_j = 1$ (both locations are cases) and location j is in the q nearest neighbors of location i.

For inference, Cuzick and Edwards (1990) provide an asymptotic normal distribution; however, Monte Carlo tests under the random labeling hypothesis are applicable for any sample size. As described in Section 5.2.3, the rank of the test statistic based on the data observed among the values based on the randomly labeled data allows calculation of the p-value associated with the test.

Different values of q may generate different results, possibly indicating the scale (in the sense of the number of nearest neighbors, not necessarily geographic distance) of any clustering observed. However, T_{q_2} is correlated T_{q_1} for $q_1 < q_2$ since the q_2 nearest neighbors include the q_1 nearest neighbors since we condition on the set of all locations, somewhat complicating any adjustment for multiple testing in the use of multiple values of q. Ord (1990) suggests the contrasts between statistics (e.g., $T_{q_2} - T_{q_1}$) which exhibit considerably less correlation and may provide more direct inference regarding the spatial scale of any clustering tendencies observed. The contrasts are interpreted as excess cases *between* the q_1 and the q_2 nearest neighbors of cases. As above, any conclusions regarding scale are with respect to the neighbor relationships, not necessarily geographic distance.

As described above, the Cuzick and Edwards (1990) and Alt and Vach (1991) approach is a general test of clustering. Cuzick and Edwards (1990) also describe its use as a focused test of clustering by considering only the q nearest neighbors to a fixed set of foci locations, and defining the test statistic as the total number cases among the q nearest neighbors *of the foci*. Inference again follows via Monte Carlo testing under the random labeling hypothesis.

Jacquez (1994) proposes an extension to the method of Cuzick and Edwards (1990) for application when case and control locations are not known exactly; rather, cases and controls are assigned to centroids of enumeration districts.

Published health-related applications of the method of Cuzick and Edwards (1990) include assessments of spatial patterns of childhood leukemia and non-Hodgkin's lymphoma (Alexander et al. 1992; Dockerty et al. 1999), assessments of rodent bites in New York City (Childs et al. 1998), and assessments of patterns of infections in cattle and horses (Singer et al. 1998; Doherr et al. 1999).

DATA BREAK: Early Medieval Grave Sites (*cont.*) We next apply the Cuzick and Edwards (1990)/Alt and Vach (1991) q nearest-neighbor statistics to the medieval grave site data. [Incidentally, the grave site data originally appear in Alt and Vach (1991) and served as the primary motivation for their approach.]

To illustrate the approach, arrows go from each affected site to each of its three nearest neighbors in Figure 6.12. The value of the test statistic T_3 is simply the number of these nearest neighbors that are also affected (cases). Note that the statistic will count some affected sites more than once (affected sites that are within the three nearest neighbors of more one affected site). For example, consider the collection of cases in the southernmost portion of the study area

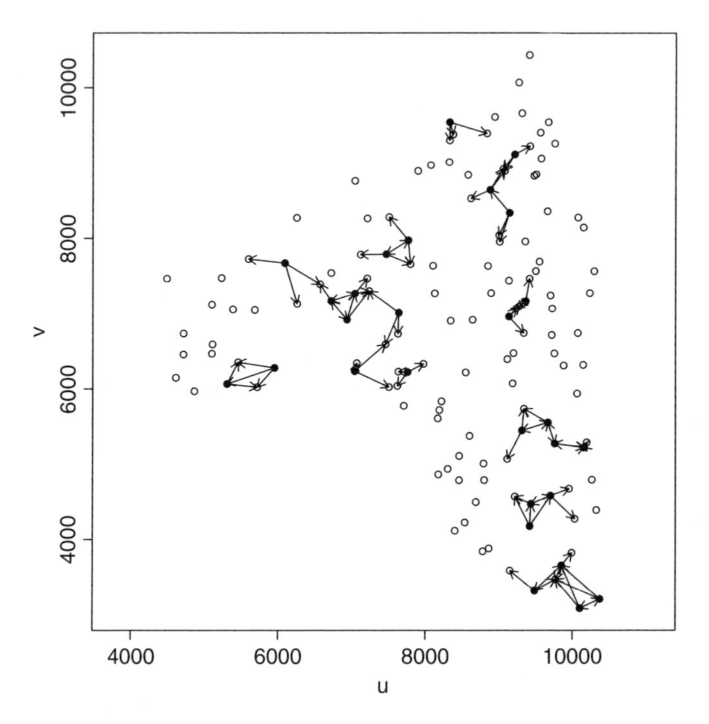

FIG. 6.12 Three nearest neighbors of each affected site for the medieval grave site data. Filled circles represent affected sites (cases), and open circles represent nonaffected sites (controls). Arrows point from each case to its three nearest neighbors.

[near location (10000,4000)]. Also note that the nearest-neighbor relationship is not reciprocal. For example, consider the three affected sites near location (6000, 6000) (recall from Figure 5.8 that the western affected site is actually two sites very close together).

Table 6.2 gives test statistics and associate p-values (based on 499 random labeling simulations) for a variety of values of q. All numbers of nearest neighbors suggest statistically significant clustering among the cases. To determine whether the tendency for clustering occurs among large or small groups of affected sites, we follow the suggestion of Ord (1990) and consider the contrasts presented in Table 6.3. Since none of the contrasts suggest significant clustering of affected sites outside the three nearest neighbors, we conclude that the significant clustering observed among collections of more than three nearest neighbors is driven primarily by clustering among the three nearest neighbors.

The medieval data set provides another interesting example of the methodology. How can we observe significant *clustering* but not find significant *clusters*? As in Section 6.4.4, the data suggest a pattern of clustering at small distances (i.e., between events falling within the three nearest neighbors of affected sites). These clusters appear to be quite small and involve only a few affected (case) sites each. Such small clusters are difficult to detect individually (without using very small

Table 6.2 Observed Test Statistics, T_q (Number of Cases within the q Nearest Neighbors of Other Cases), for the Medieval Grave Site Data[a]

Number of Nearest Neighbors (q)	T_q	Monte Carlo p-Value (Based on 499 Simulations)
3	32	0.002
5	45	0.010
7	58	0.028
9	73	0.016
11	91	0.016
13	109	0.006
15	122	0.010

[a] 499 random labeling simulations define Monte Carlo p-values.

Table 6.3 Observed Contrasts $T_{q_2} - T_{q_1}$ between Test Statistics (Number of Cases between and including the q_1 and q_2 Nearest Neighbors of Other Cases) for the Medieval Grave Site Data[a]

Contrast	Value	Monte Carlo p-Value (Based on 499 Simulations)
$T_5 - T_3$	13	0.490
$T_7 - T_5$	13	0.540
$T_9 - T_7$	15	0.258
$T_{11} - T_9$	18	0.106
$T_{13} - T_{11}$	18	0.108
$T_{15} - T_{13}$	13	0.492
$T_7 - T_3$	26	0.510
$T_9 - T_3$	41	0.314
$T_{11} - T_3$	59	0.154
$T_{13} - T_3$	77	0.066
$T_{15} - T_3$	90	0.078

[a] 499 random labeling simulations define Monte Carlo p-values.

bandwidths), but the general pattern appears for both the difference of K functions and the nearest-neighbor analysis.

With regard to the motivating question of whether this society tended to bury family members together, the results in the sections above do suggest some evidence for a general tendency for affected sites to occur together in small groups (in agreement with the original analysis of the data by Alt and Vach 1991), and also suggest particular areas as the most likely clusters. The results suggest areas for future fieldwork and detailed laboratory analysis of artifacts and remains recovered from these locations.

CASE STUDY: San Diego Asthma The medieval grave site data provide valuable insight into the mechanisms and application of the various methods presented in this chapter. However, these examples also reveal some limitations in application of the methods to relatively small data sets (only 30 case events). We now apply the same methods to a much larger public health data set, drawn from a study reported by English et al. (1999).

The data involve the point locations of 3302 cases and 2289 controls and reflect a subset of the original data used for a spatial substudy. Cases and controls were drawn from the MediCal paid claims database, maintained by the Medical Care Statistics Program of the California Department of Health Services in Sacramento, California. MediCal represents California's Medicaid program and pays for health care costs incurred by persons qualifying under public assistance, those who are "medically needy" (blind, disabled, elderly) or those who are medically indigent. For potential cases, English et al. (1999) consider all claims from San Diego County, California paid between January 1993 and June 1994 with a diagnosis of asthma (ICD-9 code 493) for children aged less than or equal to 14 years. English et al. (1999) select study controls from a random sample of all paid claims for the same county, time period, and age group. The control set excludes pharmacy claims (no ICD-9 diagnoses), asthma and respiratory diagnoses, and subsequent paid claims from the same person occurring in the study period). Additional details appear in English et al. (1999).

The spatial data structure mirrors that of the medieval grave site data, with point locations and corresponding case–control labels. Precise residential locations were masked geographically to preserve confidentiality by shifting each location by the same small distance and direction (Armstrong et al. 1999).

Figures 6.13 and 6.14 illustrate the point locations in the data. The polygon outline represents the boundary used for intensity (density) function estimation and K- function estimation. The western coast corresponds to the Pacific coastline, but the eastern edge is selected primarily for convenience and to avoid large empty areas. For the two point process approaches (intensity estimation and K functions), we ignore the few cases and controls residing in the more rural locations in the eastern part of the study area.

Both cases and controls exhibit spatial patterns relating to the heterogeneous distribution of children at risk. This spatial pattern reflects the distribution of children aged $\leq$14 years presenting paid claims to MediCal during the study period. We note that this probably does not reflect the spatial distribution of *all* children aged $\leq$14 years during the study period, so our inference is based on spatial patterns of asthma in children within the population of MediCal paid claims for the study period.

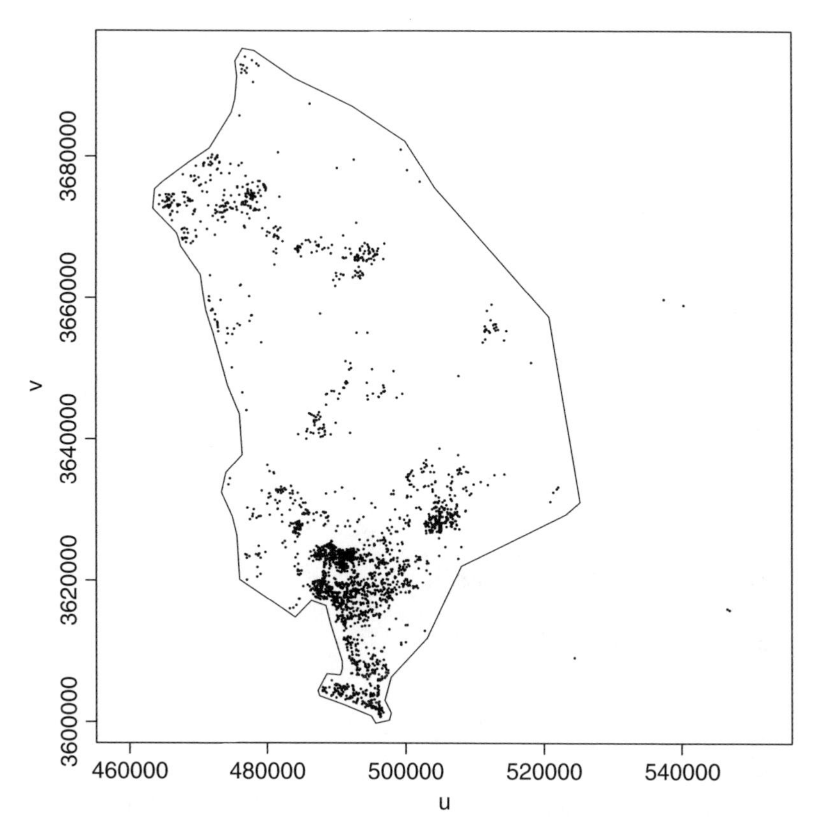

FIG. 6.13 Residence locations for 3302 MediCal claims for asthma diagnoses aged 0–14 years (cases) in San Diego County for 1993 (see text for details). The polygon defines the study area used for the ratio of intensity (density) functions and the local rate estimates.

Due to the strong background pattern, we begin by estimating the log relative risk function based on kernel density estimation. Figures 6.15 and 6.16 use Gaussian kernels with bandwidths of 2000 and 4000 distance units, respectively. For reference, the cross-validation approach defined by Kelsall and Diggle (1995b) suggests a bandwidth in the range of 3500 distance units. The top surface plots have the same vertical range, indicating the relative change in smoothness due to the increasing bandwidth. Collections of "+" and "−" symbols indicate areas where the estimated log relative risk surface is above or below (respectively) the pointwise tolerance intervals defined by 500 random labeling simulations. Both bandwidths suggest areas of local deviation from the random labeling null hypothesis, including an area of reduced risk along the eastern border. As one might expect, a higher bandwidth results in a smoother relative risk surface and larger, more connected areas of high risk. Compared to a bandwidth of 4000 units, setting the bandwidth to 2000 units provides more local detail but considerably more variation in the log relative risk surface.

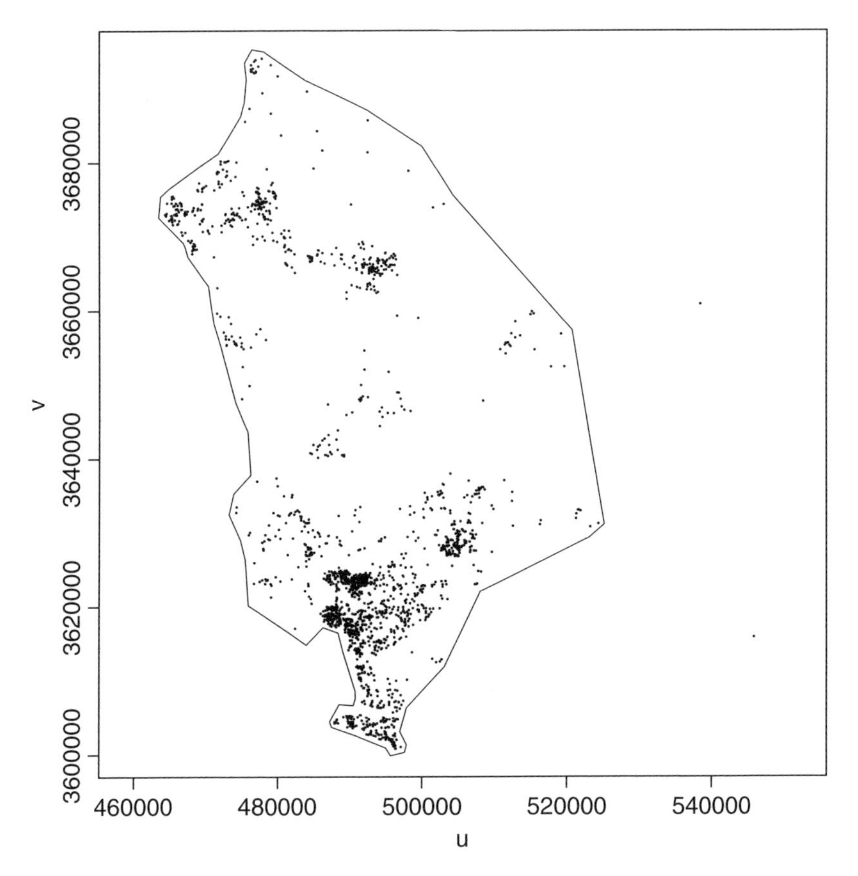

FIG. 6.14 Residence locations for 2289 MediCal nonrespiratory controls aged 0–14 years in San Diego County for 1993 (see text for details). The polygon defines the study area used for the ratio of intensity (density) functions and the local rate estimates.

Figure 6.17 reproduces the bottom plot in Figure 6.16, adding case and control locations indicating potential clusters near urban concentration of San Diego itself and near the central portion of the study area. The log relative risk surface with bandwidth 2000 units subdivides the northern cluster into smaller east and west components, and substantially reduces the suggestion of the southern cluster. We present both to illustrate the dependence of results on bandwidth and to provide comparison for the results below.

We next explore second-order properties of the case and control patterns for evidence of *clustering*. Figure 6.18 indicated the $\widehat{L}$ plots for cases and controls revealing a clear separation indicating increased clustering in the cases compared to that observed in the controls. To assess the significance of this, we display 95% tolerance envelopes based on 499 simulations under a random labeling hypothesis. The median of the simulated values corresponds to the K function of the entire set of locations (cases and controls), and the tolerance envelopes indicate that the

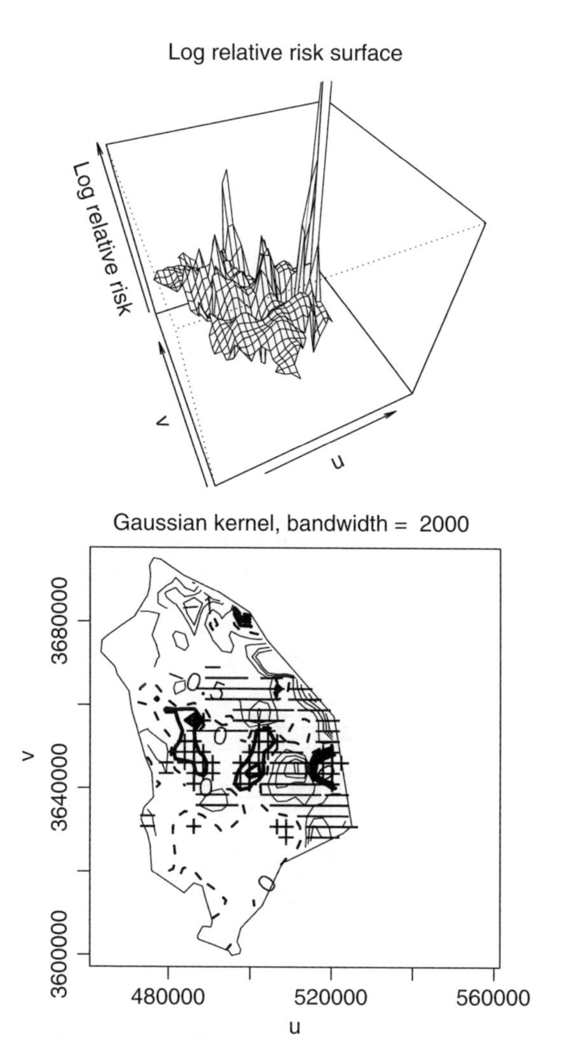

FIG. 6.15 Estimated log relative risk surface for San Diego asthma data based on a ratio of case and control density estimates (Gaussian kernels, bandwidth = 2000). The symbol "+" denotes areas with log relative risk above the upper 95% pointwise tolerance bound, and the symbol "−" denotes areas with log relative risk below the lower 95% based on 500 random labeling simulations.

observed separation between the K functions is far beyond what we would expect under random labeling.

Figure 6.19 presents the results in terms of the difference between the case and control K functions $[\widehat{KD}(\cdot)]$ further illustrating significantly more clustering among the cases than among the controls.

Next, we apply the method of Rushton and Lolonis (1996) to the San Diego data using grid spacing of 1332 units, a circle radius of 1066 units (approximate distances based on transformation from latitude and longitude), and calculating the

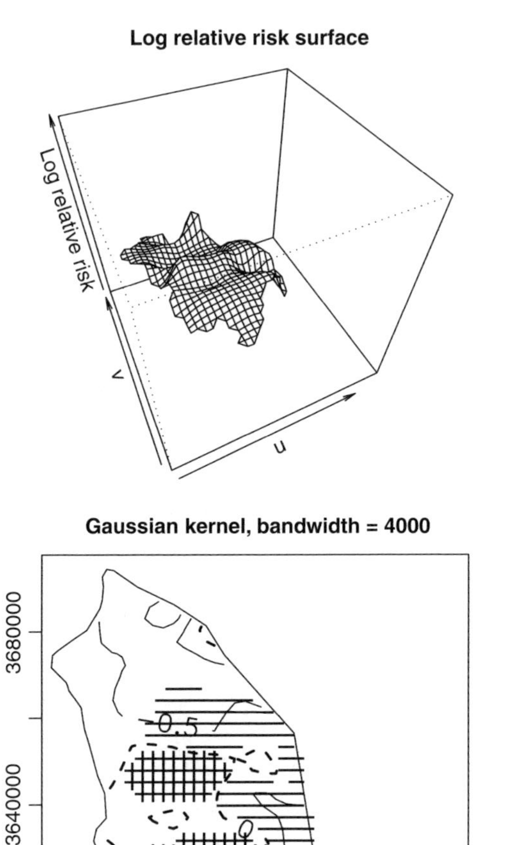

FIG. 6.16 Estimated log relative risk surface for San Diego asthma data based on a ratio of case and control density estimates (Gaussian kernels, bandwidth = 4000). The symbol "+" denotes areas with log relative risk above the upper 95% pointwise tolerance bound, and the symbol "−" denotes areas with log relative risk below the lower 95% based on 500 random labeling simulations.

local case proportion only for circles containing at least 10 events. As before, our choices for grid spacing, radii, and minimum denominator reflect a compromise between the grid resolution, stability of local estimates, and coverage of the study area. Figure 6.20 illustrates those circles meeting the minimum denominator criterion. Note the concentration of local estimates in areas with higher densities of both cases and controls, in particular the small coverage of the northern cluster(s) suggested by the log relative risk approach described above.

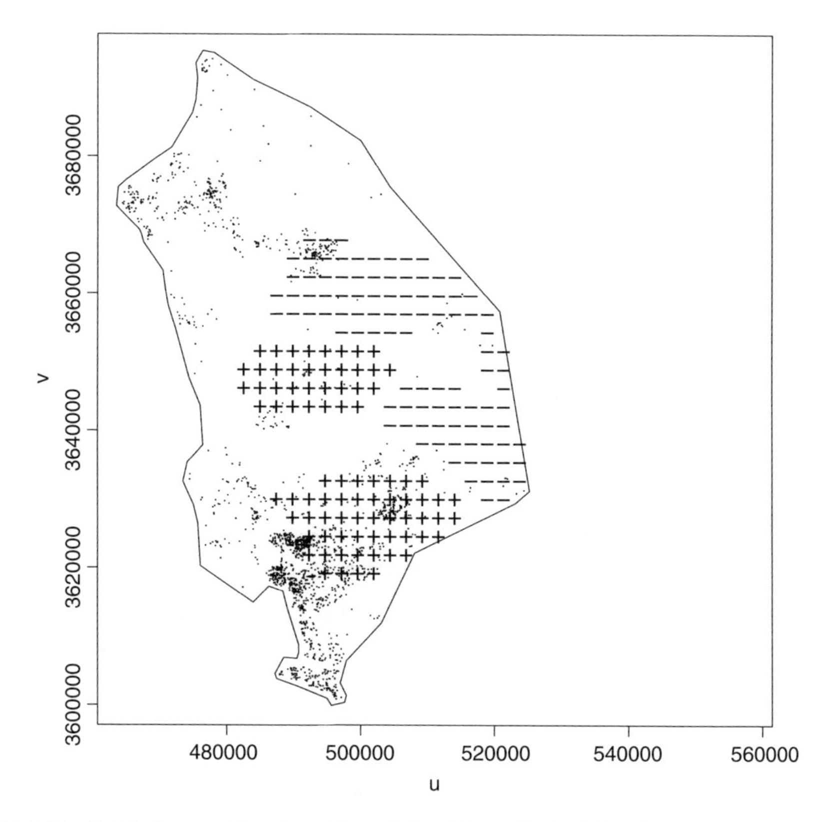

FIG. 6.17 Detail of areas with estimated log relative risk outside the 95% tolerance envelopes (Gaussian kernel, bandwidth = 4000), indicating case and control locations.

Figure 6.21 indicates local case proportions above ("+") or below ("−") the upper or lower (respectively) 90% tolerance bounds based on 500 constant case proportion simulations. The approach suggests clusters in areas corresponding to the southern cluster indicated by the ratio of density functions with bandwidth set to 4000 units. The clusters indicated here are somewhat more local due to both the radius used (limiting weight to a very local collections of cases and controls) and to the set of grid points meeting the minimum denominator criterion (10 events). This criterion results in very few estimated (or evaluated) case proportions between the collections of "+" symbols in Figure 6.21. In fact, close comparison of Figures 6.16 and 6.21 illustrates that differences between the collections of "+" symbols in the southern cluster in the two figures correspond directly to differences between the set of grid points reporting local case proportions (circles in Figure 6.20) and the set of all grid points.

Figure 6.20 suggests careful consideration of the (user-specified) lower bound on the denominator for calculating local case proportions, particularly in populations with a very heterogeneous spatial distribution. The San Diego data include concentrations of many events interspersed with empty areas containing few events,

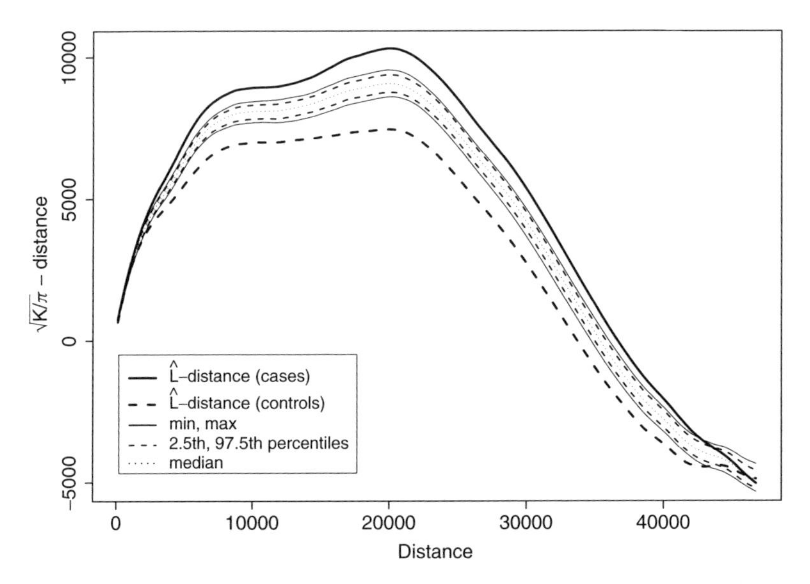

FIG. 6.18 $\widehat{L}$ plots for cases (thick solid line) and controls (thick dashed line) in the San Diego asthma data. Thin solid lines represent the minima/maxima envelope, thin dashed lines represent the 95% tolerance envelope, and the thin dotted line represents the median $\widehat{L}$ plot, all based on 500 random labeling simulations.

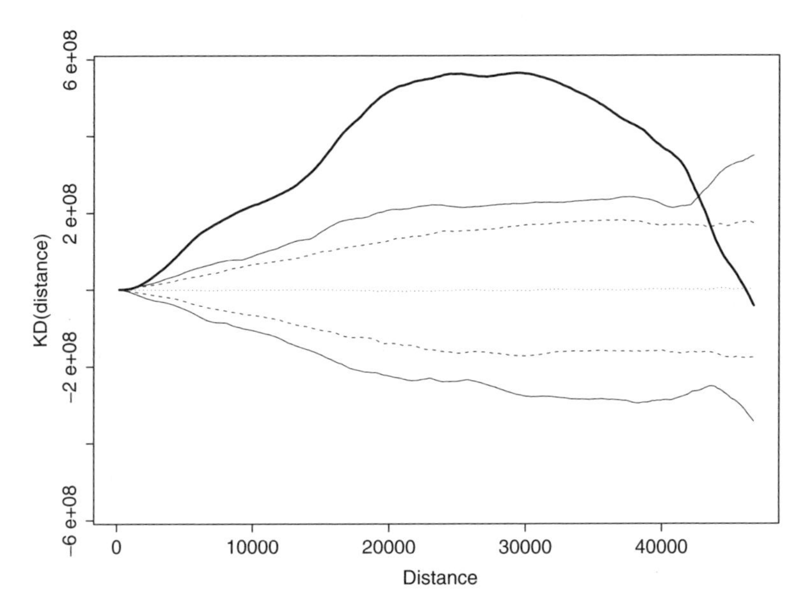

FIG. 6.19 The difference between case and control K functions for the San Diego asthma data (thick line). Thin solid lines represent the minima/maxima envelope, thin dashed lines the 95% tolerance envelope, and the thin dotted line the median difference, all based on 500 random labeling simulations.

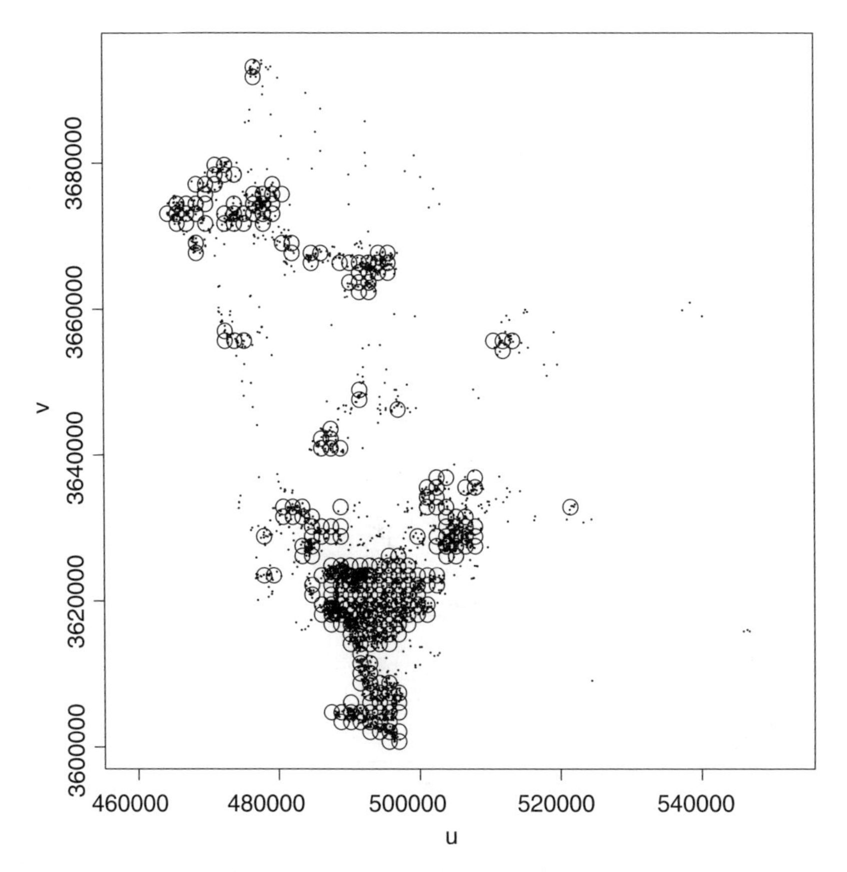

FIG. 6.20 Circles of radius approximately 1070 units, indicating grid points meeting criteria of at least 10 case and control locations. Local case/(case + control) ratios (Rushton and Lolonis 1996) calculated only for the circles shown.

again reflecting a combination of the population distribution in general and local concentrations of paid MediCal claims within San Diego county. As with our analysis of the medieval grave site data, more general kernel intensity (density) estimation may provide a more robust approach to identifying areas of excess risk than the current implementation of local case proportions found in the DMAP package. The local case proportion approach involves calculations better suited to current GIS environments, although some GISs incorporate density estimation techniques. However, as noted by Rushton and Lolonis (1996), Monte Carlo simulation remains an open area for development in the GIS arena.

Figure 6.22 illustrates the most likely cluster identified by the spatial scan statistic ($p < 0.001$). The most likely cluster appears in an area consistent with areas suggested by both the ratio of intensity (density) functions and the local case proportions. Note that our spatial scan statistic analysis considers only circular potential clusters, and given the highly heterogeneous spatial distribution of the population at

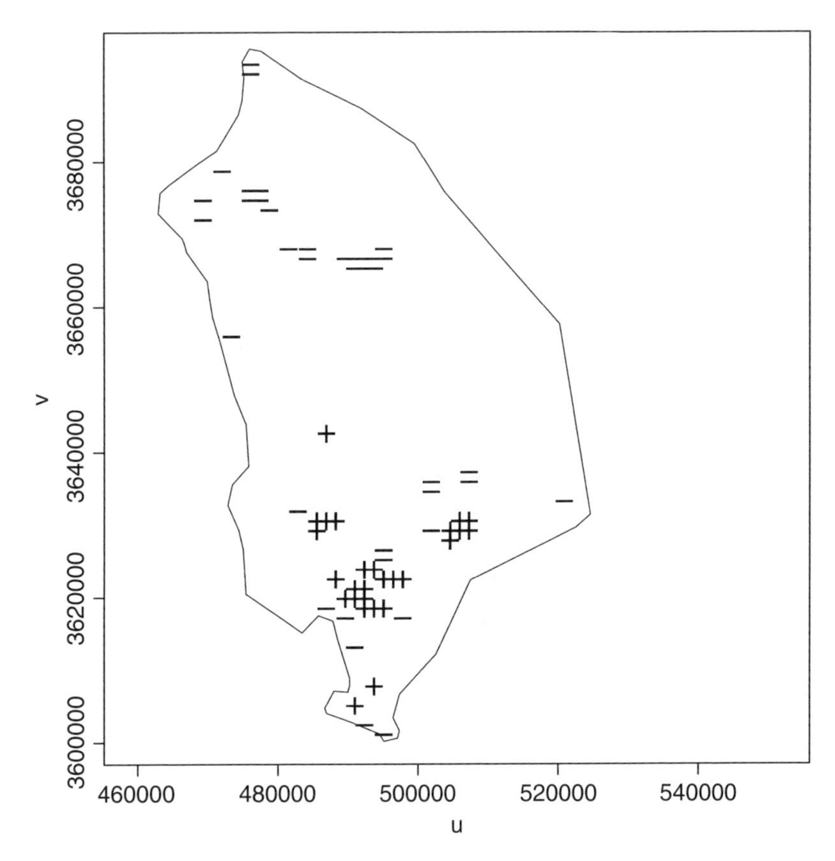

FIG. 6.21 Areas above or below 90% range of simulated case/(case + control) ratios, based on 500 constant case proportion simulations.

risk and the general shapes for clusters suggested by the ratio of intensity (density) functions and the local case proportions, elliptical or perhaps more complex shapes for potential clusters may be desirable.

Table 6.4 presents results for the data based on the q-nearest-neighbor test of *clustering* developed by Cuzick and Edwards (1990) and Alt and Vach (1991). The total number of cases within the q nearest neighbors of other cases exceeded all values generated under the random labeling hypothesis, suggesting strong evidence for clustering among the case locations. These results echo those the difference in K-function results: The overall pattern of cases is more clustered than one would expect from a random sample of 3308 cases from the 5581 total event locations.

Both the q-nearest-neighbor analysis and the comparisons of K functions indicate very strong evidence for clustering of the cases above and beyond that observed in the controls. Furthermore, the clustering pattern extends across both large distances (K functions) and large numbers of nearest neighbors (q nearest neighbors). The log relative risk surface, the local case proportions, and the spatial scan statistic suggest similar areas for the most likely clusters. As these occur in or near areas

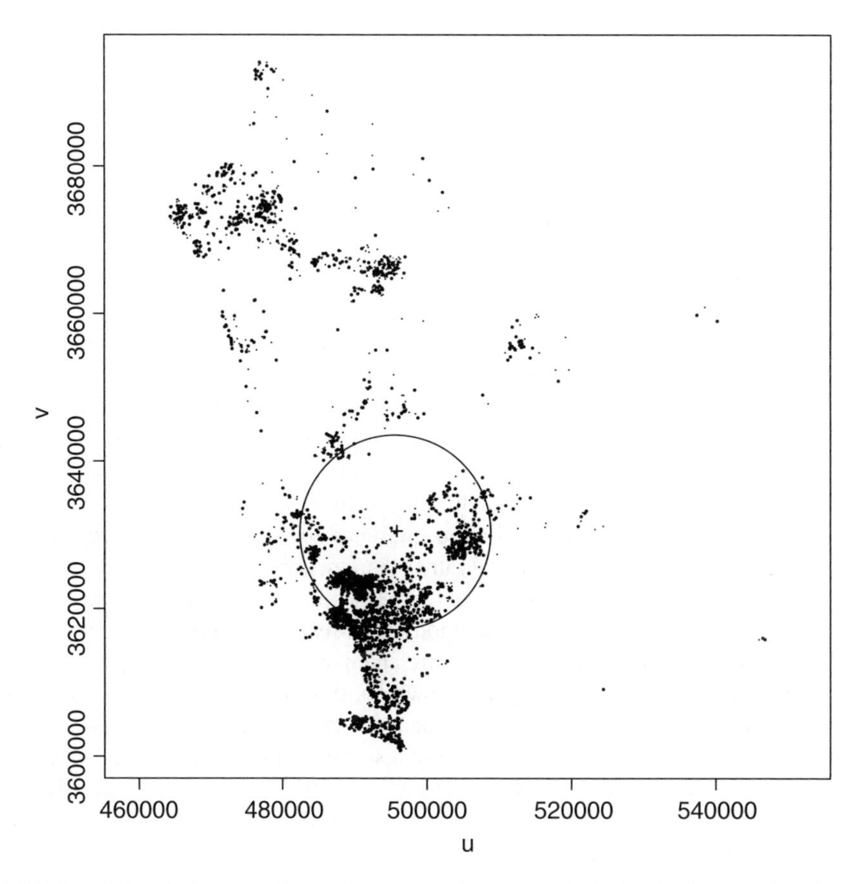

FIG. 6.22 Most likely cluster detected by the spatial scan statistic for the San Diego asthma data.

Table 6.4 ***q*-Nearest-Neighbor Statistics for the San Diego Asthma Data**[a]

Test Statistic	Value	Monte Carlo p-Value (Based on 499 Simulations)
T_9	18072	<0.00
T_{20}	40172	<0.00
T_{100}	199313	<0.00
$T_{20} - T_9$	22100	<0.00
$T_{100} - T_9$	181241	<0.00
$T_{100} - T_{20}$	159141	<0.00

[a]499 random labeling simulations define Monte Carlo p-values.

containing some of the highest densities of events (MediCal claims), perhaps a more focused analysis of these areas (with smaller bandwidths) would provide additional insight into local variations in the risk of a paid MediCal claim associating with asthma rather than nonrespiratory ailments in children aged 0–14 years.

6.7 FURTHER READING

The methods described in this chapter illustrate several types of approaches used to investigate clustering and to detect clusters in case–control point data. Diggle (2000) and Wakefield et al. (2000b) provide additional reviews of point process methods applied to disease clusters and clustering.

There is a wide and growing literature on statistical modeling and inference for point processes building from the basic extensions outlined at the end of Chapter 5. Stoyan et al. (1995), Barndorff-Neilsen et al. (1999), and Lawson and Denison (2002) provide texts focusing on such models. In general, Geyer (1999) provides a very general framework for likelihood inference for spatial point processes.

Finally, we concentrate on *general* rather than *focused* approaches in the sections above. The addition of foci of suspected increases in relative risk allows construction of models and refinement of methods to assess clustering or detect clusters only near the foci. The spatial scan statistic and q-nearest-neighbor approaches can be readily applied in the situation where we consider only potential clusters (radii or nearest neighbors) of the foci rather than the cases. Local case proportions and ratios of intensity (density) functions may also be adapted to the focused setting. Diggle (1990), Diggle et al. (2000), and Lawson (2001, Chapter 7) specifically consider such focused approaches, and Lawson and Waller (1996) provide a review of point process methods for focused tests.

6.8 EXERCISES

6.1 Contrast the goals of identifying clusters and identifying clustering. What sort of conclusions does each approach provide when applied to disease incidence data?

6.2 Using the medieval grave site data given in Table 5.2, construct kernel intensity (density) estimates for the affected and nonaffected sites based on a variety of bandwidths. For what bandwidths do the kernel estimates seem similar? For what bandwidths do the kernel estimates differ?

6.3 Construct log relative risk surfaces for the medieval grave site data, and identify areas exceeding the pointwise 90% tolerance surfaces using simulations under the random labeling hypothesis for a variety of bandwidths. For what range of bandwidths does the log relative risk surface exceed the pointwise tolerance limits for the area indicated by "+" symbols in Figure 6.3? How stable is the area indicated by "−" in Figure 6.3 for the same range of bandwidths?

6.4 Create a cluster in the medieval grave site data by selecting a set of nearby locations. Reassign any nonaffected sites in your cluster to "affected," and keep the same affected/nonaffected ratio by reassigning as "nonaffected" the same number of affected sites randomly selected from those outside your cluster. Create log relative risk surfaces for Gaussian kernels and bandwidths of 350 and 700 units. Does the approach detect your cluster?

6.5 Create a cluster as in Exercise 6.4. Also create a separate data set containing two clusters, and keep the two clusters close to the same size (i.e., construct both clusters with approximately the same radius). For both data sets, estimate the K functions for affected and nonaffected sites. Does the difference between these K functions detect your cluster(s) as evidence of clustering? Compare the results between the two data sets.

6.6 Calculate $E\left(T_q\right)$ and $\text{Var}\left(T_q\right)$ under the random labeling hypothesis for the test statistic defined in Section 6.6.3.

6.7 Create a data set contain a single cluster as in Exercises 6.4 and 6.5. Does the q-nearest-neighbor approach described in Section 6.6.3 detect your cluster? Repeat with two clusters. Do contrasts between test statistics identify the scale of your clusters correctly?

CHAPTER 7

Spatial Clustering of Health Events: Regional Count Data

The species Homo sapiens *has a powerful propensity to detect patterns, even when no patterns exist.*

Julian Bond, economist, quoted in Fienberg and Kaye (1991)

The statistical methods for detecting disease clustering and disease clusters presented in Chapter 6 draw fairly directly from the concepts and theory of spatial point processes introduced in Chapter 5. Many times, however, access to point data is either strictly or practically impossible. As mentioned in Chapters 2 and 3, confidentiality restrictions often limit release of point-level disease or census data, and many official agencies release disease, census, or other data only as summary counts for a particular set of *enumeration districts*. These regions partition the study area, assigning each location to one region only. In the United States, states are divided into counties which are divided into census tracts. Census tracts are divided into block groups, which in turn are divided into census blocks. In this chapter we turn attention to statistical approaches for detecting clustering and/or clusters in disease incidence data available as counts of cases from a set of geographic regions. We use the term *regions* throughout to refer to the enumeration districts partitioning the study area and the term *area* to refer to the entire study area or a particular collection of regions.

7.1 WHAT DO WE HAVE AND WHAT DO WE WANT?

In Sections 6.1 and 6.2 we introduce general issues that arise in specifying the null and alternative hypotheses in tests to detect disease clusters or tests to identify disease clustering. Many of the ideas apply to both point and regional count data. However, the use of counts raises some additional analytic and inferential complications, three of which we outline below. As a result, methods proposed to detect clusters and/or clustering in regional count data often take a slightly different form than those proposed for point data.

Applied Spatial Statistics for Public Health Data, by Lance A. Waller and Carol A. Gotway
ISBN 0-471-38771-1

First and foremost, we only view patterns in regional count data through the filter of the aggregation system. That is, we cannot observe spatial patterns at a scale smaller than that defined by the smallest set of units for which data are available. For example, in a set of census tract incidence data, we cannot explore the distribution of cases *within* tracts without additional information or assumptions.

Second, aggregate data yield *ecological analyses*, that is, analyses based on grouped data as defined in Section 2.7.4. Such analyses always contain the potential for ecological fallacy wherein analysts extrapolate associations between outcomes and potential risk factors observed in groups of people to similar associations at the individual level. Furthermore, spatial analyses of regional count data are subject to the modifiable areal unit problem (MAUP), defined in Section 4.5, where observed associations between variables can change with different aggregations of individuals into different sets of regions. The MAUP is particularly an issue if the data contain (or are suspected of containing) small clusters associated with increased local risk. If enumeration district boundaries divide a particular cluster between two or more regions, any statistical evidence of the cluster can be diluted across these boundaries and can appear much weaker than an assessment based on point data.

Finally, as we saw in Chapter 4, regional counts must also balance the *small-number problem* with the *spatial scale* of the data. This balance is crucial when investigating hypotheses concerning disease clustering. Recall that the small-number problem occurs when one subdivides the study area into very small regions and observes the incidence of a rare disease over a relatively short period. In such instances, expected numbers of cases per region can be so small that any single observed case appears suspicious (i.e., as a "cluster"). We cannot detect meaningful increases in risk in such regions without an appreciable increase in the total number of persons at risk or cases observed in each region, thereby arguing for fewer, larger regions observed over a longer study period. In contrast, the spatial scale of the data defines the geographic resolution. In this case, smaller regions provide more local information, arguing for many small regions. The balance between the two issues manifests itself as a trade-off between geographic resolution (where we want many small areas) and the statistical stability of estimates associated with these areas (where we want stable local estimates).

As a result of these three interweaving issues, the particular set of regions within a data set provides a lower bound to the observable spatial scale of any pattern and must provide a context within which to interpret any analytic results (Waller and Turnbull 1993). For example, statistically significant clustering at the census tract level does not necessarily imply significant clustering at the block group level, and vice versa.

7.1.1 Data Structure

The basic form of the data involves a set of *counts observed* (one count for each region) and a matching set of *counts expected* reporting the number of cases we expect in each region, under the null hypothesis. We base statistical inference on comparisons between these two sets of counts. More formally, we often assume that the data represent a set of counts arising from a heterogeneous Poisson process (i.e., the data $Y_1, Y_2, \ldots, Y_N$ in regions $1, 2, \ldots, N$ are mutually independent Poisson random variables). Furthermore, we assume that we observe fixed (nonrandom) population counts for each region, denoted $n_1, n_2, \ldots, n_N$. As in the empirical Bayes smoothing approaches defined in Section 4.4.3, these population counts are used in determining the number of cases expected in each region, under a null hypothesis of no clusters/clustering, denoted $E_1, E_2, \ldots, E_N$.

7.1.2 Null Hypotheses

Like the methods defined in Chapter 6, many of the methods build on a probability model based on the assumptions of an underlying heterogeneous Poisson spatial point process (cf. Section 5.2.4). In particular, many methods model the regional counts as independent Poisson random variables based on one of the basic properties of a spatial Poisson process: event counts from nonoverlapping regions follow independent Poisson distributions where the underlying intensity function defines the expected values (and variances). Some analysts prefer the binomial distribution as a probabilistic model for regional counts, since the Poisson distribution assigns a nonzero positive probability of observing more cases than persons at risk in each region. However, for rare diseases, this probability is very small, so the practical difference between the Poisson and binomial distributions is often negligible. In addition, since we continue to advocate the use of Monte Carlo hypothesis tests, the choice between an underlying binomial or Poisson distribution governs the underlying simulation, but not the general structure of the analytic approaches, as outlined below.

In some instances we may want to condition on the total number of cases in the study area, yielding a multinomial distribution for the set of counts. Since we consider the population sizes $n_1, n_2, \ldots, n_N$ fixed, the total population size in the study area,

$$n_+ = \sum_{i=1}^{N} n_i,$$

is also fixed. If we condition on Y_+, the total number of cases observed, we are in effect setting the individual disease risk $r = Y_+/n_+$, which is assumed fixed for everyone under the constant risk null hypothesis. Although there can be motivation for conditioning on the total number of cases (or equivalently, the assumed constant disease risk), analysts should realize that conditioning on the total can subtly change the question addressed (e.g., from "Is there clustering among leukemia cases in upstate New York?" to "Is there clustering among 592 cases distributed at random to people in upstate New York?" [cf. Table 6.1 and Bithell (1995)].

For the most part, methods to assess clusters and clustering in count data assume some background information on the entire population rather than a set of controls. This is due primarily to the wide availability of regional census data. For many countries, the census provides readily available data giving detailed background information on the population at risk within a specific set of defined regions.

Since regional count methods for assessing clustering or detecting clusters typically use observed incident disease counts and census-based population counts for the same set of regions, most assess the constant risk hypothesis (people are equally likely to contract the disease regardless of location) by comparing the counts observed to their corresponding counts expected based on a global incidence rate (proportion) applied to local population counts. (Here the term *global rate* refers to the rate observed across the entire data set, and *local population count* refers to the population size observed within a single enumeration district.) Since the comparison group (census data) typically includes all persons at risk (including the cases), application of the random labeling hypothesis (fixing the case and control locations and randomly assigning the case and control labels) is less straightforward for regional count data than for point data.

As noted above, the constant risk hypothesis assumes a constant disease risk, r, giving $E_i = rn_i$ for $i = 1, 2, \dots, N$. The counts expected may also be standardized in the manner discussed in Section 2.3. For example, if we have age-specific rates r_j for age groups $j = 1, \dots, J$, and population sizes n_{ij} for the same age groups within each region, we can define an age-adjusted expected count via $E_i = \sum_j r_j n_{ij}$, for $i = 1, \dots, N$.

Simulation of regional count data sets under the constant risk null hypothesis differs somewhat from approaches defined for complete spatial randomness, heterogeneous Poisson processes, or the random labeling hypothesis. Rather than simulate event locations as points, we simply simulate the counts directly, based on the properties of a heterogeneous spatial Poisson process (i.e., we simulate Y_i using a Poisson random number generator with mean E_i). For a heterogeneous Poisson process, recall that Y_i is independent of Y_j for $i \neq j$. If we wish to condition on the total number of cases Y_+, we simply draw regional counts $(Y_1, Y_2, \dots, Y_N)$ based on a multinomial distribution with cell probabilities $(n_1/n_+, n_2/n_+, \dots, n_N/n_+)$.

7.1.3 Alternative Hypotheses

Under a heterogeneous Poisson process, our observed regional counts should appear (1) independent, (2) Poisson distributed, with (3) expectations (and variances) E_i for $i = 1, \dots, N$. These three components represent areas for potential deviation from a heterogeneous Poisson process, and these (individually and in combination) represent alternative hypotheses for many of the statistical tests of disease clustering and clusters proposed for regional count data. Although only the third component relates directly to the constant risk hypothesis per se, the literature contains many different statistical assessments of clustering and clusters, each building on different deviations from the components noted above. Some estimate and assess measures of correlation between observations, some assess the accuracy of a Poisson distribution (usually through assessments of over- or underdispersion expressed through apparent differences between the mean and variance), and many tests compare observed to expected counts or rates in a manner very similar to goodness-of-fit statistics. We focus primarily on the first and last of these types of tests, deferring discussion of tests of over- and underdispersion to the references cited in Section 7.8.

The use of correlation as a measure of clustering or as an approach to detect clusters merits some clarification, particularly for chronic (noninfectious) diseases. A spatial Poisson process, the assumed probability model for our null hypothesis, generates independent events. Conceptually with an infectious disease, we tend to attribute deviations from independence to the direct relationship between cases (e.g., a large number of influenza cases in one week generates a similar or even greater number of cases the following week). With a chronic (noninfectious) disease, we typically think of clusters and/or clustering resulting from putative environmental causes. Such an exposure–disease link tends to suggest a local increase in the number of cases observed in areas with higher exposure over that expected under a constant risk, but maintains independence between individual cases.

Does this mean that any correlation-based alternative implies an infectious nature to the disease? Not necessarily. At the risk of being overly simplistic, suppose that we expect to observe the same number of cases in every region of the study area (i.e., the constant risk hypothesis applies to a set of regions each containing the same population size). Next, suppose that we observe a collection of three contiguous regions each containing twice the number of cases expected. This deviation could be caused by a *trend* in the true (unknown) means of the Poisson counts for these regions or by *correlation* between the counts. Recall from Section 5.4.4 that it is mathematically impossible from a single data realization to distinguish between heterogeneously distributed independent events and homogeneously distributed dependent events. The practical implication is that a method assuming independence identifies the deviating regions as evidence of a trend, while a method assuming no trend identifies the deviation as correlation. Both methods may "notice" the deviation, but each summarizes the pattern in a different way. As a result, we may find some approaches more appropriate (and possibly more statistically powerful) in some situations than in others.

Often, assessing deviation from a heterogeneous Poisson process in only one category (correlation, Poisson, or expectation) may be inadequate for detecting clusters or clustering. Rogerson (1999) provides an excellent example illustrating this point, which we paraphrase here. A purely goodness-of-fit approach (e.g., Pearson's χ^2 statistic) compares observed to expected counts without regard to location. In our simplistic example from the preceding paragraph, the value of such a statistic is identical (provides the same evidence of lack of fit), regardless of the relative location of the three deviant observations. That is, the statistic's value is the same whether the three outlying observations are next to one another, or separated. Surely, we would prefer an approach where deviations proximate to each other suggest greater evidence of a cluster. Similarly, a statistic measuring the amount of correlation assesses similarity between neighboring observations, not necessarily their deviation from expectation. That is, an estimate of the degree of autocorrelation will not provide us directly with an assessment of the relative risk of disease within a particular cluster compared to outside the cluster. Neither goodness of fit nor autocorrelation is entirely satisfactory without some input from the other approach. We review approaches from both perspectives as well as some approaches seeking to combine both goals in the sections below.

Finally, the distinctions defined in Section 6.2 between *tests of clustering* and *tests to detect clusters*, and between *general* and *focused tests* (Besag and Newell 1991), still apply. These distinctions define the sorts of alternative hypotheses of primary interest in the application of a particular analytic technique. As a reminder, recall that methods assessing clustering address global patterns of correlation or fit across the study area, while methods to detect clusters involve local assessments of these same quantities. General tests assess clusters and clustering *anywhere* and focused tests assess clusters and clustering around foci of suspected increased risk.

7.2 CATEGORIZATION OF METHODS

Following the format of Chapter 6, we consider tests of disease clusters and clustering for regional count data in categories based on the statistical strategy for detecting clusters and clustering:

- Methods based on scanning local rates
- Methods based on global indexes of spatial autocorrelation
- Methods based on local indexes of spatial autocorrelation
- Methods based on goodness-of-fit tests
- Methods combining goodness of fit and indexes of spatial autocorrelation

We begin with methods extended directly from those introduced in Chapter 6, then branch into tests particularly addressing deviations from a heterogeneous Poisson process based primarily on either spatial correlation or lack of correspondence between observed and (constant risk) expected values, then conclude with approaches combining autocorrelation and fit.

7.3 SCANNING LOCAL RATES

The *geographical analysis machine* (GAM) of Openshaw et al. (1988) introduced in Section 6.5.3 provides an exploratory tool for both case–control point data and regional data. Recall that to implement the GAM, we construct circles of various distances, count the number of cases and the number of people at risk within the circle, calculate a local incidence proportion (rate), and display those circles with local incidence proportions exceeding some user-specified threshold.

The use of regional count data requires some additional specification not needed in the analysis of case–control point data regarding assignment of cases and people at risk to particular circles (e.g., should all or a fraction of the cases in a region intersecting the edge of a circle be included within the circle?). We take care to specify how each approach outlined below addresses this issue.

7.3.1 Goals

The goal for methods based on scanning local rates remains the same for regional data as for point data [outlined in Section 6.5; i.e., to identify areas with unusually high (or perhaps unusually low) local incidence proportions (rates)]. The motivation for overlapping circles is similar to the smoothing methods of Chapter 4 (i.e., to combine information from neighboring areas in order to stabilize local estimates). As such, these methods are primarily tests to detect individual clusters rather than tests of overall clustering. However, as we note below, summarizing local deviations over the study area often also provides a general test of clustering.

7.3.2 Assumptions

Recall from Section 6.5.3 that the GAM was intended as an exploratory device, not a statistical assessment of clusters (Openshaw 1990). However, the GAM received much statistical criticism motivating development of several statistical approaches seeking to provide local inference based on GAM-type operations. Overlapping circles and spatially heterogeneous population distributions yield correlated incidence proportions with differing variances, respectively, considerably complicating our desire to assign statistical significance to each local estimate.

The distributional building blocks for constructing inference involve the null hypothesis based on mutually independent Poisson counts with a constant individual risk of disease (i.e., a Poisson count Y_i with expectation $E_i = rn_i$ for each region). Although the counts themselves are independent under the null hypothesis, neighboring local incidence proportions calculated for overlapping circles share a large number of the same counts and are correlated. Several of the approaches described below use Monte Carlo simulation to generate (simulated) data sets based on the underlying independent counts and calculate the local incidence proportions (rates) within the user-defined circles for each simulated data set. The local incidence proportion (rate) estimates are correlated *within* each data set but are *independent* between them, allowing a local Monte Carlo hypothesis test at each location. Such tests allow us to calculate a Monte Carlo significance value corresponding to the local incidence proportion observed in each circle.

Population heterogeneity complicates inference since often each local incidence proportion derives from a different number of people at risk, yielding different expectations and variances for each local incidence proportion. These heterogeneous distributions make statistical comparisons between local incidence proportions difficult. Some methods detailed below improve comparability through revising the circles to collections of regions containing the same number of cases or number at risk (i.e., controlling the numerator or the denominator of the incidence proportion, respectively).

We describe four related approaches below. The first and last represent direct generalizations of point methods introduced in Chapter 6, and the other two explore statistical versions of the GAM.

7.3.3 Method: Overlapping Local Rates

Recall the method of Rushton and Lolonis (1996) defined in Section 6.5.4. In this approach, based on GIS-friendly operations, we define a set of grid points covering the study area and calculate local incidence proportions within circles centered at the grid points. Also recall that we typically use circle radii slightly smaller than our user-defined grid spacing. To apply the approach to rates, we count a region as falling within the circle if the region's centroid falls within the circle. Other definitions for including regions are possible, such as including cases from regions having any portion within the circle, or including only a fraction of the observed cases and persons at risk from any region intersecting the circle. Note that the latter choice requires an additional choice regarding what fraction to include. Including a fraction of cases and people at risk proportional to the fraction of the geometric area of the region falling within the circle requires an accompanying assumption of a homogeneous population density within the region which may be reasonable in some settings and not in others. In addition, the proportion of area falling within a circle may also depend on the choice of map projection, possibly resulting in similar but slightly different assignment of cases to circles in different projections.

To assess the statistical significance of the local incidence proportions, Rushton and Lolonis (1996) utilize Monte Carlo tests at each location based on an overall constant risk hypothesis where cases are assigned to regions according to the incidence proportion observed for the entire study area, and the total number of cases in the study area varies between iterations.

DATA BREAK: New York Leukemia Data To illustrate the methods defined in this chapter, we consider the New York leukemia data introduced in the data break following Section 4.4.5. Recall that the data include the number of cases of leukemia (all types) diagnosed in people residing in an eight-county region of upstate New York for the years 1978–1982. The original data appearing in Turnbull et al. (1990) and Waller et al. (1992, 1994) involve counts for block groups in seven of the eight counties, and counts for census tracts only in Broome County (southeastern corner of the study area). For illustration, we consider the data aggregated to the census tract level for all eight counties, leading to 592 cases in 281 regions.

Figure 7.1 provides a contour plot of the local rate surface estimated for the New York data defined by the method of Rushton and Lolonis (1996). Census tract centroids appear as filled circles and grid points as small "×" symbols. Circle radii are slightly smaller than the grid spacing. Note that circles for many grid points will contain no tract centroids, and these circles are not considered in the analysis. Furthermore, we calculate local rates only for grid points with corresponding circles containing at least 500 persons at risk, indicated by the larger "×" symbols in Figure 7.1. (For visual simplicity, the contours derive from interpolation between those grid points meeting our measurement criterion.) Under the constant risk hypothesis, we expect to observe approximately 0.25 case in 500 people at risk. This choice of a lower limit for the population size results in many local estimates based on zero observed cases. As noted in Section 6.5.4, the choice of grid spacing and circle radius require a compromise between local detail in the surface and stability of the local incidence proportions (rates).

We note some areas with slightly increased local incidence proportions in the central portion of the study area, and a visually striking area of nested contours

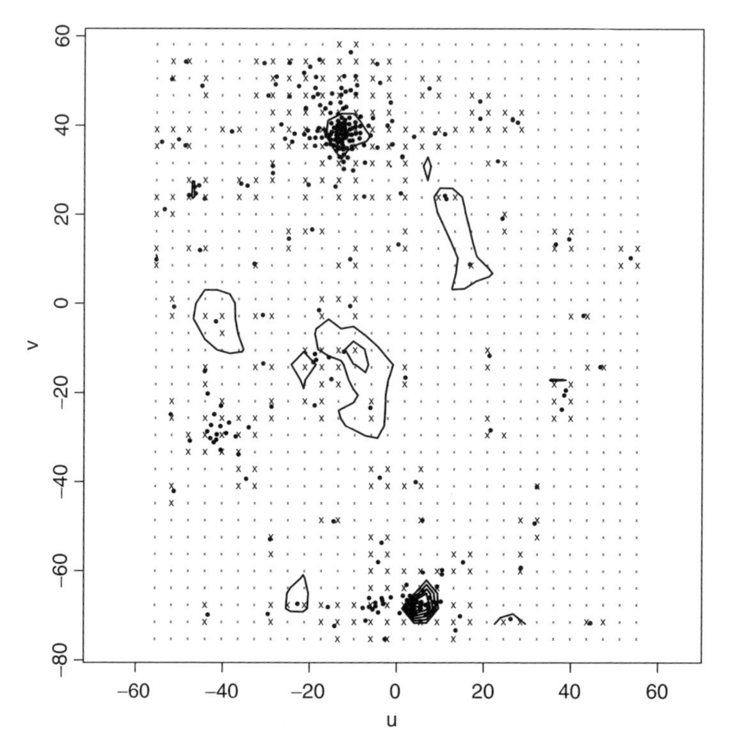

FIG. 7.1 Local case proportions for the tract-level New York leukemia data. Filled circles denote census tract centroids (data locations), small "×" symbols denote the grid considered, larger "×" symbols denote grid points meeting the minimum population size of 500 people (1980 census). Contour lines correspond to the smoothed relative risk surface.

in Figure 7.1 corresponding to a locally increased incidence proportion in the city of Binghamton, located in the south-central portion of the study area. However, based on 999 simulations, no location exhibits a statistically significant deviation from the constant risk hypothesis.

We note that our assessment omits many of the rural tracts, due to our selection of grid spacing and a 500-person lower bound for each circle. Lowering the population size threshold for the same grid spacing and radius could be counterproductive since, coupled with the rarity of the disease, it would probably increase the number of local rate estimates of zero. Monte Carlo tests for grid points with rate estimates of zero make little sense (a zero observed rate will never appear significantly high!). As a result, our selections for grid spacing, circle radius, and population lower bound in this example are in no sense optimal. We also need to interpret our results with even greater care since (1) each local incidence proportion derives from a different number of people at risk; and (2) conducting many significance tests using the same data alters the overall type I error level (i.e., the more tests we make, the greater the chance that we will find at least one test to be significant). This is often referred to as the *multiple testing problem*. The methods described in

Sections 7.3.4 to 7.3.6 address one or both of these problems. However, the results in Figure 7.1 provide an initial view of the data and highlight areas of suggestively (although not statistically significantly) increased local incidence.

7.3.4 Method: Turnbull et al.'s CEPP

The heterogeneous population density provides a statistical complication in the interpretation of incidence proportions (rates) based on local aggregations of regional counts. The use of a fixed geographic distance in the circles for both the GAM of Openshaw et al. (1988) and the approach of Rushton and Lolonis (1996) generates collections of circles with varying numbers of incident cases (the numerator) and varying numbers of people at risk (the denominator). One way to increase comparability between local rates is to limit attention to circles containing a constant number of people at risk. In this spirit, Turnbull et al. (1990) introduce a *cluster evaluation permutation procedure* (CEPP), requiring the user to define a population size n^* of interest. The user then considers (again overlapping) collections of n^* persons at risk, centered at each region. These collections vary in geographic size but maintain a constant population size at risk, so observed counts are identically distributed. However, since these collections of cases and people overlap, the counts are not independently distributed.

For a fixed population radius n^*, the CEPP builds a circle containing n^* persons at risk around each region in the data set. Note that the CEPP does not examine all collections of n^* persons at risk, or even all geographically contiguous collections of n^* persons at risk. Instead, the CEPP examines disease counts observed from each collection of the n^* persons at risk residing in a particular region and its nearest surrounding regions. That is, for region i, we aggregate region i and the regions nearest region i until we reach a collection of n^* persons at risk.

Usually, we define the population radius to be larger than the region-specific population size. To achieve an at-risk population size of n^*, we typically need to add only a fraction of the persons and cases in the most distant of the nearby regions added to a particular circle. In practice, the choice of what fraction of cases to include in the circle imposes some additional assumptions on the analysis. For example, if n_j denotes the population size of the most distant region added to the circle around region i, we need to include $(n^* - n_{+,i})/n_i$ persons at risk, where $n_{+,i}$ is the sum of the population sizes of region i and regions nearer than region j. Including the same fraction of the number of cases observed in region j to the circle centered at region i assumes a homogeneous risk within region j. Often, this is a reasonable assumption to make, since we have no information regarding the distribution of cases within each region, but acknowledging such assumptions provides a clearer interpretation of results. In addition, specifying such assumptions allows us to conduct sensitivity analyses wherein we measure the impact of various case allocation strategies on the final results (cf. Waller et al. 1992).

Monte Carlo simulations based on the constant risk hypothesis provide a means for "pointwise" significance testing for each circle in precisely the same manner as described for the method of Rushton and Lolonis (1996) in Sections 6.5.4 and 7.3.3.

That is, we can generate simulated data sets based on the constant risk hypothesis, then consider a Monte Carlo test for counts observed within each region's circle. However, such an approach still suffers from the problem of multiple testing and is further complicated by correlations between the multiple tests.

Rather than focus on multiple tests each centered at different regions, Turnbull et al. (1990) focus attention on the maximum number of cases observed in any collection of n^* persons at risk. Since all circles are based on the same number of persons at risk, comparing counts corresponds to comparing incidence proportions (ignoring risk variations due to age and other risk factors, for simplicity's sake), and the highest count corresponds to the highest local incidence proportion observed in any of the circles. The question of interest becomes: Is the highest observed count higher than we would anticipate under the constant risk hypothesis?

To assess this question, Turnbull et al. (1990) consider the following Monte Carlo test: For each simulated data set, we find the highest count observed in any circle of n^* persons at risk and compare our maximum count observed to the distribution of the maxima from the constant risk simulations. Note that the maximum from any given simulated data set may occur at any location in the study area, so we are comparing our maximum incidence proportion observed to the maximum incidence proportions in each of the simulated values rather than to the incidence proportion for the same set of n^* people in each simulation. This results in a single test statistic (the maximum incidence proportion observed) and single reference distribution approximated by the histogram of maximum incidence proportions observed in each of the simulated data sets.

The simulation approach of Turnbull et al. (1990) addresses two inferential problems. First, the approach avoids multiple testing since we use a single test statistic, and each Monte Carlo realization produces an independent comparison value. Second, the approach differs from the pointwise Monte Carlo test of the maximum incidence proportion (i.e., comparing the maximum count observed to the simulation values for the same circle), since we compare the value observed to the maximum observed for *any* circle in each simulation. This distinction avoids the "Texas sharpshooter" problem of identifying the maximum observed, then conducting a local hypothesis test for counts (or incidence proportions) observed in that particular circle (similar to shooting the side of a barn, then painting a bull's-eye around the bullet hole).

DATA BREAK: New York Leukemia Data (*cont.*) We illustrate the CEPP approach via application to the tract-level New York leukemia data [the original analysis of the block group-level data appears in Turnbull et al. (1990)]. Figure 7.2 illustrates the variable geographic extent of the circles (actually, aggregations of tracts) based on a constant population radius. Each circle represents a separate collection of n^* persons at risk within the analysis. As noted above, we build the circles by combining census tracts in order of intercentroid distance. Although a reasonable approach, the easternmost example in Figure 7.2 illustrates that our set of circles includes at least one noncontiguous collection of tracts. The smallest tract in this circle has a centroid closer to the centroid of the central tract for this

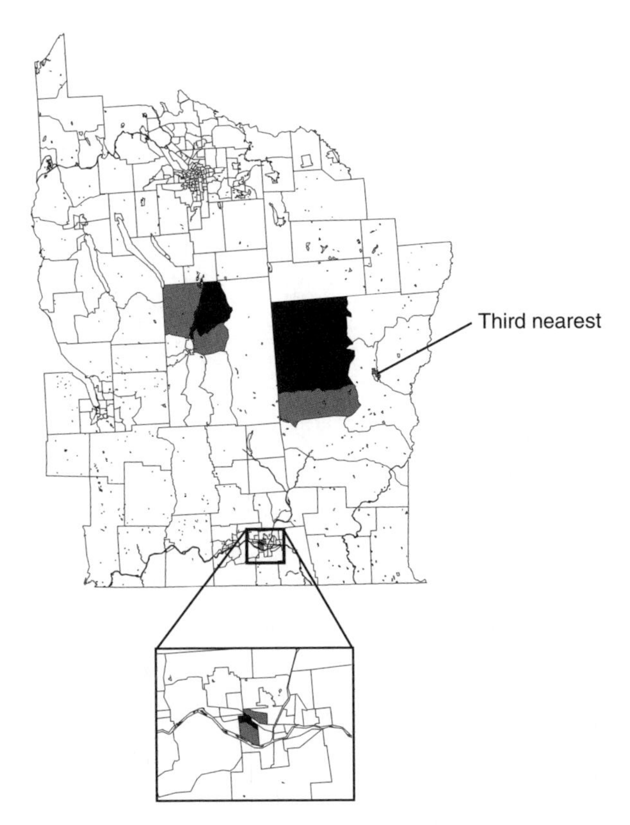

FIG. 7.2 Example of three different circles, all with a population radius of 10,000 persons at risk. The dark census tracts correspond to the central tract of each circle, and gray areas the additional tracts defining an associated circle (see text).

circle than does the centroid of the long and winding intermediary tract. We leave such circles in the analysis, but the example illustrates how aggregating irregular regions based on intercentroid distances can stretch the geometric appropriateness of the term *circle* in this context.

We consider four population radii: $n^* = 1000$, 5000, 10,000, and 40,000 persons at risk. We obtain the number of cases observed in the n^* at-risk persons centered in each tract, and find identify the maximum observed count (and its location). To assess significance, we consider 999 simulations under the constant risk hypothesis, where we allow the total number of cases to vary between simulations. For each data set simulated under the constant risk hypothesis, we store the maximum observed count occurring in any circle (again noting that the maximum count for each simulated data set could occur in any of the collections of n^* at-risk persons under consideration).

Figure 7.3 shows histograms of the maximum count based on 999 constant risk simulations for each population radius. The maximum count observed among all circles (the nearest n^* persons to each census tract) appears as a vertical line,

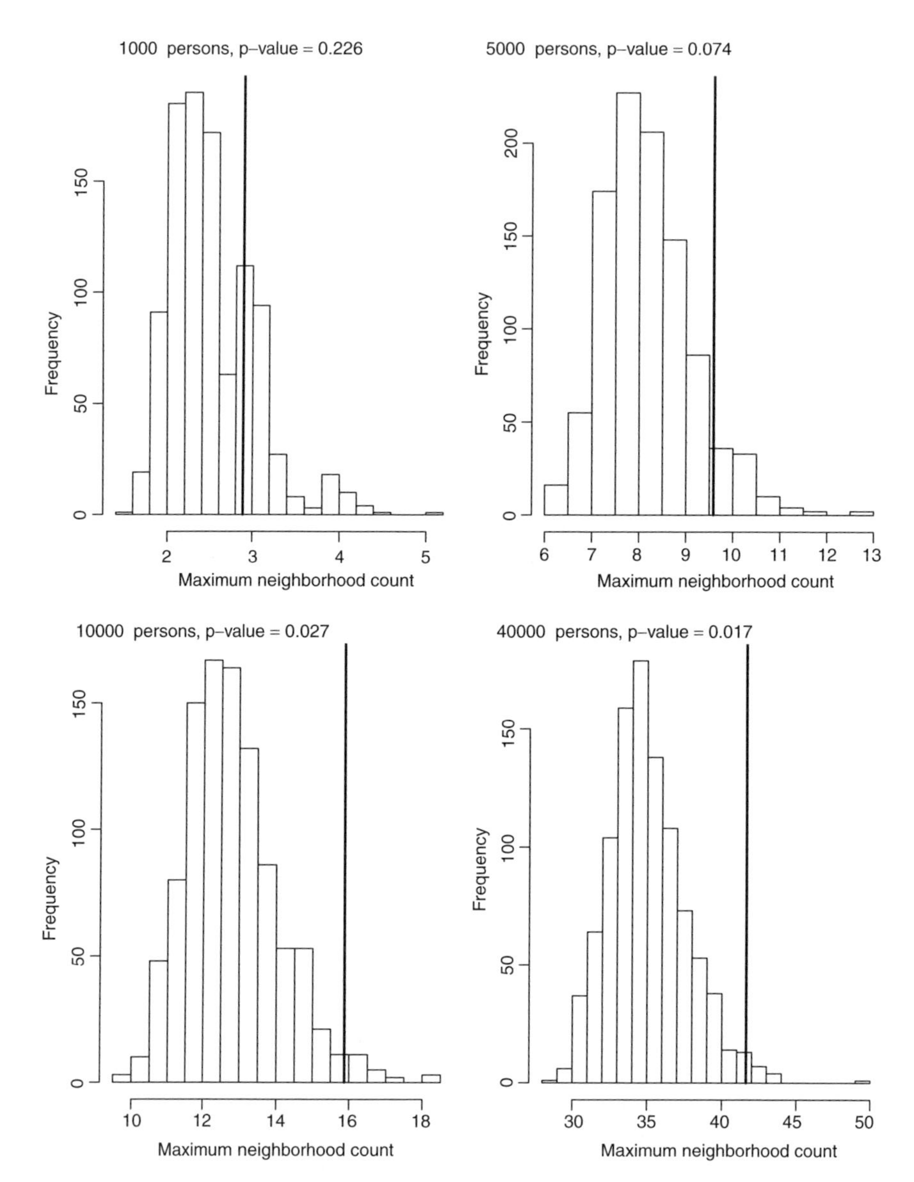

FIG. 7.3 Histograms and associated p-values (based on 999 constant risk simulations) of the maximum case count observed among all circles of the same population radius, applying the cluster evaluation permutation procedure to the tract-level New York leukemia data (see text). The vertical line denotes the maximum count observed among all circles.

and the one-sided p-value represents the proportion of maximum counts from the simulated data sets exceeding the maximum observed. Naturally, the maximum count observed increases as we increase n^* (the number at risk in each circle), although we could divide by the number at risk for comparability. We note that the

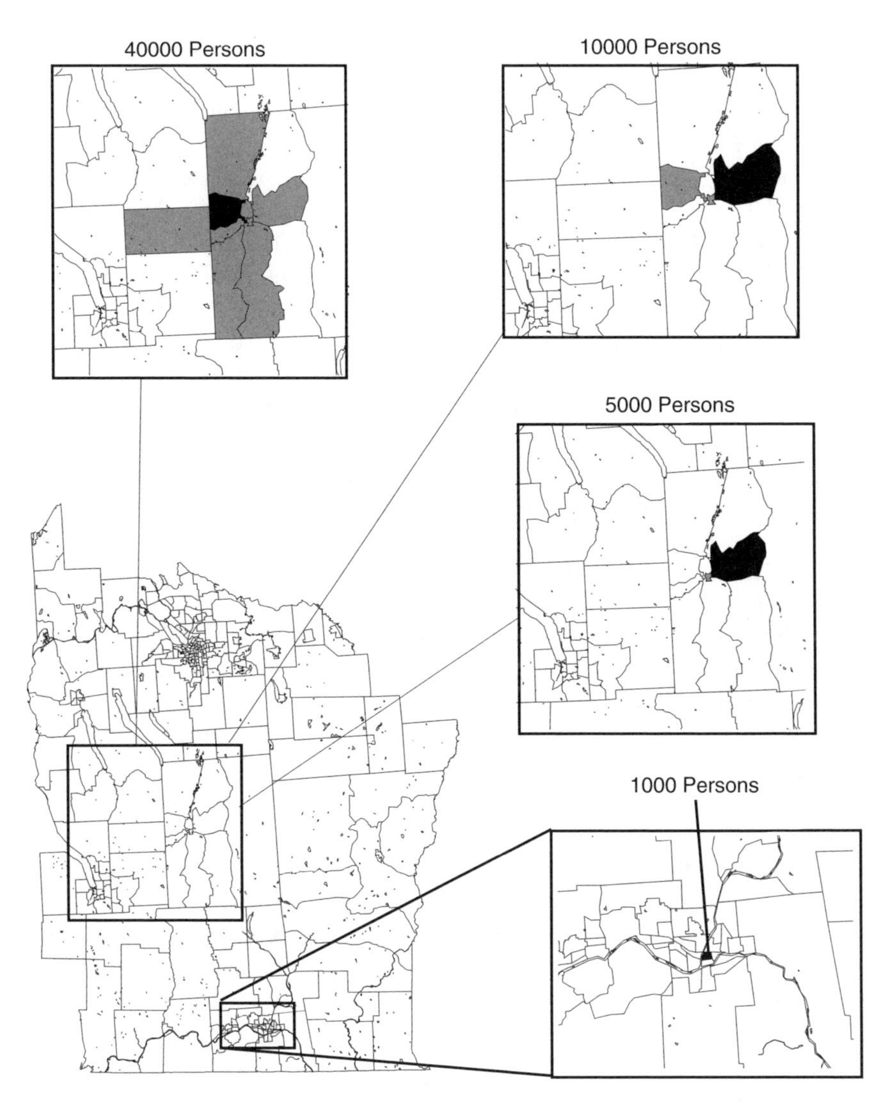

FIG. 7.4 Collections of tracts containing the maximum disease count observed using the cluster evaluation permutation procedure for each of several population radii (see text).

maximum number of cases observed is not statistically significant for population radii $n^* = 1000$ or 5000 persons but is for the two larger population radii.

Figure 7.4 illustrates the location of the tracts containing the maximum observed count for each value of n^*, the population radius. We shade the central tract black, and other tracts contributing cases and population at risk to this tract's circle, gray. Note that the maximum occurs in different places for different population radii. For the smaller population radii ($n^* = 1000$), the most likely (but statistically non-significant) cluster is in Binghamton, but for larger population radii the most likely clusters appear near Cortland, in the center of the study area. We note that the circle associated with the maximum count observed for a population radius of 10,000 persons occurs in a somewhat noncircular circle, again based on intercentroid distance, as shown in Figure 7.2.

To emphasize again the nature of the Monte Carlo test and to contrast the method of Turnbull et al. (1990) with a local test of the count (or incidence proportion) observed for a single circle, we consider how often the overall maximum count appears in each circle under the constant risk hypothesis. We prefer analytic approaches to be "fair" under the constant risk null hypothesis, where each tract has an approximately equal chance of anchoring the circle containing the maximal count. Gangnon and Clayton (2001) refer to this feature of tests to detect clusters as *unbiased*, although we prefer the term *geographically unbiased*, to distinguish the property from the usual definition of *unbiased* from the theory of hypothesis testing (i.e., the power of an unbiased test never exceeds the significance level under the null hypothesis and always exceeds the significance level under any alternative hypothesis; cf. Lehmann 1994, Chapter 4).

Figure 7.5 indexes tracts from 1 to 281 and reports the number of times that the circle of population radius n^* centered at each tract contained the maximum count across 9999 constant risk simulations. Under an equal chance of selection we would expect each tract to contain the maximum $9999/281 = 35.6$ times. For population radii 10,000 and 40,000, we see relatively little systematic departure from this expected value. We do note an apparent reduction in the variability associated with tracts having indexes between 100 and 200. We index tracts sequentially according to their Federal Information Processing Standards (FIPS) codes, so tracts appear together in counties. Mapping the values (not shown) does not reveal clear geographic trends in the estimated probability of selection, but reveals that the tracts with reduced variance correspond to tracts in Syracuse within Onondaga County. The reason for this apparent reduction in variation in the number of times that a particular tract appears as the center of the maximum cluster could depend on a number of factors, such as the higher population density across a set of tracts, higher variation in population sizes between tracts (one tract in this area contains only nine residents), and the geographically small area associated with each tract (so overlapping circles in this area share many more tracts than do those in more rural areas).

7.3.5 Method: Besag and Newell Approach

Another approach for controlling variability in local incidence proportions (rates) within distance-based circles is to limit attention to circles containing a constant number of cases (the local incidence proportion numerator) rather than a constant population radius (the local incidence proportion denominator considered in the CEPP). That is, we now consider circles with a constant case radius rather than the CEPP's circles with a constant population radius. We use the term *case circles* to distinguish circles defined by a case radius from those defined by a distance or population radius. Besag and Newell (1991) consider such an approach, directly

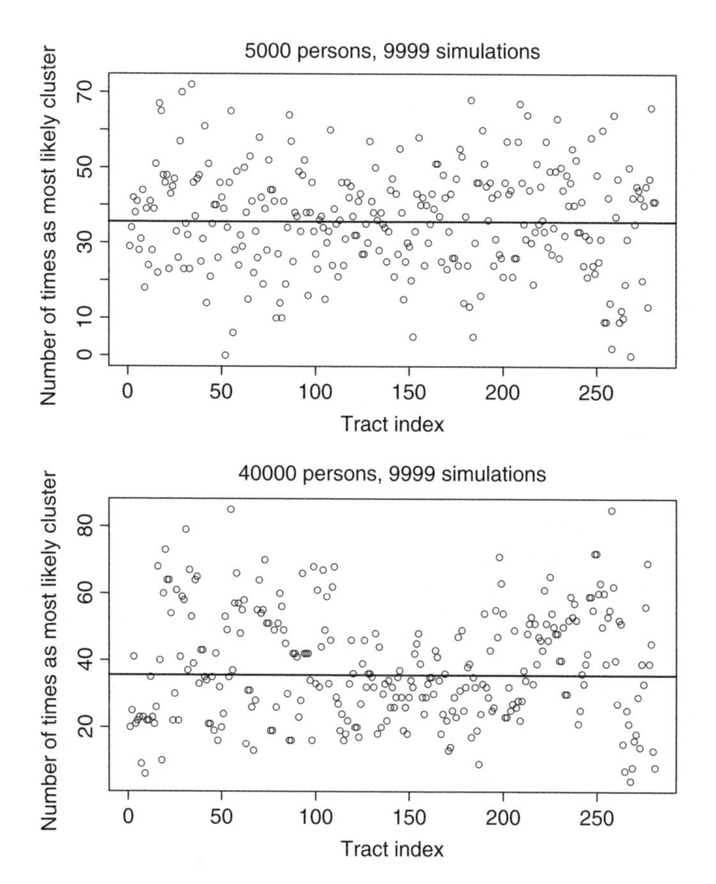

FIG. 7.5 Number of times (out of 9999 constant risk simulations) that each tract appears as the most likely cluster for population radii 10,000 (top) and 40,000 (bottom). The horizontal line denotes the number expected under a random assignment among tracts (9999/281).

addressing the question of defining the most likely clusters of c^* cases for a user-defined case radius (or cluster size) c^*.

To implement the approach of Besag and Newell (1991) we define a number of cases c^*, then consider the collections of c^* cases centered at each census region and identify the most unusual collections of c^* cases as possible clusters. As with the CEPP, the approach does not consider all collections of c^* cases nor all geographically contiguous collections of c^* cases, but rather, all collections of c^* cases observed in each region and its surrounding regions.

As proposed originally, the approach considered data aggregated to geographically small regions typically containing zero, one, or possibly two observed cases each. In this data setting, Besag and Newell (1991) center a case circle around each *case*. For data aggregated to larger regions often containing multiple cases, such a definition results in multiple case circles containing precisely the same cases for regions containing more than one case, and no case circles for regions containing no observed cases. As our example data set contains many regions with more than one case, we limit attention to a single case circle at each region. In addition, for regions containing no observed cases, we consider case circles where none of the c^* cases occur in the central region (i.e., the c^* clusters occur in a ring around the central region).

For each region we determine the number of regions in its case circle (i.e., the number of regions containing the c^* nearest cases) and assess significance based on the probability of observing c^* cases in fewer regions. That is, we calculate the probability of observing a more tightly clustered collection of the c^* cases around the region of interest.

More specifically, we order regions by their distance to the centroid of the region of interest, say region i. Next, we define n_{i,c^*} as the cumulative population size of the nearest regions (including region i) containing c^* cases. We define L_i as a random variable associated with region i representing the number of regions containing the collection of c^* nearest cases, and l_i as the observed value of L_i. For instance, if we set the case radius $c^* = 12$ and region i contains five cases, the nearest region to region i contains three cases, and the next-nearest region contains seven cases, $l_i = 3$. Besag and Newell (1991) base inference on L_i rather than the incidence proportions observed themselves, and unlike the CEPP, we do not need to add fractions of the observed cases or population size for the farthest region.

To calculate $\Pr(L_i \leq l_i)$, we define r as the overall disease incidence proportion for the region. Under the constant risk hypothesis, we assume an underlying Poisson distribution for each region, so $\Pr(L_i \leq l_i)$ corresponds to the probability (under the constant risk hypothesis) of observing c^* or more cases within n_{i,c^*} persons at risk:

$$\begin{aligned}\Pr(L_i \leq l_i) &= \sum_{j=c^*}^{\infty} \frac{\exp(-rn_{i,c^*})(rn_{i,c^*})^j}{j!}, \\ &= 1 - \sum_{j=0}^{c^*-1} \frac{\exp(-rn_{i,c^*})(rn_{i,c^*})^j}{j!}. \qquad (7.1)\end{aligned}$$

Since the method is based on the probability of observing c^* cases in fewer regions than observed, the method preforms best when we choose a case radius c^* such that most case circles cover multiple regions. See the exercises at the end of this chapter for further discussion of the relationship between the level of aggregation and the choice of the case radius c^*.

The method provides a significance value associated with each region and hence is primarily a collection of tests to detect individual clusters. If pressed for an overall test of clustering, Besag and Newell (1991) suggest the total number of clusters (for a given case radius) achieving some nominal level of significance, say 0.05, as a test statistic. We denote this number T_{BN} and note that we make no adjustment for multiple tests. An approximation of expected value of T_{BN} under the constant risk null hypothesis is the number of tests multiplied by the nominal significance level of each test. This is only an approximation, due to the discrete distribution of T_{BN}, and Besag and Newell (1991) provide a derivation of the exact expectation as follows: For each region, we apply equation (7.1) successively for $l_i = 0$, 1, and so on, until the significance level first exceeds our nominal level (e.g., 0.05), say for $l_i = l^*$. The value of equation (7.1) for $l_i = l^* - 1$ provides the true attainable significance level, denoted α_i, for the c^* cases in the ith and neighboring regions. The exact expectation of T_{BN} under the constant risk null hypothesis is given by

$$E(T_{BN}) = \sum_{i=1}^{N} \alpha_i.$$

Waller et al. (1994) point out that the accuracy of the approximation depends not only on the case radius c^*, but also on the level of aggregation (population size of the regions) in the data. Simulations under the constant risk hypothesis provide Monte Carlo tests for the value of T_{BN} observed.

Finally, we may obtain a focused version of the method of Besag and Newell (1991) by limiting attention to the c^* nearest cases to each *focus* instead of each *case* or each *region*. We start by finding the nearest c^* cases to each focus, and determine whether these collections of cases represent unusual aggregations compared to the local populations at risk. We obtain significance values associated with each focus using equation (7.1) as before.

DATA BREAK: New York Leukemia Data (*cont.*) We now apply the method of Besag and Newell (1991) to the tract-level New York leukemia data. [For application to the block-group-level data, see Waller et al. (1992, 1994) and Waller and Turnbull (1993).] For comparability with the results of the CEPP of Turnbull et al. (1990), we consider case radii (cluster sizes) of 6, 12, 17, and 23 cases, corresponding to the nearest integer number of cases expected in 1000, 5000, 10,000, and 40,000 persons at risk, under a constant risk hypothesis based on the incidence proportion (rate) observed in the entire study area.

Figure 7.6 illustrates the most significant clusters for each cluster size, those with the lowest associated local p-value calculated using equation (7.1). We use the term *local p-value* since the significance values correspond to the collection of (at least) c^* cases in the tracts nearest to each tract centroid. Besag and Newell (1991) suggest mapping all clusters attaining some nominal significance level (e.g., 0.05 or 0.01). We limit our attention to the most significant clusters, primarily for space reasons. Figure 7.6 resembles Figure 4.21, the probability map for the same data. Both figures display local Poisson probabilities, but Figure 4.21 presents values for each region separately, while Figure 7.6 seeks to increase comparability and stability (at the cost of independence between local tests) by combining cases and at-risk populations across local collections of regions.

Table 7.1 provides additional detail regarding the most significant clusters illustrated in Figure 7.6. First we note that due to the aggregations of cases into tracts, each case circle may contain more than c^* cases. Recall that unlike the approach of Turnbull et al. 1990, the farthest tract is added to each tract in its entirety rather than

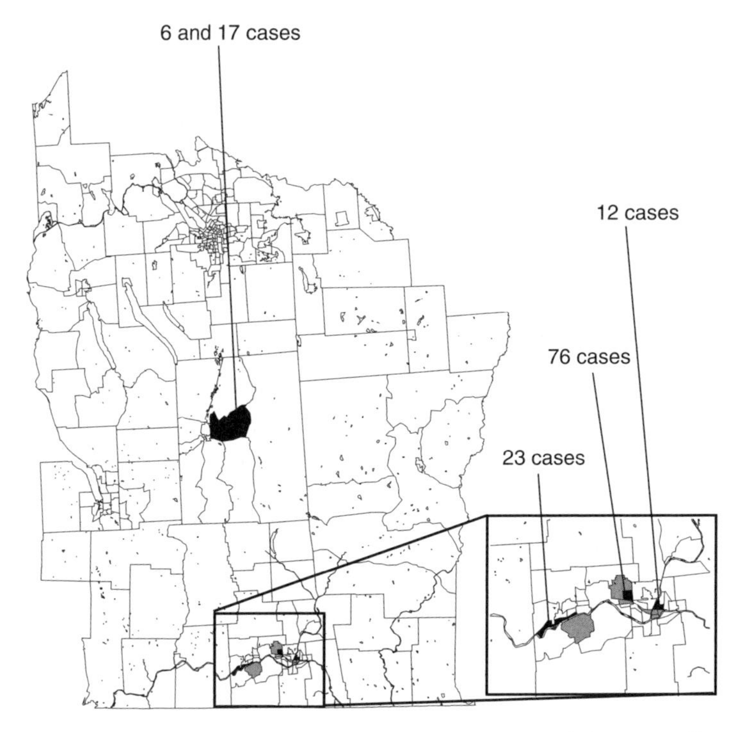

FIG. 7.6 Most significant clusters from the method of Besag and Newell, based on collections of 6, 12, 17, 23, and 76 cases (see text).

Table 7.1 Values Observed and Local Significance of the Most Locally Significant Clusters in the New York Leukemia Data as Determined by the Method of Besag and Newell[a]

Case Radius, c^*	Cases Observed	Cumulative Population Size, n_{i,c^*}	Local p-Value
6 cases	8.18	2,921	0.002
12 cases	12.21	8,876	0.002
17 cases	17.69	11,268	<0.001
23 cases	25.46	19,615	<0.001

[a]Local significance is determined by the collection of c^* cases nearest to each tract centroid (see text).

as a fraction. Also, the most significant cluster need not be the cluster exhibiting the maximum observed local incidence proportion. Finally, we note the local p-values defined by equation (7.1) differ from the p-value associated with the maximum incidence proportion observed in the CEPP of Turnbull et al. (1990). Recall that the p-value associated with the maximal incidence proportion for the CEPP reflects the probability of observing a *maximal* incidence proportion (anywhere) higher than the value observed under the constant risk hypothesis. In comparison, the local p-values of the method of Besag and Newell (1991) parallel those of the GAM of Openshaw et al. (1988) and the method of Rushton and Lolonis (1996) representing the probability of observing a more extreme local incidence proportion, thereby providing a separate p-value for each location measured.

7.3.6 Method: Spatial Scan Statistics

Although the approach of Turnbull et al. (1990) introduces a novel approach for assessing the statistical significance of the maximum local incidence proportion, inference remains linked to the user's choice of a population radius. The user's choice of bandwidth for kernel smoothing, distance radius for the approach of Rushton and Lolonis (1996), and case radius for the approach of Besag and Newell (1991) each provides a similar context for the interpretation of associated results. None of these methods provide a straightforward manner for comparisons across radii (bandwidth values). The spatial scan statistic defined by Kulldorff (1997) and introduced for point data in Section 6.5.5 aims to address this particular issue and provide inference across a range of cluster radii.

As a brief review of the material in Section 6.5.5, Kulldorff (1997) builds the spatial scan statistic from results of Loader (1991) and Nagarwalla (1996) regarding links between variable-width scan statistics and likelihood ratio statistics. Furthermore, Kulldorff (1997) notes that methods such as those proposed by Turnbull et al. (1990) and Rushton and Lolonis (1996) correspond to fixed-window spatial scan statistics and may be viewed as special cases of his general approach.

Implementation of the spatial scan statistic for regional count data mirrors that for case–control point data, replacing controls by census-based regional population counts. Recall that the primary goal of a scan statistic is to find the collection of cases (among the collections considered) least consistent with the null hypothesis (i.e., the most likely cluster) and to provide a significance value representing the detected cluster's "unusualness." In a regional count setting, Kulldorff (1997) considers distance-based circles with radii ranging from the smallest observed distance between a pair of regions (e.g., intercentroid distance) to a user-defined upper bound (e.g., one-half the width of the study area). A region contributes all of its cases and individuals at risk to the circle if the region's centroid falls within the circle. As illustrated in the preceding sections, collections of irregular regions with centroids within a given circle may not appear "circular" on the map. However, we retain the term *circle* here since each collection of regions arises from the region centroids falling within a distance-based circle rather than a population- or case-based circle. More recent implementations of the spatial and space-time scan statistic allow for distance-based linear and elliptical clusters, but not clusters based on population or case radii, as far as we are aware.

At each possible radius in the user-defined interval (e.g., at each observed intercentroid distance) and for each circle having that radius, we calculate a likelihood ratio statistic testing the constant risk hypothesis versus the specific alternative that risk within regions having their centroid within the circle differs from the risk in the rest of the study area. With regional data we observe counts rather than individual cases or controls, so we base the likelihood ratio in terms of the Poisson distribution rather than the Bernoulli case described for case–control point data in equation (6.7). In this setting, the scan statistic involves the number of cases observed in regions defining the circle of interest, Y_{in}, the number expected within this circle under the null hypothesis, E_{in}, and the corresponding number of cases observed and expected occurring outside the circle, denoted Y_{out} and E_{out}, respectively. Under the constant risk hypothesis, the expected counts consist of age-standardized values or of regional population sizes multiplied by an estimate of the overall risk. Therefore, the spatial scan statistic is proportional to

$$\max \left(\frac{Y_{\text{in}}}{E_{\text{in}}} \right)^{Y_{\text{in}}} \left(\frac{Y_{\text{out}}}{E_{\text{out}}} \right)^{Y_{\text{out}}}. \tag{7.2}$$

The Monte Carlo assessment of significance for the maximum observed count in the approach of Turnbull et al. (1990) provides direct motivation for inference of the spatial scan statistic (Kulldorff 1997). As before, we generate independent data sets under the null hypothesis, calculate the likelihood ratio statistic for each circle, and store the maximum statistic value, regardless of where it may occur. Statistics are correlated between circles *within* each simulation, but the maximum values are independent *between* simulations, providing a valid p-value for the most likely cluster, provided that one interprets the p-value as the probability of observing a more extreme maximal statistic *anywhere* in the study area (rather than the significance of observing the maximum at a particular location).

DATA BREAK: New York Leukemia Data (*cont.*) The methods of Rushton and Lolonis (1996) and Turnbull et al. (1990) suggest the possibility of a geographically small local increase in the Binghamton area in the southern portion of the study area, and the possibility of a less pronounced but geographically larger increase in the central portion of the study area (Cortland County). In both cases, for the geographic and population radii considered, the test statistic values observed are not unusual when compared to the distribution of values obtained by repeatedly assigning the 592 cases at random to the 1,057,673 people at risk (a Monte Carlo test under the constant risk assumption, where the total number of cases observed varies between simulations). It appears that the most likely clusters in the observed data are not much different than those we would expect to observe by chance. These methods indicate little evidence of significant *clusters* in the data.

We next apply the spatial scan statistic to the data. Figure 7.7 reveals three suggestive clusters, labeled A, B, and C. Table 7.2 provides summary information on the three clusters, including the number of cases observed and expected under the constant risk hypothesis. The ratio of cases observed to cases expected provides the standardized morbidity ratio (SMR), as defined in Section 2.3.2, providing an estimate of the relative risk of leukemia, comparing people residing inside each cluster to those residing outside that particular cluster.

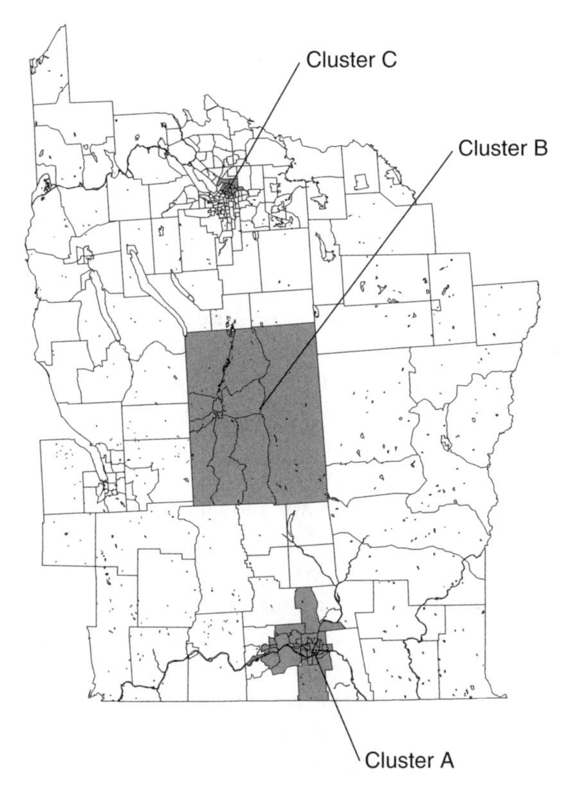

FIG. 7.7 Spatial scan statistic results for the New York leukemia data (281 tracts). Shading represents the census tracts (1980 Census) included in each potential cluster. Details regarding clusters A, B, and C appear in Table 7.2.

Table 7.2 Spatial Scan Statistic Results for New York Leukemia Data (281 Tracts)[a]

Cluster	Cases Observed	Cases Expected	Relative Risk (SMR)	Population Size	p-Value
A	117	70.61	1.657	135,295	0.001
B	47	25.31	1.857	48,820	0.050
C	44	23.83	1.846	45,667	0.101

[a]Clusters A, B, and C are shown in Figure 7.7. Significance (p-values) based on 999 constant risk simulations (see text).

Cluster A has the highest corresponding likelihood ratio statistic and represents the collection of cases least consistent with the constant risk null hypothesis (i.e., the most likely cluster in the data). This cluster corresponds to the area of the highest local risk estimated by the method of Rushton and Lolonis (1996) (see Figure 7.1). The associated p-value of 0.001 reported in Table 7.2 reveals that the maximum likelihood ratio test statistic observed was significantly higher than the maximum likelihood ratio statistics observed for 9999 simulations under the constant risk hypothesis.

We note that the number at risk in cluster A is considerably larger than any of the population radii considered in the preceding data breaks using the approaches of Turnbull et al. (1990) and Besag and Newell (1991). The scan statistic radii include those comparable to the population and case radii considered above, but the scan statistic suggests much larger radii for the most suspicious clusters. For comparison, applying the CEPP with population radius 135,000 yields a maximum disease count of 120 occurring in the circles based on four tracts in the same area as cluster A. (These four circles overlap and contain many of, if not precisely, the same tracts.) The maximum count observed exceeds all 999 maxima for data simulated under the constant risk hypothesis. Furthermore, applying the method of Besag and Newell (1991) with a case radius of 76 cases (the number expected in 135,000 persons at risk under the constant risk hypothesis) yields 77 cases observed among 85,271 persons at risk with location shown in Figure 7.6 and a local p-value less than 0.001.

Clusters B and C represent the second- and third-highest observed likelihood ratio statistics, under a constraint of considering the likelihood ratio statistics from nonoverlapping clusters. Since many of the potential clusters overlap, neighboring likelihood ratio statistics are often very similar since they contain many of the same cases and persons at risk. There are a variety of ways to constrain consideration of the next-most-likely clusters, and as long as the same constraints apply to each simulated data set, the Monte Carlo inference remains valid (subject to the constraint).

Cluster B corresponds exactly to the tracts in Cortland County. The fairly regular shape of the county and the collection of census tracts and their associated centroids around a central tract allow our circular potential clusters to include this rectangular area. Note that cluster B overlaps the most likely cluster defined by the CEPP for a population radius of 40,000 people (see Figure 7.4), but cluster radii based on population size and on distance result in slightly different clusters.

The p-values associated with clusters B and C rank the second- and third-highest likelihood ratio statistics observed for 9999 constant risk simulations. The precise questions addressed by these p-values are rather specific and differ somewhat from the sort of questions that are of interest to health officials and the public. For instance, compare the following statements:

1. "The secondary cluster at location B appears statistically significantly higher than we would expect the highest cluster to appear under a hypothesis of constant risk."
2. "The secondary cluster also exhibits an observed incidence proportion significantly higher than expected from national incidence proportions."

Generally, interested parties prefer an answer to statement 2, but our Monte Carlo ranking provides a statistical answer to statement 1.

7.4 GLOBAL INDEXES OF SPATIAL AUTOCORRELATION

We now move from methods that smooth local incidence proportions (rates) to methods that summarize the extent of observed spatial similarity between nearby regions. Griffith (1992) describes several interpretations of spatial autocorrelation, including the notion of *self-correlation.* Under this interpretation, the term *spatial autocorrelation* implies correlation among the same type of measurement taken at different locations. A *global index of spatial autocorrelation* provides a summary over the entire study area of the level of spatial similarity observed among neighboring observations. Statistical indexes of autocorrelation appear in a wide variety of applications, and Cliff and Ord (1973, 1981) are two classic references on the theory and application of these indexes.

7.4.1 Goals

The goal of a global index of spatial autocorrelation is to summarize the degree to which similar observations tend to occur near each other. Typically, extreme values of the index in one direction suggest positive spatial autocorrelation, while extreme values in the opposite direction suggest negative spatial autocorrelation. Since global indexes are by definition summaries over the study area, most applications of global indexes of spatial correlation in the assessment of disease patterns result in tests of *clustering* rather than tests to detect individual *clusters.* As discussed in Section 7.1.3, autocorrelation among disease counts or incidence proportions may reflect real association between cases due to infection, or perceived association based on a spatial aggregation of similar values.

7.4.2 Assumptions and Typical Output

Most indexes of autocorrelation share a common basic structure. In this structure, we calculate the similarity of values at locations i and j, then weight this similarity by the proximity of locations i and j. High similarities with high weight (i.e., similar values close together) lead to high values of the index, while low similarities with high weight (i.e., dissimilar values close together) lead to low values of the index. Following Lee and Wong (2001, pp. 79–80), let sim_{ij} denote the similarity between data values Y_i and Y_j, and let w_{ij} denote a weight describing the proximity between locations i and j, for i and $j = 1, \ldots, N$. Most global indexes of spatial autocorrelation build on the basic form

$$\frac{\sum_{i=1}^{N}\sum_{j=1}^{N} w_{ij}\text{sim}_{ij}}{\sum_{i=1}^{N}\sum_{j=1}^{N} w_{ij}}, \tag{7.3}$$

the weighted average similarity between observations. The geography and statistical literature often refer to statistics of this form as *general cross-product statistics*, introduced by Mantel (1967) as a test statistic for comparing two matrices. The matrices of interest here are the matrix of fixed weights w_{ij} and the matrix of observed similarity values sim_{ij} for $i, j = 1, \ldots, N$. Various indexes adjust the average similarity by different multiplicative constants to rescale or otherwise normalize the index, but the basic structure remains the same. Many statistics fall into this category, including the q-nearest-neighbor methods described for point data in equation (6.9) of Section 6.6.3.

The basic form in equation (7.3) is similar to the locally weighted-average smoothers presented in Section 4.4.1. However, the two approaches differ with respect to the weights w_{ii} controlling the impact of the value observed in region i on the weighted average for region i. When calculating a spatially averaged *incidence proportion* to stabilize the incidence proportion estimate for region i, we typically assume that the data observed in region i should substantially contribute to this weighted average and hence set $w_{ii} > 0$. In contrast, when calculating a spatially weighted average *similarity* of nearby observations as in equation (7.3), we typically omit the similarity of the ith region with itself and set $w_{ii} = 0$. For the remainder of this chapter, we assume that $w_{ii} = 0$.

We note that the measure of similarity sim_{ij} depends on random variables defining observations, and the w_{ij} are fixed quantities based on the underlying geography of the regions. As such, the sim_{ij} define the distributional structure of the index, and the w_{ij} define the spatial structures of correlation that a particular index (i.e., a particular combination of sim_{ij} and w_{ij}) is best suited to detect. Therefore, different measures of similarity define different index classes (e.g., Moran's I and Geary's c, as defined below), while different measures of proximity lead to different applications within the class of index.

Spatial Proximity Matrices We often report our collection of weights w_{ij} as a *spatial proximity matrix* (also called *spatial connectivity* or *spatial weight matrixes*; see, e.g., Cliff and Ord 1981; Haining 1990; Bailey and Gatrell 1995, pp. 261–262). The (i, j)th element of a spatial proximity matrix W, denoted w_{ij}, quantifies the spatial dependence between regions i and j, and collectively, the w_{ij} define a neighborhood structure over the entire area (cf. Section 4.4.1). Perhaps the simplest neighborhood definition is provided by the *binary connectivity matrix*, whose elements are

$$w_{ij} = \begin{cases} 1 & \text{if regions } i \text{ and } j \text{ share a boundary} \\ 0 & \text{otherwise.} \end{cases} \tag{7.4}$$

Note that this choice of proximity measure necessarily results in a symmetric spatial proximity matrix since $w_{ij} = w_{ji}$. As noted above, we set $w_{ii} = 0$ for $i = 1, \ldots, N$.

As in Section 4.4.1, many other choices of spatial proximity measures can be considered. For instance, we may want to expand our idea of a neighborhood to include regions that are close, but not necessarily adjacent. Thus, we could use

$$w_{ij} = \begin{cases} 1 & \text{if the centroid of region } j \text{ is one of the } q \text{ nearest} \\ & \text{to the centroid of region } i \\ 0 & \text{otherwise.} \end{cases} \tag{7.5}$$

The regions for which $w_{ij} = 1$ in equation (7.5) are called the *q nearest neighbors* of region i, and the resulting spatial proximity matrix is not necessarily symmetric (i.e., w_{ij} need not be equal to w_{ji}).

Instead of specifying a certain number of nearest neighbors, we can define the neighbors by some parametric function of distance. For example, if d_{ij} is the distance (Euclidean, city-block, or any other distance metric) between the centroids of regions i and j, we could choose

$$w_{ij} = \begin{cases} 1 & \text{if } d_{ij} < \delta \\ 0 & \text{otherwise} \end{cases} \tag{7.6}$$

or

$$w_{ij} = \begin{cases} d_{ij}^{-\alpha} & \alpha > 0 \\ 0 & \text{otherwise} \end{cases} \tag{7.7}$$

for some power α. Both approaches yield symmetric weights.

As a final example, we could define neighborhood structure based on the fraction of region i's border that is shared with region j; that is,

$$w_{ij} = \begin{cases} \dfrac{l_{ij}}{l_i} & \text{if regions } i \text{ and } j \text{ share a boundary} \\ 0 & \text{otherwise,} \end{cases}$$

where l_{ij} is the length of the common boundary between regions i and j and l_i is the perimeter of region i (Cliff and Ord 1981, pp. 17–18). Such a structure may arise as a model of the flow of goods, people, or possibly disease between regions. If such commodities flow out from a region uniformly with respect to direction, neighboring regions covering a greater proportion of the common border will receive more of region i's output. Note that in this case the spatial proximity matrix W is not symmetric.

Sometimes, we may want to adjust for the total number of neighbors in each region and employ a *row standardized matrix* where we divide each w_{ij} by the sum of neighbor weights for region i giving a matrix W_{std}, where

$$w_{\text{std},ij} = \frac{w_{ij}}{\sum_{j=1}^{N} w_{ij}}.$$

If region i has four neighbors, each receives weight $\frac{1}{4}$. Note that W_{std} need not be symmetric, and is not symmetric in most situations where the regions are of different spatial support (e.g., irregularly shaped regions).

Null Distributions Inference for a global index of spatial autocorrelation derives from the null distribution (i.e., the distribution of the index under the null hypothesis).

Observed values of the index falling in the tails of this distribution suggest significant spatial autocorrelation. Thus, identification of the appropriate null distribution is critical for accurate statistical conclusions.

Cliff and Ord (1973) define distributional properties for global indexes of spatial autocorrelation under a null hypothesis of independent observations under two different assumptions. The first, termed the *normality assumption*, assumes that all observations follow identical and independent Gaussian (normal) distributions. With the normality assumption, the values observed represent a single observation from an infinite set of possible realizations. If we were to simulate such a process (by generating independent Gaussian observations at each location), the sum of the values is not constrained, hence the normality assumption is often referred to as *normality sampling* or *free sampling*. The second assumption, termed the *randomization assumption*, assesses the distribution of the autocorrelation index under random assignment of the values observed to locations (similar to a generalization of *random labeling* where we assign N labels to locations rather than just two). With the randomization assumption, the set of observations remains the same in each randomization. The values are simply reassigned among the (fixed) locations, so some texts refer to randomization as *nonfree sampling*. In both settings, under the additional assumption that the mean and variance of the data are both constant across the regions, Cliff and Ord (1973, Chapter 2) prove the global indexes of spatial autocorrelation have asymptotic Gaussian (normal) distributions as the number of regions (N) increases. Upton and Fingleton (1985) suggest that the asymptotic approximations are accurate for $N > 20$ regions, although Tiefelsdorf and Boots (1995) indicate that the appropriateness of the asymptotic distribution is a function of the spatial proximity matrix W as well as the number of regions.

As noted in Section 7.1.3, our null hypothesis of no clustering (or no clusters), operationalized through the constant risk hypothesis, typically assumes Poisson-distributed regional counts with heterogeneous expected values (due to varying population sizes across regions) in addition to the assumed independence between regional counts. The discrete nature of the data and the relatively small counts expected violate any assumption of normality, and heterogeneous population sizes violate any assumption of constant variance among incidence proportions (even under the constant risk hypothesis). As a result, the normality assumption is inappropriate for most public health (and many geographical) applications. In addition, variation in the expectations and variances of counts (and in the variances of incidence proportions) renders the randomization assumption inappropriate (Besag and Newell 1991). Results in Walter (1992a,b) suggest that population heterogeneity can lead to inflated type I error levels, causing us to reject the null hypothesis of no clustering more often than we should.

Since the standard approximations to the null distribution of global indices of spatial autocorrelation may be inappropriate for assessing clustering in heterogeneously distributed Poisson data, we again turn to Monte Carlo hypothesis tests as defined in Section 5.2.3 and described by Besag and Newell (1991, p. 146). We simply calculate the value of the autocorrelation index for each of a number of data sets simulated under the constant risk hypothesis and distributional assumptions more appropriate to our application, and compare the index observed to the distribution defined by the simulated values.

In the sections below, we define two common global indexes of spatial autocorrelation, Moran's I and Geary's c, illustrate them on the New York leukemia data introduced in Chapter 4, and contrast Monte Carlo results with naive inference based on the normalization and randomization assumptions.

7.4.3 Method: Moran's I

The first index we consider is *Moran's I* (Moran 1950). Moran's I is widely used, and variations of it relate to likelihood ratio tests and best invariant tests for particular models of correlation for normally distributed random variables [cf. Haining (1990, p. 146) and Tiefelsdorf (2000) for discussion].

Moran's I follows the basic form [equation (7.3)] for global indexes of spatial autocorrelation with similarity between regions i and j defined as the product of the respective difference between Y_i and Y_j with the overall mean:

$$\text{sim}_{ij} = (Y_i - \overline{Y})(Y_j - \overline{Y})$$

where $\overline{Y} = \sum_{i=1}^{N} Y_i/N$. In addition, we divide this basic form by the sample variance observed in the Y_i's, yielding

$$I = \left(\frac{1}{s^2}\right) \frac{\displaystyle\sum_{i=1}^{N}\sum_{j=1}^{N} w_{ij}(Y_i - \overline{Y})(Y_j - \overline{Y})}{\displaystyle\sum_{i=1}^{N}\sum_{j=1}^{N} w_{ij}}, \tag{7.8}$$

where

$$s^2 = \frac{1}{N}\sum_{i=1}^{N}(Y_i - \overline{Y})^2.$$

Thus, I is a random variable having a distribution defined by the distributions of and interactions between the Y_i. We obtain the value of I observed by inserting observations into equation (7.8). When neighboring regions tend to have similar values (i.e., the pattern is clustered), I will be positive. If neighboring regions tend to have different values (i.e., the pattern is regular), I will be negative. When there is no correlation between neighboring values, the expected value of I is

$$E(I) = -\frac{1}{N-1}, \tag{7.9}$$

approaching zero as N increases. Unlike a traditional correlation coefficient, values for Moran's I need not be constrained to the interval $[-1, 1]$. Usually, $|I| < 1$, unless regions with extreme values of $Y_i - \overline{Y}$ are heavily weighted. The theoretical upper bound is

$$|I| \leq \frac{N}{\sum_{i \neq j} \sum_{j=1}^{N} w_{ij}} \left\{ \frac{\sum_{i \neq j} \left[\sum_{j=1}^{N} w_{ij}(Y_i - \overline{Y}) \right]^2}{\sum_{i=1}^{N} (Y_i - \overline{Y})^2} \right\}^{1/2}$$

(cf. Cliff and Ord 1981, p. 21; Haining 1990, p. 234; Bailey and Gatrell 1995, p. 270).

Moran's I is very similar to Pearson's correlation coefficient, a measure of association between N observed values of random variables X and Y. Recall that the definition of Pearson's correlation coefficient is

$$\frac{\sum_{i=1}^{N} \frac{(X_i - \overline{X})(Y_i - \overline{Y})}{N}}{\sqrt{\sum_{i=1}^{N} \frac{(X_i - \overline{X})^2}{N}} \sqrt{\sum_{i=1}^{N} \frac{(Y_i - \overline{Y})^2}{N}}}.$$

Replacing X_i by Y_j, comparing Y_j to the overall mean $\overline{Y}$, and weighting elements by their proximity as defined by the W matrix yields

$$\frac{\sum_{i=1}^{N} \sum_{j=1}^{N} w_{ij} \frac{(Y_i - \overline{Y})(Y_j - \overline{Y})}{\sum_{i=1}^{N} \sum_{j}^{N} w_{ij}}}{\sqrt{\sum_{i=1}^{N} \frac{(Y_i - \overline{Y})^2}{N}} \sqrt{\sum_{j=1}^{N} \frac{(Y_j - \overline{Y})^2}{N}}}.$$

The two terms in the denominator are identical; hence, Moran's I reflects a spatially weighted form of Pearson's correlation coefficient.

We can judge the significance of any observed value of I by comparing it to its expected value of $-1/(N-1)$, but we must also account for the expected variability in the I statistic under the appropriate null hypothesis. This is where the distributional assumptions about the data become very important. With the randomization assumption, data values are reassigned among the N fixed locations, providing a randomization distribution against which we can judge our observed value. If our observed value of I lies in the tails of this distribution, we reject the assumption of independence among the observations and conclude that there is significant spatial autocorrelation in the data. If we rely instead on the normality assumption, we compare the z-score $z = [I - E(I)]/\sqrt{\text{Var}(I)}$ to a standard normal distribution where $E(I)$ is as given in equation (7.9) and Var(I) is given by

$$\text{Var}(I) = \frac{N^2 S_1 - N S_2 + 3S_0^2}{(N-1)(N+1)S_0^2} - \left(\frac{1}{N-1}\right)^2,$$

with $S_0 = \sum_{i=1}^N \sum_{j=1}^N w_{ij}$, $S_1 = 1/2 \sum_{i=1}^N \sum_{j=1}^N (w_{ij} + w_{ji})^2$, and $S_2 = \sum_{i=1}^N (w_{i+} + w_{+j})^2$, with $w_{i+} = \sum_{j=1}^N w_{ij}$ and $w_{+i} = \sum_{j=1}^N w_{ji}$ (Cliff and Ord 1981, Chapter 2).

Application of Moran's I to public health regional count data merits some thought. Note that in the definition of Moran's I in equation (7.8), we assess the spatial similarity of deviations of each regional count Y_i with the overall mean regional count $\overline{Y}$. Does spatial variation in deviations from the mean regional count really assess clustering? Due to the spatial heterogeneity of regional at-risk population sizes inherent in regional public health data, observed spatial similarity in regional deviations from the mean regional count may simply be due to variations in the regional at-risk population size. For example, suppose that regions with large population sizes tend to occur near each other. Under the constant risk hypothesis, regions with higher-than (overall)-average population sizes will tend to have higher-than-average observed counts, elevating the value of Moran's I. In short, we may observe high values of Moran's I [as defined in equation (7.8)] even when the constant risk hypothesis is satisfied. Any autocorrelation in the data may simply be due to relationships among the population sizes and not to any spatial pattern in the disease counts.

We could replace regional disease counts with regional crude incidence proportions (rates), seeking to remove or at least lessen the impact of population heterogeneity. Consideration of incidence proportions (rates) removes heterogeneity in the value expected under the constant risk hypothesis since comparison of regional incidence proportions to the overall mean incidence proportion makes more sense than comparison of regional counts to the overall mean count. However, the variances of the local incidence proportions depend on the regional at-risk population sizes, which remain heterogeneous. Oden (1995), Waldhör (1996), and Assunção and Reis (1999) each propose adaptations of Moran's I for incidence proportions and provide derivations of the associated null distribution in the presence of heterogeneous regional population sizes.

We could also adjust Moran's I for regional counts by comparing the observed count in region i with its expectation under the constant risk hypothesis, rather than comparing the count to the overall mean count. Walter (1992a) suggests modifying equation (7.8) as follows:

$$I_{\text{cr}} = \frac{\sum_{i=1}^N \sum_{j=1}^N w_{ij} \dfrac{Y_i - rn_i}{\sqrt{rn_i}} \dfrac{Y_j - rn_j}{\sqrt{rn_j}}}{\sum_{i=1}^N \sum_{j=1}^N w_{ij}}, \tag{7.10}$$

where n_i denotes the population size for region i, and r denotes the overall disease incidence proportion (rate) specified a priori or estimated by the total number of cases observed divided by the total number of persons at risk. Note that we replace the scaling factor s^2 with the product of the region-specific (Poisson) standard deviations, to emphasize variation around each regional expectation rather than around an overall mean count. Equation (7.10) reflects a weighted cross-product of "observed minus expected" elements bearing resemblance to goodness-of-fit statistics, a similarity we return to in subsequent sections.

The statistic I_{cr} represents an assessment of *residual* spatial autocorrelation, or autocorrelation among deviations of values observed from local expectations based on some model of disease incidence (here the constant risk assumption serves as our model). Cliff and Ord (1973, 1981) and Tiefelsdorf (2000) explore the application of Moran's I to linear regression residuals (an application we return to in Chapter 9) and provide the relevant theory and asymptotics for inference based on identically distributed Gaussian residuals.

Here I_{cr} corresponds to Moran's I applied to the *Pearson residuals* from a generalized linear model (GLM) for Poisson outcomes with local mean equal to rn_i (McCullagh and Nelder 1989, p. 37). Jacqmin-Gadda et al. (1997) provide some relevant theoretical results for a general version of equation (7.10), where we replace the value expected under the constant risk hypothesis with the expectation of Y_i under any generalized linear model (in practice, typically a logistic or a Poisson regression model) fit to the data. Jacqmin-Gadda et al. (1997) show that this more general statistic corresponds to a score test of correlation among GLM model residuals comparing a null hypothesis of no correlation with a particular correlation model defined by the user's choice of weights w_{ij}. The converse implies that if the user has a particular correlation structure of interest, we can define specific weights making the generalization of I_{cr} a score test for that particular alternative. Score tests are locally most powerful tests (cf. Cox and Hinkley 1974); that is, score tests have optimal statistical power (probability of detecting deviations from the null when an alternative hypothesis holds) for small deviations from the null toward the alternative of interest. Theoretically, these score tests have asymptotic (N going to infinity) Gaussian distributions, but to our knowledge, the sensitivity of the asymptotic distribution of I_{cr} (or generalizations thereof) to the number of regions (N), the rarity of the disease (r), or the specification of the spatial weights (w_{ij}'s) remains largely unexplored [with the exception of the work of Jacqmin-Gadda et al. (1997)].

To conclude our discussion of Moran's I, even if we accept the statistic as a meaningful indicator of spatial similarity, we find that both the normality and the randomization assumptions are generally inappropriate for testing clustering with heterogeneous count data or incidence proportions. However, the simplicity of simulating statistically independent Poisson variables under the constant risk hypothesis that accounts for the differing at-risk population sizes provides straightforward application of Monte Carlo hypothesis tests (Besag and Newell 1991, p. 146). These allow us to compare our observed value of Moran's I (or any other index of spatial autocorrelation) against more appropriate null distributions, and we compare and contrast such approaches in the data break below.

DATA BREAK: New York Leukemia Data (*cont.*) We illustrate the use (and misuse) of Moran's I using census tract counts from the New York leukemia data described previously. For simplicity, we limit attention to the binary connectivity matrix with elements $w_{ij} = 1$ if regions i and j share any portion of their borders with one another. (These are often called *adjacency weights*.)

Table 7.3 gives Moran's I for both leukemia counts and the local incidence proportions (crude rates). The expectation of I under the null hypothesis of independence is $-1/(N-1) = -1/280 \approx -0.00357$ for all three outcomes (since this expectation depends only on the number of regions, not the measurements under consideration).

Even though we argue against their use above, we present p-values associated with the normality and randomization assumptions for comparison with the p-value based on a Monte Carlo test using the constant risk hypothesis based on 9999 simulations where we generate independent Poisson counts with mean rn_i (the overall incidence proportion times the population size) for each region i. Note that we simulate counts based on these expectations but apply Moran's I as defined in equation (7.8), comparing each regional count to the overall mean regional count.

For counts, Table 7.3 reveals a substantial difference in significance levels based on the (incorrect) normality and randomization assumptions and that based on constant risk. Figure 7.8 illustrates the source of the difference. The top histogram shows the distribution of Moran's I values under randomization, where we reassign observed counts at random among the 281 regions (which makes little sense with heterogeneous population densities, as noted above). The bottom histogram illustrates the distribution of Moran's I under the constant risk hypothesis and reveals a considerable shift away from the usual null distribution of Moran's I for independent, identically distributed (i.i.d.) regional random variables. We see more positive values of Moran's I than we would expect for i.i.d. counts. However, since we simulated the data, we know that our counts are independent and differ

Table 7.3 Moran's I Values for Incidence Counts and Proportions Observed for Leukemia (All Types), 1978–1982, for an Eight-County Region of Upstate New York[a]

Outcome	I	Null Distribution	p-Value
Count	0.110	Normality	<0.001
		Randomization	0.002
		Constant risk (Poisson)	0.143
Incidence proportion	0.039	Normality	0.119
		Randomization	0.106
		Constant risk (Poisson)	0.143

[a] Significance values are calculated from the standard Gaussian distribution for the normality assumption and based on 9999 simulations each under randomization and the constant risk hypotheses (see text).

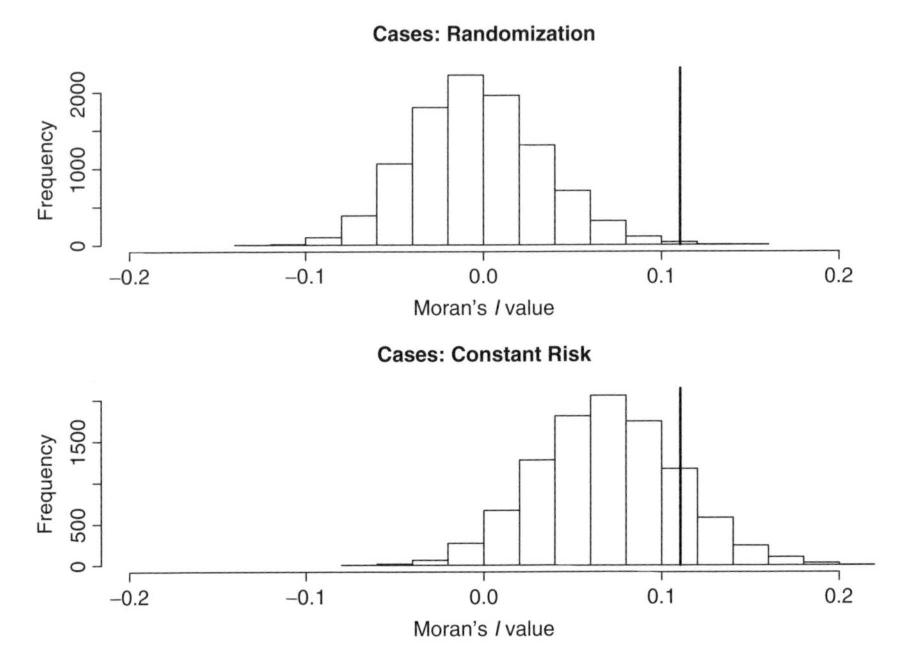

FIG. 7.8 Histograms of 9999 values of Moran's I for upstate New York leukemia incidence counts simulated under the randomization assumption (top) and the constant risk hypothesis (bottom). The thick vertical line represents the observed value of Moran's I for the New York leukemia data.

in distribution only through their associated means and variances. This observation suggests that the spatial structure in the population sizes (hence expected counts) induces measurable positive spatial correlation among the observed counts, even under the constant risk hypothesis. The key to interpretation is our understanding of the null distributions. Our data are inconsistent with the normality and randomization assumptions, but when we think about these assumptions, we wouldn't expect our data to satisfy them. On the other hand, the Monte Carlo test of the constant risk hypothesis acknowledges the impact of the heterogeneous regional population sizes and suggests that the data do not contain significant spatial clustering of deviations of counts from the overall mean count. In effect, we find a Monte Carlo approximation to the distribution of Moran's I *conditional* on the spatial heterogeneous regional population distribution in order to turn attention away from the heterogeneous spatial population pattern and toward spatial patterns in local deviations from this process.

As we noted in the description of Moran's I, assessing spatial patterns in deviations of regional incidence *proportions* (rates) from the overall mean regional incidence proportion may be preferable to comparing regional *counts* to the overall mean regional count when we have heterogeneous population sizes. Table 7.3 provides the p-values associated with the normality and randomization assumptions, and that obtained from Monte Carlo simulation under the constant risk hypotheses when applying Moran's I to the local incidence proportions (rates). Figure 7.9

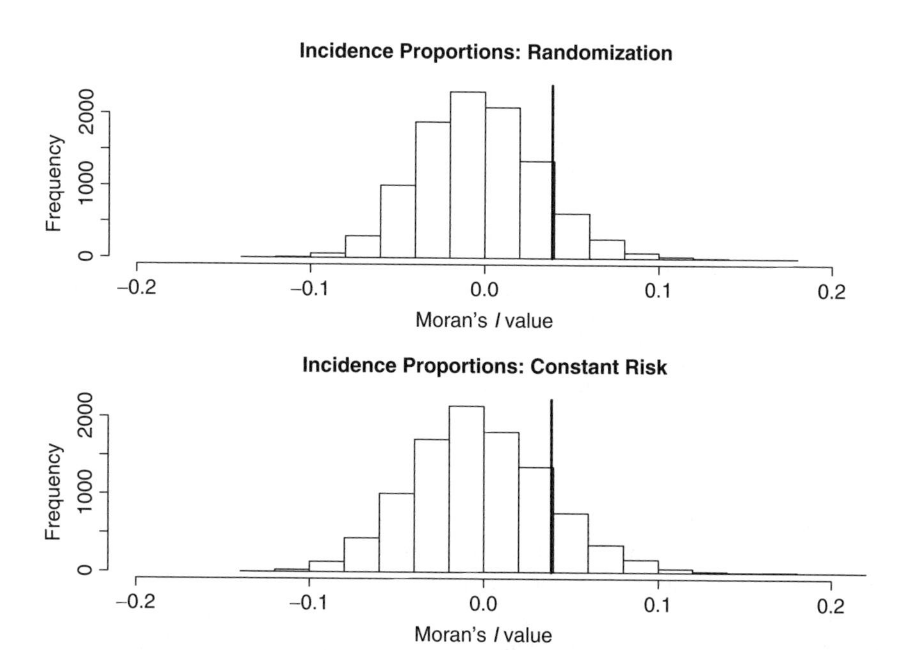

FIG. 7.9 Histograms of 9999 values of Moran's I for upstate New York leukemia incidence proportions (rates) simulated under the randomization assumption (top) and the constant risk hypothesis (bottom). The thick vertical line represents the observed value of Moran's I for the New York leukemia data.

illustrates histograms comparing the null distribution of Moran's I under the randomization assumption to that obtained with the constant risk simulations. The histograms do not shift as dramatically for incidence proportions (rates) as they did for counts since we adjust for heterogeneous population sizes by dividing each count by the regional population size. However, as noted in Chapter 4, the heterogeneities in population size affect the statistical stability (variation) of local estimates of estimation, and these heterogeneous variances result in a slight shift and wider tails in the histogram based on constant risk simulations. As we expect, we observe less difference between the distribution of Moran's I for incidence proportions (rates) under the constant risk hypothesis and those under the normality and randomization assumptions than we do between the corresponding distributions for Moran's I for counts. Finally, we note that under the Monte Carlo test we obtain nearly identical inference, regardless of our choice to work with counts or incidence proportions.

To account more directly for population heterogeneity, we apply I_{cr} to the New York leukemia data. Recall that I_{cr} summarizes the spatial similarity in the discrepancy of each regional count with its expectation under the constant risk hypothesis. Monte Carlo tests based on 9999 simulations yield a p-value of 0.001 for the constant risk hypothesis, suggesting significant clustering of standardized deviations of the regional counts observed from their values expected under constant risk.

To summarize, the example illustrates several applications of Moran's I and variants thereof to data with a heterogeneously distributed population at risk. We find the normality and randomization assumptions inappropriate in such a situation and illustrate how naive application may yield misleading results. Monte Carlo testing based on the constant risk hypothesis suggests little statistical evidence of significant spatial correlation of deviations of regional counts from the overall mean regional count, little statistical evidence for significant spatial correlation of deviations of regional incidence proportions (rates) from the overall mean incidence proportion (rate), but we do find strong statistical evidence for spatial correlation of standardized deviations from regional expected counts under the constant risk hypothesis. How are these results mutually compatible?

Note our application of Moran's I [equation (7.8)] to counts and incidence proportions assumed both a single reference mean and a single reference variance, the latter estimated by s^2 and assumed homogeneous across the study area. Our application of I_{cr} [equation (7.10)] allows for heterogeneity in regional variation from the regional mean, based on an assumed underlying Poisson probability distribution. The specification of regional variations appears to provide additional local precision in assessing the spatial similarity of statistically unusual counts. The example illustrates the importance of assessing the particular question addressed by a statistical test, and the importance of aligning the statistical methodology with appropriate assumptions based on the structure of the data.

Finally, our analysis suggests evidence of *clustering* (based on I_{cr}) but does not identify the locations of any particular *clusters* driving the pattern observed. We investigate methods to identify the location of clusters based on components of Moran's I in Section 7.5.

7.4.4 Method: Geary's *c*

A second popular global index of spatial autocorrelation derives from equation (7.3), where we measure similarity between observations via

$$\text{sim}_{ij} = (Y_i - Y_j)^2.$$

If regions i and j have similar values (e.g., counts or incidence proportions), sim_{ij} will be small. We build a global index of spatial autocorrelation based on a weighted average of the similarity values observed for all pairs of regions assigning weights by spatial proximity (i.e., assigning higher weights for closer pairs of observations). Geary (1954) scales this weighted average by a measure of overall variation around the mean regional observation $\overline{Y}$, yielding a statistic now called *Geary's contiguity ratio*, or *Geary's c*, defined as

$$c = \frac{N-1}{2\sum_{i=1}^{N}(Y_i - \overline{Y})^2} \frac{\sum_{i=1}^{N}\sum_{j=1}^{N} w_{ij}(Y_i - Y_j)^2}{\sum_{i=1}^{N}\sum_{j=1}^{N} w_{ij}}. \tag{7.11}$$

Geary's c ranges in value from 0 to 2, with 0 indicating perfect positive spatial correlation ($Y_i = Y_j$ for any pair of regions with nonzero w_{ij}), and 2 indicating perfect negative spatial autocorrelation. Geary's c does not correspond directly to a correlation coefficient, but instead, corresponds to the Durbin–Watson *d statistic*, used to test for serial autocorrelation in regression and time series.

In contrast to Moran's I, low values of Geary's c denote positive autocorrelation and high values indicate negative correlation. Also, under the null hypothesis of spatial independence, and assuming constant means and variances, the expected value of Geary's c is equal to 1 under either the normality or the randomization assumptions. Again, these assumptions (and the assumptions of constant means and variances across regions) are often inappropriate in the analysis of regional health data with heterogeneous population sizes, and we contrast these with a Monte Carlo implementation based on the constant risk hypothesis in the data break below.

We can also adjust Geary's c for counts in a manner similar to the modification of Moran's I denoted I_{cr} and defined in equation (7.10). The key is to replace each regional count Y_i by a standardized value (thereby adjusting values Y_i and Y_j to have comparable variance) and to remove the overall measure of variation around the mean regional count. We leave precise specification and implementation of such an adjustment as an exercise.

DATA BREAK: New York Leukemia Data (*cont.*) Table 7.4 provides the observed value of Geary's c for the New York leukemia regional counts and incidence proportions (rates). Due to the nature of Geary's c, low values denote positive autocorrelation and we perform a lower-tail test to test against an alternative of positive spatial autocorrelation. We report lower-tail probabilities as p-values (the probability, under the null hypothesis, of observing a value of the test statistic less than that computed from the observed data).

Table 7.4 Geary's c Values for Observed Incidence Counts, Population Sizes (1980 Census), and Incidence Proportions for Leukemia (All Types) 1978–1982 for an Eight-County Region of Upstate New York[a]

Outcome	c	Null Distribution	p-Value
Count	0.874	Normality	0.003
		Randomization	0.006
		Constant risk	0.176
Incidence proportion	0.925	Normality	0.054
		Randomization	0.289
		Constant risk	0.129

[a] Significance values calculated from the Gaussian distribution for the normality assumption and based on 9999 simulations each for the randomization assumption and the constant risk hypotheses (see text).

As with Moran's I, we present p-values based on naive (and incorrect) application of Geary's c based on the normality and randomization assumptions and contrast this with Monte Carlo tests based on the constant risk hypothesis. Applying Geary's c to the count data, we find that both the normality and randomization null hypotheses report strong statistical evidence for positive spatial correlation, but the Monte Carlo constant risk test moderates our enthusiasm for such a conclusion. Applying the statistic to the incidence proportions, we find that p-values based on normalization and on randomization are quite different from each other. This suggests that the incidence proportions observed appear to exhibit positive spatial autocorrelation compared to i.i.d./Gaussian (normal) random variables but not when compared to random allocation of the observed incidence proportions among the 281 census tracts. The difference here may be due to the spatially heterogeneous distribution of the population at risk.

As above, we note that neither the normality nor the randomization assumptions are appropriate for determining the null distribution, and we find the Monte Carlo tests based on the constant risk hypothesis to provide fairly consistent inference for both counts and incidence proportions. In short, we find suggestive but not statistically significant evidence of greater positive spatial autocorrelation than would be expected under the constant risk hypothesis given the spatial distribution of the population at risk.

Finally, we note that Moran's I, Geary's c, and all other global indexes of spatial autocorrelation (typically, general cross product statistics) are tests of *clustering* and provide a single p-value summarizing spatial autocorrelation observed across all regions in the study area. To use tests of spatial autocorrelation to detect *clusters*, we next consider *local* indicators of spatial autocorrelation.

7.5 LOCAL INDICATORS OF SPATIAL ASSOCIATION

As their name implies, global indicators of spatial association assess patterns of spatial similarity summarized (often through weighted averages) over the entire study area. When such indexes indicate positive spatial autocorrelation, this autocorrelation may arise from a number of sources. If the index compares regional counts or incidence proportions to an overall mean regional count or proportion, a spatial trend in expectation can result in index values suggesting spatial similarity. In addition, and more to our interest, local pockets of mutually similar deviations from the overall mean regional count or proportion may drive the value of the index. Such collections reflect our intuitive definition of disease clusters. As noted in our motivation and description of the adjusted I_{cr} statistic defined in equation (7.10), removing trend and spatial heterogeneities in regional variances can reduce the influence of overall trends and variance heterogeneities on the index, thereby making the adjusted index more responsive to clusters than to trends.

Even adjusted for trends and variance heterogeneities, global indexes remain global and only detect spatial associations averaged over the entire study area. Therefore, such indexes may have little statistical power to detect a single cluster within a study area otherwise following the null hypothesis. In addition, a global index can suggestion *clustering* but cannot identify individual *clusters*. These issues led Getis and Ord (1992), Anselin (1995), and Ord and Getis (1995) to consider local forms of the global indexes, which Anselin (1995) termed *local indicators of spatial association* (LISAs).

7.5.1 Goals

Anselin (1995) outlines the goals and structure of the class of LISAs. The main purpose of such indicators is to provide a local measure of similarity between each region's associated value (in our case, a count or an incidence proportion) and those of nearby regions. We can map each region's LISA value to provide insight into the location of regions with comparatively high or low local association with neighboring values.

Anselin (1995) also formally links LISAs with corresponding global indicators by requiring that the LISA values from each region sum to a global indicator of spatial association (up to a multiplicative constant). This connection defines LISAs as components of a global index, and provides a means for partitioning a test of *clustering* (the global index) into a set of tests to detect *clusters* (the LISAs). As a result, most LISAs are defined as local versions of well-known global indexes. One of the most popular LISAs is a local version of Moran's I, which we consider in some detail below.

7.5.2 Assumptions and Typical Output

Anselin (1995), Ord and Getis (1995), and Getis and Ord (1996) provide detailed overviews of LISAs and their application, which we review briefly here. Getis and Ord (1996) trace the basic idea to Mantel (1967)'s derivation of the general cross-product statistic defined in Section 7.4.2, and give the basic form of the LISA for region i as

$$\sum_{j=1}^{N} w_{ij} \ \text{sim}_{ij}.$$

Although not required, many applications use *row-standardized weights*, so the weights w_{ij}, $j = 1, \ldots, N$, sum to 1, and there is some comparability between regions with different numbers of neighbors. This form represents the ith summand in the numerator of the basic structure of a global indicator of spatial association (the denominator is the sum of the weights and is a multiplicative constant). Hence, the sum of such local indicators will equal (up to a multiplicative constant) a global indicator, meeting the requirement of Anselin (1995). As defined in Section 7.4.2, sim_{ij} represents a measure of similarity between regional observations and in our case is a function of the regional count or incidence proportion (rate).

As noted above, we consider the proximity weights to be fixed quantities and the similarity measurements sim_{ij} to be functions of the observations at locations i and j. Since we consider these observations to represent observed values of random variables, the distribution of these variables defines the distribution of the sim_{ij}

values, which in turn define the distribution of each local indicator. The distribution of each LISA allows probability statements such as the probability of any LISA exceeding a specified critical value.

The null hypotheses for LISAs mirror those for general indicators of spatial association, namely that the Y_i represent independent observations. Most analytic results for LISAs involve independent, identically distributed (i.i.d.) Gaussian (normal) regional random variables, but even in this case analytic solutions are complicated (cf. Tiefelsdorf and Boots 1995, 1996; Tiefelsdorf 2000). Anselin (1995) applies a randomization assumption, which applies most accurately to i.i.d. data as noted in Section 7.4. In our data break below we repeat our pattern in Section 7.4 and contrast Monte Carlo tests based on the randomization assumption and the (in our setting) more appropriate constant risk hypothesis.

The typical output of a LISA analysis involves the values of the LISAs themselves, typically mapped to indicate areas with high values, suggesting stronger local correlation than others. We note that high LISA values may be due to aggregations of high counts or proportions, aggregations of low counts or proportions, or aggregations of moderate counts or proportions. As a result, high values of a LISA suggest clusters of similar (but not necessarily large) counts or proportions across several regions, and low values of a LISA suggest an outlying cluster in a single region (different from most or all of its neighbors).

Other typical output includes maps of p-values associated with the probability of exceeding the observed value of each regional LISA, under a given set of assumptions that determines the distribution of the LISA under the null hypothesis. Calculations of p-values or any other probability statements are complicated by the following four issues [compiled from similar lists in Getis and Ord (1996) and Tiefelsdorf (2000)]:

1. The analytic distributional properties of LISAs remain largely unknown, with the recent exception of the work of Tiefelsdorf and colleagues (cf. Tiefelsdorf and Boots 1995, 1996; Tiefelsdorf 1998, 2000, 2002), who provide approaches for obtaining the exact distribution of local (and global) Moran's I under assumed Gaussian (normal) distributions in all regions.
2. The multiple testing problem of conducting a separate statistical test for each region.
3. The correlation between neighboring LISAs, which share observed counts or incidence proportions (rendering the typical Bonferroni adjustment for multiple tests very conservative).
4. The problem of conducting many tests, each based on a relatively small sample size (resulting in spurious significant results within the type I error rate of each test), and relatively unstable tests on very discrete outcomes (resulting in the observable type I error rates varying between regions).

We use Monte Carlo testing in our development to address the distribution of LISAs based on heterogeneous non-Gaussian random variables, thereby addressing issue 1, but the other issues remain in most applications of LISAs to public health data.

As a final general consideration, Anselin (1995), Ord and Getis (1995), and Tiefelsdorf (2000, pp. 133–134) provide derivations of the distribution of the local indicator for each region *conditional* on a known or estimated background spatial trend (or more generally, a known or estimated spatial process). As discussed in Section 7.4.3, by conditioning on known heterogeneities in either the mean (trend) or variance (e.g., due to heterogeneous population sizes in the constant risk hypothesis), local deviations from local expectations (e.g., clusters) drive the value of the index more than deviations from a the overall (global) regional mean value. See Anselin (1995), Ord and Getis (1995), and Tiefelsdorf (2000, pp. 133–134) for further discussion of the conditional distribution of local Moran's I and analytic results for regional values following Gaussian (normal) distributions.

7.5.3 Method: Local Moran's *I*

Probably the most widely used family of LISAs is the local version of Moran's I, defined for the ith region as

$$\begin{aligned} I_i &= \sum_{j=1}^{N} w_{ij} \ \text{sim}_{ij} \\ &= \sum_{j=1}^{N} w_{ij}(Y_i - \overline{Y})(Y_j - \overline{Y}) \\ &= (Y_i - \overline{Y}) \sum_{j=1}^{N} w_{ij}(Y_j - \overline{Y}). \end{aligned}$$

Most authors (e.g., Anselin 1995; Lee and Wong 2001) divide each deviation from the overall mean by the overall variance of the Y_i values, yielding

$$I_{i,\text{std}} = \frac{Y_i - \overline{Y}}{s} \sum_{j=1}^{N} w_{ij} \frac{Y_j - \overline{Y}}{s}, \tag{7.12}$$

where s represents the square root of the sample variance of the Y_i's, and the "std" subscript represents the use of the standardized difference of each regional observation from the overall regional mean. Tiefelsdorf (2000, pp. 134–136) presents an application of $I_{i,\text{std}}$ (assuming that each Y_i follows a Gaussian (normal) distribution) to health data in an analysis of regional patterns of bladder cancer incidence proportions among men and women in the former German Democratic Republic.

With heterogeneous population sizes yielding local Poisson distributions with heterogeneous expected counts and variances under the constant risk hypothesis, we can follow equation (7.10) and define an adjusted local Moran's I statistic for the constant risk hypothesis:

$$I_{i,\text{cr}} = \frac{Y_i - rn_i}{\sqrt{rn_i}} \sum_{j=1}^{N} w_{ij} \frac{Y_j - rn_j}{\sqrt{rn_j}}, \tag{7.13}$$

where, as before, r denotes the assumed constant risk and n_i denotes the population size in region i.

DATA BREAK: New York Leukemia Data (*cont.*) To illustrate the use of LISAs, we apply local Moran's I, I_{std}, and our modification for the constant risk hypothesis I_{cr} to the New York leukemia data using row-standardized adjacency weights. Figure 7.10 provides choropleth maps of local values for these three LISAs. We divide the 281 census tracts into quintiles of I_{cr}, then use the same intervals for all three maps, using darker shades of gray to indicate increasing positive values, and more densely striped areas to indicate increasing (absolute) values of negative correlation. The maps of I_{std} and I_{cr} show some similarities, with the highest fifth of values concentrated primarily near Binghamton in the south, Cortland in the center, and Syracuse in the north-central sections. However, they differ with respect to the extent of these concentrated values. The values of I_{std} for the

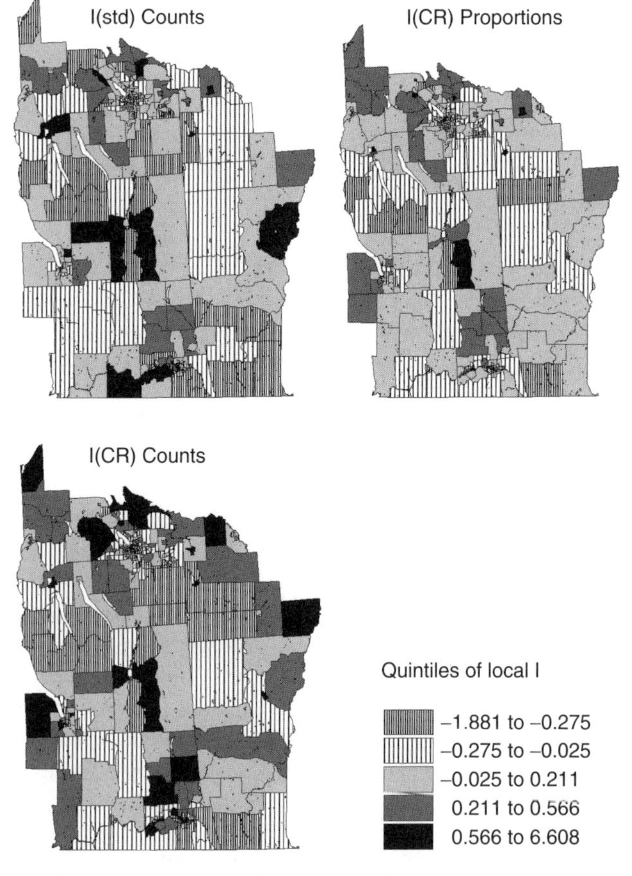

FIG. 7.10 Maps of I_{std} for counts (top left) and incidence proportions (top right), and a map of I_{cr} for counts (bottom left) based on the New York leukemia data.

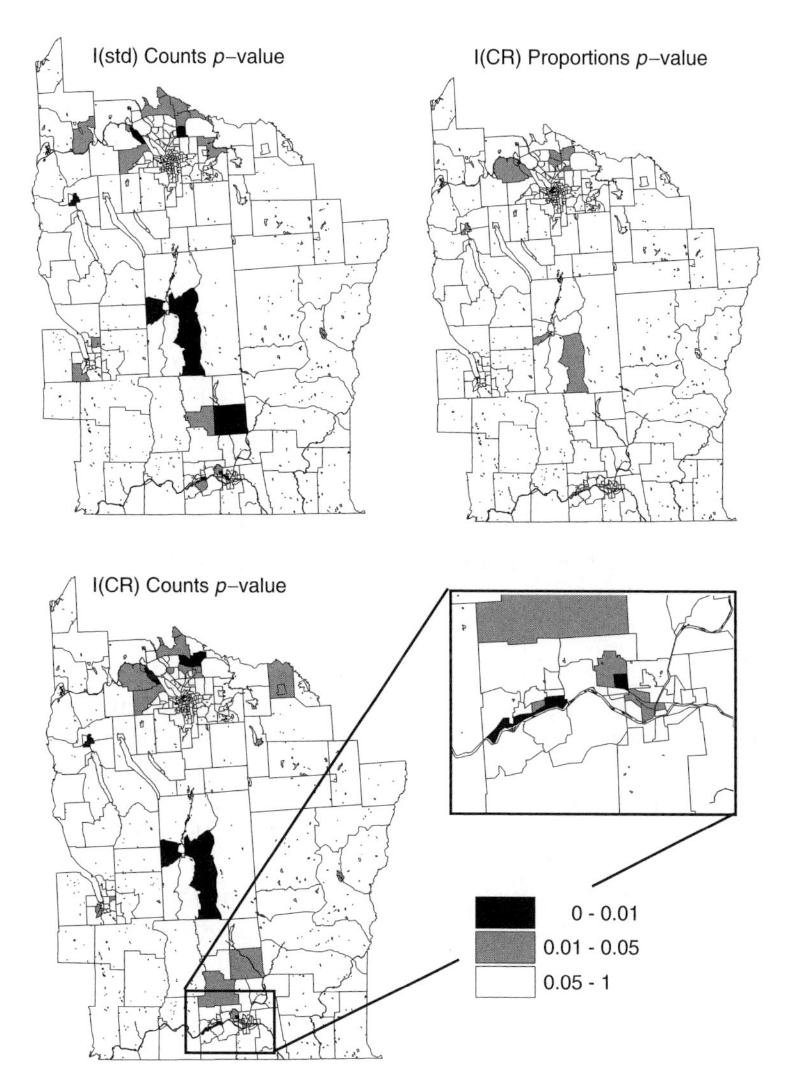

FIG. 7.11 Maps of p-values for I_{std} based on counts (top left) and incidence proportions (top right), and a map of p-values for I_{cr} based on counts (bottom left). Inset (bottom right) shows p-values for I_{cr} within tracts in the area of Binghamton, New York.

incidence proportions (rates) are less extreme than those for counts as evidenced by fewer tracts in the highest and lowest quintiles of I_{cr}; however, the highest values occur in similar areas.

Figure 7.11 presents the p-values based on 999 simulations under the constant risk hypothesis. We make no adjustment for multiple testing and simply indicate those tracts where the associated LISA value results in a p-value less than 0.05 or less than 0.01. As in Figure 7.10, the LISA values for incidence proportions are less extreme than those for counts. The statistics I_{std} and I_{cr} highlight similar areas (again, Binghamton, Cortland, and Syracuse) with some outlying rural areas also indicated. The figures illustrate little qualitative difference between conclusions drawn for I_{std} and I_{cr} in this data set, when we base p-values for both on Monte Carlo tests under the constant risk hypothesis. Whether this similarity holds more broadly remains to be seen.

7.6 GOODNESS-OF-FIT STATISTICS

In the preceding two sections, we found that indexes of spatial association based on spatial versions of familiar correlation coefficients often involve weighted averages of "observed minus expected" terms. In equations (7.10) and (7.13) we used this format to adjust the statistics to allow for heterogeneities in trend (expected values) and variances (due to varying population sizes) to better match the constant risk hypothesis. Many other tests of clustering and/or tests to detect clusters involve similar tests but are not necessarily derived as indexes of autocorrelation. We consider goodness-of-fit statistics and spatially weighted versions of such statistics here, illustrating a certain similarity with indexes of autocorrelation when applied to assess disease clustering.

7.6.1 Goals

The goal of any goodness-of-fit statistic is to summarize deviation between observed data and their expected values under some probabilistic model. The model may be as simple as comparing all observations to a constant value (usually estimated by the sample mean), or may involve more complex modeling (e.g., a heterogeneous Poisson process with an estimated intensity function, depending on covariate values).

One of the (if not *the*) original goodness-of-fit test is *Pearson's* χ^2 *statistic* defined for a 2×2 contingency table as

$$\chi^2 = \sum_{i=1}^{N} (O_i - E_i)^2 / E_i, \tag{7.14}$$

where N is the number of cells, O_i corresponds to the value observed in cell i of the contingency table, and E_i is the value expected in cell i based on independence between rows and columns. In traditional contingency table analysis, the E_i are based on binomially (or multinomially) distributed cell counts, and a test of independence between rows and columns is based on expected relationships among the E_i under this null hypothesis.

We can heuristically apply these ideas to the spatial case by thinking of regional data from irregular regions as a large contingency table (here, map) of cell counts, not necessarily constrained to be in rows and columns. In our setting, we replace the null hypothesis of independence between rows and columns with the constant risk hypothesis based on Poisson-distributed counts. This heuristic development requires a few modifications for use with a single set of spatial data, but the basic structure and purpose of the test statistic remains the same.

7.6.2 Assumptions and Typical Output

In general, Pearson's χ^2 statistic measures any deviation from expectation and takes no account of spatial patterns among these deviations; that is, if we were to randomly reassign the counts or rates to different regions, the value of χ^2 would remain the same. Therefore, the use of goodness-of-fit statistics to assess spatial pattern often incorporates some sort of spatial weighting to deviations from expectation, thereby limiting attention of the test to alternatives consistent with some sort of spatial pattern. In other words, the characteristic making a goodness-of-fit test appropriate for assessing spatial clustering is the consideration of particular alternative hypotheses, specifically those suggesting a spatial pattern in deviations from expectation.

Most goodness-of-fit tests assume statistically independent regional counts under both the null and alternative hypotheses, thereby distinguishing them from indexes of spatial association that assume independence under the null hypothesis, but not under the alternative. That is, usual applications of goodness-of-fit tests typically quantify spatial dependence in a different way than do indexes of spatial association. When applying goodness-of-fit tests as that tests of clustering or to detect clusters, we typically maintain the assumption of regional independence under the null hypothesis of interest (e.g., the constant risk hypothesis), and often under the alternative hypotheses defining clusters or clustering as well. Although we focus discussion below on independent counts under the constant risk hypothesis, this need not apply strictly, and Waller et al. (2003) illustrate the use of Monte Carlo tests based on Pearson's χ^2 statistic for a null hypothesis containing positive spatial correlation.

Under a null hypothesis with independent counts, inference for goodness-of-fit tests typically draws from the distribution of a sum of independent, standardized regional observations. Pearson's χ^2 statistic is an example of this approach. We subtract the expectation (under the null hypothesis) and divide by the standard deviation to create a sum of i.i.d. random variables. In the case of Pearson's χ^2 statistic, this leads to an asymptotic χ^2 distribution with $N - 1$ degrees of freedom, but modifications of the statistic may complicate distributional results. Monte Carlo tests of the constant risk hypothesis are straightforward and we continue our use of such tests in the development below.

The typical output of a goodness-of-fit test is a single p-value summarizing the evidence for deviation of observed values from those expected under the null hypothesis, summarized across all regions. As such, these typically provide general tests of clustering, although we also present some focused tests among the methods outlined below.

7.6.3 Method: Pearson's χ^2

To start our discussion of goodness-of-fit statistics, we consider whether Pearson's χ^2 statistic as defined in equation (7.14) provides a reasonable test of clustering. Rogerson (1999) observes that Pearson's statistic seeks to detect any sort of deviation from the null hypothesis and, as a result, makes no distinction between nonspatial and spatially structured collections of deviations. To repeat a simple example from

Section 7.1.3, suppose that only three regions in a study area have large deviations of observed from expected values. The value of Pearson's χ^2 statistic is unchanged whether these three regions are contiguous (perhaps suggesting a small cluster) or widely separated.

Rogerson (1999) also notes that indexes of spatial association (which *do* assess whether similar deviations occur near each other) may not provide a completely satisfactory means of detecting clustering since most indexes of spatial association only compare deviations between pairs of regions and do not assess the magnitude of lack of fit within each region (since typically, the spatial weight $w_{ii} = 0$). Thus, as we saw in Section 7.4, violations in model assumptions can affect the validity of spatial autocorrelation statistics, but these assumptions often go unchecked in the analysis.

As a compromise between these extremes, Rogerson (1999) explores a spatial χ^2 statistic building on an earlier adjustment to Moran's I for heterogeneous population density proposed by Oden (1995), and an index of clustering originally proposed for temporal data by Tango (1984), who later extended the index to the spatial setting (Tango 1995). Based on Tango's development of the basic statistic, its generalization to heterogeneous time intervals, and its extension to a spatial setting, we refer to the test as *Tango's index.*

7.6.4 Method: Tango's Index

Tango (1984) introduces an index of disease *clustering* in time using interval count data, based on equal-length time intervals subdividing the entire study period with event counts observed for each interval. He later generalizes the index for applications involving unequal time intervals and/or interval-specific covariates (Tango 1990b). Finally, and most directly applicable to our interest, Tango (1995) recasts the generalized statistic in a spatial setting. We present this version of Tango's index here.

First, rather than the set of regional *counts* $Y_1, \ldots, Y_N$, we consider the set of regional *proportions*,

$$\left(\frac{Y_1}{Y_+}, \ldots, \frac{Y_N}{Y_+}\right),$$

where $Y_+ = \sum_{i=1}^{N} Y_i$, the total number of observed cases. Note that the elements of this set of values reflect the proportion of cases in each region, not the incidence proportion (rate) in each region. The former divides by the total number of cases, while the latter divides by the population size of the corresponding region.

Next, we obtain the vector of expected proportions under the constant risk null hypothesis, namely the vector of population proportions

$$\left(\frac{n_1}{n_+}, \ldots, \frac{n_N}{n_+}\right),$$

where $n_+ = \sum_{i=1}^{N} n_i$ denotes the total population at risk.

Note that Tango's index assumes that both Y_+ and n_+ are known. When we condition a set of independent Poisson counts on their total, the distribution of the set of counts follows a multinomial distribution. Thus, under the constant risk hypothesis, the population proportions provide the expected cell probabilities for a multinomial distribution. Tango's index compares the case proportions observed to those expected under the constant risk null hypothesis.

We define *Tango's index* as

$$T_{\text{ti}} = \sum_{i=1}^{N} \sum_{j=1}^{N} w_{ij}^* \left(\frac{Y_i}{Y_+} - \frac{n_i}{n_+} \right) \left(\frac{Y_j}{Y_+} - \frac{n_j}{n_+} \right), \tag{7.15}$$

where the w_{ij}^* denote spatially defined weights providing a measurement of the "closeness" between regions i and j. Tango (1995) considers spatial weights, w_{ij}^*, defined by the value of a monotonically decreasing function of the distance d_{ij} between the centroids of regions i and j. The choices of d_{ij} and w_{ij}^* define the clustering alternatives of interest. Tango (1995) suggests

$$w_{ij}^* = \exp\left(-d_{ij}/\kappa\right)$$

as a good starting point, where κ represents a tuning parameter that increases sensitivity of the test to large or small clusters, corresponding to large or small values of κ, respectively.

We note that Tango's index is similar in spirit to a weighted version of the Pearson's χ^2 goodness-of-fit test in the sense that the index is a sum of weighted "observed minus expected" elements. Tango's index also closely resembles the global indices of spatial association defined in Section 7.4; in particular, it appears to fit the basic form of such indexes defined in equation (7.3). However, in Tango's index, we typically assign a nonzero value to w_{ii}^*, for $i = 1, \ldots, N$; therefore, Tango's index summarizes both the squared deviation of the case proportions observed to those expected under the null hypothesis *and* the cross-product terms defining a measure of spatial similarity (sim_{ij}) in equation (7.3). Recall that we often assume that $w_{ii} = 0$ for $i = 1, \ldots, N$ in global indexes of spatial association, giving the motivation to distinguish (in notation) the weights w_{ij}^* in equation (7.15) from the weights w_{ij} in equation (7.3). By its structure, Tango's index provides a compromise between a goodness-of-fit test ignoring spatial pattern and a global index of spatial association ignoring local fit (Rogerson 1999).

To see this feature of Tango's index more clearly, Rogerson (1999) splits the right-hand side of equation (7.15) into two pieces:

$$\begin{aligned} T_{\text{ti}} &= \sum_{i=1}^{N} \sum_{j=1}^{N} w_{ij}^* \left(\frac{Y_i}{Y_+} - \frac{n_i}{n_+} \right) \left(\frac{Y_j}{Y_+} - \frac{n_j}{n_+} \right) \\ &= \sum_{i=1}^{N} w_{ii}^* \left(\frac{Y_i}{Y_+} - \frac{n_i}{n_+} \right)^2 + \sum_{i=1}^{N} \sum_{j \neq i} w_{ij}^* \left(\frac{Y_i}{Y_+} - \frac{n_i}{n_+} \right) \left(\frac{Y_j}{Y_+} - \frac{n_j}{n_+} \right), \end{aligned} \tag{7.16}$$

where often $w_{ii}^* = 1$ for $i = 1, \ldots, N$. Rogerson (1999) thereby clearly represents Tango's index as the sum of two terms, the first directly measuring goodness of fit in each region, the second measuring spatial similarity between regions.

Rogerson's representation of Tango's index as the sum of a goodness-of-fit component and a spatial autocorrelation component provides important insight into the sorts of deviation from the null hypothesis likely to set off the clustering "alarm." Tango's index may be large (indicating clustering) due to either a lack of fit *within* regions (poor fit), spatial similarity in deviations from expectation (spatial autocorrelation) *between* regions, or both. In the extreme case, if we obtain a significant value of Tango's index comprised entirely of large goodness-of-fit terms, we conclude that the constant risk hypothesis does not hold. On the other hand, if we obtain a significant value of Tango's index comprised entirely of large spatial autocorrelation terms, we conclude that proportions associated with regions that are close together are more alike than those farther apart. Both of these conclusions may be interpreted as evidence of clustering.

Rogerson's summation representation of Tango's index also provides insight into the impact of the choice of spatial weights (the w_{ij}^*) on the performance of the statistic. For instance, suppose that we choose weights based on a particular distance threshold, d_{ij}^* (e.g., we define the neighbors of region i to be any region j with its centroid within a prespecified distance, say d_{ij}^*, of the centroid of region i, for all regions i). If we choose our threshold distance d_{ij}^* to be smaller than the minimum intercentroid distance in our data set, we remove the spatial autocorrelation term from equation (7.16) and Tango's index becomes a goodness-of-fit test. This feature becomes particularly important for distance-based weights (e.g., distance threshold or distance decay) in sets of regions of varying geographic support (e.g., varying geographic sizes), as we illustrate in the data break below.

In his discussion of Tango's index, Rogerson (1999) suggests defining w_{ij}^* by

$$\frac{\exp(-d_{ij}/\kappa)}{\sqrt{(n_i/n_+)(n_j/n_+)}} \tag{7.17}$$

so the first (goodness of fit) term in equation (7.16) more closely matches Pearson's χ^2 (each term now represents the ratio between the squared deviation of the proportion observed from the proportion expected, divided by the proportion expected), and the second term (a global cross-product index of spatial association) more closely resembles Moran's I with

$$\text{sim}_{ij} = \left(\frac{Y_i}{Y_+} - \frac{n_i}{n_+}\right)\left(\frac{Y_j}{Y_+} - \frac{n_j}{n_+}\right).$$

Rogerson's weights also link Tango's index with a statistic proposed by Oden (1995), a connection meriting further discussion. Oden (1995) proposes an adjustment to Moran's I for application to counts, proportions, or rates based on regions with heterogeneous population sizes. Using Rogerson's weights with Tango's index in equation (7.16) provides the dominant term in Oden's population-adjusted statistic. Oden notes that equation (7.16) corresponds to a spatial version of Pearson's

χ^2 statistic for testing a null hypothesis of homogeneous proportions, and notes that such a statistic can detect clustering *within* regions via local lack of fit as well as clustering *between* regions via the index of spatial association. Oden (1995) notes that spatial variability in the proportions (which probably contributes to significant lack of fit) is viewed as evidence of clustering, since this spatial variation suggests within-region disease aggregations even if the rates have no spatial pattern. However, since Moran's I does not consider local lack of fit, Assunção and Reis (1999) argue that direct comparisons between Oden's adjustment (and, by extension, Tango's index) and Moran's I are inappropriate since the null hypotheses associated with the various statistics differ in their inclusion (for Oden and Tango) or exclusion (for Moran) of local lack of fit as evidence against the null hypothesis of "no clustering." Assunção and Reis (1999) make an important point regarding comparison between tests of clustering, echoing the central issue raised in Sections 6.2 and 7.1: What question do we wish to address with a statistical test of clustering? Oden (1995) and Rogerson (1999) argue for a combination of local lack of fit and spatial autocorrelation since disease clustering may result in either or both aspects, depending on the spatial scale of clustering and the spatial scale of data aggregation.

The next step in applying Tango's index is to determine its distribution under the constant risk hypothesis. Whittemore and Keller (1986), Whittemore et al. (1987), and Rayens and Kryscio (1993) explore the distributional properties of Tango's index applied to temporal clustering. These authors show that the index is a member of the class of *U statistics*, a family of nonparametric tests, including the Wilcoxon rank-sum test (Cox and Hinkley 1974, pp. 198–202). The theory of U statistics suggests an asymptotic Gaussian (normal) distribution for Tango's index. However, Tango (1990a) and Rayens and Kryscio (1993) note that this asymptotic derivation applies most directly under increasing values of the number of time intervals, and the convergence with respect to increasing values of Y_+ (the total number of observed cases) is often too slow to be useful in disease-clustering investigations. In our spatial setting, this corresponds to asymptotics based on increasing the number of geographic regions rather than being based on increasing numbers of cases observed. The second setting may be more natural in the clustering application, where we observe cases over a longer period of time (Y_+ increasing) rather than over a greater number of regions (N increasing).

Two options allow us to improve on the asymptotic Gaussian distribution for typical clustering applications. First, we could apply a Monte Carlo testing approach, where we simulate regional counts conditional on the fixed total Y_+ (i.e., each simulation assigns a total of Y_+ cases to the regions where the probability of each case falling in region i is n_i/n_+ for $i = 1, \dots, N$). Second, Tango (1990a) derives an approximate chi-square distribution for his index, based on adjustments for the substantial amount of skewness in the distribution of T_{ti}. Tango (1990a) shows this chi-square approximation to be adequate for sample sizes with as few as one case expected per region. Although at first glance the notation may appear somewhat dense, any statistical package allowing basic matrix operations (e.g., transpose and trace) allows quick calculation of the approximation, which performs well in practice for a variety of sample-size configurations with respect to both number of cases and number of regions (Rayens and Kryscio 1993).

We apply the chi-square approximation as follows. Let $\boldsymbol{W}^*$ denote the matrix of weights w^*_{ij} for $i, j = 1, \ldots, N$, and $\boldsymbol{p}$ the vector of expected proportions:

$$\boldsymbol{p} = \left(\frac{n_1}{n_+}, \ldots, \frac{n_N}{n_+}\right).$$

Next, consider the standardized statistic

$$T^*_{\text{ti}} = \frac{T_{\text{ti}} - E(T_{\text{ti}})}{\sqrt{\text{Var}(T_{\text{ti}})}}$$

with expectation and variance (under the constant risk hypothesis) given by

$$E(T_{\text{ti}}) = \frac{1}{Y_+}\text{tr}(\boldsymbol{W}^*\boldsymbol{V}_{\boldsymbol{p}})$$

and

$$\text{Var}(T_{\text{ti}}) = \frac{2}{Y_+}\text{tr}[(\boldsymbol{W}^*\boldsymbol{V}_{\boldsymbol{p}})^2],$$

where

$$\boldsymbol{V}_{\boldsymbol{p}} = \text{diag}(\boldsymbol{p}) - \boldsymbol{p}\boldsymbol{p}'$$

is the asymptotic variance of $\boldsymbol{r}$ (Agresti 1990, pp. 423–424), diag($\boldsymbol{p}$) denotes a matrix with the elements of $\boldsymbol{p}$ along the diagonal and zeros elsewhere, tr($\cdot$) denotes the trace function (the sum of the diagonal elements of a matrix), and $\boldsymbol{p}'$ denotes the transpose of vector $\boldsymbol{p}$. Tango's chi-square approximation (Tango 1990a, 1995) requires calculation of the skewness, sk(T_{ti}), of T_{ti} via

$$\text{sk}(T_{\text{ti}}) = 2\sqrt{2}\frac{\text{tr}[(\boldsymbol{W}^*\boldsymbol{V}_{\boldsymbol{p}})^3]}{(\text{tr}[(\boldsymbol{W}^*\boldsymbol{V}_{\boldsymbol{p}})^2])^{1.5}}.$$

Tango (1995) derives the asymptotic chi-square distribution

$$(\text{df}_{\text{ti}}) + T^*_{\text{ti}}\sqrt{2(\text{df}_{\text{ti}})} \overset{a}{\sim} \chi^2_{\text{df}_{\text{ti}}}, \tag{7.18}$$

where $\text{df}_{\text{ti}} = 8/[\text{sk}(T_{\text{ti}})]^2$ denotes the degrees of freedom adjusted for skewness.

In summary, Tango's index offers a straightforward general-purpose test of spatial clustering which incorporates aspects of tests of goodness of fit and general indexes of spatial association. Furthermore, Tango's index allows us to "tune" the test to particular types of clustering (e.g., single clusters at prespecified places, or focused clusters around putative sources of increased risk) through our choice of the distance measure d_{ij} and the spatial weights w^*_{ij}, as illustrated in the data break below. Tango's index can also be modified to provide local indexes similar to the LISAs discussed in Section 7.5 [see Rogerson (1999) and the exercises at the end of the chapter).

DATA BREAK: New York Leukemia Data (*cont.*) We illustrate the application of Tango's index using the New York leukemia data. Table 7.5 provides the value of Tango's index T_{ti} observed and its standardized value T^*_{ti} based on Tango's weights $w^*_{ij} = \exp(-d_{ij}/\kappa)$ for various values of κ. We present p-values based on Tango's chi-square approximation and Monte Carlo p-values based on 9999 simulations under the constant risk hypothesis. We observe fairly close agreement between both sets of p-values, and note a rather dramatic decrease in p-values as we increase κ.

What happens as we increase κ? First, note that $w^*_{ii} = 1$ for all values of κ, so that the goodness-of-fit component of Tango's index T_{ti} remains constant across values of κ. Hence, the difference between values of Tango's index for different values of κ derives entirely from differences in the spatial autocorrelation component. Changing the weight matrix $\boldsymbol{W}^*$ changes the skewness of T_{ti}, which in turn reduces the degrees of freedom $\mathrm{df}_{\mathrm{ti}}$ dramatically for Tango's chi-square approximation, resulting in much smaller p-values.

To see the impact of the choice of weights on the goodness-of-fit and spatial autocorrelation components of T_{ti} [defined in equation (7.16)], Figure 7.12 plots the two components against each other for the data observed and for 999 simulations under the constant risk hypothesis. We note that the two components of Tango's index are not necessarily independent (i.e., they are not orthogonal contrasts; cf. Best and Rayner 1991), so plotting each pair of components provides insight into their joint distribution. The plots indicate an increasing impact of the spatial autocorrelation term as we increase κ but also reveal that the statistic observed suggests clustering both within and between tracts through evidence for both poor fit and spatial autocorrelation.

To press the point further, for $\kappa = 1$, w^*_{ij} is appreciably greater than zero only for very close pairs of tracts, effectively limiting consideration of spatial association

Table 7.5 Tango's Index for the New York Leukemia Data Using Weights $w^*_{ij} = \exp(-d_{ij}/\kappa)$, Where d_{ij} Represents the Distance between Centroids of Tracts i and j[a]

κ	Tango's Index, T_{ti}	Standardized Statistic (T^*_{ti})	$\mathrm{df}_{\mathrm{ti}}$	Chi-Square p-Value	Monte Carlo p-Value
1	0.0029	36.40	29.27	0.171	0.181
10	0.0056	20.84	5.56	0.001	0.003
15	0.0062	20.38	4.79	0.001	0.002
20	0.0065	20.09	4.38	0.001	0.001

[a]We calculate the chi-square p-value using Tango's adjusted chi-square approximation (see text) and the Monte Carlo p-value based on 9999 simulations under the constant risk hypothesis with a fixed total number of cases.

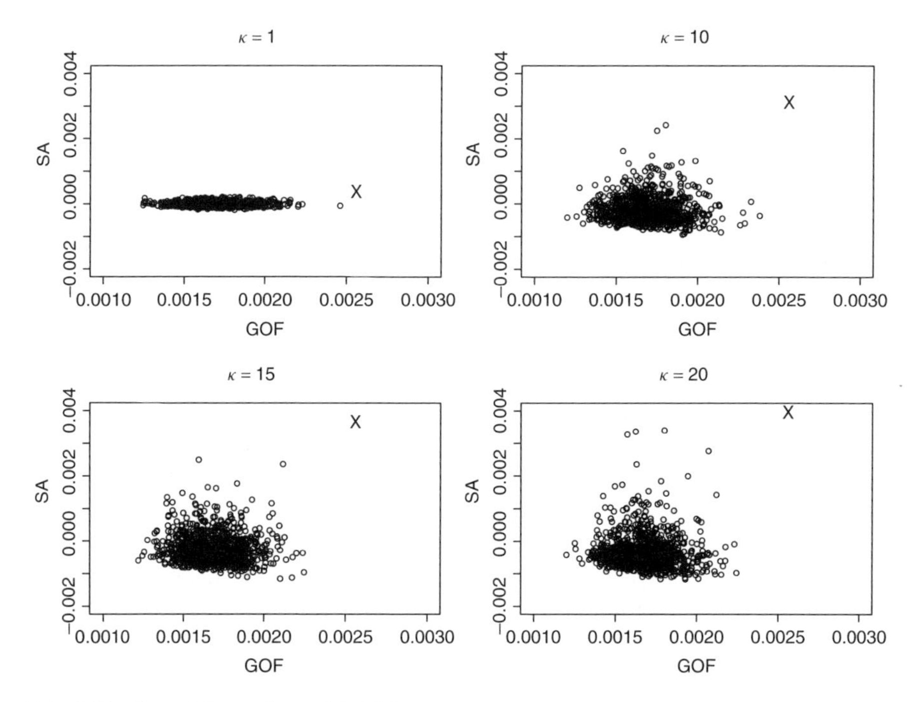

FIG. 7.12 Plots of the goodness of fit (GOF) versus the spatial autocorrelation (SA) terms for Tango's index, based on equation (7.16). The "×" denotes the components of the value of Tango's index observed for the New York leukemia data, based on weights $w^*_{ij} = \exp(-\kappa/d_{ij})$ for $\kappa = 1$, 10, 15, and 20. The open circles represent GOF and SA components of Tango's index based on 999 simulations under the constant risk hypothesis (see text).

to tracts within Syracuse in the north and Binghamton in the south. For $\kappa = 10$ all tracts assign weight greater than 0.05 to at least one other tract, and we see a jump in the value of T_{ti}, coupled with increased skewness leading to the reduction in the significance value observed.

Table 7.6 gives the observed test statistic values and associated significance levels for Tango's index applied to the New York leukemia data using Rogerson's weights, i.e.,

$$w^*_{ij} = \frac{\exp(-d_{ij}/\kappa)}{\sqrt{p_i p_j}}.$$

The results of Tables 7.5 and 7.6 are qualitatively similar. Since the proportion of the overall population residing in each of the 281 census tracts is relatively small, Rogerson's weights are much larger in magnitude than Tango's weights (although the standardization within Tango's index somewhat mitigates this discrepancy). However, we do note another difference in the two weighting schemes. Tango's weights will assign the same value of w^*_{ij} to any pairs of tracts separated by the same distance d_{ij}. In contrast, Rogerson's weights adjust the distance-based component, $\exp(-d_{ij}/\kappa)$, by the proportion of the population in tracts i and j.

Table 7.6 Tango's Index for the New York Leukemia Data Using Weights $w^*_{ij} = \exp(-d_{ij}/\kappa) \,/\, \sqrt{p_i p_j}$[a]

κ	Tango's Index (Rogerson's Weights) T_{ti}	Standardized Statistic T^*_{ti}	df_{ti}	Chi-Square p-Value	Monte Carlo p-Value
1	0.821	33.94	25.95	0.135	0.147
10	1.460	17.46	4.65	0.003	0.006
15	1.533	16.64	4.23	0.003	0.006
20	1.576	16.25	4.00	0.003	0.006

[a] d_{ij} represents the distance between centroids of tracts i and j, and p_i denotes the proportion of the study area population residing in tract i. The degrees of freedom df_{ti} reflect an adjustment for the skewness of the distribution of T_{ti}. We calculate the chi-square p-value using Tango's adjusted chi-square approximation (see text) and the Monte Carlo p-value, based on 9999 simulations under the constant risk hypothesis with a fixed total number of cases.

As a result, two different pairs of tracts, each separated by distance d_{ij}, may receive different weights w^*_{ij} if the population proportions are different within the respective tracts.

Figure 7.13 indicates the goodness-of-fit and spatial autocorrelation components of Tango's index, based on Rogerson's weights. As in Figure 7.12, we observe the impact of the changing weights on the relative impact of the two components. Figure 7.13 also reveals that Rogerson's weights tend to result in a few very high lack-of-fit values under the constant risk hypothesis, due primarily to a few regions with very small population sizes (found in the city of Syracuse in these data). As a result, the joint distribution of the two components of Tango's index is somewhat more complicated.

For both sets of weights, Tango's index suggests evidence of *clustering* in the data. Figures 7.12 and 7.13 suggest somewhat stronger evidence of clustering across tracts than within tracts, due to the goodness-of-fit and spatial autocorrelation components of Tango's index.

7.6.5 Method: Focused Score Tests of Trend

Up to this point, we describe primarily *general* tests of clustering and/or algorithms to detect clusters anywhere in the study area. We now turn to the problem of assessing *focused* clustering/clusters. Recall that for focused tests, we have a predefined set of *foci* or locations of putative increased disease risk. Our examples involve point locations, but foci could also be lines (e.g., highways or power lines) or areas (e.g., agricultural fields treated with particular pesticides). Our interest involves the question: Is there evidence of increased disease incidence in areas exposed to the foci?

To maintain a proper inferential setting for the focused tests outlined here, it is important that foci be identified prior to assessment of the most likely general clusters. The "Texas sharpshooter" phenomenon of shooting the barn first, then painting

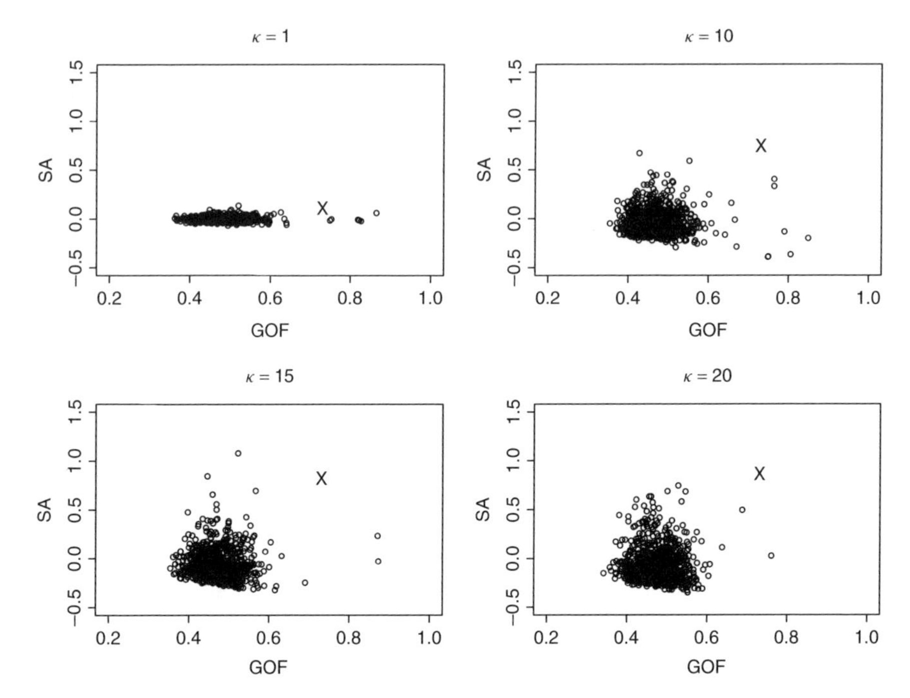

FIG. 7.13 Plots of the goodness of fit (GOF) versus the spatial autocorrelation (SA) terms for Tango's index, based on equation (7.16). The "×" denotes the components of the value of Tango's index observed for the New York leukemia data, based on weights proposed by Rogerson (1999) for $\kappa = 1$, 10, 15, and 20. The open circles represent GOF and SA components of Tango's index based on 999 simulations under the constant risk hypothesis (see text).

a bull's-eye around the bullet hole again provides an extreme example of the fallacy of identifying a significant local cluster, identifying nearby putative sources of increased risk, then testing for significant clustering around these sources. Although we may find such an approach tempting (particularly if we have ready access to multiple layers of GIS data pertaining to possible foci), this sequential nature of cluster, then foci identification redefines the null and alternative hypotheses, and as a result, the interpretation of significance values. By identifying foci near the most unusual observed local collections of cases, we tip the balance in favor of detecting focused clustering, even if there is no association between the disease and the foci.

For instance, in the tests below, we define a set of foci and wish to assess the conceptual null hypothesis defined in Section 6.2:

H_0: There are no clusters of cases *around the foci.*

Contrast this notion with the Texas sharpshooter conceptual null hypothesis:

H_0: There are no clusters of cases *around the foci nearest the most likely clusters.*

In this admittedly oversimplified example, we observe that the second hypothesis suffers from both convoluted English and convoluted logic, considerably complicating the interpretation of any claims of statistical significance.

With this in mind, we assume that we have identified a set of foci based on our knowledge or suspicions regarding possible causes of the disease under study. Such foci generally define sources of known or suspected exposure to particular substances putatively associated with disease outcome. For example, if the outcome of interest is leukemia, we may be interested in sources of possible exposure to known leukemogens such as benzene or ionizing radiation, or to substances whose leukemogenic properties are subject to ongoing study and debate (e.g., trichloroethylene or electromagnetic fields).

Often, we define the foci as a set of *locations* (points, lines, or areas) representing the source of suspected exposures. Information regarding the magnitude of exposures may be nonexistent, or may include emission levels from each focus or monitored exposure values (typically, at a different set of locations). With nonexistent exposure levels, we often use increasing distance from the foci as a surrogate for decreasing exposure, or at least decreasing *potential* of exposure. The presence of reported emission levels or monitored exposure levels requires interpolation of exposure values to nonmonitored sites, as discussed in Chapters 4 and 8. Here we describe tests based on minimal exposure data (focus locations only), but these could be modified to include exposure estimates (and associated estimates of uncertainty), if such data are available.

Waller et al. (1992, 1994) and Lawson (1993) consider focused tests based on the following operationalization of the constant risk null hypothesis:

$$H_0 : Y_i \stackrel{\text{ind}}{\sim} \text{Poisson}(rn_i), \tag{7.19}$$

where, as before, Y_i represents the number of cases observed in region i, r denotes the hypothesized constant individual-level risk of disease, and n_i denotes the population size in region i. The hypothesis defined in equation (7.19) derives from an assumption of an underlying heterogeneous Poisson process generating case locations.

Both Waller et al. (1992) and Lawson (1993) consider the following alternative hypothesis:

$$H_A : Y_i \stackrel{\text{ind}}{\sim} \text{Poisson}(rn_i(1 + \varpi_i \varepsilon)), \tag{7.20}$$

where ϖ_i represents exposure to the foci experienced by residents of region i and ε represents a small, positive constant. The only difference between the hypotheses defined in equations (7.19) and (7.20) is the multiplicative increase in individual-level risk associated with living in region i. That is, the probability that a person in region i will contract the disease during the time period of interest is r under the (constant risk) null hypothesis and $r(1 + \varpi_i \varepsilon)$ under the alternative hypothesis; therefore, the relative risk of disease comparing people residing in region i to people with no exposure is $1 + \varpi_i \varepsilon$.

The exposure value ϖ_i is fairly general and may be used to represent a variety of types of focused clusters. Setting $\varpi_i = 1$ for regions within a given distance of the foci and $\varpi_i = 0$ for all other regions gives an example of a *hot spot cluster* (cf. Wartenberg and Greenberg 1990) wherein all persons residing within the cluster experience the same increase in risk, and people outside the cluster experience no increase in risk. Setting ϖ_i to a distance–decay function represents decreasing exposure with increasing distance from the foci, resulting in what Wartenberg and Greenberg (1990) refer to as a *clinal cluster*, a cluster where risk decreases smoothly with exposure to the focus. In addition, since the null and alternative hypotheses defined in equations (7.19) and (7.20) both assume independent disease counts, ϖ_i is not limited to spatially defined risk patterns, and by an appropriate choice of ϖ_i the alternative could represent any classification of regions by exposure, even those with little or no spatial pattern of exposure (e.g., smoking habits by census tract). Since alternative hypotheses need not be spatial, the tests defined below are equivalent to a widely used class of trend tests for Poisson random variables (cf. Rothman 1986, pp. 346–349; Breslow and Day 1987).

Waller et al. (1992) and Lawson (1993), independently, developed score tests of the null hypothesis given in equation (7.19) based on the alternative hypothesis defined in equation (7.20). Score tests provide statistical hypothesis tests based on the derivative of the likelihood function (cf. Cox and Hinkley 1974, p. 315), and are asymptotically equivalent to likelihood ratio tests. In addition, score tests have some optimal statistical power properties; namely, if a uniformly most powerful (UMP) test against a certain family of alternative hypotheses exists, the score test is equivalent to the UMP test. As mentioned briefly above, if a UMP test does not exist (as is often the case), score tests retain certain optimal *local* power properties (e.g., they are "locally most powerful" rather than UMP), where here the term *local* refers to small deviations from the null hypothesis, not small geographic distances. In the case of alternatives defined by equation (7.20), local alternatives for a fixed set of ϖ_i values represent small values of ε, yielding small increases in risk for regions with high exposure.

Since the alternative hypothesis defined in equation (7.20) ignores spatial autocorrelation, the test represents a goodness-of-fit test comparing the counts observed to those expected under the null hypothesis. The test statistic is a weighted sum of deviations of observed case counts from those expected under the constant risk hypothesis, with the weight for region i given by the exposure, ϖ_i.

The score test statistic is

$$T_{\mathrm{sc}} = \sum_{i=1}^{N} \varpi_i (Y_i - r n_i),$$

the sum of each region's deviation from expectation weighted by the region's exposure. Waller et al. (1992, 1994) use ϖ_i defined by the inverse distance of each region from the foci, while Lawson (1993) develops tests for a wide variety of exposure values. For inference, we typically standardize T_{sc} by noting that the expectation of T_{sc} is zero under the null hypothesis, then dividing by the square root of the variance of T_{sc} under the null hypothesis which, if r is known, is

$$\text{Var}(T_{sc}) = r\left(\sum_{i=1}^{N} \varpi_i^2 n_i\right).$$

If r is unknown, we estimate it using the maximum likelihood estimate of r,

$$\widehat{r} = \frac{Y_+}{n_+},$$

where Y_+ and n_+ denote the total number of cases observed and the total population size, respectively. In this case, the variance of T_{sc} is

$$\text{Var}(T_{sc}) = \widehat{r}\left(\sum_{i=1}^{N} \varpi_i^2 n_i\right) - \frac{Y_+}{n_+^2}\left(\sum_{i=1}^{N} \varpi_i n_i\right)^2.$$

Based on the theory of score tests, we compare the observed value of the standardized statistic

$$T_{sc}^* = \frac{T_{sc}}{\sqrt{\text{Var}(T_{sc})}}$$

to a standard normal distribution. The normal approximation follows asymptotic results based on an increasing number of regions (N). Monte Carlo tests remain an option if the appropriateness of the approximation is in question, particularly for a small number of regions, or for a very rare disease (i.e., very small value of r leading to very small expected counts in each region). As an alternative to Monte Carlo tests, Waller and Lawson (1995) provide an algorithm for determining the exact distribution of T_{sc}^* using numerical inversion of the statistic's characteristic function. Since the number of Monte Carlo simulations required for accurate estimates increases as we estimate probabilities further into the tail of the distribution, we may find increased computational efficiency in the calculation of tail probabilities under the exact approach.

Tango (1995) notes that T_{sc} based on $\widehat{r} = Y_+/n_+$ yields

$$\begin{aligned} T_{sc} &= \sum_{i=1}^{N} \varpi_i \left[Y_i - n_i\left(\frac{Y_+}{n_+}\right)\right] \\ &= Y_+ \sum_{i=1}^{N} \varpi_i \left(\frac{Y_i}{Y_+} - \frac{n_i}{n_+}\right), \end{aligned} \tag{7.21}$$

indicating that T_{sc} provides a score test comparing regional proportions of cases and proportions of population at risk as well as a test comparing observed and expected counts. As a result of equation (7.21), the score test statistic bears some resemblance to the goodness-of-fit portion of Tango's index; that is, $\sum_{i=1}^{N} w_{ii}^* (Y_i/Y_+ - n_i/n_+)^2$ if we define weights w_{ii}^* based on the product of the total number of cases Y_+ and the exposure associated with region i, and weights $w_{ij}^* = 0$ for $i \neq j$. Like Pearson's χ^2, Tango's index assesses squared deviations from expectation. The score test can be defined equivalently through squared deviations (cf. Lawson 1993), but there are some interpretative advantages to using T_{sc}. In particular, squared deviations provide the same contribution regardless of whether observed counts are above or below their respective null expectations. Through the sign of its components, the statistic T_{sc} indicates which regions exceed expectation. As a result, we can use a two- or one-tailed test of significance with T_{sc}, depending on whether we desire inference on any deviation from expectation or only increases above expectation, respectively.

DATA BREAK: New York Leukemia Data (*cont.*) We now illustrate the focused score test using the New York leukemia data set. Foci include inactive hazardous waste sites documented as containing trichloroethylene (TCE) (New York State Department of Environmental Conservation 1987). In general, the epidemiologic links between TCE exposure and human cancer are weak or nonexistent [see Bogan and Gold (1997), particularly their review of epidemiologic findings on page 27]. Exposure to TCE was one of the motivating concerns driving the highly visible investigation of childhood leukemia in Woborn, Massachusetts in the 1980s (Lagakos et al. 1986), reviewed in the book and motion picture *A Civil Action* (Harr 1995). In fact, the events in Massachusetts motivated the state of New York to explore proactive methods of cluster investigation, and part of this effort led to the original analyses of the New York leukemia data. We note that the results below do not represent a thorough assessment of biological associations between TCE exposure and leukemia (nor would any spatial analysis based on observational data); rather, the results provide an illustration of the methods above.

Waller et al. (1992, 1994) consider 11 (then inactive, or not accepting new materials) waste sites, each documented with the New York State Department of Environmental Conservation as containing TCE (generally in addition to other contaminants). Table 7.7 gives the coordinates (in kilometers) and name of each site, as reported originally by Waller et al. (1992).

The locations of the TCE sites appear in Figure 7.14. We note that many of the sites appear along the Susquehanna River passing through an industrial area in and near Binghamton. As an aside, the original report (New York State Department of Environmental Conservation 1987) provides a street address for each site. Waller et al. (1992) "geocoded" these addresses by hand by locating each site to the extent possible along roads labeled on U.S. Geological Survey (USGS) 7.5° × 7.5° quadrangle topographic maps of the area. The x and y coordinates (not to be confused with the number of cases in region i, Y_i) in Table 7.7 are defined by the 1980 U.S. Census and represent deviations from the geographic centroid of the study area in the east-west and north-south directions. Global positioning system (GPS) data (much less expensive to obtain today than in the mid-1980s)

Table 7.7 Location of 11 Inactive Hazardous Waste Sites Containing Trichloroethylene in Upstate New York

x	y	Name
−0.14	−67.19	Monarch Chemicals
−4.47	−67.65	IBM Endicott
11.98	−71.61	Singer
13.03	−75.34	Nesco
−46.60	24.43	GE Auburn
9.30	−5.82	Solvent Savers
−19.04	−15.37	Smith Corona
−19.41	−67.39	Victory Plaza
−17.97	−67.16	Hadco
−41.99	−30.90	Morse Chain
−30.37	−14.39	Groton

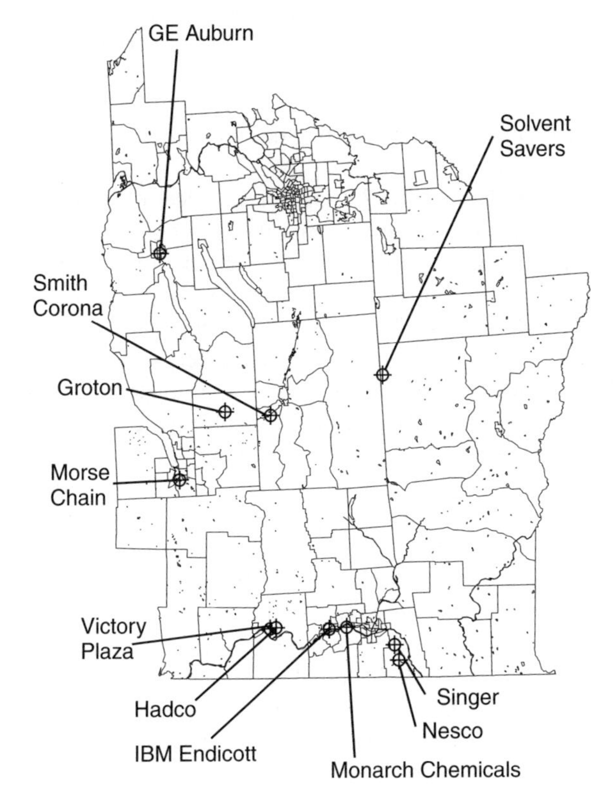

FIG. 7.14 Location of 11 inactive hazardous waste sites containing trichloroethylene in upstate New York.

Table 7.8 Standardized Score Test Statistics for the New York Leukemia Data[a]

Site	T^*_{sc} (r Known)	p-Value (r Known)	T^*_{sc} (r Unknown)	p-Value (r Unknown)
Monarch Chemicals	4.13	<0.0001	4.69	<0.0001
IBM Endicott	3.40	0.0003	3.57	0.0002
Singer	2.47	0.0067	2.87	0.0020
Nesco	2.47	0.0068	2.86	0.0021
GE Auburn	2.43	0.0075	2.49	0.0063
Solvent Savers	0.60	0.2731	1.63	0.0518
Smith Corona	2.80	0.0025	3.26	0.0006
Victory Plaza	1.96	0.0254	2.41	0.0080
Hadco	1.28	0.1009	1.50	0.0669
Morse Chain	0.01	0.4974	0.01	0.4974
Groton	0.86	0.1947	0.93	0.1772
All sites	2.27	0.0117	2.27	0.0117

[a] Exposure surrogates defined by the inverse distance to each site and the inverse distance to the nearest site ("All sites"). Values of the test statistic and the associated standard normal p-value based on treating the overall disease incidence proportion as known (center columns) or unknown (right columns).

would provide much more accurate location data and would improve the geographic precision of the analysis.

We note that the results in Table 7.8 suggest statistically significant focused clustering around many of the sites and around the set of sites as a whole (based on using the inverse distance to the nearest site as an exposure surrogate). However, the results do not necessarily indicate a statistically significant link between exposure to TCE and incidence of leukemia for several reasons. First, recall that our data do not include detailed exposure measurements; rather, we use the inverse distance between TCE sites and census tract centroids as a surrogate for exposure. Although this provides some insight into the general geographic pattern of leukemia incidence around the TCE sites, it is not a necessarily accurate assessment of individual-level exposure. Second, we calculate expected incidence proportions based on the overall five-year incidence proportion of leukemia in the study area, without adjustments for common risk factors such as age or occupation. Waller and McMaster (1997) present results based on indirect age standardization for the tracts in Broome County with little change in results. Occupational adjustments are important (since occupational use provides an important route of exposure), but such adjustments are difficult due to the lack of detailed, individual-level data. Ahrens et al. (2001) take a step in this direction by incorporating aggregate occupational information from the 1980 U.S. Census (e.g., proportions of residents employed in each of several job classes) in a generalized linear model that explains much of the suspicious spatial pattern suggested above.

The modeling results of Ahrens et al. (2001) provide an important step into understanding the reasons behind the spatial patterns observed throughout the data breaks in this chapter and highlight that all tests of clustering and tests to detect clusters provide only an initial component to describing and understanding spatial patterns of disease. Application of the score test based on more realistic exposure surrogates would likely provide additional insight into the patterns observed above.

7.7 STATISTICAL POWER AND RELATED CONSIDERATIONS

In the sections above we present a variety of statistical hypothesis tests for detecting clusters or clustering in spatially referenced public health data. Which method do we use? Statisticians often turn to assessments of statistical power to decide between competing hypothesis tests. Briefly, power represents the probability of detecting departures from the null hypothesis given that the data, in fact, arise under some alternative hypothesis. In our setting, statistical power represents the probability of detecting clusters or clustering when we should (i.e., when such features are present). Although the term *power* is related with a type II error (failing to reject a null hypothesis that is false), the probability of making a type I error (rejecting the null hypothesis when it is true) is also important. We want the probability of both types of errors to be small, but for a given sample size, there is typically a trade-off between them. Thus, although most of the discussion below focuses on the power of tests under alternatives of clustering, we note that inflated type I error rates can be particularly serious, requiring unnecessary and expensive cluster investigations.

7.7.1 Power Depends on the Alternative Hypothesis

In many statistical testing situations, there is a clear alternative hypothesis or family of alternative hypotheses (e.g., a shift in the mean response, or model parameters not equal to zero). However, as detailed in Sections 6.2 and 7.1, there is no general family of alternatives capturing all possible cluster/clustering scenarios, and individual tests vary with respect to the types of null and alternative hypotheses of interest. Examples of null hypotheses include the constant risk hypothesis and the random labeling hypothesis. Examples of families of alternative hypotheses include general and focused alternatives and cluster and clustering alternatives. Even among these families, important distinctions between types of clusters/clustering could occur (e.g., "hot-spot" clusters/clustering as addressed by the spatial scan statistic and the clinal clusters/clustering as addressed by Tango's index and the focused score test).

A particularly important distinction occurs between lack-of-fit alternatives that maintain independence between regional counts but do not follow the constant risk hypothesis and spatial autocorrelation alternatives that contain correlated counts that may or may not follow a constant risk model. Kulldorff et al. (2003) refer to lack-of-fit alternatives as first-order clustering (since clusters/clustering occur due to deviations from the expected regional mean values) and spatial autocorrelation alternatives as second-order clustering (since clustering occurs due to correlation between counts). The terms relate to first- and second-order properties of the assumed underlying spatial point process driving the observed pattern of regional counts. As noted in Chapter 5, it is impossible to distinguish between first- and second-order patterns from a single data realization, so the distinction between alternatives is somewhat vague [e.g., tests developed to detect first-order clustering will have power to detect second-order clustering, but power properties may not always translate easily (or even intuitively) between different families of alternatives]. For example, many indices of spatial correlation (e.g., Moran's I and Geary's c), developed for second-order clustering, have power against first-order clusters as well. McMillen (2003) provides an excellent example where such indexes suggest autocorrelation among model residuals arising from a local lack of fit. In this case, the test attributes the observed pattern to autocorrelation rather than its true cause (a missing indicator of increased local intensity).

As a result of the wide variety of situations encompassed in our conceptual notions of cluster and clustering, different tests address different particular aspects, and no single test will serve as the "most powerful" in all situations. Rather, we may seek tests with optimal (or at least comparatively high) power for certain specific cluster/clustering scenarios, using families of statistical tests with known theoretical power advantages such as likelihood ratio tests or score tests. Examples of these approaches include the spatial scan statistic (based on likelihood ratio tests for hot-spot clusters) and the focused score test [based on focused clusters defined by the family of alternatives given in equation (7.20)]. Such approaches yield competitive power results for the family of alternatives under consideration, but the power under other cluster/clustering scenarios often remains unexplored.

7.7.2 Power Depends on the Data Structure

In addition to the particular alternative hypothesis or hypotheses, the structure of the data also affects the ability of any given test to detect clusters/clustering. Two data features particularly important in the analysis of regional count data are the level of aggregation in the data and the amount of population heterogeneity (numbers and demographics of the population at risk) between regions.

Aggregation and the population composition and density affect the number of cases expected under the constant risk assumption (or any other null hypothesis). Areas with more people at risk have higher local sample sizes, often yielding higher power to detect a given local increase in relative risk (for first-order alternatives). As a result, most (if not all) tests to detect clusters have spatially heterogeneous power (i.e., the power to detect a cluster depends on where the cluster occurs). In other words, there is not a single summary power value for a test to detect clusters when applied to a study area with spatially heterogeneous population density. Geographic variation in power is noted by some authors (cf. Waller and Poquette 1999; Gangnon and Clayton 2001) and explored in some depth by Rudd (2001). The power of tests of *clustering* will also depend on the location of clusters in heterogeneous population densities, but the extent of the impact is less clear given the summary nature of such tests.

7.7.3 Theoretical Assessment of Power

In some settings, exact or approximate theoretical distributional results under particular alternative hypotheses allow direct calculation of power or approximations to power. For instance, Rayens and Kryscio (1993) report that Tango's chi-square approximation (defined in Section 7.6.4) remains appropriate for any alternative hypotheses defined by an alternative set of expected proportions, provided that one assumes that the incidence counts in different regions remain independent. That is, the chi-square approximation allows power calculations for lack-of-fit (first-order) alternatives but not for spatial autocorrelation (second-order) alternatives. As another example of theoretical power assessments, Waller and Lawson (1995) consider numerical approximations to the distribution of the focused score test under the lack-of-fit alternatives defined by equation (7.20). Finally, Waller and Poquette (1999) extend the results of Waller and Lawson (1995) to explore the impact of misspecified exposure values (ϖ_i) on the statistical power of the focused score test (e.g., assessing the power of the test based on inverse-distance exposure surrogates to detect alternatives based on exponential decay distance–exposure relationships).

Generally, such theoretical assessments of power rely on asymptotic approximations (e.g., the chi-square and normal approximations used in the references above), and one must always assess the appropriateness of these approximations in any given data setting. In the disease cluster/clustering literature, most theoretical approaches assess power for lack-of-fit alternatives (based on independent regional counts with nonconstant risk) rather than spatially autoregressive alternatives (based on dependent regional counts), although Cline and Kryscio (1999) provide algorithms to determine the distributions of Tango's index, Pearson's χ^2, and similar statistics under alternative hypotheses generated under a family of contagion models yielding dependent region counts.

7.7.4 Monte Carlo Assessment of Power

Since theoretical assessments of power are often elusive, especially for spatial autocorrelation (second-order) alternatives, Monte Carlo methods play an important role. Since omnibus power results covering all possible cluster/clustering alternatives are unavailable (and probably unattainable), power comparisons typically focus on certain collections of alternative hypotheses of interest. This collection of alternative hypotheses defines the probability model(s) underlying the generation of simulated data sets containing clusters and/or clustering.

A Monte Carlo assessment of statistical power typically involves the following steps:

1. Find the critical value for the test statistic under the null distribution. Either use a theoretical null distribution (e.g., find the 95th percentile of the null distribution), or approximate the critical value using Monte Carlo methods. That is, generate a large number of data sets under the null hypothesis and calculate the test statistic T for each. Find the critical value under the null distribution (e.g., the 95th percentile of the T values associated with the simulated data sets). Note that accurate estimation of extreme percentile values generally requires a large number of simulations.
2. Generate a large number of data sets under a particular *alternative* hypothesis (e.g., containing a hot-spot cluster with a doubling of the relative risk for

people residing within the cluster). Calculate the test statistic T for each data set and estimate the power using the proportion of test statistic values exceeding the critical value found in step 1.

Often, we repeat the process for several related alternative hypotheses and then describe the relationship of power across the alternatives considered. For example, Waller (1996) considered hot-spot clusters with increasing relative risk associated with people residing in the hot spot, and plotted the associated power versus relative risk (within the hot spot) to explore the detectable effect size for several tests. For second-order alternatives, Anselin and Rey (1991) simulate data sets containing spatial correlation and plot power values versus the correlation parameter.

Such Monte Carlo power assessments provide important information regarding the performance of tests to detect clusters/clustering. However, Kulldorff et al. (2003, p. 666) correctly note that these assessments are "tedious, time consuming, and unglamorous to perform." Conclusions are limited to the particular alternative hypotheses under consideration and may not correspond to the alternatives of interest in other settings. As a result, power assessments for various tests are not directly comparable since the assessments occur for different families of alternatives. For example, there is currently a wide gap in the literature between power assessments based on first-order alternatives (primarily for tests of disease clusters/clustering; cf. Waller and Lawson 1995; Waller 1996; Kulldorff et al. 2003) and those based on second-order alternatives (primarily for general and local indexes of spatial autocorrelation applied to linear regression residuals; cf. Anselin and Rey 1991; Anselin and Florax 1995; Anselin et al. 1996).

7.7.5 Benchmark Data and Conditional Power Assessments

To address some of the variation in the power literature for tests of clusters/clustering, Kulldorff et al. (2003) propose the creation and use of *benchmark data sets* incorporating a wide variety of types of clusters and clustering made available through the Internet to allow researchers to compare and contrast the performance of new and existing methods on the same sets of data. The idea is similar to the use of *phantoms* (items of a particular shape and/or composition) to test imaging hardware and software. Kulldorff et al. (2003) constructed over 1,000,000 simulated data sets generated under 51 different clustering models (some first and some second order) set in the counties of the northeastern United States. These data are freely available to assess performance of tests. One advantage of the use of benchmark data sets is that we may compare the power of any particular test to that reported for any other test previously assessed on the same data sets without reevaluation of the tests assessed previously. This allows a growing collection of comparable power results based on the same underlying data structure and cluster models.

Although benchmark data sets will provide valuable comparisons between methods, the comparisons are not global, even within a particular family of alternatives, since power depends on the level of aggregation and the population heterogeneity. In particular, power comparisons based on test performance on the counties in the northeastern United States may not translate to the relative performance of the same tests applied to different data settings. As a result, power comparisons cannot entirely replace Monte Carlo power comparisons conducted on the particular study area of interest (Waller and Poquette 1999).

In conclusion, power provides a yardstick for comparing the statistical performance of various tests, but the comparisons are valid only within the family of alternatives considered and within the particular structure of the data at hand.

DATA BREAK: New York Leukemia Data (*cont.*) After all of the analyses in this chapter, we return to our original question of interest: Are there clusters of elevated leukemia rates in upstate New York? The honest answer is "possibly." We give this rather tentative answer since any answer must depend on our beliefs about the validity of the test statistics, the types of clusters they detect (often defined by user-specified parameters such as n^* in CEPP and κ in Tango's test), and the degree to which our data support the assumptions the test statistics require and provide sufficient statistical power to detect the deviations observed.

The traditional spatial autocorrelation statistics are not statistically significant, yet we raised some question regarding their meaning when applied to counts and rates, particularly those arising from differing population sizes. In contrast, I_{cr}, a statistic adjusting for population heterogeneity, indicates significant spatial clustering measured as spatial correlation among population-adjusted counts and rates. Tango's index indicates significant clustering for $\kappa \geq 10$, yet it is difficult to determine if this is solely the result of spatial autocorrelation or is due partially to the addition of many more terms in the index and/or the increased influence of neighboring values.

Scanning local rates suggests particular clusters near Binghamton, Syracuse, and Cortland, but as we noted in Chapter 4, the rate estimates associated with each region may not be stable. These statistics also depend on the radii of the scanning circles. Scanning local counts using either the CEPP statistic or Besag and Newell's test indicates clusters near Binghamton and Cortland, but these locations depend on what we assume for either the population radius (n^* in CEPP) or the case radius (c^* in Besag and Newell's test). Scan statistics indicate similar areas, but for wide radii, including many people. The LISAs highlight similar areas (near Binghamton, Cortland, and Syracuse) as pockets of local positive spatial autocorrelation, yet differ in construction and interpretation from other tests used to identify particular clusters.

Although we would like to take some comfort from the fact that all of these tests and the local smoothing in Chapter 4 indicate roughly the same areas as potentially higher-than-expected risk, these approaches still make some common assumptions and may be sensitive to violations of them. For instance, the assumption of Poisson counts that we have made throughout this analysis may not realistic since it implicitly assumes that $E(Y_i) = \text{Var}(Y_i)$, an assumption violated by many count data sets, even in nonspatial settings. To our knowledge, the effect of any *overdispersion* [a term used for cases where $E(Y_i) < \text{Var}(Y_i)$] on the type I error levels or the power of any of these test statistics has not been widely investigated. Finally, as we noted above, we must temper any interpretation of unusual clusters until we account for spatial patterns in important covariates possibly affecting local leukemia rates (cf. Chapter 9).

Although we want to put our interpretation of these statistics in context, it is easy to be just as critical of any statistical application, particularly with observational data. Our focus here and throughout this chapter is to stress the importance of key issues (e.g., clustering vs. clusters, the effect of population heterogeneity, and distributional assumptions) so that we may make more valid interpretations and conclusions. The key questions "What do we have?" and "What questions can we answer?" drive all of the discussion above and provide a yardstick for the application of any of the methods described here. We revisit these issues in Chapter 9.

7.8 ADDITIONAL TOPICS AND FURTHER READING

The sections above provide an introduction to various tests to detect disease clusters and/or clustering. However, the methods above only highlight a fraction of the methods proposed and applied in this arena. We present tests representing a variety of approaches to the cluster/clustering detection problem and illustrate their application. However, there are several other approaches and we list some of these here briefly, providing references for the interested reader.

7.8.1 Related Research Regarding Indexes of Spatial Association

Our overview of indexes of spatial autocorrelation is brief and focuses on application as tests of disease clustering and to detect disease clusters. This application represents only a fraction of the use of such statistics, and there is a wide literature regarding the theory and application of such indexes. Particularly relevant to the study of public health data are recent results pertaining to spatial autocorrelation indexes applied to regions with heterogeneous population sizes. Relevant references include Getis and Ord (1992, 1996), Oden (1995), Waldhör (1996), and Assunção and Reis (1999).

In addition, other recent research explores approaches other than Monte Carlo for obtaining the exact distribution of spatial autocorrelation indexes for Gaussian (Tiefelsdorf and Boots 1995, 1996; Hepple 1998; Tiefelsdorf 1998, 2000, 2002) and Poisson or binomial (Hill 2002) data. Although such methods based on characteristic function inversion and saddlepoint approximations offer some computational improvements over Monte Carlo tests, the details of these methods fall beyond the scope of this text.

7.8.2 Additional Approaches for Detecting Clusters and/or Clustering

Tests of Overdispersion As noted in Section 7.1.3, deviations from the Poisson distribution may offer evidence of clustering or local clusters. One approach to assess the adequacy of the Poisson distribution is to explore the similarity between the sample mean and variance. Another is to formally test for overdispersion, as in Potthoff and Whittinghill (1966a,b), Breslow (1984), Muirhead and Ball (1989), Dean (1992), and Muirhead and Butland (1996).

Other Modifications to Pearson's χ^2 Hook and Carothers (1997) propose a Monte Carlo test of clustering based on the maximum summand in Pearson's χ^2. Since simulations compare the observed maxima, the inferential procedure avoids the multiple comparisons problem in precisely the same manner as the CEPP of Turnbull et al. (1990) and the spatial scan statistic of Kulldorff (1997), defined in Sections 7.3.4 and 7.3.6, respectively.

Also, Best and Rayner (1991) propose an alternative approach to Tango's statistic based on collections of the orthogonal components of Pearson's χ^2 statistic to test for temporal clustering, arguing that these components offer score tests with optimal power properties for particular clustering alternatives. However, as illustrated in Best and Rayner (1992) and Tango (1992), the interpretation of the components of Pearson's χ^2 requires some care, as some types of clustering appear significant in some components of Pearson's χ^2 but not in other components.

Stone's Tests The focused score tests of Section 7.6.5 provide one means of constructing statistical tests of fit for particular alternatives of interest. Another approach is to use likelihood ratio tests [i.e., compare the likelihood of the data under the null hypothesis to that under the alternative hypothesis (or hypotheses) of interest]. In this setting, Stone (1988) develops a set of hypothesis tests of focused clustering designed specifically to compare the constant risk hypothesis to the alternative hypothesis where risks decrease monotonically as exposure to the focus (or foci) decrease. The tests do not require specification of a precise or even parametric exposure–disease relationship in the alternative (as in the focused score tests); rather, they only depend on an assumption that region-specific disease risk either stays the same or decreases as regions experience less exposure to the focus (or foci). This feature has lead to widespread application of Stone's tests (and variants thereof) by the Small Area Health Statistics Unit (SAHSU) in the United Kingdom (cf. Elliott et al. 1992, 1996; Morris and Wakefield 2000). However, calculation and application of Stone's statistic typically involve fitting isotonic (order-constrained) regression models and falls somewhat outside the scope of this text. Variants and extensions of Stone's approach appear in Lumley (1995) and Morton-Jones et al. (1999, 2000).

Weighted Likelihood Ratio Tests Gangnon and Clayton (2001) extend the likelihood ratio structure of the spatial scan statistic and present weighted likelihood ratio tests, illustrating the approach on the block-group-level New York leukemia data.

Bayesian Cluster Detection Gangnon and Clayton (2000) define a Bayesian approach to cluster detection based on model averaging ideas, also illustrated on the block-group-level New York leukemia data.

Classification Methods A separate usage of the term *clustering* appears in the statistical classification literature wherein one seeks to partition each of a set of observations into separate clusters or collections of observations more like one another than like the observations in other clusters. In this setting, every observation is assigned to one and only one cluster. Such methods have been applied to geographically referenced regional count data and provide inference somewhat related to the cluster/clustering methods of this chapter. Such approaches appear in Schlattman and Böhning (1993), Knorr-Held and Rasser (2000), and Knorr-Held and Best (2001).

7.8.3 Space–Time Clustering and Disease Surveillance

We end with what historically appeared first. Much of the initial interest in the development of tests to detect disease clusters or clustering occurred in the setting of detecting clusters in space *and* time. That is, a cluster consists of cases near other cases in both space and time. We focus on spatial clusters in this and preceding chapters, but acknowledge a wide literature on the detection of space–time clusters. Key early references include Ederer et al. (1964), Knox (1964), and Mantel (1967).

Recent increased interest in bioterrorism and emerging infectious diseases has lead to increased efforts to detect *emerging* clusters (i.e., spatially proximate cases that are occurring now). Kulldorff (2001), Rogerson (2001), Lazarus et al. (2002), and Mostashari et al. (2003) provide related developments in this area.

7.9 EXERCISES

7.1 Consider regions with 50, 500, and 5000 people at risk, respectively. Find the Poisson probability of observing more cases than people at risk for diseases with individual risks of 0.1, 0.01, 0.001, and 0.0001.

7.2 We note some similarities between assessments of overlapping local incidence proportions and ratios of kernel intensity estimates for point data in Section 6.5.4. Do such similarities extend to the analysis of regional count data? How would we implement kernel estimates? Discuss.

7.3 Replicate the assessment of geographic unbiasedness reported in the data break following Section 7.3.4. Can you quantify a reason for the apparent reduced variation indicated in Figure 7.5?

7.4 Derive the likelihood ratio statistic associated with each potential cluster in the spatial scan statistic, where regional counts are assumed to follow independent Poisson distributions under both the null (no clusters) and alternative (single cluster) hypotheses, where the only difference between the hypotheses is with regard to the expected value of the counts inside and outside the potential cluster.

7.5 Use equation (7.1) to relate the choice of the case radius c^* in the method of Besag and Newell (1991) to the population size of a particular region (say, region i). For a given population size in region i, are there case radii that cannot be declared significance at a given level of significance (say, 0.05)? What does this suggest about possible choices for c^*?

7.6 In Geary's c statistic, the scaling factor preceding the weighted average of sim_{ij} in equation (7.11) summarizes variation of regional count around the mean regional count. As mentioned with respect to Moran's I, variability around the mean regional count is not appropriate when we have heterogeneous regional population sizes. Define an adjustment to Geary's c similar to the adjusted Moran's I statistic I_{cr} defined in equation (7.10) and apply it to the New York leukemia data. Compare your results to those reported in Table 7.4.

7.7 Divide the unit square into a 4×4 grid of regions. Generate 100 events from a homogeneous Poisson process on the unit square and create aggregate counts in each region. Calculate Tango's statistic and the spatial scan statistic for your data. Create a cluster within two adjacent regions by selecting several cases at random from the regions outside the cluster and adding them to two adjacent regions. Increase the number of cases moved to the cluster until the scan statistic and Tango's statistic become significant. How many cases did you need to move to the two regions? Can you phrase this cluster "size" in terms of relative risk? What does this suggest regarding the size of clusters detectable by the scan statistic and Tango's statistic in your data?

7.8 For the New York leukemia data in Table 7.9, plot Tango's and Rogerson's weights versus distance for several values of κ. Will the different weighting schemes affect the type of clustering detected by Tango's index? If so, how?

Table 7.9 New York Leukemia Data[a]

x	y	Pop.	Cases	x	y	Pop	Cases
4.069	−67.353	3540	3.083	4.639	−66.862	3560	4.083
5.709	−66.978	3739	1.087	7.614	−65.996	2784	1.065
7.316	−67.318	2571	3.060	8.559	−66.934	2729	1.064
9.207	−67.179	3952	2.092	10.180	−66.879	993	0.023
8.698	−68.307	1908	2.045	7.405	−68.078	948	0.022
7.335	−68.351	1172	1.027	6.644	−67.644	1047	3.025
5.556	−67.778	3138	5.073	5.403	−68.525	5485	4.128
3.892	−68.166	5554	6.130	4.320	−69.593	2943	2.069
6.726	−69.763	4969	5.116	8.341	−68.803	4828	4.113
4.319	−40.067	2618	0.061	5.888	−48.612	2244	0.053
−3.922	−39.102	2039	1.048	−3.473	−53.637	1425	0.033
−4.243	−57.960	5262	1.123	10.472	−59.754	4126	1.097
10.429	−60.770	4133	2.097	6.029	−60.332	3974	1.093
9.294	−63.504	3036	4.071	15.301	−57.990	4364	2.102

(*continued overleaf*)

Table 7.9 (*continued*)

x	y	Pop.	Cases	x	y	Pop	Cases
28.533	−59.213	4965	1.116	44.542	−71.661	2635	1.062
26.200	−70.753	5911	7.138	14.651	−70.153	5834	1.137
13.633	−73.304	6204	5.145	5.520	−71.256	5007	1.117
6.220	−64.636	5594	5.131	2.294	−63.134	1198	0.028
−1.307	−65.936	5088	7.119	−3.056	−67.421	3107	4.073
−3.228	−66.656	2851	0.067	−3.376	−66.134	3725	3.087
−7.735	−68.314	5505	4.129	−6.265	−66.089	8122	0.190
−4.848	−67.158	5146	7.120	−4.788	−67.943	2143	2.050
−6.278	−68.079	3912	0.092	−5.496	−68.645	3256	6.076
3.106	−65.587	3909	5.091	2.420	−66.551	3106	1.073
2.739	−67.014	3433	5.080	2.646	−67.673	4048	1.095
1.476	−65.563	2630	3.062	0.728	−69.439	12221	9.286
−4.198	−69.329	5963	6.140	−7.078	−71.146	3857	3.090
−2.693	−75.291	5197	2.122	−50.243	36.814	10494	3.839
−48.713	54.252	3571	0.626	−44.846	48.834	1322	0.232
−51.984	50.333	2235	0.392	−54.284	36.220	3905	1.684
−48.719	35.411	6501	1.139	−45.506	26.448	5163	4.905
−44.249	23.500	6021	2.055	−46.511	26.100	7398	8.296
−47.855	24.276	5200	6.911	−53.546	21.137	5616	1.984
−46.274	24.648	6810	7.193	−55.482	9.899	2919	3.511
−45.278	11.980	1765	0.309	−32.888	8.954	3117	0.546
−30.870	−2.614	4278	0.750	−41.620	−4.037	1817	3.318
−51.202	−0.781	1762	0.309	42.713	−2.720	5780	1.703
21.226	−11.684	4189	0.509	38.318	−20.559	4141	4.504
38.701	−19.448	3941	5.479	46.626	−14.208	5802	4.705
37.769	−23.729	7710	2.938	21.514	−28.348	2376	1.289
32.135	−41.099	7278	2.885	31.607	−49.284	8127	3.988
1.862	−16.601	5532	3.340	−10.903	−0.588	2592	1.159
−17.986	−1.508	5653	6.347	−18.630	−12.635	5105	7.314
−18.906	−11.309	4421	2.272	−15.73	−12.060	3242	2.199
−12.310	−10.786	2921	8.180	−6.136	−23.354	3711	5.228
−15.148	−16.950	4855	1.298	−19.260	−13.129	6438	7.396
−18.944	−22.815	4350	4.267	26.365	41.438	5170	2.476
27.552	40.655	2940	3.271	26.373	41.236	2700	0.249
18.846	45.413	3766	0.347	18.898	41.544	4773	0.440
7.169	48.289	6557	2.604	10.795	38.083	2519	0.232
8.497	38.279	4295	1.396	10.823	24.177	2599	3.239
11.161	23.461	3281	4.302	23.025	31.970	6250	2.576
24.096	19.087	6677	0.615	16.640	8.843	3245	4.299
36.296	13.316	3725	1.343	39.356	14.481	4616	1.425
53.509	10.264	2037	0.188	−15.326	40.508	9	0.000
−13.793	41.011	3704	4.056	−12.939	41.735	1702	0.026
−12.226	41.264	4193	3.063	−13.906	40.029	1401	1.021
−13.351	40.456	3268	2.049	−12.758	40.442	1612	0.024
−12.147	40.364	2705	4.041	−11.244	40.312	3927	2.059
−9.848	40.709	4330	6.065	−14.694	39.499	143	1.002

Table 7.9 (*continued*)

x	y	Pop.	Cases	x	y	Pop	Cases
−13.917	39.117	99	0.001	−13.303	39.395	1475	0.022
−12.970	39.858	2766	3.042	−12.276	39.573	2636	4.040
−12.173	38.934	3132	3.047	−11.109	39.123	2603	5.039
−10.519	39.400	2973	1.045	−9.809	39.762	3156	0.048
−8.752	39.839	4807	1.073	−16.723	38.980	2587	2.039
−15.217	38.544	1997	3.030	−14.159	38.501	1211	2.018
−12.996	38.885	2549	1.038	−11.893	38.702	2231	0.034
−16.457	38.264	2225	3.034	−16.375	37.649	2291	0.035
−15.444	38.028	1189	0.018	−14.124	37.801	2621	2.040
−13.363	38.134	914	2.014	−12.743	37.939	1409	0.021
−12.224	38.122	1268	0.019	−11.479	37.992	1437	0.022
−10.724	37.938	3359	2.051	−9.753	38.180	2662	2.040
−8.704	38.332	2356	0.036	−15.727	37.105	503	1.008
−15.397	36.783	2852	1.043	−14.469	36.803	5883	2.089
−13.954	37.319	2446	0.037	−13.265	36.954	717	1.011
−12.722	36.979	2579	2.039	−12.024	37.260	9393	4.142
−11.158	36.577	2193	2.033	−10.470	36.651	4524	0.068
−8.878	37.115	5469	7.083	−16.433	35.815	2014	1.030
−15.426	35.799	1661	0.025	−14.754	35.563	3213	0.048
−13.920	35.189	3061	2.046	−13.832	36.218	3525	1.053
−12.852	36.222	3128	0.047	−12.634	35.421	4144	0.063
−11.764	34.930	2912	0.044	−10.617	35.288	1689	1.025
−10.592	34.676	2720	0.041	−14.111	34.358	2670	5.040
−13.321	34.785	3108	4.047	−12.558	34.582	3072	0.046
−13.447	32.917	4149	2.063	−12.469	33.387	3635	3.055
−11.562	32.740	2801	5.042	−12.506	31.784	3097	0.047
−4.891	53.764	2154	0.032	−10.943	56.410	3290	1.05
−9.834	51.064	5935	0.090	−4.197	49.537	3095	2.047
−9.488	49.009	2677	0.040	−9.754	47.072	4443	0.067
−10.954	47.897	2095	0.032	−12.085	47.577	5875	2.089
−13.100	46.879	3234	0.049	−15.175	47.155	7914	3.119
−13.057	48.404	4740	1.072	−18.973	48.402	8140	1.123
−18.418	47.007	4081	1.062	−21.552	51.780	2668	0.040
−20.175	53.142	1733	2.026	−18.852	50.853	6762	4.102
−12.434	51.045	4889	0.074	−18.052	54.741	2802	0.042
−24.874	54.020	1704	2.026	−30.753	53.944	5743	3.087
−22.711	48.810	2345	0.035	−27.924	50.923	4105	1.062
−28.128	49.183	2514	0.038	−24.891	46.477	6261	0.094
−29.806	46.681	3810	0.057	−38.079	38.625	5885	3.089
−26.755	40.217	2397	0.036	−25.887	37.029	1298	0.020
−24.213	36.358	5311	3.080	−23.675	38.145	4774	1.072
−21.451	37.998	4629	1.070	−20.238	37.167	4429	2.067
−20.627	38.879	1495	1.023	−21.121	43.888	3092	2.047
−18.195	39.401	2729	1.041	−18.463	38.801	4411	4.067
−18.940	37.247	4713	3.071	−17.473	37.273	3583	4.054
−17.892	44.541	2849	2.043	−19.460	46.367	5520	2.083

(*continued overleaf*)

Table 7.9 (*continued*)

x	y	Pop.	Cases	x	y	Pop	Cases
−15.544	45.000	4629	2.070	−16.679	43.819	4437	1.067
−15.545	42.823	3823	0.058	−13.259	45.162	2406	3.036
−11.959	44.163	3169	3.048	−12.618	43.821	4354	2.066
−13.802	42.558	1576	2.024	−11.201	41.737	4637	5.070
−6.841	39.955	3412	1.051	−8.644	41.997	3073	0.046
−5.825	41.656	4837	2.073	−6.325	37.769	6146	5.093
−7.852	35.601	4813	4.073	−4.732	35.064	3077	2.046
−7.625	31.607	1510	0.023	−1.213	35.810	4709	3.071
−1.369	35.773	4927	0.074	1.035	32.848	2510	3.038
1.028	32.994	5241	0.079	3.692	37.486	859	1.013
−1.368	41.001	3640	1.055	−2.432	39.997	4101	2.062
−1.698	45.139	2502	0.038	0.683	24.737	4492	0.068
−7.767	24.012	4488	4.068	−14.328	26.250	596	0.009
−20.450	26.646	5424	2.082	−10.325	29.876	1214	1.018
−12.444	30.194	2779	1.042	−15.661	32.754	5690	2.086
−19.003	35.414	2717	0.041	−28.670	29.259	4310	1.065
−28.688	30.852	1870	1.028	−35.983	26.866	2786	1.042
−34.554	26.419	5009	2.076	−24.898	14.560	1596	0.024
−19.610	16.637	2112	0.032	−10.921	9.999	2409	1.036
0.175	13.306	1811	0.027	−14.565	−48.845	6006	4.085
−29.003	−52.870	4919	1.889	−15.798	−68.106	7023	2.269
−14.282	−72.352	9084	4.641	−22.738	−67.371	4364	6.788
−29.470	−69.684	6999	2.265	−43.339	−69.836	11417	5.063
−30.749	−13.465	5213	4.060	−44.146	−15.211	3916	1.045
−40.460	−22.936	887	0.010	−43.466	−20.207	475	0.005
−51.912	−24.866	7041	2.081	−43.550	−28.728	3476	1.04
−40.564	−27.572	3404	6.039	−38.618	−26.765	2630	3.03
−39.284	−29.119	1777	1.020	−41.395	−29.395	13015	3.149
−41.510	−30.601	4358	3.050	−42.080	−31.169	3880	3.045
−42.878	−30.248	5630	1.065	−47.493	−30.821	971	0.011
−40.500	−32.883	5613	1.064	−36.439	−33.877	524	0.006
−37.096	−29.876	884	1.010	−34.078	−27.819	3025	0.035
−28.790	−23.104	7723	1.089	−34.646	−39.355	5203	3.060
−51.142	−42.100	4401	1.051	−41.960	−24.820	1010	0.012
−42.675	−27.313	2029	2.023				

[a] x and y denote coordinates of the centroid of each of 281 census tracts in an eight-county region of upstate New York. "Pop." denotes the 1980 U.S. Census population size of each tract, and "cases" denotes the number of leukemia cases assigned to each tract (see text for explanation of fractional cases).

7.9 For the New York leukemia data, simulate 1000 data sets under multinomial sampling (592 cases in each simulation). Compare Tango's χ^2 approximation and the Monte Carlo distribution of the test statistic under the constant risk hypothesis. Compare the distributions when we only have half as many cases (but the same population proportions).

7.10 Rogerson (1999) proposes a local form of Tango's index, defined as

$$R_i = \frac{1}{\sqrt{n_i/n_+}}\left(\frac{Y_i}{Y_+} - \frac{n_i}{n_+}\right)\sum_{j=1}^{N} \frac{\exp(-d_{ij}/\kappa)}{\sqrt{n_i/n_+}}\left(\frac{Y_j}{Y_+} - \frac{n_j}{n_+}\right)$$

for $i = 1, \ldots, N$. Does R_i satisfy the criteria for local indicators of spatial association (LISAs) outlined in Section 7.5?

Based on Tango's chi-square approximation, Rogerson (1999) suggests comparing each R_i to a chi-square distribution with one degree of freedom. Are negative values of R_i possible? What does this suggest regarding the chi-square approximation? Outline a Monte Carlo approach for obtaining p-values for each R_i.

Apply R_i to the New York leukemia data for different values of κ and discuss the results. Compare your Monte Carlo approach to the chi-square approximation. Is the chi-square approximation appropriate for R_i in these data? Which tracts contain the most suggestive values of R_i?

Using Monte Carlo simulation, assess the appropriateness of the normal approximation to the distribution of the focused score test under the constant risk hypothesis for:

(a) The entire New York leukemia data set

(b) The first 51 elements of the New York leukemia data set (Broome County)

(c) The first 51 elements with 70 observed cases

(d) The first 51 elements with 30 cases

How robust does the approximation appear to be?

CHAPTER 8

Spatial Exposure Data

I speculate. Mapmakers are entitled to do so, since they readily acknowledge that they are rarely in possession of all the facts. They are always dealing with secondary accounts, the tag ends of impressions. Theirs is an uncertain science.

James Cowan, *A Mapmaker's Dream, the Meditations of Fra Mauro, Cartographer to the Court of Venice*, 1996, Warner Books, p. 11

We now turn to a different aspect of the spatial analysis of public health data: spatial exposure information. When analyzing spatial patterns of disease, we may also want to study spatial patterns of potential exposures. In fact, we often need to consider spatial exposure information to understand the observed spatial variation in disease. As we noted in Chapter 1, Palm (1890) was among the first to link the spatial distribution of a disease (rickets in Great Britain) to a spatial exposure when he noted that sunlight deficiency was an important component in the etiology of this disease. Spatial analysis also led Blum (1948) and Lancaster (1956) to identify sunlight as a causal factor in skin cancer. While latitude is a surrogate for sunlight that is easily recorded, other studies may require exposure assessment and maps that are based on field measurements. This is particularly true in environmental health applications in which environmental measures (e.g., air pollution, groundwater contamination) are thought to exacerbate disease. Spatial exposure assessment is also important from a health policy standpoint since environmental monitoring data often formulate regional air and water quality standards.

Maps of both disease and potential exposures form the basis for *geographical correlation studies* that attempt to draw inferences about disease risk in relation to spatially varying risk factors. We discuss statistical methods for such studies in Chapter 9. In this chapter we focus on the exposure component alone and statistical methods for mapping spatial exposure data. We will borrow much of the methodology from the field of *geostatistics*, a field of statistics concerned with the study of spatial data that have a continuous spatial index (i.e., data can be observed at any location within a domain of interest, at least conceptually). This is in contrast to aggregated spatial data (discussed in Chapter 7), which are associated with areal

Applied Spatial Statistics for Public Health Data, by Lance A. Waller and Carol A. Gotway
ISBN 0-471-38771-1

regions for which there is no opportunity for measurement between locations. In geostatistics, the locations of the data are assumed to be fixed and known, not random as is the case with spatial point patterns discussed in Chapters 5 and 6. In using geostatistical methodology, we seek a general statistical model to infer the characteristics of the spatial process that gives rise to the data we observe. Much of the material in this chapter draws heavily from that in Cressie (1993) and from Carol Gotway's coursework and interaction with Noel Cressie as one of his first Ph.D. students in spatial statistics, and his continued long-term mentoring as an incredible resource on spatial statistics.

8.1 RANDOM FIELDS AND STATIONARITY

Suppose that we have spatial exposure data $Z(\boldsymbol{s}_1), Z(\boldsymbol{s}_2), \ldots, Z(\boldsymbol{s}_N)$ that represent observations of a variable Z at spatial locations $\boldsymbol{s}_1, \boldsymbol{s}_2, \ldots, \boldsymbol{s}_N$. The spatial locations may be aligned on a regular grid or distributed irregularly throughout some domain of interest, D. We restrict our attention to two dimensions, so each location is a two-dimensional vector, $\boldsymbol{s} = (x, y)$, referencing a point in the plane.

In geostatistical applications, the data are assumed to be a partial realization of a random process (called a *stochastic process* or *random field*)

$$\{Z(\boldsymbol{s}) : \boldsymbol{s} \in D\}$$

where D is a fixed subset of $\Re^2$, and the spatial index, $\boldsymbol{s}$, varies continuously throughout D. Thus, for a fixed location $\boldsymbol{s}$, $Z(\boldsymbol{s})$ is a random variable to which the laws of probability apply; for a fixed realization of this process, we observe a function of space: namely, the data at locations $\boldsymbol{s}_1, \boldsymbol{s}_2, \ldots, \boldsymbol{s}_N$. The data are only a partial realization of a spatial function since we cannot, for practical reasons, observe the process at every point in D.

This model for spatial data makes traditional statistical inference difficult since we do not have independent replication. As mentioned in Chapter 5, a facsimile of replication is provided by the concept of *stationarity*. With a random field, if

$$E[Z(\boldsymbol{s})] = \mu \qquad \text{for all } \boldsymbol{s} \in D \tag{8.1}$$

(i.e., the mean of the process does not depend on location) and

$$\operatorname{Cov}\big(Z(\boldsymbol{s}_i), Z(\boldsymbol{s}_j)\big) = C(\boldsymbol{s}_i - \boldsymbol{s}_j) \qquad \text{for all } \boldsymbol{s}_i, \boldsymbol{s}_j \in D \tag{8.2}$$

(i.e., the covariance depends only on the difference between locations $\boldsymbol{s}_i$ and $\boldsymbol{s}_j$, *not on the locations themselves*), then $Z(\cdot)$ is said to be *second-order stationary*. The function $C(\cdot)$ defined by equation (8.2) is called the *covariance function* and is one measure of spatial autocorrelation. Thus, through the assumption of stationarity, the process essentially repeats itself in space, providing the replication necessary for estimation and inference. If, in addition, $C(\boldsymbol{s}_i - \boldsymbol{s}_j)$ is a function only of the distance between s_i and s_j and not direction, the process is called *isotropic*. If $C(s_i - s_j)$ depends on both distance and direction, the spatial process is called *anisotropic*. The notions of stationarity and isotropy correspond conceptually to those defined for spatial point processes in Chapter 5, although equations (8.1) and (8.2) phrase the concepts directly in terms of the Z process.

We do not need stationarity to work with random fields and geostatistics, but it provides a convenient place to begin our development of geostatistical methods for public health data. Methods for handling nonstationary exposure data are described in Section 9.2.

8.2 SEMIVARIOGRAMS

We have seen in Chapter 7 that one of the fundamental attributes of spatial data is spatial autocorrelation: observations closer together tend to be more alike than observations farther apart. In geostatistics, this idea of autocorrelation is quantified through a function called a *semivariogram*.

Suppose that in addition to the constant mean assumption given in equation (8.1), $\{Z(s) : s \in D\}$ also satisfies

$$\text{Var}(Z(s_i) - Z(s_j)) = 2\gamma(s_i - s_j), \quad s_i, s_j \in D. \tag{8.3}$$

Then $Z(\cdot)$ is said to be *intrinsically stationary* and the function $2\gamma(\cdot)$ defined by equation (8.3) is called a *variogram*. If a process is intrinsically stationary [i.e., it satisfies equations (8.1) and (8.3)], $2\gamma(\boldsymbol{h})$ is a function of the *spatial lag,* $\boldsymbol{h} = \boldsymbol{s} - \boldsymbol{u}$, *but not of the locations* $\boldsymbol{s}$ *and* $\boldsymbol{u}$. Note that the definition of intrinsic stationarity is very similar to that of second-order stationarity, where the former is defined in terms of the variogram and the latter in terms of the covariance function. In fact, the variogram is a generalization of the covariance function, and under the assumption of second-order stationarity, the two functions are related, as we shall see below.

The function $\gamma(\cdot)$ is called a *semivariogram*, as it is one-half the variogram. The semivariogram is central to the field of geostatistics. Although many authors use the terms *variogram* and *semivariogram* interchangeably, they clearly differ: One is twice the other. This may not matter in some calculations, but in others the distinction can be crucial. Since we have seen too many studies (and even theoretical results) off by a factor of 2, we will distinguish the variogram from the semivariogram and use just the latter term.

The semivariogram is a function of the spatial process and as such satisfies certain properties:

(i) $\gamma(-\boldsymbol{h}) = \gamma(\boldsymbol{h})$ [i.e., the autocorrelation between $Z(\boldsymbol{s})$ and $Z(\boldsymbol{u})$ is the same as that between $Z(\boldsymbol{u})$ and $Z(\boldsymbol{s})$].

(ii) $\gamma(\boldsymbol{0}) = 0$, since by definition, $\text{Var}(Z(\boldsymbol{s}) - Z(\boldsymbol{s})) = 0$.

(iii) $\gamma(\boldsymbol{h})/\|\boldsymbol{h}\|^2 \longrightarrow 0$ as $\|\boldsymbol{h}\| \longrightarrow \infty$, where $\|\boldsymbol{h}\|$ denotes the length of the vector $\boldsymbol{h}$.

(iv) $\gamma(\cdot)$ must be *conditionally negative definite*; that is,

$$\sum_{i=1}^{m}\sum_{j=1}^{m} a_i a_j \gamma(\boldsymbol{s}_i - \boldsymbol{s}_j) \leq 0 \tag{8.4}$$

for any finite number of locations $\{\boldsymbol{s}_i : i = 1, \ldots, m\}$ and real numbers $\{a_1, \ldots, a_m\}$ satisfying $\sum_{i=1}^{m} a_i = 0$. This condition is the analog of the positive-definite condition for covariance functions and variance–covariance matrices, ensuring that all variances are nonnegative.

(v) If the spatial process is isotropic, $\gamma(\boldsymbol{h}) \equiv \gamma(h)$, where $h = \|\boldsymbol{h}\|$ (i.e., the semivariogram is a function of distance alone).

A graph of a semivariogram plotted against separation distance, $\|\boldsymbol{h}\|$, conveys information about the continuity and spatial variability of the process. This graph starts at zero, and if observations close together are more alike than those farther apart, increases as the separation distance increases. In this way, increasing variation in pairwise differences with increasing distance reflects decreasing spatial autocorrelation, since $Z(\boldsymbol{s})$ and $Z(\boldsymbol{u})$ can vary more with respect to each other as locations $\boldsymbol{s}$ and $\boldsymbol{u}$ move farther apart. Often, the semivariogram will level off to nearly a constant value (called the *sill*) at a large separation distance (called the *range*). Beyond this distance, observations are spatially uncorrelated, reflected by a (near) constant variance in pairwise differences. These properties are depicted in Figure 8.1. Note that if the spatial process is not isotropic, the semivariogram and the information it conveys will differ with direction and we can envision several graphs like Figure 8.1, one for each direction. If there is no autocorrelation between $Z(\boldsymbol{s})$ and $Z(\boldsymbol{u})$, the semivariogram will be a horizontal line.

The shape of the semivariogram near the origin is of particular interest since it indicates the degree of smoothness or spatial continuity of the spatial variable under study. A parabolic shape near the origin arises with a very smooth spatial variable

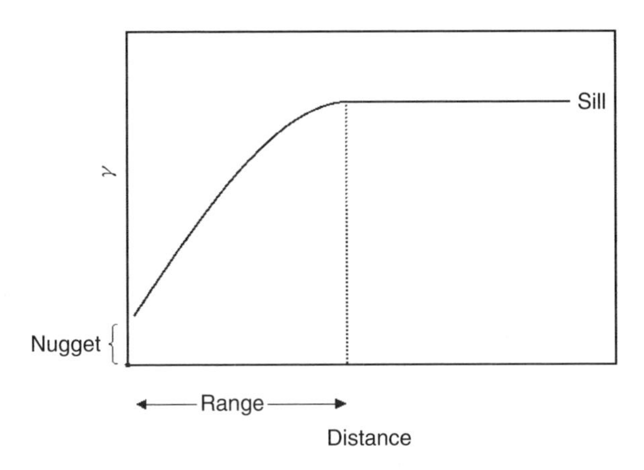

FIG. 8.1 Typical semivariogram.

that is both continuous and differentiable. A linear shape near the origin reflects a variable that is continuous but not differentiable, and hence less regular. A discontinuity, or vertical jump, at the origin [i.e., $\lim_{\boldsymbol{h}\to\boldsymbol{0}} \gamma(\boldsymbol{h}) = c_0 > 0$] indicates that the spatial variable is not continuous and has highly irregular spatial variability. This discontinuity is called the *nugget effect* in the geostatistical literature. If the process has a large nugget effect, two observations fairly close together have very different values. This is often due to measurement error, but can also simply indicate a spatially discontinuous process. (The term *nugget effect* comes from mining. In mining gold ore, we may not find ore at one location, but then at a nearby location find a gold nugget.) The nugget effect is a discontinuity; by definition [see equation (8.3)] the semivariogram at the origin (i.e., at zero separation distance) is always zero.

8.2.1 Relationship to Covariance Function and Correlogram

The covariance function defined in equation (8.2) is related to the semivariogram in the following way. If $Z(\cdot)$ is second-order stationary [i.e., satisfied equations (8.1) and (8.2)], then

$$\gamma(\boldsymbol{h}) = C(\boldsymbol{0}) - C(\boldsymbol{h}).$$

If $C(\boldsymbol{h}) \longrightarrow 0$ as $\|\boldsymbol{h}\| \longrightarrow \infty$, then $\gamma(\boldsymbol{h}) \longrightarrow C(\boldsymbol{0})$. So $C(\boldsymbol{0})$ is the variance of $Z(\boldsymbol{s})$ and the sill of the semivariogram. When there is a nugget effect, the *partial sill* is defined as the difference between the process variance (sill) and the nugget effect, or $C(\boldsymbol{0}) - c_0$. The term *relative nugget effect* refers to the percentage of the total sill comprised of the nugget effect. Formally, the *range* of the semivariogram in the direction $\boldsymbol{r}_0/\|\boldsymbol{r}_0\|$ is the smallest length $\|\boldsymbol{r}_0\|$ such that $\gamma(\boldsymbol{r}_0(1+\varepsilon)) = C(\boldsymbol{0})$ for any $\varepsilon > 0$ (i.e., for any distance larger than $\|\boldsymbol{r}_0\|$, the semivariogram equals the sill). Practically, for any fixed direction, it is the minimum distance, r, for which $\gamma(r) = C(0)$.

Sometimes, particularly if we are comparing two spatial processes, it is useful to use a measure of correlation instead of covariance. Thus, we can define the spatial *correlogram* as

$$\rho(\boldsymbol{h}) = C(\boldsymbol{h})/C(\boldsymbol{0}).$$

The definition of $\rho(\boldsymbol{h})$ is analogous to that of a typical correlation [i.e., scaled so that $|\rho(\boldsymbol{h})| \leq 1$].

Since these functions are all related, why do we use the semivariogram instead of a covariance function? Theoretically, the class of intrinsically stationary processes (those with a valid semivariogram) is more general than the class of second-order stationary processes (those with a valid covariance function). But only barely, and processes that have a semivariogram but not a covariance function rarely arise in public health applications. The curious can refer to Cressie (1993, p. 68) for an example of a process (Brownian motion) for which $\gamma(\cdot)$ is defined but $C(\cdot)$ is not. A practical reason for preferring the semivariogram to the covariance function is that estimation of the semivariogram from the data observed is more reliable than estimation of the covariance function, since estimation of the semivariogram does not require estimation of the mean (see Cressie 1993).

8.2.2 Parametric Isotropic Semivariogram Models

There are many parametric functions that satisfy the properties of the semivariogram (see, e.g., Journel and Huijbregts 1978; Chilès and Delfiner 1999). We say that a semivariogram model is valid in d dimensions (i.e., in $\Re^d$) if it satisfies the conditional negative-definite property defined in Section 8.2 [equation (8.4)]. A closer look at some of these will give us a better understanding of the semivariogram and its relationship to the spatial process of interest. We also use these as models for the empirical semivariogram in Section 8.2.4. Since these are isotopic models, we write them in terms of a generic lag distance, denoted h. Graphs of these theoretical semivariograms illustrate their differences (Figure 8.2).

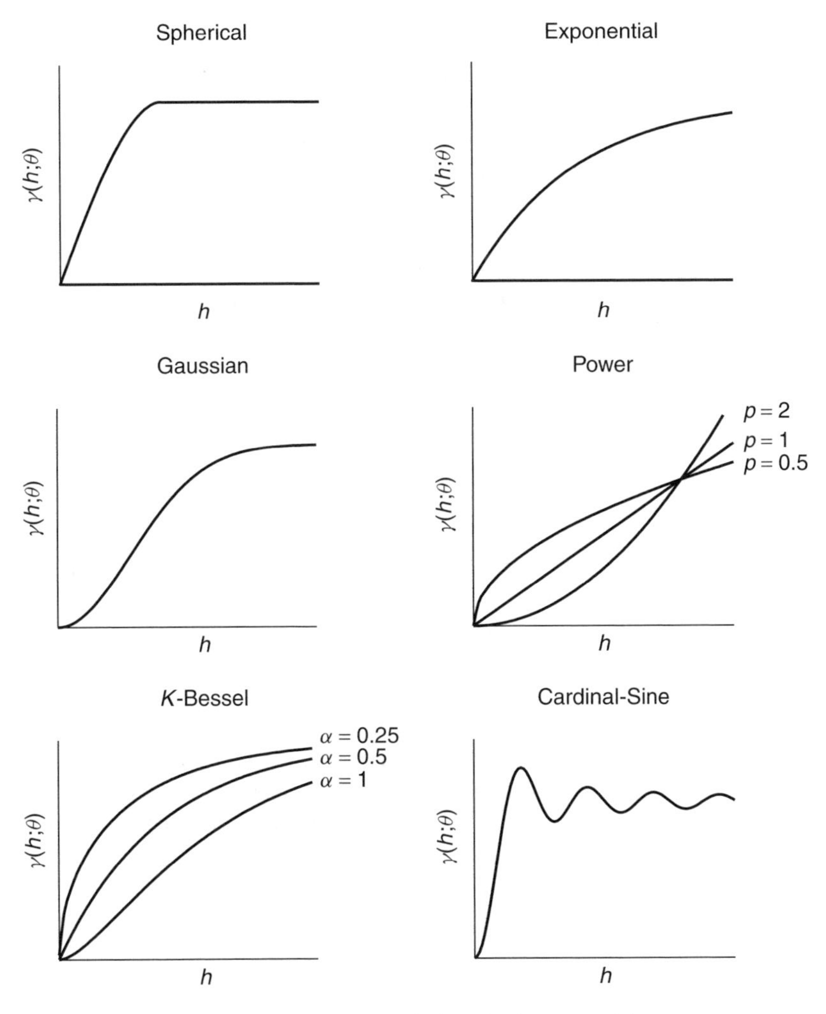

FIG. 8.2 Selected theoretical semivariogram models.

- *Spherical:*

$$\gamma(h;\boldsymbol{\theta}) = \begin{cases} 0, & h = 0 \\ c_0 + c_s\left[(3/2)(h/a_s) - (1/2)(h/a_s)^3\right], & 0 < h \leq a_s \\ c_0 + c_s, & h > a_s, \end{cases} \tag{8.5}$$

where $\boldsymbol{\theta} = (c_0, c_s, a_s)'$; $c_0 \geq 0$, $c_s \geq 0$, $a_s > 0$. It is valid in $\Re^d, d = 1, 2, 3$. The spherical semivariogram is nearly linear near the origin. The parameter c_0 measures the nugget effect, c_s is the partial sill (so $c_0 + c_s$ is the sill), and a_s is the range.

- *Exponential:*

$$\gamma(h;\boldsymbol{\theta}) = \begin{cases} 0, & h = 0 \\ c_0 + c_e\left[1 - \exp(-h/a_e)\right], & h > 0, \end{cases} \tag{8.6}$$

where $\boldsymbol{\theta} = (c_0, c_e, a_e)'$; $c_0 \geq 0$, $c_e \geq 0$, $a_e > 0$. It is valid in $\Re^d, d \geq 1$. The exponential semivariogram rises more slowly from the origin than does the spherical semivariogram. As with the spherical model, c_0 is the nugget effect and c_e is the partial sill (so $c_0 + c_e$ is the sill). However, this model approaches the sill asymptotically, so the range is not a_e, since $\gamma(a_e) \neq c_0 + c_e$. The "effective range" (traditionally defined as the distance at which the autocorrelation is 0.05) is $3a_e$.

- *Gaussian:*

$$\gamma(h;\boldsymbol{\theta}) = \begin{cases} 0, & h = 0 \\ c_0 + c_g\left\{1 - \exp[-(h/a_g)^2]\right\}, & h > 0, \end{cases}$$

where $\boldsymbol{\theta} = (c_0, c_g, a_g)'$; $c_0 \geq 0$, $c_g \geq 0$, $a_g > 0$. It is valid in $\Re^d, d \geq 1$. The Gaussian semivariogram model is parabolic near the origin, indicative of a very smooth spatial process. Many argue that such processes rarely arise in practice, although the Gaussian model is often deemed best by automatic model-fitting criteria. This is a valid semivariogram model; however, its use can often lead to singularities in spatial prediction equations (Davis and Morris 1997). Wackernagel (1995) calls it "pathological" since it corresponds to a deterministic process and thus contradicts the underlying randomness assumption in geostatistics. Although we do not take such an extreme view, we do recommend that the Gaussian semivariogram model only be used with caution and never without a lot of closely spaced data to assess behavior near the origin. Similar to the previous models, c_0 measures the nugget effect and c_g is the partial sill (so $c_0 + c_g$ is the sill). The effective range is $\sqrt{3}\, a_g$.

- *Power:*

$$\gamma(h;\boldsymbol{\theta}) = \begin{cases} 0, & h = 0 \\ c_0 + bh^p, & h > 0, \end{cases}$$

where $\boldsymbol{\theta} = (c_0, b, p)'$; $c_0 \geq 0, b \geq 0, 0 \leq p < 2$. It is valid in $\Re^d, d \geq 1$. Models in this family do not have a sill or a range, so spatial correlation does not level off for large lag distances. They play an important role in fractal processes and the estimation of the fractal dimension [see Gallant et al. (1994) for a comparative overview of fractal dimension estimation]. The linear model, obtained by taking $p = 1$, is the most common member of this class.

- *Stable:*

$$\gamma(h; \boldsymbol{\theta}) = \begin{cases} 0, & h = 0 \\ c_0 + c_t \{1 - \exp[(-h/a_t)^\alpha]\}, & h > 0, \end{cases}$$

where $\boldsymbol{\theta} = (c_0, c_t, a_t, \alpha)'$; $c_0 \geq 0, c_t \geq 0, a_t > 0, 0 \leq \alpha \leq 2$. It is valid in $\Re^d, d \geq 1$. Near the origin, models in the stable semivariogram family have the same behavior as models in the power family. The behavior near the origin is determined by α. However, they do reach a sill (c_0 measures the nugget effect and c_t is the partial sill, so $c_0 + c_t$ is the sill). As with the exponential model that is a member of this family, models in this family approach the sill asymptotically, so the range is not a_t. The effective range depends on both a_t and α. Given a_t, models with smaller values of α will approach the sill more slowly.

- *K-Bessel (Matérn):*

$$\gamma(h; \boldsymbol{\theta}) = \begin{cases} 0, & h = 0 \\ c_0 + c_k \left[1 - \dfrac{1}{2^{\alpha-1}\Gamma(\alpha)}\left(\dfrac{h}{a_k}\right)^\alpha K_\alpha \dfrac{h}{a_k}\right], & h > 0, \end{cases}$$

where $\boldsymbol{\theta} = (c_0, c_k, a_k, \alpha)'$; $c_0 \geq 0, c_k \geq 0, a_k > 0, \alpha \geq 0$, $K_\alpha(\cdot)$ is the modified Bessel function of the second kind of order α, and $\Gamma(\cdot)$ is the gamma function. It is valid in $\Re^d, d \geq 1$. This family of models has long been referred to as the *K-Bessel model* in geostatistics, due to its dependence on $K_\alpha(\cdot)$. Recently, statisticians rediscovered the utility of this family and renamed it the *Matérn class*, based on its initial presentation by Matérn (1960). Here, c_0 measures the nugget effect and c_k is the partial sill (so $c_0 + c_k$ is the sill). Models in this family approach the sill asymptotically. As in the stable family, the behavior near the origin is determined by α, and the parameter a_k controls the range. The Gaussian semivariogram model is obtained in the limit by letting $\alpha \to \infty$, and the exponential semivariogram corresponds to the case where $\alpha = \frac{1}{2}$. An advantage of this family of models (and the stable family) is that the behavior of the semivariogram near the origin can be estimated from the data rather than assumed to be of a certain form. However, the computation of $K_\alpha(\cdot)$ needed for this estimation is cumbersome and, as for the Gaussian model, requires some closely spaced data.

- *Cardinal-Sine:*

$$\gamma(h;\boldsymbol{\theta}) = \begin{cases} 0, & h = 0 \\ c_0 + c_w\left(1 - \dfrac{a_w}{h}\sin\dfrac{h}{a_w}\right), & h > 0, \end{cases}$$

where $\boldsymbol{\theta} = (c_0, c_w, a_w)'$; $c_0 \geq 0$, $c_w \geq 0$, $a_w > 0$. It is valid in $\Re^d$, $d = 1, 2, 3$. The cardinal-sine model is one member of a family of models called *hole-effect* models that are parameterized by a more general form called the *J-Bessel model* [see Chilès and Delfiner (1999) for the equation of the J-Bessel model]. These models, and the cardinal-sine model in particular, are useful for processes with negative spatial autocorrelation or processes with cyclical or periodic variability. It reaches a maximum and then continues to oscillate around the sill with a period of a_w.

There are many more parametric semivariogram models not described here [see, e.g., Armstrong (1999), Chilès and Delfiner (1999), and Olea (1999) for several others]. In addition, the sum of two semivariogram models that are both valid in $\Re^d$ is also a valid semivariogram model in $\Re^d$, so more complex processes can be modeled by adding two or more of these basic semivariogram models (Christakos 1984). Semivariogram models created this way are referred to as models of *nested structures.* Note that a model valid in $\Re^{d_2}$ is also valid in $\Re^{d_1}$, where $d_2 > d_1$, but the converse is not true. An important example is the piecewise linear or "tent" function:

$$\gamma(h;\boldsymbol{\theta}) = \begin{cases} 0, & h = 0 \\ c_0 + c_s h, & 0 \leq h \leq a_s \\ c_0 + c_s, & h > a_s, \end{cases} \tag{8.7}$$

where $\boldsymbol{\theta} = (c_0, c_s, a_s)'$; $c_0 \geq 0$, $c_s \geq 0$, $a_s \geq 0$. This model is a valid semivariogram in $\Re^1$ but not in $\Re^2$. Thus, this model should not be used with spatial processes.

8.2.3 Estimating the Semivariogram

The semivariogram can be estimated easily from data $\{Z(\boldsymbol{s}_i) : i = 1, \ldots, N\}$ under the assumption of intrinsic stationary so that equations (8.1) and (8.3) hold. Using rules of expectation, we can write the variogram as

$$\begin{aligned} 2\gamma(\boldsymbol{h}) &= \mathrm{Var}(Z(\boldsymbol{s}+\boldsymbol{h}) - Z(\boldsymbol{s})) \\ &= E[(Z(\boldsymbol{s}+\boldsymbol{h}) - Z(\boldsymbol{s}))^2] - [E(Z(\boldsymbol{s}+\boldsymbol{h}) - Z(\boldsymbol{s}))]^2. \end{aligned}$$

From equation (8.1), $E[Z(\boldsymbol{s}_i)] = \mu$ for all i, so the second term is zero. Thus, to estimate the variogram we need only estimate $E[(Z(\boldsymbol{s}+\boldsymbol{h}) - Z(\boldsymbol{s}))^2]$. Since expectations are just statistical averages, one way to estimate this term is to average all observed squared differences $[Z(\boldsymbol{s}_i) - Z(\boldsymbol{s}_j)]^2$ for pairs of observations taken the same distance apart in the same direction (i.e., for all $\boldsymbol{s}_i, \boldsymbol{s}_j$ such that $\boldsymbol{s}_i - \boldsymbol{s}_j = \boldsymbol{h}$). This is the rationale behind the *method of moments estimator* of the semivariogram, given by

$$\widehat{\gamma}(\boldsymbol{h}) = \frac{1}{2|N(\boldsymbol{h})|} \sum_{N(\boldsymbol{h})} [Z(\boldsymbol{s}_i) - Z(\boldsymbol{s}_j)]^2, \qquad \boldsymbol{h} \in \Re^2, \tag{8.8}$$

where $N(\boldsymbol{h})$ is the set of distinct pairs separated by $\boldsymbol{h}$ [i.e., $N(\boldsymbol{h}) = \{(\boldsymbol{s}_i, \boldsymbol{s}_j) : \boldsymbol{s}_i - \boldsymbol{s}_j = \boldsymbol{h},\ i, j = 1, \dots, N\}$ and $|N(\boldsymbol{h})| =$ the number of distinct pairs in $N(\boldsymbol{h})$].

Equation (8.8) gives what is often referred to as the *classical semivariogram estimator*. It gives point estimates of $\gamma(\cdot)$ at observed values of $\boldsymbol{h}$. If the process is isotropic, we need only consider pairs lagged $||\boldsymbol{h}||$ apart. If the process is anisotropic, the semivariogram can be estimated in different directions by selecting a particular direction and averaging pairs of data lagged $||\boldsymbol{h}||$ apart in that particular direction.

If we have data on a regular grid, we can easily define the lag distances, $||\boldsymbol{h}||$, and the directions using the grid. With irregularly spaced data, there may be only one pair of locations that is $\boldsymbol{h}$ apart (two for $\|\boldsymbol{h}\|$). Averages based on only one or two points are poor estimates with large uncertainties. We can reduce this variation and increase the accuracy of our point estimates by allowing a *tolerance* on the lags. Thus, we will define *tolerance regions* and group the sample pairs into these regions prior to averaging. This is analogous to the procedure used in making a histogram, adapted to two dimensions (see Figure 8.3). We average the pairwise squared differences for pairs of points in the tolerance regions to produce point estimates of the semivariogram at the average lag distances in each region. Each region should be small enough so that we retain enough spatial resolution to define the structure of the semivariogram, but also large enough so that we base each point estimate on a relative large number of paired differences. Typically, one specifies tolerance regions through the choice of five parameters: the direction of interest; the *angle tolerance*, which defines a sector centered on the direction of interest; the *lag spacing*, which defines the distances at which the semivariogram is estimated; the *lag tolerance*, which defines a distance interval centered at each lag; and the total number of lags at which we wish to estimate the semivariogram. Tolerance regions should include at least 30 pairs of points each to ensure that the empirical semivariogram at each point is well estimated (Journel and Huijbregts 1978). Usually, a set of directions and associated angle tolerances are chosen together so that they completely cover two-dimensional space. For example, we might choose the four main directions east-west, north-south, northeast-southwest, and northwest-southeast, and an angle tolerance of 22.5°. This partitions the space into four sectors that cover the plane completely. A more complete analysis of potential anisotropies might specify directions every 10° with a 5° angle tolerance. An isotropic semivariogram results when the angle tolerance is 90°, so we use all pairs to estimate the semivariogram. In a similar fashion, one typically defines distance classes by specifying the lag spacing and lag tolerance (directly analogous to the class spacing and number of

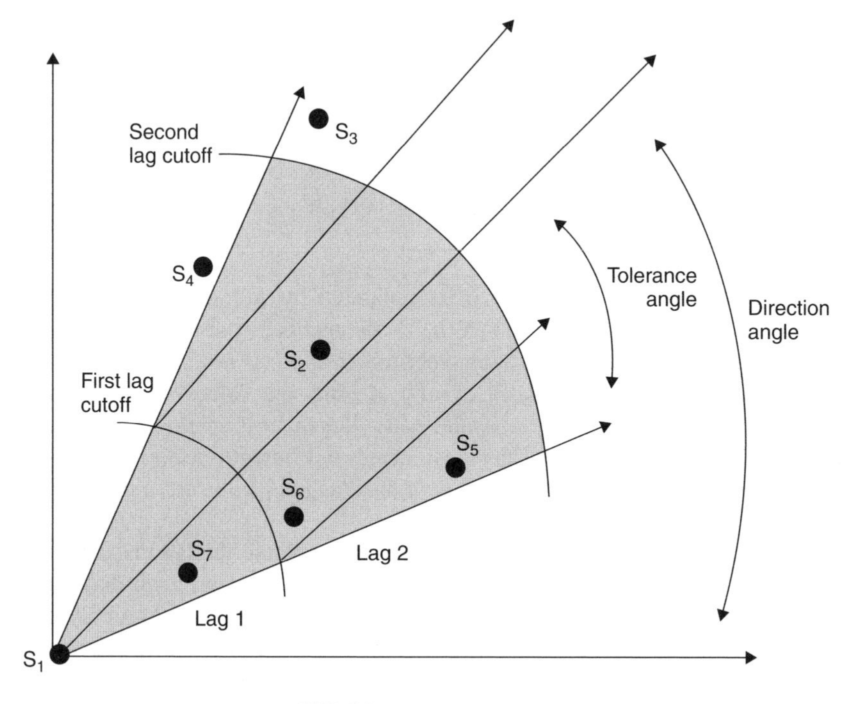

FIG. 8.3 Tolerance regions.

classes in a histogram). As a rule of thumb, one should construct these intervals so that the total number of lags is between 10 and 20 in order to see the structure of the semivariogram. Finally, note that estimates of the semivariogram at large lags rely only on points at the opposite ends of the domain. This usually results in very few pairs of data locations and wide variation in the estimates. Thus, in practice, we usually take the maximum lag distance to be about half the maximum separation distance (Journel and Huijbregts 1978). One should be careful of the use of very short maximum lag distances. The semivariogram is a picture of your data *spatially*: the sill and the range, if they exist, provide estimates of the process variance and the zone of influence of the observations, and information at larger lags can indicate large-scale trends that may be important to interpret.

DATA BREAK: Smoky Mountain pH Data The pH of a stream can affect organisms living in the water, and a change in the stream pH can be an indicator of pollution. Values of pH can range from 0 to 14, with 7 considered neutral; values less than 7 are termed *acidic* while pH values greater than 7 are called *alkaline*. Acidic stream water (with pH < 5) is particularly harmful to fish. In a study of the chemical properties of streams in the mid-Atlantic and southeastern United States, Kaufman et al. (1988) measured water pH at many locations within the Great Smoky Mountains. The locations of these measurements are shown in Figure 8.4. The relative variation in the pH values is also indicated in Figure 8.4,

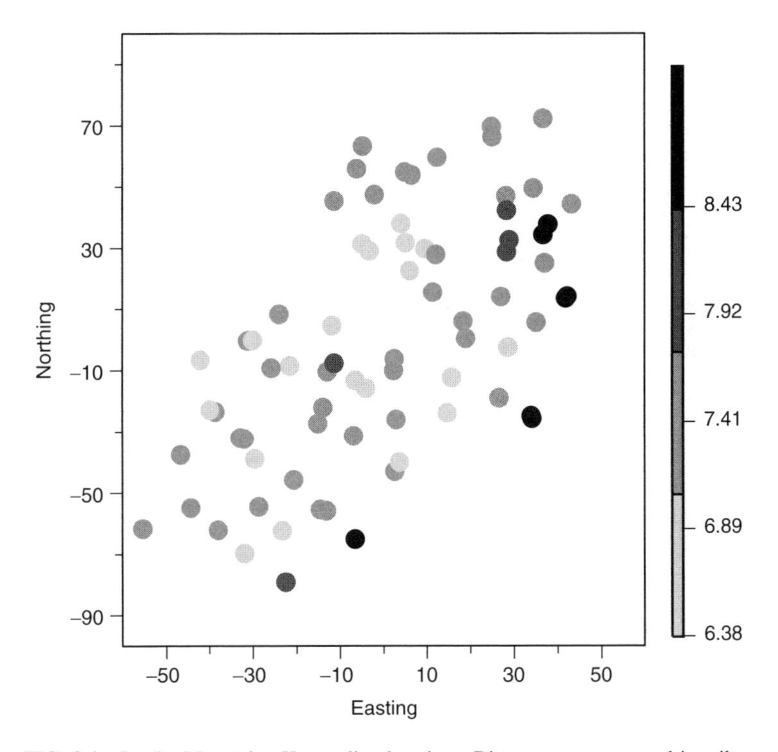

FIG. 8.4 Smoky Mountain pH sampling locations. Distances are measured in miles.

with the darker circles indicating higher values of pH. Initially, we assume that the water pH process is isotropic and estimate what is called an *omnidirectional* semivariogram. Here, we are simply concerned with the distances between points and not in directional variation. Since the data do not lie on a regular grid, we will have to define tolerance regions (which for an omnidirectional semivariogram are tolerance intervals on the lag distances) for semivariogram estimation.

We begin with the following specifications as a starting point: Let the maximum lag distance be one-half the maximum separation distance, which in our case is $\sqrt{(43.2+55.4)^2+(72.3+79.2)^2}/2 = 90.4$ miles; set the number of lags equal to 20 (arbitrarily chosen); take the lag spacing = maximum lag distance/number of lags, or 4.5 miles; and set the lag tolerance = lag spacing/2, in this case 2.3 miles. Using these defaults with the pH values, we obtain the empirical semivariogram in shown Figure 8.5. The distance column gives the average distance between locations in each tolerance interval. It is also common simply to use the midpoint of each tolerance interval to indicate the spacing of the intervals. Notice that the estimates of the semivariogram at the first few lags are based on only a few pairs of observations and may not be very accurate. Also, the empirical semivariogram is a bit noisy and we may be able to obtain a clearer structure by taking a larger tolerance interval of, say, 10 miles. We may also want to extend the maximum

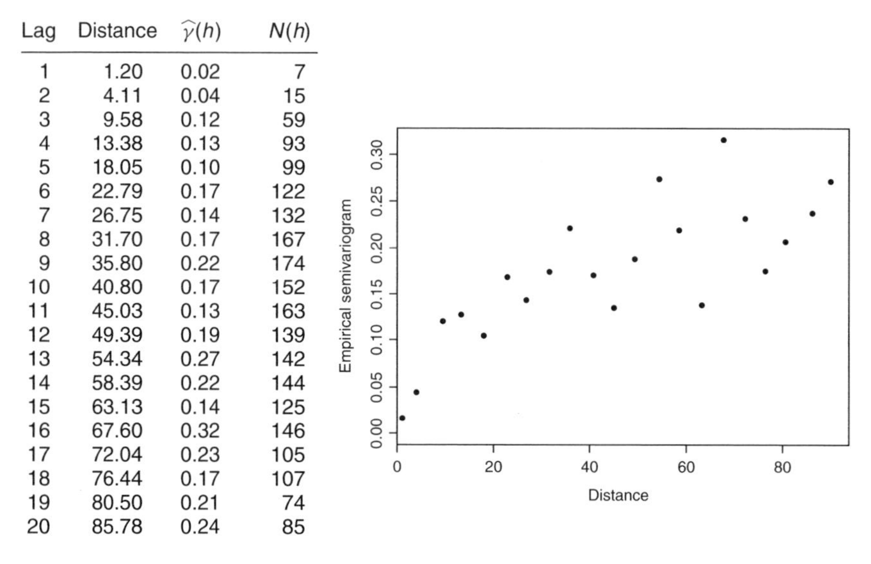

Lag	Distance	$\widehat{\gamma}(h)$	$N(h)$
1	1.20	0.02	7
2	4.11	0.04	15
3	9.58	0.12	59
4	13.38	0.13	93
5	18.05	0.10	99
6	22.79	0.17	122
7	26.75	0.14	132
8	31.70	0.17	167
9	35.80	0.22	174
10	40.80	0.17	152
11	45.03	0.13	163
12	49.39	0.19	139
13	54.34	0.27	142
14	58.39	0.22	144
15	63.13	0.14	125
16	67.60	0.32	146
17	72.04	0.23	105
18	76.44	0.17	107
19	80.50	0.21	74
20	85.78	0.24	85

FIG. 8.5 Empirical semivariogram of pH values. The lag spacing is 4.5 miles.

lag distance to be sure that there is a well-defined sill. The resulting empirical semivariogram is shown in Figure 8.6.

The latter empirical semivariogram shows a much clearer relationship. It is always a good idea to experiment with several choices for the maximum lag distance and lag spacing. Semivariogram estimation is a mixture of both science and art. The goal is accurate estimation, a clear structure, and at least a total of 10 to 20 lags for modeling and inference. The guidelines presented here should work well in many applications. However, in others, the empirical semivariogram may appear erratic for many reasonable choices of the lag spacing and lag tolerance. Common problems with semivariogram estimation and more complex solutions are discussed in Section 8.4.1.

8.2.4 Fitting Semivariogram Models

The empirical semivariogram, $\widehat{\gamma}(\cdot)$, is not guaranteed to be conditionally nonnegative definite. This is not a problem if we limit ourselves to inferences about the spatial continuity of the process, but it can lead to problems when used for spatial prediction and mapping where we need reliable estimates of prediction uncertainty. Thus, we will need to find a valid theoretical semivariogram function that closely reflects the features of our empirical semivariogram. We limit our choices to a parametric family of theoretical variograms (like those described in Section 8.2.2) and seek to find the parameter estimates that best fit the data.

Nonlinear Least Squares Regression The idea here is to select a theoretical semivariogram family and find a vector of parameters $\widehat{\boldsymbol{\theta}}$ that makes this theoretical

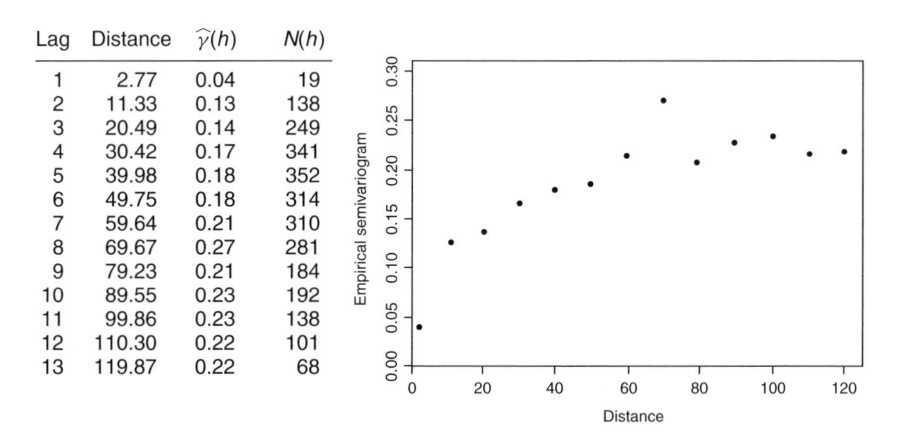

Lag	Distance	$\widehat{\gamma}(h)$	$N(h)$
1	2.77	0.04	19
2	11.33	0.13	138
3	20.49	0.14	249
4	30.42	0.17	341
5	39.98	0.18	352
6	49.75	0.18	314
7	59.64	0.21	310
8	69.67	0.27	281
9	79.23	0.21	184
10	89.55	0.23	192
11	99.86	0.23	138
12	110.30	0.22	101
13	119.87	0.22	68

FIG. 8.6 Empirical semivariogram of pH values. The lag spacing is 10 miles.

model "close" to the empirical semivariogram. Let $\widehat{\gamma}(\cdot)$ be the *empirical semivariogram* estimated at K lags, $h(1), \ldots, h(K)$ and let $\gamma(h; \boldsymbol{\theta})$ be the *theoretical semivariogram* model whose form is known up to $\boldsymbol{\theta}$. Since the relationship between $\widehat{\gamma}(h)$ and h is usually nonlinear, nonlinear least squares regression can be used to estimate $\boldsymbol{\theta}$.

Nonlinear ordinary least squares (OLS) finds $\widehat{\boldsymbol{\theta}}$ minimizing the squared vertical distance between the empirical and theoretical semivariograms, that is, minimizing

$$\sum_{j=1}^{K} \left[\widehat{\gamma}(h(j)) - \gamma(h(j); \boldsymbol{\theta})\right]^2 .$$

However, the estimates $[\widehat{\gamma}(h(j))]$ are correlated and have different variances, violating the general assumptions underling OLS theory. The usual statistical adjustment to OLS when observations are correlated and heteroskedastic is generalized least squares (GLS). Cressie (1985) applied nonlinear GLS to semivariogram estimation, finding $\widehat{\boldsymbol{\theta}}$ minimizing the objective function

$$[\hat{\boldsymbol{\gamma}} - \boldsymbol{\gamma}(\boldsymbol{\theta})]' \boldsymbol{V}(\boldsymbol{\theta})^{-1} [\hat{\boldsymbol{\gamma}} - \boldsymbol{\gamma}(\boldsymbol{\theta})],$$

where $\hat{\boldsymbol{\gamma}} = [\widehat{\gamma}(h(1)), \ldots, \widehat{\gamma}(h(K))]'$ with variance–covariance matrix $\boldsymbol{V}(\boldsymbol{\theta})$ and $\boldsymbol{\gamma}(\boldsymbol{\theta}) = \left[\gamma(h(1); \boldsymbol{\theta}), \ldots, \gamma(h(K), \boldsymbol{\theta})\right]'$. Since $\boldsymbol{V}(\boldsymbol{\theta})$ depends on $\boldsymbol{\theta}$ and $\boldsymbol{\theta}$ is unknown, this estimator is computed iteratively from starting values (one for each parameter in $\boldsymbol{\theta}$) that are improved (using, e.g., the Gauss–Newton algorithm) until the objective function is minimized. Taking $V(\boldsymbol{\theta}) \equiv I$ gives the OLS estimator, and taking $V(\boldsymbol{\theta}) \equiv \mathrm{diag}\{\mathrm{Var}[\hat{\gamma}(h(1))], \ldots, \mathrm{Var}[\hat{\gamma}(h(K))]\}$ gives a nonlinear weighted least squares (WLS) estimator.

Determining the elements of $\boldsymbol{V}(\boldsymbol{\theta})$ requires knowledge of the fourth-order moments of $\mathbf{Z}$. Although these have been derived (see Cressie 1985), they are tedious to compute. Cressie (1985) showed that a nonlinear WLS estimator based on

$$\mathrm{var}[\widehat{\gamma}(h(j))] \approx 2[\gamma(h(j);\boldsymbol{\theta})]^2/N(h(j)) \tag{8.9}$$

yields an estimation procedure that often works well in practice. Thus, weighting the OLS objective function inversely proportional to the (approximate) variance of the empirical semivariogram estimator gives an estimator of $\boldsymbol{\theta}$ that minimizes the weighted regression sum of squares:

$$\mathrm{WRSS}(\boldsymbol{\theta}) = \frac{1}{2}\sum_{j=1}^{K} \frac{N(h(j))}{[\gamma(h(j);\boldsymbol{\theta})]^2} \left[\widehat{\gamma}(h(j)) - \gamma(h(j);\boldsymbol{\theta})\right]^2. \tag{8.10}$$

This approach is an approximation to WLS and offers a pragmatic compromise between OLS and GLS. It gives more weight where there is more "data" [large $N(h(j))$] and near the origin [small $\gamma(\boldsymbol{h};\boldsymbol{\theta})$], thus improving on OLS. Although it will not be as efficient as GLS, the ease of computation is a definite advantage. It can be used even when the data are not Gaussian, and empirical studies have shown (e.g., Zimmerman and Zimmerman 1991) this approach to be fairly accurate in a variety of practical situations.

An approximation to the covariance matrix of $\widehat{\boldsymbol{\theta}}$ can also be obtained from the regression, based on the matrix of partial derivatives of $\gamma(\boldsymbol{h};\boldsymbol{\theta})$ with respect to each parameter in $\boldsymbol{\theta}$. Approximate confidence limits are then $\widehat{\boldsymbol{\theta}} \pm t_{K-g,1-\alpha/2}\mathrm{s.e.}(\widehat{\boldsymbol{\theta}})$, where $\mathrm{s.e.}(\widehat{\boldsymbol{\theta}})$ is the standard error of $\widehat{\boldsymbol{\theta}}$, $t_{K-g,1-\alpha/2}$ is the $1-\alpha/2$ percentage point of a t-distribution with $K-g$ degrees of freedom, and $g=\dim(\boldsymbol{\theta})$. Textbooks on nonlinear regression (e.g., Seber and Wild 1989) provide the theoretical and computational details of nonlinear regression.

Maximum Likelihood Estimation If the data, $\mathbf{Z}$, follow a multivariate Gaussian distribution with mean $\mathbf{1}\mu$ (here $\mathbf{1}$ is a vector of 1's) and variance–covariance matrix $\Sigma(\boldsymbol{\theta})$, likelihood-based techniques can be used to estimate $\boldsymbol{\theta}$. Maximizing the multivariate Gaussian likelihood with respect to $\boldsymbol{\theta}$ yields the maximum likelihood estimator (MLE) of $\boldsymbol{\theta}$. With restricted maximum likelihood (REML), the likelihood derived from error contrasts (or differences) of the data is maximized. Since maximizing the likelihood is equivalent to minimizing twice the negative log likelihood, in practice, the following objective functions are minimized:

$$\begin{aligned}\text{ML:}\quad l(\boldsymbol{\theta}) &= \log(|\Sigma(\boldsymbol{\theta})|) + (\mathbf{Z}-\mathbf{1}\mu)'\Sigma(\boldsymbol{\theta})^{-1}(\mathbf{Z}-\mathbf{1}\mu) + N\log(2\pi)\\ \text{REML:}\quad l_R(\boldsymbol{\theta}) &= (N-1)\log(2\pi) + \log(|\Sigma(\boldsymbol{\theta})|) + \log(|\mathbf{1}'\Sigma(\boldsymbol{\theta})^{-1}\mathbf{1}|)\\ &\quad + \mathbf{Z}'\{\Sigma(\boldsymbol{\theta})^{-1} - \Sigma(\boldsymbol{\theta})^{-1}\mathbf{1}(\mathbf{1}'\Sigma(\boldsymbol{\theta})^{-1}\mathbf{1})^{-1}\mathbf{1}'\Sigma(\boldsymbol{\theta})^{-1}\}\mathbf{Z}.\end{aligned}$$

An approximate covariance matrix of $\widehat{\boldsymbol{\theta}}$ can be obtained as the inverse of the Fisher information matrix. Approximate confidence limits are then $\widehat{\boldsymbol{\theta}} \pm z_{1-\alpha/2}\mathrm{s.e.}(\widehat{\boldsymbol{\theta}})$, where $\mathrm{s.e.}(\widehat{\boldsymbol{\theta}})$ is the standard error of $\widehat{\boldsymbol{\theta}}$, and $z_{1-\alpha/2}$ is the $1-\alpha/2$ percentage point of a standard normal distribution. Searle et al. (1992) is a good reference text for the computational details and distributional properties of likelihood-based estimators.

Empirical Model Comparison A major advantage of statistical approaches to fitting semivariogram models (as opposed to fitting them "by eye" as is often done in many disciplines) is the availability of objective criteria for comparing the fits of two or more competing models. Although the details depend on whether nonlinear least squares (NLS) or likelihood-based (LB) approaches are used to estimate the model parameters, such criteria take three broad forms.

1. *Single-parameter tests.* These are *Wald tests* for each parameter computed as $\widehat{\theta_i}/\text{s.e.}(\widehat{\theta_i})$. For NLS, this test statistic is compared to a t-distribution on $K - g$ degrees of freedom, and for LB tests, it is compared to a standard normal distribution. Such tests are similar to the familiar significance tests for individual parameters in a linear regression.
2. *Full and reduced model tests.* The best-fitting model should have the smallest value of the objective function [either $\text{WRSS}(\boldsymbol{\theta})$, $l(\boldsymbol{\theta})$, or $l_R(\boldsymbol{\theta})$]. The question is whether or not the difference in these criteria between two models is "significant." When the two candidate models are nested (i.e., one is a special case of the other obtained by putting one or more of the parameters equal to zero), formal tests can be made.

   Consider comparing two models of the same form, one based on parameters $\boldsymbol{\theta}_1$ and a larger model based on $\boldsymbol{\theta}_2$, with $\dim(\boldsymbol{\theta}_2) > \dim(\boldsymbol{\theta}_1)$ (i.e., $\boldsymbol{\theta}_1$ is obtained by setting some parameters in $\boldsymbol{\theta}_2$ equal to zero). With NLS, the test statistic for testing $H_0 : \gamma(h;\boldsymbol{\theta}) = \gamma(h;\boldsymbol{\theta}_1)$ vs. $H_1 : \gamma(h;\boldsymbol{\theta}) = \gamma(h;\boldsymbol{\theta}_2)$ is (Webster and McBratney 1989)

$$\frac{\text{WRSS}(\boldsymbol{\theta}_1) - \text{WRSS}(\boldsymbol{\theta}_2)}{\dim(\boldsymbol{\theta}_2) - \dim(\boldsymbol{\theta}_1)} \bigg/ \frac{\text{WRSS}(\boldsymbol{\theta}_2)}{K - \dim(\boldsymbol{\theta}_2)}, \tag{8.11}$$

   and the test is made by comparing this statistic to an F distribution with $(\dim(\boldsymbol{\theta}_2) - \dim(\boldsymbol{\theta}_1), K - \dim(\boldsymbol{\theta}_2))$ degrees of freedom. With REML, the comparable test is based on comparing

$$l_R(\boldsymbol{\theta}_2) - l_R(\boldsymbol{\theta}) \tag{8.12}$$

   to a χ^2 with $\dim(\boldsymbol{\theta}_2) - \dim(\boldsymbol{\theta}_1)$ degrees of freedom. [An analogous test can be done for ML using $l(\boldsymbol{\theta})$.] An important exception occurs when the parameters to be tested lie on the boundary of the parameter space. In such cases, the test statistic in equation (8.12) is a mixture of χ^2 distributions. Such boundary exceptions arise in practice when testing whether variance components (e.g., nugget and sill) are equal to zero. If we are testing only one of these variance components against 0, the test statistic has a distribution that is a 50:50 mixture of a degenerate χ^2 that places all mass at {0} and a

χ^2 with $\dim(\boldsymbol{\theta}_2) - \dim(\boldsymbol{\theta}_1)$ degrees of freedom (Self and Liang 1987; Littell et al. 1996). Thus, to make the test, simply divide by 2 the p-value obtained from a χ^2 with $\dim(\boldsymbol{\theta}_2) - \dim(\boldsymbol{\theta}_1)$ degrees of freedom.

3. *Penalized objective functions.* The tests described above should be used with caution. Wald tests can be unreliable with small samples and for variance components that have a skewed distribution. The full and reduced F-test is based on assumptions of independence and normality, assumptions not met by the empirical semivariogram. Moreover, when the models are not nested (e.g., we want to compare the fit of a spherical to that of an exponential), full and reduced tests are not applicable, even for likelihood-based methods. Thus, rather than relying on a statistical test, we should simply choose the model that has the smallest value for the objective function. Since the value of this function is reduced by increasing the number of parameters in the model, other criteria that penalize the objective functions for additional parameters have been developed. Akaike's information criterion (AIC) (Akaike 1974) is perhaps the most commonly used of these. This criterion was originally developed for likelihood methods and then adapted to regression fitting of semivariogram models by Webster and McBratney (1989):

$$\text{AIC}(\boldsymbol{\theta}) = K \log\left(\frac{\text{WRSS}(\boldsymbol{\theta})}{K}\right) + 2p \qquad \text{(NLS)} \qquad (8.13)$$

$$\text{AIC}(\boldsymbol{\theta}) = l_R(\boldsymbol{\theta}) + 2p, \qquad \text{(REML)} \qquad (8.14)$$

where p is the number of parameters in the model. We should prefer the model with the smallest AIC value.

Practical Notes on Model Fitting There are many different ways to parameterize each semivariogram model (particularly the exponential, Gaussian, and K-Bessel models), and different computer software programs may use slightly different forms. Also, some programs simply ask for or return "the range" and "the sill," which may or may not be one of the parameters of the model. It is a good idea to check the software manual or online help for the equation of each model to be sure of the exact form of the models you are using.

Good starting values are very important in iterative fitting methods. We recommend using a parameter search to determine good starting values, even if you feel your initial values are very close. If convergence is still a problem, using a different optimization approach (e.g., use of the Marquardt method in NLS or Fisher scoring in LB methods) may be helpful (Seber and Wild 1989). NLS can be affected adversely by a noisy semivariogram, so you may need to try a different lag spacing to define the structure of the semivariogram more clearly. LB methods are based on a covariance function, not on a semivariogram, and they do not calculate an empirical covariance function analogous to equation (8.8). They also use all the data to estimate the model parameters, whereas the empirical semivariogram is often estimated only for lags less than half the maximum separation distance. Thus, judging the model fits from LB approaches by superimposing the fitted model on the empirical semivariogram can be misleading.

Finally, remember that although the semivariogram is estimated from the data available, it is describing the variability *of a spatial process*. So even though a particular model is deemed best for a particular data set by a statistical comparison, it may not be the best choice. For example, the Gaussian model is often selected as best with automatic fitting criterion, but it also corresponds to a process that is often unrealistically smooth. Ultimately, the final choice of model should reflect both the results of the statistical model fitting procedure and an interpretation consistent with the scientific understanding of the process being studied.

DATA BREAK: Smoky Mountain pH Data (*cont.*) To continue our Smoky Mountain pH data break, consider fitting a theoretical semivariogram model to the empirical semivariogram shown in Figure 8.6. The semivariogram appears to reach a definite sill, but we do not have a lot of information about the shape of the semivariogram near the origin or the value of the nugget effect. In the absence of such information, a model that is approximately linear near the origin is a good choice since it does not assume that the process is too smooth. Thus either an exponential model or a spherical model might be a good choice. The

Table 8.1 Weighted Nonlinear Least Squares Fit of the Exponential Model to the Empirical Semivariogram in Figure 8.6[a]

Parameter	Estimate	Approximate Standard Error	Approximate 95% Confidence Limits
a_e	34.432	12.352	(6.909, 61.955)
c_e	0.191	0.025	(0.137, 0.246)
c_0	0.057	0.025	(0.002, 0.111)

$\text{WRSS}(\widehat{\boldsymbol{\theta}}) = 26.81$ with 10 degrees of freedom

[a]WRSS is the weighted residual sum of squares as discussed in the text.

Table 8.2 Weighted Nonlinear Least Squares Fit of the Spherical Model to the Empirical Semivariogram in Figure 8.6[a]

Parameter	Estimate	Approximate Standard Error	Approximate 95% Confidence Limits
a_s	110.312	31.939	(39.138, 181.521)
c_s	0.185	0.026	(0.126, 0.243)
c_0	0.084	0.016	(0.048, 0.121)

$\text{WRSS}(\widehat{\boldsymbol{\theta}}) = 29.28$ with 10 degrees of freedom

[a]WRSS is the weighted residual sum of squares as discussed in the text.

values of pH may have some measurement error associated with them, so we initially include a nugget effect in both models. The NLS fit statistics for the exponential model are shown in Table 8.1, and those for the spherical model are given in Table 8.2. (These results depend on the options used in the NLS fitting. We compared the results from three different software packages using their default options and obtained different results from each. Hence your results may differ from those presented here, but they should be close.) The fitted models are superimposed on the empirical semivariogram in Figures 8.7 and 8.8.

Since the models contain the same number of parameters, comparing AIC criteria computed from equations (8.13) is the same as comparing the weighted residual sums of squares [shown as $\text{WRSS}(\widehat{\boldsymbol{\theta}})$ in each table]. Since the fit to the exponential model has the smallest WRSS, this model fits the empirical semivariogram better than the spherical model.

We have several criteria to help us decide whether or not a nugget effect is needed. First, the Wald confidence limits do not contain zero, indicating that the nugget effect is significantly different from 0. Refitting the model without a nugget effect gives WRSS $= 36.89$, much higher than WRSS $= 26.81$ for the full model. The full and reduced F statistic is then $(36.89 - 26.81)/1/(26.81/10) = 3.76$ on (1,10) degrees of freedom, giving a corresponding p-value for the test of 0.08. Although this is not technically significant at 0.05, it is significant at 0.10 and provides some evidence against our null hypothesis of a zero nugget effect. Finally, a comparison of the AIC criteria gives AIC $= 15.41$ for the full model and AIC $= 17.56$ for the reduced model. Taken together, these statistics lead us to conclude that including a nugget effect probably results in a better-fitting model.

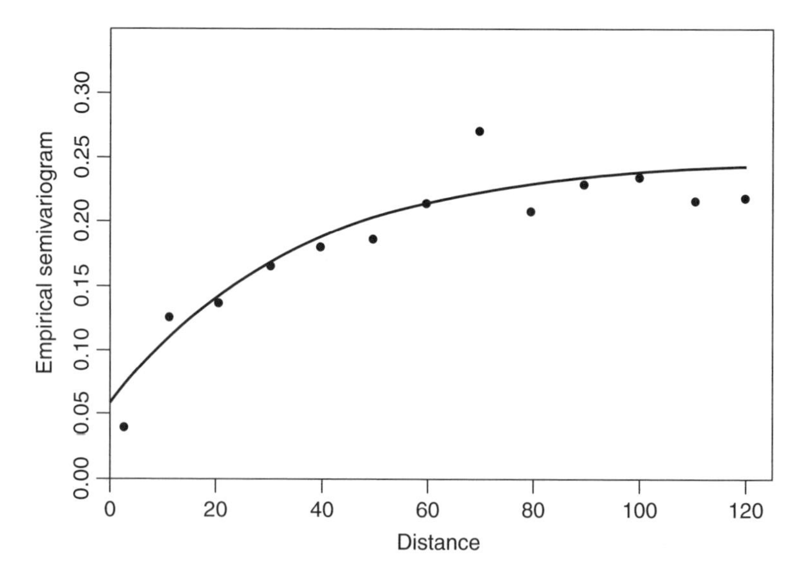

FIG. 8.7 Exponential model fit to the empirical semivariogram of pH values.

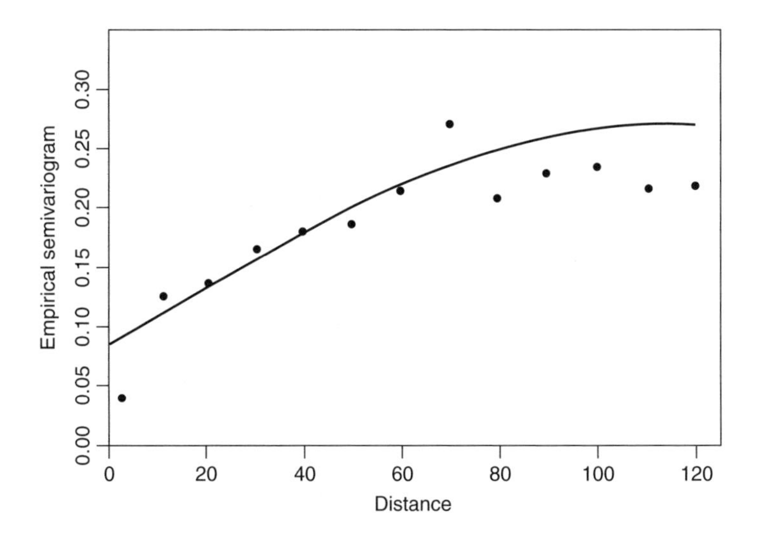

FIG. 8.8 Spherical model fit to empirical semivariogram of pH values.

8.2.5 Anisotropic Semivariogram Modeling

The nature of the semivariogram may change with direction. Then $\gamma(\boldsymbol{h})$ will be a function of both the magnitude and direction of the lag vector $\boldsymbol{h}$. Such spatial processes are referred to as *anisotropic*. Anisotropies result from the differential behavior of a physical process. For example, the pH of a stream may vary with the direction of stream flow. Although anisotropic processes are probably more common than isotropic ones, they receive less attention in the literature because they are more difficult mathematically and require more data for inference.

Since we must refer to direction as well as distance, we need a way to describe directions succinctly. The term *northwest* is too vague, and notation such as "N30°E" can be too cumbersome. In this book, we report directions as an angle, ϕ, measured in degrees counterclockwise from east. This allows the use of standard geometrical definitions.

Geometric Anisotropy Geometric anisotropy is a particular type of anisotropy characterized by two properties: (1) the directional semivariograms have the same shape and sill but different ranges; and (2) the semivariogram in direction ϕ has the maximum range of any direction, $a_{\max}$, and perpendicular to this direction, the semivariogram in direction $\phi \pm 90°$ has the minimum range of any direction, $a_{\min}$, and all the ranges delineate an ellipse with major and minor radii equal to $a_{\max}$ and $a_{\min}$, respectively. This is depicted graphically in Figure 8.9. To work with anisotropy we need to construct anisotropic semivariogram models that are conditionally negative definite. To do this, we adapt the isotropic semivariogram models described in Section 8.2.2 using elliptical geometry. Eriksson and Siska (2000) provide an excellent discussion of anisotropy, and our presentation draws greatly from their work.

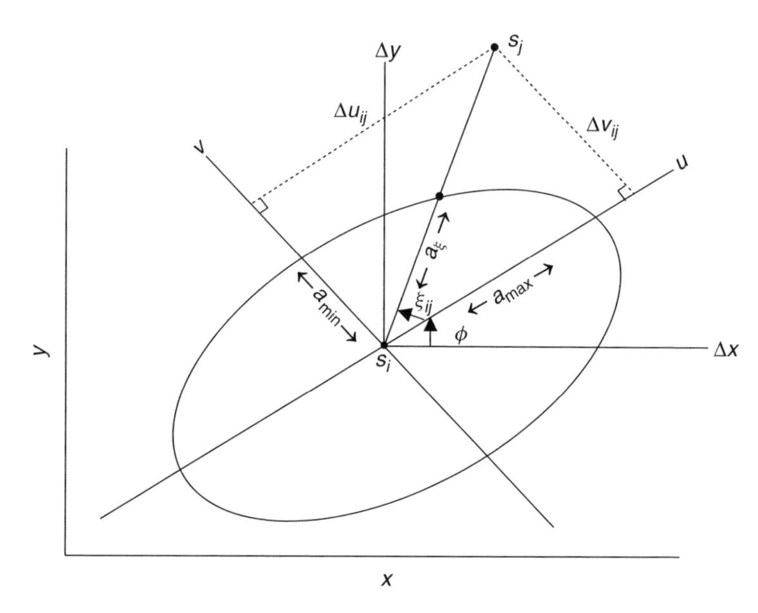

FIG. 8.9 Geometric anisotropy. The maximum range is in the direction ϕ. The points s_i and s_j are separated by a distance h_{ij} in the direction $\eta_{ij} = \xi_{ij} + \phi$. [Adapted from Eriksson and Siska (2000).]

Let u and v be the axes defined by the major and minor axes of the ellipse and convert these to rectangular coordinates:

$$u = a_\xi \cos \xi, \qquad v = a_\xi \sin \xi, \qquad \text{with } a_\xi = \sqrt{u^2 + v^2}.$$

Here ξ is the angle between the vector $\overrightarrow{s_i s_j}$ and the u-axis relative to the (u, v) coordinate system and a_ξ is the range (length) in the direction ξ. Then, substituting into the equation of an ellipse, $u^2/a_{\max}^2 + v^2/a_{\min}^2 = 1$, gives

$$\frac{a_\xi^2 \cos^2 \xi}{a_{\max}^2} + \frac{a_\xi^2 \sin^2 \xi}{a_{\min}^2} = 1.$$

So, relative to the u, v coordinate system, the range in direction ξ is

$$a_\xi = a_{\max} a_{\min} \Big/ \sqrt{a_{\min}^2 \cos^2 \xi + a_{\max}^2 \sin^2 \xi}\,. \tag{8.15}$$

With respect to the original x, y coordinate system, the vector $\overrightarrow{s_i s_j}$ makes an angle $\eta_{ij} = \xi_{ij} + \phi$ which, with respect to the u, v system, is the same as the angle $\xi_{ij} = \eta_{ij} - \phi$. Thus, the range in direction η_{ij} is

$$a_{\eta_{ij}} = a_{\max} a_{\min} \Big/ \sqrt{a_{\min}^2 \cos^2(\eta_{ij} - \phi) + a_{\max}^2 \sin^2(\eta_{ij} - \phi)}\,.$$

This now plays the role of the usual range parameter in an isotropic semivariogram model. For example, using a spherical model with unit sill and zero nugget effect, a geometric anisotropic model can be written as

$$\gamma(h, \eta; \boldsymbol{\theta}) = \begin{cases} 0 & \text{for } h = 0 \\ \frac{3}{2}\left(\frac{h\sqrt{a_{\min}^2 \cos^2(\eta - \phi) + a_{\max}^2 \sin^2(\eta - \phi)}}{a_{\max} a_{\min}}\right) & \\ -\frac{1}{2}\left(\frac{h\sqrt{a_{\min}^2 \cos^2(\eta - \phi) + a_{\max}^2 \sin^2(\eta - \phi)}}{a_{\max} a_{\min}}\right)^3 & \\ \quad \text{for } 0 \le h \le a_{\max} a_{\min} / \sqrt{a_{\min}^2 \cos^2(\eta - \phi) + a_{\max}^2 \sin^2(\eta - \phi)} & \\ 1 & \text{otherwise} \end{cases} \tag{8.16}$$

where $\boldsymbol{\theta} = (a_{\min}, a_{\max}, \phi)'$.

Unfortunately, few books or papers ever write anisotropic models in this form. Instead they usually describe a method of rotation and shrinkage and a "reduced distance" notation. The idea here is first to rotate the coordinate axes so they are aligned with the major and minor axes of the ellipse. Then shrink the axes so that the ellipse is now a circle with radius 1. This can be done using

$$\begin{aligned} \boldsymbol{h}' &= \begin{bmatrix} 1/a_{\max} & 0 \\ 0 & 1/a_{\min} \end{bmatrix} \begin{bmatrix} \cos\phi & \sin\phi \\ -\sin\phi & \cos\phi \end{bmatrix} \begin{bmatrix} \Delta x_{ij} \\ \Delta y_{ij} \end{bmatrix} \\ &\equiv \begin{bmatrix} 1/a_{\max} & 0 \\ 0 & 1/a_{\min} \end{bmatrix} \begin{bmatrix} \Delta u_{ij} \\ \Delta v_{ij} \end{bmatrix}, \end{aligned} \tag{8.17}$$

where Δu_{ij} and Δv_{ij} are distance components of $\boldsymbol{s}_i - \boldsymbol{s}_j$ in the u and v directions relative to the u and v axes, and Δx_{ij} and Δy_{ij} are the same distance components in the x and y directions relative to the x and y axes. After transformation, the ellipse is now a circle with radius 1, so isotropic semivariogram models can be used with the transformed distances. Continuing with our example of a spherical model without a nugget effect, the value of the anisotropic model in various directions is equal to the value of the isotropic semivariogram with range 1 using

$$||\boldsymbol{h}'|| = \sqrt{\frac{\Delta u_{ij}^2}{a_{\max}^2} + \frac{\Delta v_{ij}^2}{a_{\min}^2}}. \tag{8.18}$$

The quantity $||\boldsymbol{h}'||$ given in equation (8.18) is called the *reduced distance*. Then, the values of the anisotropic semivariogram model given in equation (8.16) are equal to

$$\mathrm{Sph}_1(||\boldsymbol{h}'||) = \begin{cases} 0, & ||\boldsymbol{h}'|| = 0 \\ (3/2)||\boldsymbol{h}'|| - (1/2)||\boldsymbol{h}'||^3, & 0 \leq ||\boldsymbol{h}'|| \leq 1 \\ 1, & \text{otherwise,} \end{cases} \tag{8.19}$$

where $\mathrm{Sph}_a(\cdot)$ denotes an isotropic spherical semivariogram model with zero nugget effect, unit sill, and range a (Isaaks and Srivastava 1989). In this formulation the dependence on direction is not obvious but is implicit in the reduced distance (each pair of points may have different distance components). A geometric argument for the use of the reduced distance can be found in Eriksson and Siska (2000).

Zonal Anisotropy The term *zonal anisotropy* refers to the case where the sill changes with direction but the range remains constant. This type of anisotropy is common with three-dimensional spatial processes, where the vertical direction (depth, height, or time) behaves differently from the two horizontal directions. To model zonal anisotropy, assume that in the direction ϕ, the sill is $c_{\max}$, the sill in the direction perpendicular to ϕ is $c_{\min}$, and denote the constant range by a. This type of anisotropy is usually modeled using the sum of two isotropic semivariogram models, referred to as *structures*. (Recall from Section 8.2 that the sum of two valid semivariograms is also a valid semivariogram.) The first structure is an isotropic model with sill $c_{\min}$ and range a. The second structure is a contrived geometric model with sill $c_{\max} - c_{\min}$. The range in the direction of maximum sill is taken to be the common range a and the range in the direction of minimum sill is set to a very large value so that this structure does not contribute to the overall model in the direction of minimum sill. For example, suppose that the maximum sill is 9 in the direction ϕ and that the smallest sill of 5 is observed in the perpendicular direction. Assume that a spherical model can be used to fit both directions and that the constant range is 100. Then the values for the zonal model can be computed from

$$5 \cdot \mathrm{Sph}_1(h/100) + 4 \cdot \mathrm{Sph}_1(||\boldsymbol{h}'||) \quad \text{with} \quad ||\boldsymbol{h}'|| = \sqrt{\frac{\Delta u_{ij}^2}{100} + \frac{\Delta v_{ij}^2}{100{,}000}}.$$

In the direction of minimum sill, the first component of the reduced distance used in the second structure is zero and the contribution of the second term is negligible because of the large range in this direction. Hence we obtain a spherical model with range 100 and a sill of 5. In the direction of maximum sill, both structures contribute to the computations, but the second component of the reduced distance used in the second structure is negligible. Thus, the values can be obtained using $5 \cdot \mathrm{Sph}_1(h/100) + 4 \cdot \mathrm{Sph}(h/100) = 9 \cdot \mathrm{Sph}(h/100)$.

Detecting Anisotropy There are two primary tools used to explore anisotropy. The first is a contour or image map of the empirical semivariogram surface. This map is constructed by partitioning the domain into cells of length Δx in the x direction and Δy in the y direction (so the "pixels" are rectangular tolerance regions). To calculate the empirical semivariogram for locations separated by $\mathbf{h} = (h_x, h_y)$, we average the pairs separated by $h_x \pm \Delta x$ in the x direction and by $h_y \pm \Delta y$ in the y direction. Then we draw a contour or image map depicting the empirical semivariogram as a function of the x and y distances. The center of the map corresponds to (0,0), with distances increasing in each direction from this central point. If the process is isotropic, no strong directional trends will be evident in the map and we should see circular contours. Elliptical contours indicate anisotropy and the direction of maximum range or sill will be indicated by a trough of low values connected in a particular direction. This type of map is a good visual tool for detecting anisotropy and suggesting plausible anisotropic models.

Contour plots can be difficult to use for modeling where we need more precise values for the nugget effect, ranges, and the sills. Directional empirical semivariograms are used to determine these. Directions of interest may be indicated by the contour map of the semivariogram surface, determined from scientific information, or investigated systematically going from 0° in increments of d°. Once a suite of directional semivariograms is estimated from the data, the first place to start is to see if the process exhibits geometric anisotropy. Fix a common nugget effect and sill and then record the range in each direction. It may be useful to plot the length of each range as a line in the direction of interest; this plot is called *a rose diagram* (Isaaks and Srivastava 1989). If geometric anisotropy is present, the diagram will resemble an ellipse and the quantities for constructing a model of geometric anisotropy can be read easily from this diagram. The same may be done to investigate zonal anisotropy by fixing the range and the nugget effect and plotting the sills.

When investigating anisotropy, patience, creativity, and flexibility are key. The ellipses are based on semivariograms estimated from the data, and perfectly defined ellipses are rare. Investigations of anisotropy split the data set, so directional semivariograms based on a much reduced sample size are consequently noisier. In many applications, there will not be enough data to investigate anisotropy adequately, and some compromises will have to made (e.g., consider only a few directions, use large angle tolerances, assume isotropy). The semivariogram surface could show several directions of anisotropy, and the directional semivariograms may indicate both zonal and geometric anisotropy. An irregular domain can make an isotropic process appear anisotropic. One of the advantages of interactive semivariogram modeling, such as that done by ESRI's Geostatistical Analyst (Johnston et al. 2001), is that it can show hypothetical fits of an anisotropic model to several directions simultaneously. When the anisotropy is complicated, it may be easier to consider a trend process model (see the data break following Section 9.1.2) since systematic large-scale trends in the data can manifest themselves as directional spatial autocorrelation. The difference between trend and anisotropy is subtle, and it can simply be one of interpretation and preference (Zimmerman 1993; Gotway and

Hergert 1997). Remember that all models are abstract approximations of reality; the goal is not *the* model, but *a good* model that is defensible, parsimonious, and reflects understanding of the spatial processes under study.

DATA BREAK: Smoky Mountain pH Data (*cont.*) In this portion of our data break, we investigate anisotropy in the pH data. First, consider the semivariogram surface displayed as an image map in Figure 8.10. This map was based on a lag spacing of 12 miles (with a tolerance of ±6 miles) in both the x and y directions. We initially chose a lag spacing of 10 miles based on the omnidirectional semivariogram (Figure 8.6), but this resulted in too few pairs for estimation in certain directions. After experimenting with several different choices for the lag spacing, including choices that allowed different spacings in the x and y directions, we decided that this lag spacing gave the best balance between reliable estimation and map detail. From Figure 8.10 we can see a trough of low values oriented at about 70°, indicating strong spatial continuity in this direction (i.e., low variance of pairwise differences for observations in the "trough").

To explore this pattern further, we estimated four directional semivariograms, starting with direction 70° and rotating counterclockwise 45°, using an angle tolerance of ±22.5°. We considered only four directions since, with only 75 data points, restricting semivariogram estimation to data within small sectors may result in poor estimates. Figure 8.11 indicates anisotropy, with the 70° direction showing the largest range and smallest sill and the 160° direction showing the smallest range and highest sill. Thus, there is evidence of anisotropy, but the type of anisotropy is not immediately apparent. Since the sill and range depend on each other, fixing one of these parameters allows us to vary the other. Since geometric anisotropy is the simplest type of anisotropy, we start by fixing a common nugget effect and sill

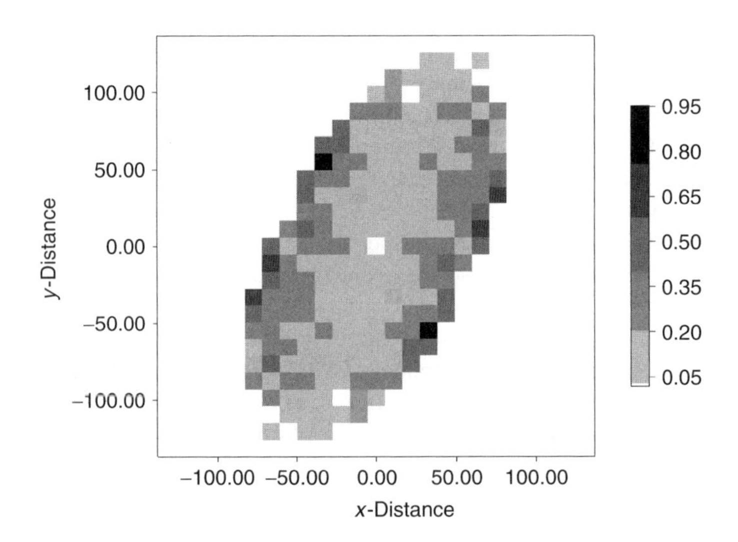

FIG. 8.10 Empirical semivariogram contour map for Smoky Mountain pH data.

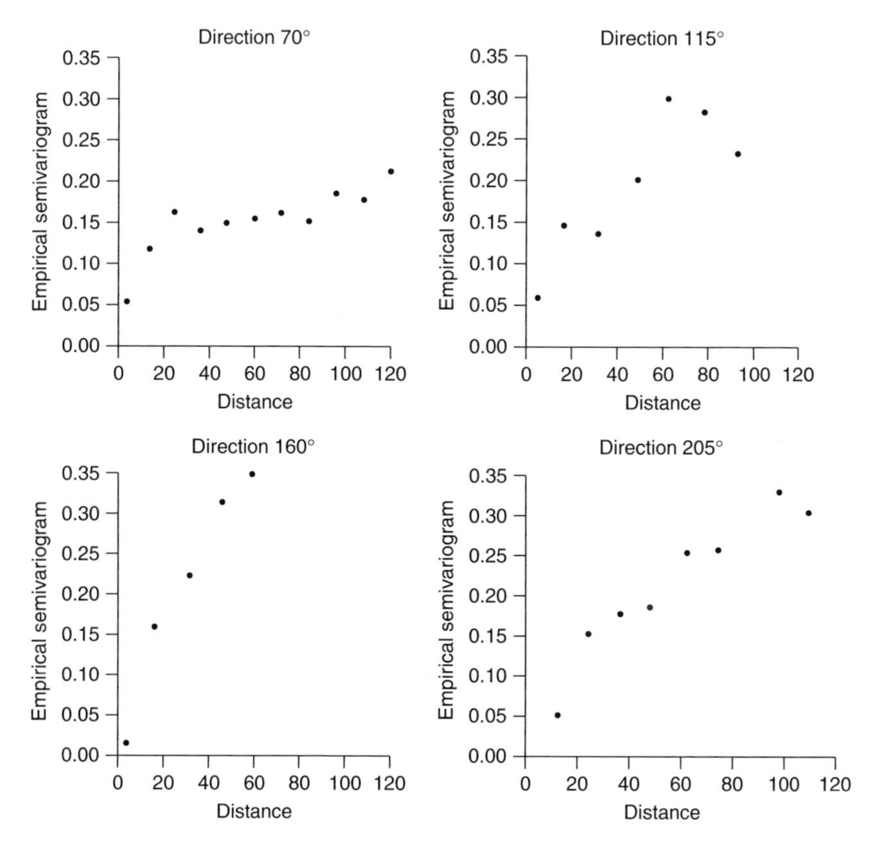

FIG. 8.11 Empirical directional semivariograms for Smoky Mountain pH data.

and then vary the ranges to see if a geometrically anisotropic model can adequately fit these empirical semivariograms. We initially chose a common nugget effect of 0 since the 160° direction does not show a nugget effect and WLS estimation will be easier without this extra parameter. Then, fixing $\phi = 70°$ and $c_0 = 0$, we used the estimates from all four directions to fit an exponential model with range given in equation (8.15) using WLS. This gave $\hat{c}_e = 0.2725$, $\hat{a}_{\max} = 36.25$, and $\hat{a}_{\min} = 16.93$, and the resulting fits are shown in Figure 8.12. Considering that we have only 75 data points, the overall fit seems adequate, although the fit to the 70° direction could be improved by including a nugget effect, but only at the expense of the fit in the 160° direction. Although we did have evidence of anisotropy, the fit of the isotropic model from Table 8.1 to these directions seems almost equally adequate. The isotropic model fit seems better in the 70° and 115° directions, but worse in the 160° and 205° directions. However, the isotropic model is a much simpler model. To help decide if a geometrically anisotropic model is better, we can compare the AIC criteria from fitting this model to that obtained by refitting an isotropic model to the directional semivariograms. This gives AIC = 67.95 for the

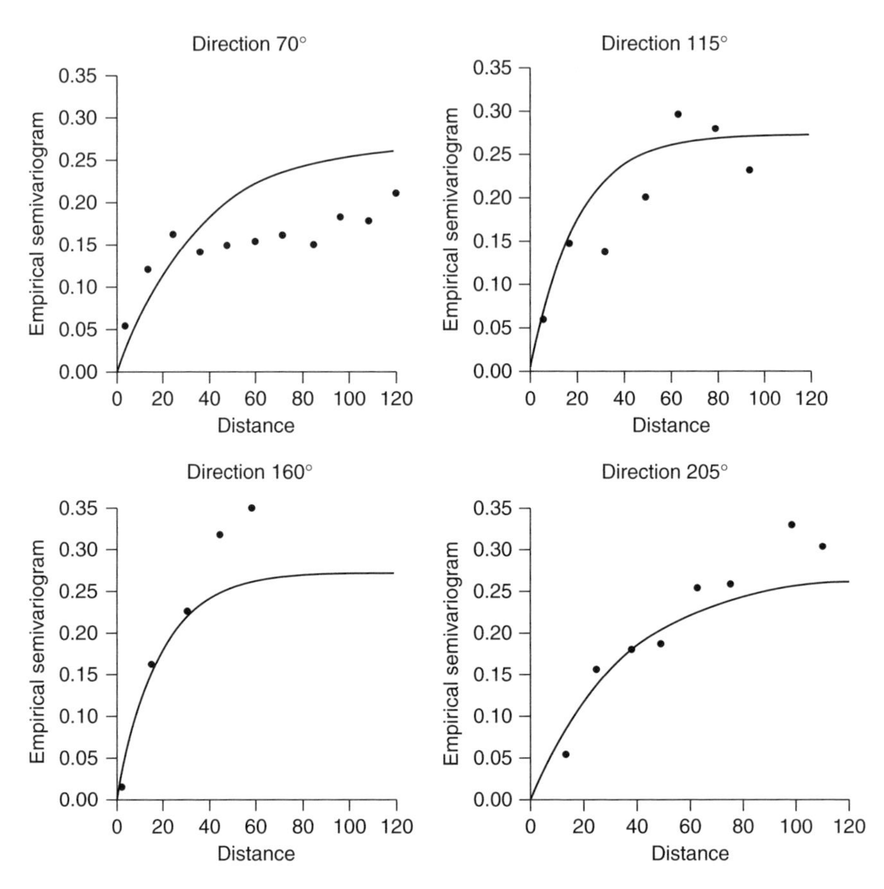

FIG. 8.12 Empirical directional semivariograms and fitted models for Smoky Mountain pH data. The solid curve is the fit of the geometric anisotropic model, and the dashed curve shows the fit of the isotropic model.

geometrically anisotropic model and AIC = 72.99 for the isotropic model. Even if we further penalize the geometrically anisotropic model for estimation of ϕ, it appears that this model gives a slightly better fit than the isotropic model. Knowledge of stream flow or other stream parameters affecting pH would also be helpful in deciding between the two models.

In this analysis we assumed that the pH process was anisotropic and estimated the direction of maximum continuity (range for geometric anisotropy and sill for zonal anisotropy) "by eye" using the empirical semivariogram surface in Figure 8.10. Instead of considering just four directions defined by nonoverlapping sectors, we could have estimated empirical semivariograms every 20° (or so) using an angle tolerance of 22.5° or even 45°, allowing the binning sectors to overlap. This would have allowed us to construct a rose diagram of the ranges in each direction and permitted a more refined estimate of the direction of maximum range, although the notion of "different directions" in the case of overlapping sectors and large angle tolerances is rather vague. More precise and objective (e.g., WLS) estimation of this direction requires many empirical directional semivariograms (i.e., measured every 10° to 20°) computed with a small angle tolerance. We usually do not have enough data to do this, and some compromise between many blurred directions and a few more precise ones must be made. This compromise must also balance precision and accuracy against the time and effort involved; obtaining good estimates of many directional semivariograms can be a tedious chore. One such compromise, based on smoothing of the semivariogram surface, is implemented with ESRI's Geostatistical Analyst (Johnston et al. 2001). A kernel smoother, similar to those described in Chapter 5, is used to smooth the semivariogram values in each cell of the semivariogram surface, borrowing strength from values in neighboring cells. Locations are weighted based on their distance from the center of each cell. A modified weighted least squares algorithm, implemented in stages, can then be used to fit an anisotropic model to the smoothed surface. Using this approach with the pH data, we obtained WLS estimates $\hat{\phi} = 69.6^\circ$, $\hat{c}_0 = 0.0325$, $\hat{c}_e = 0.2015$, $\hat{a}_{\max} = 44.9$, and $\hat{a}_{\min} = 16.65$. These values, computed from the empirical semivariogram surface, are subject to errors induced by the rectangular binning and the smoothing, but are obtained quickly and objectively (and the fit is not all that different from that obtained previously with much greater effort).

8.3 INTERPOLATION AND SPATIAL PREDICTION

In exposure assessment, we may want to predict exposure at a location where we have not recorded an observation, say at location s_0. *Interpolation* is the process of obtaining a value for a variable of interest [denoted here as $Z(s_0)$] at an unsampled location based on surrounding measurements. An example of the interpolation problem is given in Figure 8.13. Here five data values are recorded at locations s_1, s_2, s_3, s_4, and s_5, and we would like to predict the value at s_0 from these observations.

It is often useful to have a map of the spatial variation in exposure. *Gridding* refers to the systematic interpolation of many values identified by the nodes of a regular grid. These interpolated values are then displayed graphically, usually by means of a contour or surface map.

There are many methods for interpolating spatial data. These fall into two broad classes: deterministic and probabilistic. Deterministic methods have a mathematical development based on assumptions about the functional form of the interpolator. Probabilistic methods have a foundation in statistical theory and assume a statistical model for the data. When probabilistic methods are used for interpolation, they are referred to as methods for *spatial prediction*. These predictors have standard errors that quantify the uncertainty associated with the interpolated values. Deterministic interpolators do not have a measure of uncertainty associated with them. Sometimes, interpolation methods can be developed from both points of view (as with least squares regression, for example). We discuss two of the most commonly used methods: inverse distance interpolation (deterministic) and kriging (probabilistic).

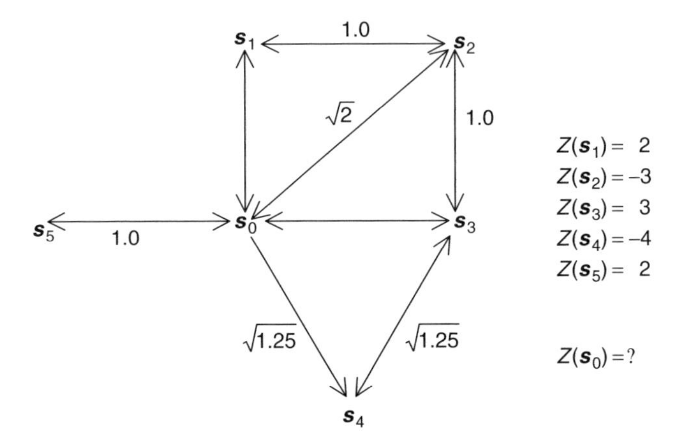

FIG. 8.13 The interpolation problem. The numbers next to each line are distances.

Cressie (1989) gives a comparative overview of many other interpolation methods not described here.

8.3.1 Inverse-Distance Interpolation

An inverse-distance interpolator is simply a weighted average of neighboring values. The weight given to each observation is a function of the distance between that observation's location and the grid point s_0 at which interpolation is desired. Mathematically, the general inverse-distance interpolator is written as

$$\hat{Z}_{\mathrm{ID}p} = \sum_{i=1}^{N} Z(s_i)\, d_{0,i}^{-p} \Bigg/ \sum_{i=1}^{N} d_{0,i}^{-p} . \tag{8.20}$$

Here $d_{0,i}$ is the distance from the grid point location s_0 to the ith data location s_i. The weighting power, p, is selected to control how fast the weights tend to zero as the distance from the grid node increases, based on assumed increasing similarity between observations taken closer together. As the power increases, the contribution (to the interpolated value) from data points far from the grid node decreases. Distance powers between 1 and 3 are typically chosen, and taking $p = 2$ gives the popular inverse-distance-squared interpolator. [See Burrough (1986) for a general discussion and illustration of these interpolators.]

As an example, consider the spatial layout in Figure 8.13. Intuitively, a good guess for the value at s_0 is 0, the average of these values. But in inverse-distance interpolation, the values at s_2 and s_4 will receive lower weight since they are farther away. Applying equation (8.20) with $p = 2$, we see that $\hat{Z}(s_0)_{\mathrm{ID}2} = 0.53$.

Most interpolation methods use only some of the "neighboring" data. The neighborhood is usually taken to be a circle centered on the grid node unless the study domain is elongated (e.g., elliptical) or the spatial process is anisotropic. If there are many points in the neighborhood, we may further restrict the calculations and use just the closest m points. (In many computer programs, defaults for m vary from 6 to 24.) These parameters (search neighborhood size, shape, and number of points used for interpolation), together with the choice of the weighting power, can affect the nature of the interpolated surface. Higher weighting powers and small search neighborhoods with few data points retained for interpolation produce very localized, choppy surfaces; lower powers of distance and large neighborhoods with many data points used for interpolation result in smoother surfaces. This idea is similar to the role of bandwidth in kernel density estimators of spatial intensity functions discussed in Section 5.2.5. Care must be taken to ensure that the interpolated values are based on enough data so that the averaging gives a fairly accurate value, particularly for grid nodes near the edges of the domain.

Inverse-distance interpolators are popular in many disciplines since they are relatively simple conceptually, require no modeling or parameter estimation, and are computationally fast. They can be exact interpolators (i.e., the interpolated surface passes through the original observations), or smoothers (i.e., predictions at observed locations are adjusted toward their neighborhood mean). However, mapped surfaces tend to have flat-topped peaks and flat-bottomed valleys giving a characteristic bull's-eye pattern produced by concentric contours around data points that can detract from the visual interpretation of the map. Also, since there is no underlying statistical model, there is no easy measure of the uncertainty associated with the value interpolated.

8.3.2 Kriging

Kriging is a geostatistical technique for optimal spatial *prediction*. We emphasize the distinction between *prediction,* which is inference on *random* quantities, and *estimation,* which is inference on *fixed but unknown* parameters. Georges Matheron, considered by many to be the founding father of geostatistics, introduced this term in one of his early works developing geostatistical theory (Matheron 1963). A Soviet scientist, L. S. Gandin, simultaneously developed the same theory in meteorology, where it is known by the name *objective analysis* (Gandin 1963). Since these beginnings, the original development of kriging has been extended in many ways. There are now many different types of kriging, differing by underlying assumptions and analytical goals. The following represents a partial list of the different types of kriging appearing in the literature, along with a brief definition:

- *Simple kriging:* linear prediction (i.e., predictor is a linear combination of observed data values) assuming a known mean
- *Ordinary kriging:* linear prediction with an constant unknown mean
- *Universal kriging:* linear prediction with a nonstationary mean structure
- *Filtered kriging:* smoothing and prediction for noisy data; also known as kriging with measurement error
- *Lognormal kriging:* optimal spatial prediction based on the lognormal distribution

- *Trans-Gaussian kriging:* spatial prediction based on transformations of the data
- *Cokriging:* multivariate linear prediction (i.e., linear prediction based on one or more interrelated spatial processes)
- *Indicator kriging:* probability mapping using indicator functions (binary data)
- *Probability kriging:* probability mapping based on both indicator functions of the data and the original data
- *Disjunctive kriging:* nonlinear prediction based on univariate functions of the data
- *Bayesian kriging:* incorporates prior information about the mean and/or covariance functions into spatial prediction
- *Block kriging:* optimal linear prediction of areal data from point data

This list is not exhaustive, and many combinations of these are possible (e.g., universal cokriging is multivariate spatial prediction with a nonstationary mean structure).

A comprehensive discussion of all of these methods is beyond the scope of this book. Instead, our discussion focuses on a few of these methods, written to balance completeness, theoretical development, and practical implementation. Our choice was indeed a struggle. Our readers are encouraged to consult other books (e.g., Journel and Huijbregts 1978; Isaaks and Srivastava 1989; Cressie 1993; Rivoirard 1994; Wackernagel 1995; Chilès and Delfiner 1999; Olea 1999; Stein 1999) to learn more about the methods and theoretical considerations we cannot discuss here.

Ordinary Kriging Assume that $Z(\cdot)$ is intrinsically stationary [i.e., has a constant unknown mean, μ, and known semivariogram, $\gamma(\boldsymbol{h})$]. Assume that we have data $\mathbf{Z} = [Z(\boldsymbol{s}_1), \ldots, Z(\boldsymbol{s}_N)]'$ and want to predict the value of the $Z(\cdot)$ process at an unobserved location, $Z(\boldsymbol{s}_0)$, $\boldsymbol{s}_0 \in D$. As with the inverse distance methods described in Section 8.3.1, the ordinary kriging (OK) predictor is a weighted average of the data:

$$\hat{Z}_{\mathrm{OK}}(\boldsymbol{s}_0) = \sum_{i=1}^{N} \lambda_i Z(\boldsymbol{s}_i). \tag{8.21}$$

However, instead of specifying an arbitrary function of distance, we determine the weights based on the data using the semivariogram and two statistical optimality criteria: unbiasedness and minimum mean-squared prediction error. For unbiasedness, the predicted value should, on average, coincide with the value of the unknown random variable, $Z(\boldsymbol{s}_0)$. In statistical terms, unbiasedness requires $E[\hat{Z}_{\mathrm{OK}}(\boldsymbol{s}_0)] = \mu = E[Z(\boldsymbol{s}_0)]$, which means that $\sum_{i=1}^{N} \lambda_i = 1$. To ensure the second optimality criterion, we need to minimize *mean-squared prediction error* (MSPE), defined as $E[\hat{Z}_{\mathrm{OK}}(\boldsymbol{s}_0) - Z(\boldsymbol{s}_0)]^2$, subject to the unbiasedness constraint. One method for solving constrained optimization problems is the method of *Lagrange multipliers*.

With this method, we need to find $\lambda_1, \ldots, \lambda_N$ and a Lagrange multiplier, m, that minimize the objective function

$$E\left[\left(\sum_{i=1}^{N} \lambda_i Z(\boldsymbol{s}_i) - Z(\boldsymbol{s}_0)\right)^2\right] - 2m\left(\sum_{i=1}^{N} \lambda_i - 1\right). \tag{8.22}$$

The second term is essentially a penalty, minimized when $\sum_{i=1}^{N} \lambda_i = 1$, thus ensuring that our overall minimization incorporates our unbiasedness constraint. Now $\sum_{i=1}^{N} \lambda_i = 1$ implies that

$$\left[\sum_{i=1}^{N} \lambda_i Z(\boldsymbol{s}_i) - Z(\boldsymbol{s}_0)\right]^2 = -\frac{1}{2}\sum_{i=1}^{N}\sum_{j=1}^{N} \lambda_i\lambda_j \left[Z(\boldsymbol{s}_i) - Z(\boldsymbol{s}_j)\right]^2 + \sum_{i=1}^{N} \lambda_i \left[Z(\boldsymbol{s}_0) - Z(\boldsymbol{s}_i)\right]^2.$$

Taking expectations of both sides of this equation gives

$$E\left[\left(\sum_{i=1}^{N} \lambda_i Z(\boldsymbol{s}_i) - Z(\boldsymbol{s}_0)\right)^2\right] = -\frac{1}{2}\sum_{i=1}^{N}\sum_{j=1}^{N} \lambda_i\lambda_j E\left[\left(Z(\boldsymbol{s}_i) - Z(\boldsymbol{s}_j)\right)^2\right] + \sum_{i=1}^{N} \lambda_i E\left[(Z(\boldsymbol{s}_0) - Z(\boldsymbol{s}_i))^2\right],$$

so that the objective function given in equation (8.22) becomes

$$-\sum_{i=1}^{N}\sum_{j=1}^{N} \lambda_i\lambda_j \gamma(\boldsymbol{s}_i - \boldsymbol{s}_j) + 2\sum_{i=1}^{N} \lambda_i \gamma(\boldsymbol{s}_0 - \boldsymbol{s}_i) - 2m\left(\sum_{i=1}^{N} \lambda_i - 1\right). \tag{8.23}$$

To minimize (8.23), we differentiate with respect to $\lambda_1, \ldots, \lambda_N$, and m in turn and set the partial derivatives equal to zero. This gives a system of equations, referred to as the *ordinary kriging equations*,

$$\sum_{j=1}^{N} \lambda_j \gamma(\boldsymbol{s}_i - \boldsymbol{s}_j) + m = \gamma(\boldsymbol{s}_0 - \boldsymbol{s}_i), \qquad i = 1, \ldots, N$$

$$\sum_{i=1}^{N} \lambda_i = 1. \tag{8.24}$$

We solve these equations for $\lambda_1, \ldots, \lambda_N$ (and m), and use the resulting optimal weights in equation (8.21) to give the ordinary kriging predictor. Note that $\hat{Z}(\boldsymbol{s}_0)$

has weights that depend on both the spatial correlations between $Z(s_0)$ and each data point $Z(s_i)$, $i = 1, \ldots, N$, and the spatial correlations between all pairs of data points $Z(s_i)$ and $Z(s_j)$, $i = 1, \ldots, N$, $j = 1, \ldots, N$.

It is often more convenient to write the system of equations in (8.24) in matrix form as

$$\boldsymbol{\lambda}_O = \boldsymbol{\Gamma}_O^{-1} \boldsymbol{\gamma}_O \tag{8.25}$$

where

$$\boldsymbol{\lambda}_O = (\lambda_1, \ldots, \lambda_N, m)'$$
$$\boldsymbol{\gamma}_O = [\gamma(s_0 - s_1), \ldots, \gamma(s_0 - s_N), 1]'$$

and the elements of Γ_O are

$$\Gamma_{O_{ij}} = \begin{cases} \gamma(s_i - s_j), & i = 1, \ldots, N \\ & j = 1, \ldots, N \\ 1, & i = N+1; j = 1, \ldots, N \\ & j = N+1; i = 1, \ldots, N \\ 0, & i = j = N+1. \end{cases}$$

So (8.25) becomes

$$\begin{bmatrix} \lambda_1 \\ \lambda_2 \\ \vdots \\ \lambda_N \\ m \end{bmatrix} = \begin{bmatrix} \gamma(s_1 - s_1) & \cdots & \gamma(s_1 - s_N) & 1 \\ \gamma(s_2 - s_1) & \cdots & \gamma(s_2 - s_N) & 1 \\ \vdots & \ddots & \vdots & \vdots \\ \gamma(s_N - s_1) & \cdots & \gamma(s_N - s_N) & 1 \\ 1 & \cdots & 1 & 0 \end{bmatrix}^{-1} \begin{bmatrix} \gamma(s_0 - s_1) \\ \gamma(s_0 - s_2) \\ \vdots \\ \gamma(s_0 - s_N) \\ 1 \end{bmatrix}.$$

Note that we must calculate $\boldsymbol{\lambda}_O$ for each prediction location, s_0. However, only the right-hand side of equation (8.25) changes with the prediction locations (through $\boldsymbol{\gamma}_O$). Since Γ_O depends only on the data locations and not on the prediction locations, we need only invert Γ_O once and then multiply by the associated $\boldsymbol{\gamma}_O$ vector to obtain a prediction for any s_0 in D.

The minimized MSPE, also known as the *kriging variance*, is

$$\begin{aligned} \sigma_k^2(s_0) &= \boldsymbol{\lambda}_O' \boldsymbol{\gamma}_O \\ &= \sum_{i=1}^{N} \lambda_i \gamma(s_0 - s_i) + m \\ &= 2\sum_{i=1}^{N} \lambda_i \gamma(s_0 - s_i) - \sum_{i=1}^{N} \sum_{j=1}^{N} \lambda_i \lambda_j \gamma(s_i - s_j), \end{aligned} \tag{8.26}$$

and the kriging standard error, $\sigma_k(\mathbf{s}_0)$, is a measure of the uncertainty in the prediction of $Z(\mathbf{s}_0)$. If we assume the prediction errors, $\hat{Z}(\mathbf{s}_0) - Z(\mathbf{s}_0)$, follow a Gaussian distribution, then a 95% prediction interval for $Z(\mathbf{s}_0)$ is

$$(\widehat{Z}(\mathbf{s}_0) \pm 1.96\sigma_k(\mathbf{s}_0)).$$

As an example, consider the spatial configuration shown in Figure 8.13. For illustration, assume a spherical semivariogram with $c_0 = 0, c_s = 1$, and $a = 1.5$. Then the ordinary kriging equations are

$$\begin{bmatrix} \lambda_1 \\ \lambda_2 \\ \vdots \\ \lambda_5 \\ m \end{bmatrix} = \begin{bmatrix} 0 & 0.852 & 0.995 & 1.00 & 0.995 & 1 \\ 0.852 & 0 & 0.852 & 1.00 & 1.00 & 1 \\ 0.995 & 0.852 & 0 & 0.911 & 1.00 & 1 \\ 1.00 & 1.00 & 0.911 & 0 & 1.00 & 1 \\ 0.995 & 1.00 & 1.00 & 1.00 & 0 & 1 \\ 1 & 1 & 1 & 1 & 1 & 0 \end{bmatrix}^{-1} \begin{bmatrix} 0.852 \\ 0.995 \\ 0.852 \\ 0.911 \\ 0.852 \\ 1 \end{bmatrix},$$

and the ordinary kriging predictor of $Z(\mathbf{s}_0)$ is $\hat{Z}_{\text{OK}}(\mathbf{s}_0) = 0.88$. Note that this is slightly larger than $\widehat{Z}(\mathbf{s}_0)_{\text{ID2}} = 0.53$, because $Z(\mathbf{s}_2) = -3$ is given smaller with kriging than it is with inverse-distance-squared interpolation. The 95% prediction interval for $Z(\mathbf{s}_0)$ is $(-1.07, 2.83)$.

The ordinary kriging predictor has the smallest mean-squared prediction error in the class of all linear unbiased predictors. Consequently, it is often referred to as the BLUP (best linear unbiased predictor). In practice, OK is also called the EBLUP ("E" for empirical) since the unknown semivariogram is estimated and modeled parametrically, as described in Sections 8.2.3 and 8.2.4. The resulting empirical semivariogram model then provides the values of $\gamma(\mathbf{s}_i - \mathbf{s}_j)$ and $\gamma(\mathbf{s}_0 - \mathbf{s}_j)$ needed to solve the ordinary kriging equations [equations (8.24)]. The ordinary kriging predictor is always the BLUP, regardless of the underlying statistical distribution of the data (i.e., the data need not be Gaussian to use OK). Prediction intervals are also valid for non-Gaussian data, although we do have to assume that the prediction *errors* are Gaussian to construct such intervals. However, OK may not always be the best predictor. In statistical prediction theory, the best predictor of $Z(\mathbf{s}_0)$ given the data is always $E[Z(\mathbf{s}_0)|Z(\mathbf{s}_1), \ldots, Z(\mathbf{s}_N)]$. For Gaussian data, this conditional expectation is a linear function of the data and is equivalent to simple kriging (kriging with a known mean). When the mean is unknown and the data are Gaussian, ordinary kriging serves as a very good approximation to this best linear predictor. However, when the data are not Gaussian, $E[Z(\mathbf{s}_0)|Z(\mathbf{s}_1), \ldots, Z(\mathbf{s}_N)]$ may not be linear, and ordinary kriging, being a linear predictor, may not provide the best approximation to this conditional mean.

As with the inverse distance methods described in Section 8.3.1, kriging is usually done locally using search neighborhoods. In fact, when kriging any particular point, there is usually no need to use data outside the range of the semivariogram because these data will have negligible weights. The use of local search neighborhoods can result in great computational savings when working with large data sets. However, the search neighborhood should be selected with care, as it will affect the characteristics of the kriged surface. Global kriging using all the data produces a relatively smooth surface. Small search neighborhoods with few data points for prediction will produce surfaces that show more detail, but this detail may be misleading if predictions are unstable. In general, try to use at least 7–12 points for each value predicted; kriging with more than 25 points is usually unnecessary. If the data are sparse or the relative nugget effect is large, distant points may have important information and the search neighborhood should be increased to include them. When the data are evenly distributed within the domain, a simple search that defines the neighborhood by the closest points is usually adequate. However, when observations are clustered, very irregularly spaced, or located on widely spaced transects, *quadrant* or *octant searches* can be useful. Here, one divides the neighborhood around each target node into quadrants or octants and uses the nearest two or three points from each quadrant or octant in the interpolation. This ensures that neighbors from several different directions, not just the closest points, will be used for prediction. It is also possible to change the search strategy node by node. It is always a good idea to experiment with several different neighborhoods and to check the results of each prediction to be sure of the calculations.

Filtered Kriging Ordinary kriging is an *exact interpolator* that *honors the data* [i.e., the kriging surface *must* pass through all data points so that $\hat{Z}(\boldsymbol{s}_i) = Z(\boldsymbol{s}_i)$ whenever a data value is observed at location $\boldsymbol{s}_i$]. However, when the data are measured with error, it would be better to predict a less noisy or filtered version of the data instead of forcing the kriged surface to honor the errors. Suppose that we can write

$$Z(\boldsymbol{s}) = S(\boldsymbol{s}) + \epsilon(\boldsymbol{s}), \quad \boldsymbol{s} \in D,$$

where $S(\cdot)$ is the true, noiseless version of the process we are studying and $\epsilon(\boldsymbol{s})$ is a measurement error process. $S(\cdot)$ need not be a smooth process; it may also exhibit small-scale or nugget variation. Cressie (1993) gives a more general model that distinguishes between several sources of variation (measurement error variation and small-scale or nugget variation being just two of these). We have adapted his development for our discussion here. We assume that $S(\cdot)$ is intrinsically stationary and that $\epsilon(\boldsymbol{s})$ is a zero-mean white noise (i.e., without spatial correlation) process, independent of $S(\cdot)$, with $\text{Var}(\epsilon(\cdot)) = \sigma^2_{\text{ME}}$. Repeated measurements at the same location allow an estimate of σ^2_{ME}. When the measurements are recorded by a laboratory instrument (e.g., chemical concentrations), the precision of the instrument may be known from validation studies and can be used to estimate σ^2_{ME} when replicates are not available. Note that $\gamma_Z(\boldsymbol{h}) = \gamma_S(\boldsymbol{h}) + \gamma_\epsilon(\boldsymbol{h})$ with $\gamma_\epsilon(\boldsymbol{h}) = \sigma^2_{\text{ME}}$ for $||\boldsymbol{h}|| > 0$ and $\gamma_\epsilon(\boldsymbol{h}) = 0$ otherwise.

The ordinary kriging predictor of $S(\boldsymbol{s}_0)$ is derived in a manner analogous to that given above. This predictor is

$$\widehat{S}(\boldsymbol{s}_0) = \sum_{i=1}^{N} \nu_i Z(\boldsymbol{s}_i),$$

with optimal weights satisfying

$$\boldsymbol{\Gamma}_O \boldsymbol{\nu}_O = \boldsymbol{\gamma}^*_O. \tag{8.27}$$

The matrix $\boldsymbol{\Gamma}_O$ is the same as in the ordinary kriging equations (8.25), with elements $\gamma_Z(\boldsymbol{s}_i - \boldsymbol{s}_j)$. The matrix $\boldsymbol{\gamma}^*_O = [\gamma^*(\boldsymbol{s}_0 - \boldsymbol{s}_1), \ldots, \gamma^*(\boldsymbol{s}_0 - \boldsymbol{s}_N), 1]'$ is slightly different since, in the minimization, the elements of this matrix are derived from $E[(Z(\boldsymbol{s}_0) - Z(\boldsymbol{s}_i))^2] = \gamma_S(\boldsymbol{s}_0 - \boldsymbol{s}_i) + \sigma^2_{\text{ME}} \equiv \gamma^*(\boldsymbol{s}_0 - \boldsymbol{s}_i)$. At prediction locations, $\boldsymbol{s}_0 \neq \boldsymbol{s}_i$, and $\gamma^*(\boldsymbol{s}_0 - \boldsymbol{s}_i) = \gamma_Z(\boldsymbol{s}_0 - \boldsymbol{s}_i)$, $i = 1, \ldots, N$. At data locations, $\boldsymbol{s}_0 = \boldsymbol{s}_i$, and $\gamma^*(\boldsymbol{s}_0 - \boldsymbol{s}_i) = \sigma^2_{\text{ME}} (\neq 0)$. Thus, this predictor "smooths" the data, and larger values of σ^2_{ME} result in more smoothing.

The minimized MSPE is given by

$$\tau^2_k(\boldsymbol{s}_0) = \sum_{i=1}^{N} \nu_i \gamma^*(\boldsymbol{s}_0 - \boldsymbol{s}_i) + m - \sigma^2_{\text{ME}}.$$

Note that this is not equal to the ordinary kriging variance, $\sigma^2_k(\boldsymbol{s}_0)$, defined in equation (8.26), unless $\sigma^2_{\text{ME}} = 0$. Prediction standard errors associated with filtered kriging are smaller than those associated with ordinary kriging (except at data locations) since $S(\cdot)$ is less variable than $Z(\cdot)$.

Software programs sometimes implement filtered kriging by putting σ^2_{ME} on the diagonal of $\boldsymbol{\Gamma}_O$ [i.e., by replacing $\gamma_Z(\boldsymbol{0}) = 0$ with σ^2_{ME}]. This gives an incorrect set of kriging equations since, by definition, the semivariogram is always 0 at the origin. The quantity $\boldsymbol{\gamma}^*(\boldsymbol{h})$ results from the minimization and is really a cross-semivariogram between $Z(\boldsymbol{s}_i)$ and $S(\boldsymbol{s}_0)$ and not the semivariogram of either $Z(\cdot)$ or $S(\cdot)$.

DATA BREAK: Smoky Mountain pH Data (*cont.*) We now use the semivariogram models developed for the Smoky Mountain pH data (beginning at the end of section 8.2) in ordinary kriging to predict the pH value anywhere in the study area. We make a map of predicted stream pH by predicting several values on a regular grid of points within the domain of interest and then drawing a contour plot. To specify the grid, we must choose the starting and ending points of the grid in both directions and the grid spacing. A general guideline is to choose about 50 grid points in the x direction and use the resulting grid spacing in this direction to specify the grid in the y direction. These specifications can then be adjusted based on the domain dimensions and the spacing of the data points in both directions. For the stream pH data, we used this guideline, taking the minimum and maximum values of easting and northing to define the beginning and ending points of the grid, and using a grid spacing of 3 miles in each direction. Since it is easier to specify the grid as a rectangle, we will make predictions on this rectangular grid and then trim them to a polygon containing the data points.

We use ordinary kriging, filtered kriging, and inverse-distance-squared interpolation to predict pH values at the grid locations. For ordinary kriging, we use the geometrically anisotropic semivariogram model developed earlier: exponential with $\phi = 70^\circ$, $\hat{a}_{\max} = 36.25$, $\hat{a}_{\min} = 16.93$, $\hat{c}_e = 0.2725$, and $c_0 = 0$. For filtered kriging, we assume a nugget effect of $\hat{c_0} = 0.0325$ as indicated by Geostatistical Analyst and assume that this nugget effect is due entirely to measurement error in the pH values. We use the same semivariogram as with ordinary kriging but adapt it to include this nugget effect: exponential with $\phi = 70^\circ$, $\hat{a}_{\max} = 36.25$, $\hat{a}_{\min} = 16.93$, $\hat{c}_e = 0.2400$, and $\hat{c_0} = 0.0325$. The search neighborhood for all approaches was taken to be an ellipse oriented in the 70° direction, with the lengths of the major and minor axes equal to $\hat{a}_{\max}$ and $\hat{a}_{\min}$, respectively, and we based each prediction on the closest eight values in this neighborhood. The results appear in Figure 8.14.

Comparing the three pH maps, we can see that the filtered kriging map is slightly smoother than the ordinary kriging map, reflecting the extra smoothing done to filter the measurement error. The bull's-eye pattern characteristic of inverse-distance approaches is evident in the inverse-distance-squared pH map. We also notice that the root mean-squared prediction errors for the filtered kriging approach are higher at and near the data locations, but lower overall, also reflecting our measurement error modeling. The root-mean-squared prediction errors closely reflect the data locations, being smaller where pH samples were taken and higher in areas where there are relatively few pH measurements.

All three pH maps depict the general spatial pattern in the Smoky Mountain pH measurements, and any one of these is a decent picture of the spatial distribution of pH values. However, they do show subtle differences, reflecting the different models of spatial dependence that we used to construct them.

The accuracy of kriged maps compared to those constructed using inverse-distance-squared interpolation depends on the statistical and spatial characteristics of the data. Kriging is often more accurate (Isaaks and Srivastava 1989; Weber and Englund 1992; Gotway et al. 1996; Zimmerman et al. 1999) and preferred in many applications since the data determine the nature of the spatial autocorrelation, and a prediction standard error is associated with each value predicted. More objective approaches that can be used to select the "best" map include *validation* and *cross validation*, where subsets of the data are withheld from the analysis and then predicted with the remaining values (see, e.g., Isaaks and Srivastava 1989).

Lognormal Kriging When the data are very skewed, a linear predictor may not be the best choice, since the best predictor, the conditional expectation mentioned at the end of the discussion of ordinary kriging, may be highly nonlinear. In addition, the empirical semivariogram may be a poor estimator of the true semivariogram. Statisticians often deal with such problems by transforming the data so that the transformed data follow a Gaussian distribution and then performing analyses with the transformed data. If we want predictions on the original scale, we can transform back, but the resulting predictions will be biased. However, in certain cases, we can adjust the back transformation so that the resulting predictions are unbiased.

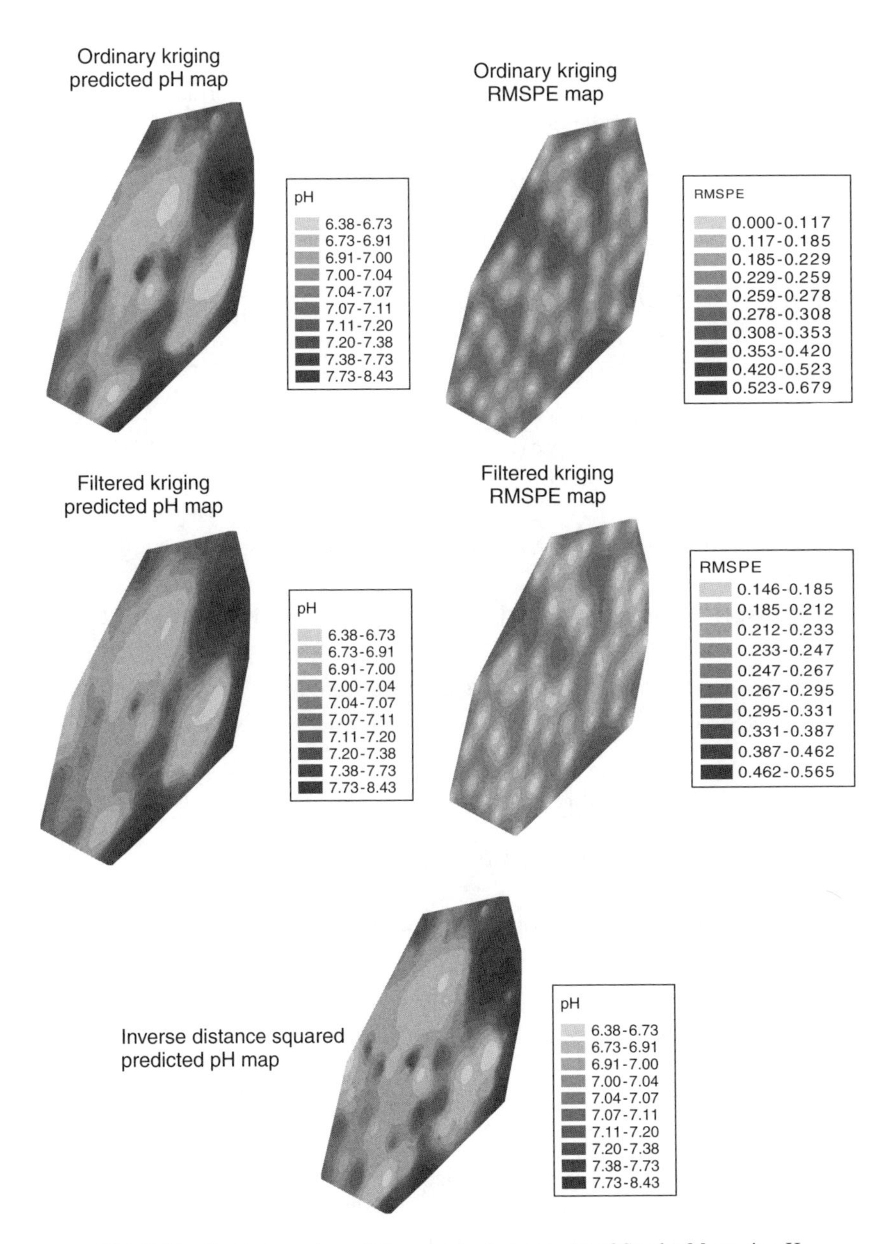

FIG. 8.14 Prediction and prediction standard error maps of Smoky Mountain pH.

With lognormal kriging, we transform the data $Z(\boldsymbol{s}_i), i = 1, \ldots, N$ to a Gaussian distribution using $Y(\boldsymbol{s}) = \log(Z(\boldsymbol{s}))$, and assume that $Y(\cdot)$ is intrinsically stationary with mean μ_Y and semivariogram $\gamma_Y(\boldsymbol{h})$. Ordinary kriging of $Y(\boldsymbol{s}_0)$ using data $Y(\boldsymbol{s}_1), \ldots, Y(\boldsymbol{s}_N)$ gives $\hat{Y}_{\text{OK}}(\boldsymbol{s}_0)$ and $\sigma^2_{Y,k}(\boldsymbol{s}_0)$, obtained from equations (8.21), (8.24) and (8.26) using $\gamma_Y(\boldsymbol{h})$. Now, if we transform predictions back to the $Z(\cdot)$

scale using the exponential function, the resulting predictor $\hat{Z}(s_0) = \exp[\hat{Y}_{\text{OK}}(s_0)]$ is biased. However, we can use the properties of the lognormal distribution to construct an unbiased predictor. Aitchison and Brown (1957) showed that if

$$\mathbf{Y} = (Y_1, Y_2)' \sim MVN(\boldsymbol{\mu}, \Sigma)$$

$$\boldsymbol{\mu} = (\mu_1, \mu_2)', \qquad \Sigma = \sigma_{ij}, i, j = 1, 2,$$

then $[\exp(Y_1), \exp(Y_2)]'$ has mean ν and covariance matrix T, where

$$\nu = (\nu_1, \nu_2)' = [\exp(\mu_1 + \sigma_{11}/2), \exp(\mu_2 + \sigma_{22}/2)]'$$

and

$$T = \begin{bmatrix} \nu_1^2[\exp(\sigma_{11}) - 1] & \nu_1\nu_2[\exp(\sigma_{12}) - 1] \\ \nu_1\nu_2[\exp(\sigma_{21}) - 1] & \nu_2^2[\exp(\sigma_{22}) - 1] \end{bmatrix}.$$

Applying this result to twice, first to $\hat{Z}(s_0)$ and then inversely to μ_Y, gives

$$E[\hat{Z}(s_0)] = E[\exp(\hat{Y}_{\text{OK}}(s_0))] = \mu_Z \exp\left\{-\sigma_Y^2/2 + \text{Var}[\hat{Y}_{\text{OK}}(s_0)]/2\right\},$$

where $\sigma_Y^2 = \text{Var}(Y(s_i))$. Then the bias-corrected predictor of $Z(s_0)$ (see Cressie 1993), denoted here as $\hat{Z}_{\text{OLK}}$ (for ordinary lognormal kriging) is

$$\begin{aligned} \hat{Z}_{\text{OLK}} &= \exp\left\{\hat{Y}_{\text{OK}}(s_0) + \sigma_Y^2/2 - \text{Var}(\hat{Y}_{\text{OK}}(s_0))/2\right\} \\ &= \exp\left\{\hat{Y}_{\text{OK}}(s_0) + \sigma_{Y,k}^2(s_0)/2 - m_Y\right\} \end{aligned} \tag{8.28}$$

where m_Y is the Lagrange multiplier on the Y scale. The bias-corrected MSPE (see, e.g., David 1988) is

$$\begin{aligned} E\left[\left(\hat{Z}_{\text{OLK}} - Z(s_0)\right)^2\right] &= \exp(2\mu_Y + \sigma_Y^2)\exp(\sigma_Y^2) \\ &\quad \cdot \left\{1 + \left[\exp(-\sigma_{Y,k}^2(s_0) + m_Y)\right]\left[\exp(m_Y) - 2\right]\right\}. \end{aligned}$$

Thus, unlike ordinary kriging, we will need to estimate μ_Y and $\sigma_Y^2(\cdot)$ as well as $\gamma_Y(\cdot)$ in order to use lognormal kriging.

The bias correction makes the lognormal kriging predictor sensitive to departures from the lognormality assumption and to fluctuations in the semivariogram. Thus, some authors (e.g., Journel and Huijbregts 1978) have recommended calibration of $\hat{Z}$, forcing the mean of kriged predictions to equal the mean of the original Z data. This may be a useful technique, but it is difficult to determine whether or not it is needed and to determine the properties of the resulting predictor. Others (e.g., Chilès and Delfiner 1999) seem to regard *mean* unbiasedness as unnecessary, noting that $\exp(\hat{Y}_{\text{OK}}(s_0))$ is *median* unbiased (i.e., $\Pr[\exp(\hat{Y}_{\text{OK}}(s_0)) > Z_0] =$

$\Pr[\exp(\hat{Y}_{\text{OK}}(s_0)) < Z_0] = 0.5$). Since the back-transformed predictor will not be optimal (have minimum MSPE), correcting for bias can be important, so we prefer to use the mean-unbiased lognormal kriging predictor given in equation (8.28).

Indicator Kriging Indicator kriging provides a simple way to make a probability map of an event of interest. Suppose that we are interested in mapping an *exceedance* probability [i.e., $\Pr(Z(s_0) > z|Z_1, \ldots, Z_N)$]. This probability can be estimated by kriging the indicator $I(Z(s_0) > z)$ from indicator data $I(Z(s_1) > z), \ldots, I(Z(s_N) > z)$ (Journel 1983), where

$$I(Z(\boldsymbol{s}) > z) = \begin{cases} 1 & \text{if } Z(s) > z \\ 0 & \text{otherwise.} \end{cases} \tag{8.29}$$

This gives an estimate of the optimal predictor, $E(I(Z(s_0) > z)|I(Z(s_i) > z)$, which for indicator data is an estimate of $\Pr(Z(s_0) > z|Z_1, \ldots, Z_N)$. The indicator kriging predictor is simply

$$\hat{I}_{\text{OK}}(\boldsymbol{s}_0) = \sum_{i=1}^{N} \lambda_i I(Z(\boldsymbol{s}_i) > z),$$

where the kriging is performed as described earlier using the semivariogram estimated and modeled from the data indicator.

As some information is lost by using indicator functions instead of the original data values, *indicator cokriging* (Journel 1983), which use k sets of indicators corresponding to various threshold levels, z_k, and *probability kriging* (Sullivan 1984), which uses both the indicator data and the original data to estimate conditional probabilities, have been suggested as better alternatives. There is no guarantee, even with these methods, that the predicted probabilities will lie in [0,1] as probabilities should. In practice, various corrections are used (see Goovaerts 1997), some of which force the kriging weights to be positive. Negative kriging weights usually occur when the influence of one data value is reduced or *screened* by a closer value. Thus, one common solution to the problem of negative probabilities with indicator kriging is to decrease the search neighborhood. This can often also correct the problem of "excessive" probabilities (those > 1). If this does not work, another common correction is to reset any unrealistic values to their nearest bound, either 0 for negative probabilities or 1 for excessive probabilities.

Kriging Areal Regions Thus far, our discussion has focused on predicting values associated with spatial *locations*. In some applications we may want to predict an average value associated with a region of interest (e.g., county, census tract) from either data at individual locations or data associated with the regions themselves. Suppose that instead of observing a realization of the process $\{Z(\boldsymbol{s}) : \boldsymbol{s} \in D\}$, data $Z(B_1), Z(B_2), \ldots, Z(B_N)$ are collected where

$$Z(B_i) = \frac{1}{|B_i|} \int_{B_i} Z(\boldsymbol{s})\, d\boldsymbol{s}.$$

Here $Z(B_i)$ is the average value of the process within region $B_i \subset D$, and $|B_i|$ is the area of $B_i, i = 1, 2, \ldots, N$. In geostatistics, B_i is called the spatial *support* of $Z(B_i)$. The support of the data reflects the size, shape, and spatial orientation of the specific regions (and not just their areas) being considered. The *change of support problem* is concerned with drawing inference on $Z(B)$ from data $Z(B_1), Z(B_2), \ldots, Z(B_N)$.

A common special case of the change of support problem is the prediction of the average value of a region, $Z(B)$, from "point" samples $Z(\mathbf{s}_1), \ldots, Z(\mathbf{s}_N)$. These samples may or may not lie within region B. We consider linear prediction using

$$\hat{Z}(B) = \sum_{i=1}^{N} \lambda_i Z(s_i), \tag{8.30}$$

and derive the optimal weights, $\{\lambda_i\}$, by minimizing the mean-squared prediction error subject to the unbiasedness constraint $E(\hat{Z}(B)) = E(Z(B))$. Since $E(Z(B)) = E(Z(\mathbf{s}_i)) = \mu$, the unbiasedness constraint implies that $\sum \lambda_i = 1$. To minimize the mean-squared prediction error, we follow a development similar to that described earlier and minimize

$$-\sum_{i=1}^{N}\sum_{j=1}^{N} \lambda_i \lambda_j \gamma(\mathbf{s}_i - \mathbf{s}_j) + 2\sum_{i=1}^{N} \lambda_i \gamma(\mathbf{s}_i, B) - 2m\left(\sum_{i=1}^{N} \lambda_i - 1\right), \tag{8.31}$$

which is analogous to equation (8.23) with $\gamma(\mathbf{s}_0 - \mathbf{s}_i)$ replaced with $\gamma(\mathbf{s}_i, B)$, the *point-to-block semivariogram*. This semivariogram can be derived from the semivariogram of the $\{Z(\mathbf{s})\}$ process as (Journel and Huijbregts 1978; Cressie 1993)

$$\gamma(\mathbf{s}, B) \equiv \int_B \gamma(\mathbf{u} - \mathbf{s}) d\mathbf{u}/|B|. \tag{8.32}$$

Differentiating equation (8.31) with respect to $\lambda_1, \ldots, \lambda_N$, and m in turn and setting each partial derivative equal to zero gives the system of equations

$$\sum_{j=1}^{N} \lambda_k \gamma(\mathbf{s}_i - \mathbf{s}_j) + m = \gamma(\mathbf{s}_i, B), \qquad i = 1, \ldots, N$$

$$\sum_{j=1}^{N} \lambda_j = 1. \tag{8.33}$$

These equations are referred to as the *block kriging equations* in geostatistics. The term *block* comes from mining applications for which this approach was developed, where the goal was the prediction of the grade of a block of ore prior to mining recovery.

The minimized mean-squared prediction error, called the *block kriging variance*, is

$$\sigma_K^2(B) = \sum_{i=1}^{N} \lambda_i \gamma(\mathbf{s}_i, B) + m.$$

The point-to-point semivariogram, $\gamma(\boldsymbol{u} - \boldsymbol{s})$, is assumed known for theoretical derivations, but is then estimated from the point data and modeled with a valid conditional nonnegative definite function (as described in Section 8.2.3). In practice, the integral in equation (8.32) is computed by discretizing B into N_u points, $\{\boldsymbol{u}'_j\}$, and using the approximation $\gamma(\boldsymbol{s}_i, B) \approx 1/N_u \sum_{j=1}^{N_u} \gamma(\boldsymbol{u}'_j, \boldsymbol{s}_i)$.

The block kriging predictor, $\hat{Z}(B)$ given in equation (8.30) with weights satisfying equations (8.33), is identical to that obtained by averaging N_u ordinary point kriging predictions at the discretized nodes $\{\boldsymbol{u}'_j\}$. However, block kriging will reduce the computational effort involved in solving many ordinary point kriging systems and will also assure the correct prediction standard error.

CASE STUDY: Hazardous Waste Site Remediation This case study is based on an investigation of dioxin-contaminated soils described by Zirschky and Harris (1986). In 1971, a truck transporting dioxin-contaminated residues dumped an unknown quantity of waste in a rural area of Missouri to avoid citations for being overweight. Although the highest concentration of wastes occurred where the waste was dumped, contamination had spread to other areas. In November 1983, the U.S. Environmental Protection Agency (EPA) collected soil samples in several areas and measured the TCDD (tetrachlorodibenzo-*p*-dioxin) concentration (in μg/kg) in each sample. Figure 8.15 shows the locations of the TCDD samples, where for illustration we have transformed the study domain by dividing the *x*-coordinate by 50 to produce a region that is almost square. The objective of the study was to determine where EPA should concentrate soil remediation efforts.

One way to address the study objective is to make a map of the TCDD concentration predicted. Since concentration values must be positive and often have skewed distributions, it is common to assume a lognormal distribution, so we will

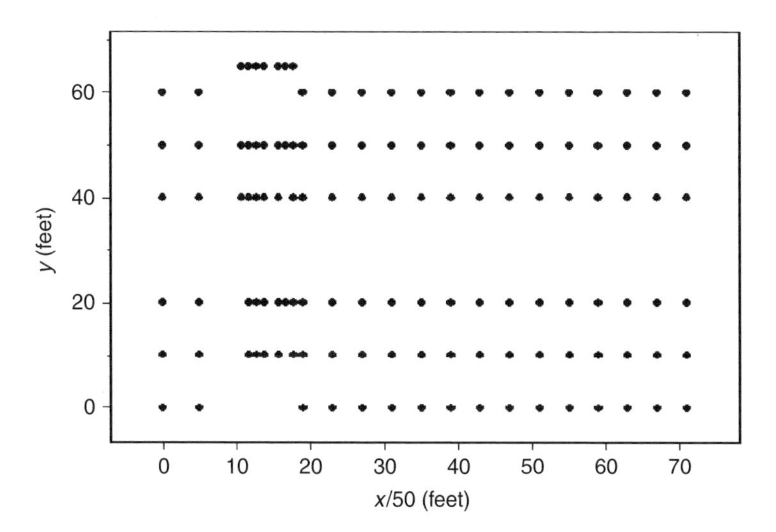

FIG. 8.15 Locations of EPA TCDD samples.

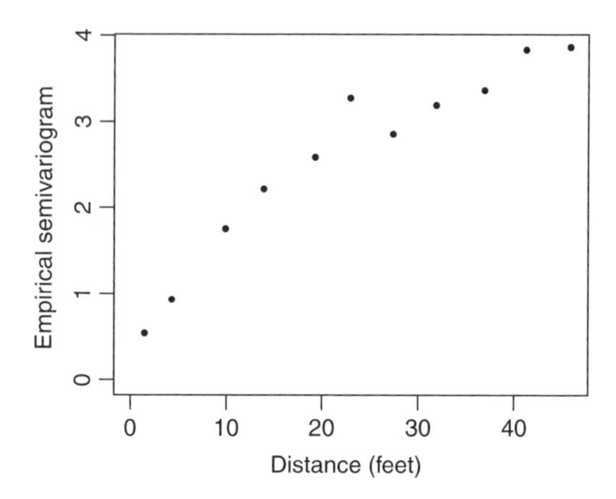

FIG. 8.16 Empirical omnidirectional semivariogram of log-TCDD data.

use lognormal kriging to make this map. The first step in lognormal kriging is to take the logarithm of the concentration data and then compute the omnidirectional semivariogram using the methods discussed in Section 8.2.3. This is shown in Figure 8.16. The initial increase in the semivariogram indicates strong spatial autocorrelation with a fairly large range and a negligible nugget effect. Given that the spill occurred along a roadway, we might expect anisotropy and can explore this using a contour map of the semivariogram surface (Figure 8.17) (see Section 8.2.5). From this figure it appears that the range of spatial autocorrelation is greatest in the east-west (0° direction), corresponding to the primary orientation of the road.

If we assume geometric anisotropy with the maximum range in the east-west direction we can fit an anisotropic model. With no other information about the laboratory process used to obtain the TCDD concentrations, we assume that the nugget effect is zero. Assuming an exponential model, we used the modified WLS approach implemented in ESRI's Geostatistical Analyst (Johnston et al. 2001) to fit a geometrically anisotropic model and obtain the estimates $\hat{a}_{\text{max}} = 18.30$, $\hat{a}_{\text{min}} = 8.18$, and $\hat{c}_e = 3.45$. Model fits to the east-west and north-south directional semivariograms are shown in Figure 8.18.

We predict values on a closely spaced regular grid superimposed on the domain depicted in Figure 8.15 using lognormal kriging. We use an elliptical search neighborhood oriented in the east-west direction with the length of the major and minor axes equal to $\hat{a}_{\text{max}} = 18.30$ and $\hat{a}_{\text{min}} = 8.18$, respectively, and retain the nearest five points from each of four quadrants for each prediction. The resulting map is shown in Figure 8.19. Based on this map, EPA should concentrate remediation efforts in the area with the highest predicted TCDD concentration, indicated by the large dark area in the center of the study domain.

An alternative approach is to recommend remediation only for those areas for which it is likely that the TCDD concentration exceeds the EPA standard. Zirschky and Harris (1986) considered 1 μg/kg as the cleanup criterion, but today, the EPA standard for disposal of sewage sludge used in agriculture is 0.3 μg/kg. We will use

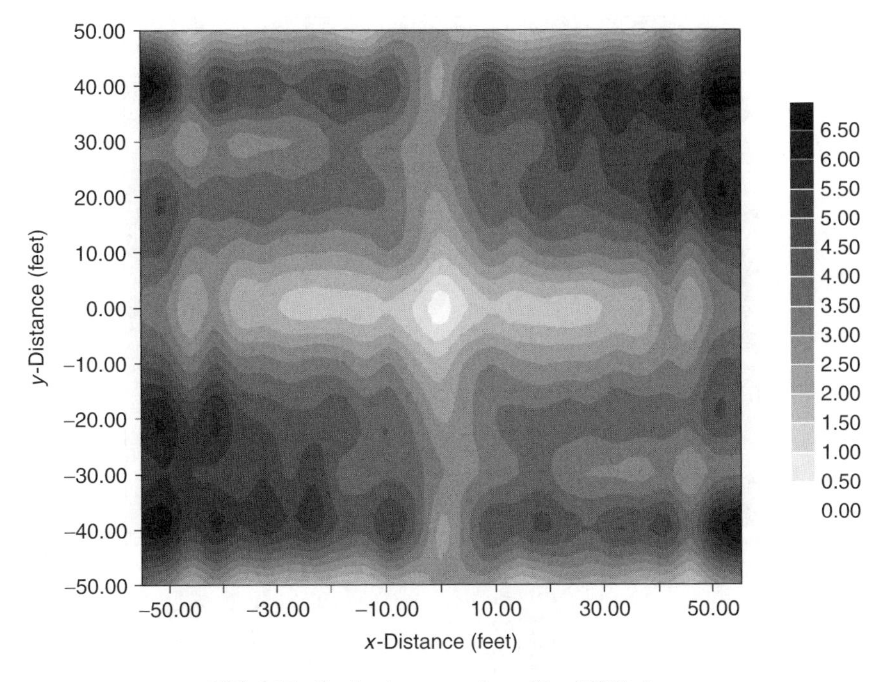

FIG. 8.17 Semivariogram surface of log-TCDD data.

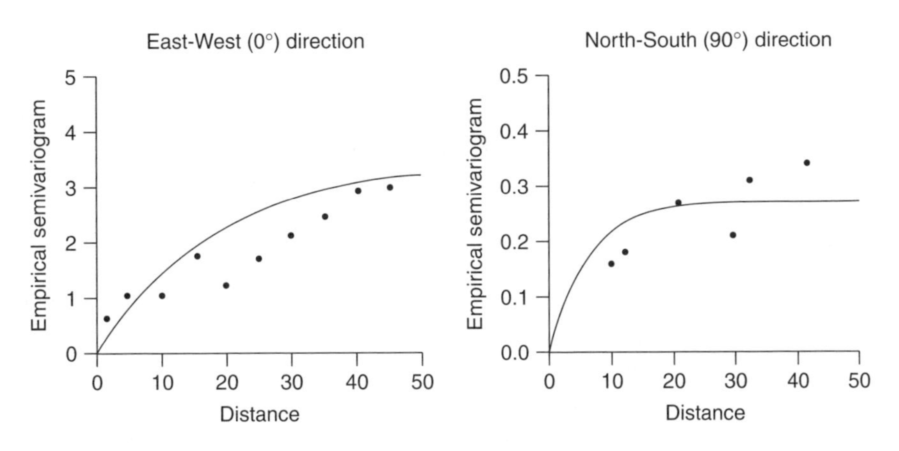

FIG. 8.18 Empirical directional semivariograms of log-TCDD data and model fit.

indicator kriging to determine areas that exceed this standard. First, we transform the data to indicators defined as

$$I(\text{TCDD}(\boldsymbol{s}) > 0.3) = \begin{cases} 1 & \text{if } \text{TCDD}(\boldsymbol{s}) > 0.3 \\ 0 & \text{otherwise.} \end{cases}$$

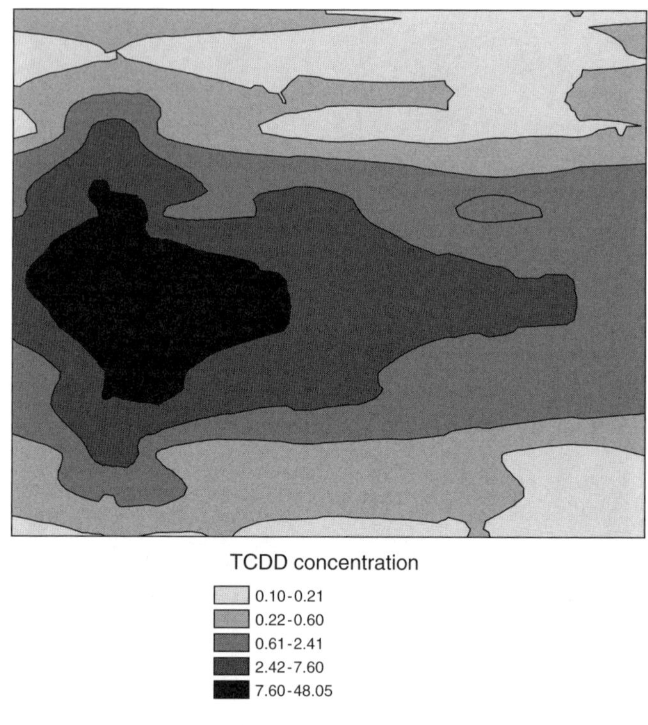

FIG. 8.19 Lognormal kriging prediction map of TCDD contamination.

The indicator process reflects the same type of anisotropy as the original concentration process, so we will consider the same type of model as used for the TCDD concentration process. Refitting this model to the indicator data, we obtain $\hat{a}_{\max} = 14.02$, $\hat{a}_{\min} = 5.57$, and $\hat{c}_e = 0.2716$. Model fits to the east-west and north-south directional indicator semivariograms are shown in Figure 8.20.

We used this fitted model to predict the indicator data on the same grid and with the same type of search neighborhood as with the original TCDD data. The resulting map, depicting the probability of exceeding the EPA standard for TCDD concentration of 0.3 μg/kg appears in Figure 8.21. This map leads to a very different remediation strategy than that inferred from the lognormal kriging map. Since most of the values that exceed our cleanup criterion of 0.3 μg/kg occur on either side of the roadway, the area with the greatest probability of exceeding this criterion occurs along the roadway as well. Thus, based on this map, we would recommend concentrating remediation efforts along a rather large swath of land centered along the roadway.

An alternative approach to constructing such a probability map is to use the lognormal kriging predictions. If we assume that the logarithms of the TCDD concentration follow a Gaussian distribution, then at each location we can calculate the probability of exceeding a threshold value. The mean and standard deviation necessary for these probabilities are the predicted value obtained from kriging and

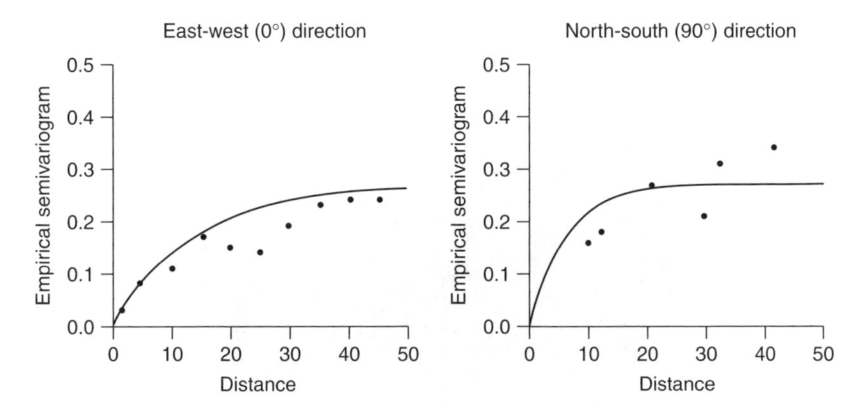

FIG. 8.20 Empirical directional indicator semivariograms and model fit.

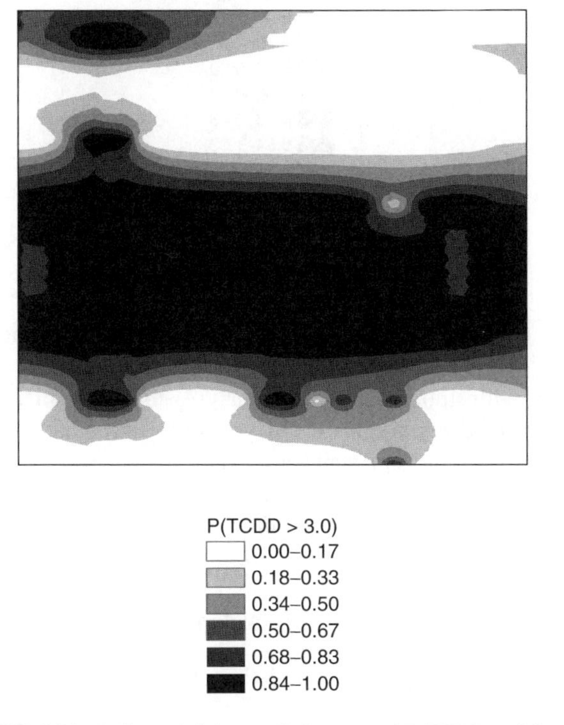

FIG. 8.21 Indicator kriging prediction map of Pr(TCDD > 0.3).

the standard error, respectively. We applied this approach to the TCDD concentration data using the same threshold of 0.3 μg/kg, and the resulting map appears in Figure 8.22. This map is similar to that made using indicator kriging, but since the actual TCDD concentration values are used in the calculations, it shows more detail.

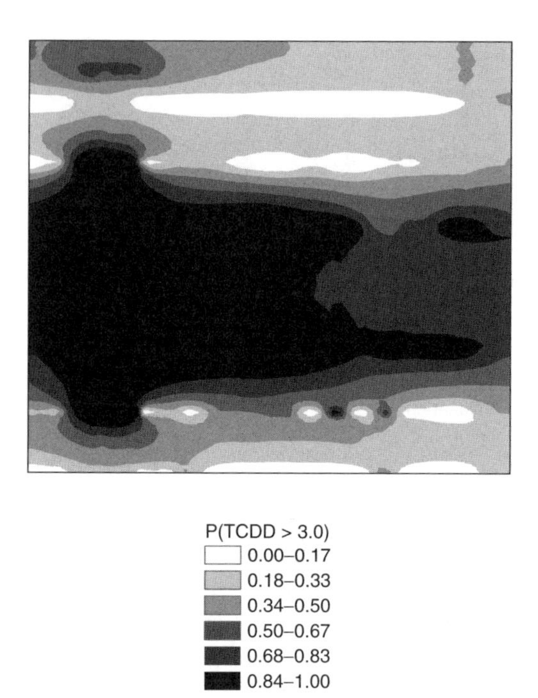

FIG. 8.22 Probability map of Pr(TCDD > 0.3) using the Gaussian distribution.

All the maps at least roughly indicate the same area of highest contamination. However, they differ greatly in the uncertainty associated with each predicted value or probability. Obtaining standard error maps for the three methods is left as an exercise.

This case study illustrates the type of analyses that geostatistical methods can provide. We would be remiss if we led you to believe that these analyses are definitive. The dioxin data represent an example of a "real" data set with many "problems" that often accompany real data. The data do not meet all of the assumptions and expectations discussed in this chapter. For example, the data are left-censored and of differing supports. In kriging the TCDD data, we essentially assumed that the spread of contamination was not affected by the placement of roadway. Nevertheless, our geostatistical methods provide valuable insight and a preliminary analysis that can form the basis for more complex models, and the case study highlights both the potential and the limitations of geostatistical analysis of environmental monitoring data.

8.4 ADDITIONAL TOPICS AND FURTHER READING

8.4.1 Erratic Experimental Semivariograms

Semivariogram estimation and modeling can be difficult, particularly if the data are noisy (either statistically or spatially), the data distribution is skewed, or there are influential observations. Good discussions of many of the common problems encountered in semivariogram estimation and model fitting, together with some suggested solutions, are given in Armstrong (1984) and Webster and Oliver (2001). Basu et al. (1997) considered the effect of influential observations on semivariogram estimation and illustrated graphical techniques for identifying such observations. Cressie and Hawkins (1980) developed several robust semivariogram estimators, using power transformations, medians, and trimmed means. One of these, based on fourth roots of squared differences, is available in many software packages as either the *robust* or the *Cressie–Hawkins semivariogram estimator*. Haining (1990) provides a good summary of robust and resistant semivariogram estimators and the results of several theoretical and empirical evaluations and comparisons.

8.4.2 Sampling Distribution of the Classical Semivariogram Estimator

Davis and Borgman (1979) tabulated the exact sampling distribution of $2\hat{\gamma}(\boldsymbol{h})$ assuming equally spaced, one-dimensional Gaussian data with a linear theoretical semivariogram. Analogous results for more general cases may be possible, but given the difficulty of this approach, attention has focused on asymptotic sampling distributions. Davis and Borgman (1982) showed that $[\hat{\gamma}(h) - \gamma(h)]/\sqrt{\mathrm{Var}(\hat{\gamma}(h))}$ converges to a standard normal distribution as the number of data values becomes large. The variance of $\hat{\gamma}(h)$ needed to compute this standardized quantity (and the covariances for the multivariate generalization needed for simultaneous confidence bands) were derived by Cressie (1985). As discussed in Section 8.2.4, these variances and covariances are not easy to obtain from the data, so approximations like the one given in equation (8.9) are used. An alternative based on iteratively reweighted generalized least squares (cf. Section 9.2) is described by Genton (1998). A comprehensive discussion and illustration of these methods and several others for assessing the uncertainty in semivariogram estimates is given in Pardo-Iqúsquiza and Dowd (2001).

8.4.3 Nonparametric Semivariogram Models

Using spectral properties of the covariance function, Shapiro and Botha (1991) introduced a nonparametric representation of the semivariogram

$$\gamma(h) = \sum_{i=1}^{k}[1 - \Omega_d(ht_i)]p_i,$$

where the values t_i are the *nodes* of the semivariogram, $\{p_i\}$ are nonzero weights and

$$\Omega_d(x) = \left(\frac{2}{x}\right)^{(d-2)/2} \Gamma\left(\frac{d}{2}\right) J_{(d-2)/2}(x),$$

where d is the spatial dimension ($d = 2$ for two-dimensional space), $\Gamma(\cdot)$ is the gamma function, and $J_m(x)$ is the Bessel function of the first kind of order m. The idea here is to build more flexible semivariogram models by adding several valid semivariograms together. This is the same idea behind the nested structure models in geostatistics that we described briefly in Section 8.2.2.

Given the nodes, constrained nonlinear least squares (constrained so that $p_i \geq 0$) can be used to estimate the weights. Various methods have been suggested for determining the number of nodes and their placement. Cherry et al. (1996) suggest using many nodes (e.g., 200) and placing half of them at equally spaced increments in [0,4] and the other half in equally spaced increments in [4.16, 20]. Ecker and Gelfand (1997) recommend using a small number of nodes (e.g., 5), spaced equally in an interval determined by the number of desired sign changes in the Bessel function and use a Bayesian approach to infer either the placement of the nodes when the weights are equal to $1/k$, or to infer the weights when the placement of the nodes is specified.

Although nonparametric semivariogram families provide a flexible alternative to parametric models, they have two main drawbacks (other than the subjectivity required in determining the nodes): their inability to fit a nugget effect and their difficulty in modeling anisotropy. Ecker and Gelfand (1999) overcome the latter difficulty by extending their Bayesian approach to geometrically anisotropic data. Ver Hoef and Barry (1996) overcome both problems using a family of semivariograms based on integration of a moving-average function over white noise random processes.

8.4.4 Kriging Non-Gaussian Data

As we discussed in Section 8.3.2, linear predictors such as ordinary and universal kriging may not be the best choice for spatial prediction with non-Gaussian data. Based on the ideas behind lognormal kriging, Cressie (1993) derives a trans-Gaussian predictor using a general transformation to a Gaussian distribution [e.g., $Y(s) = \phi(Z(s))$]. He uses a second-order Taylor series expansion to adjust for bias in the back transformation. Gotway and Stroup (1997) extend universal kriging to the class of generalized linear models that account for variance-to-mean relationships in the data (e.g., models for Poisson data for which the mean equals the variance). Diggle et al. (1998) had a similar goal but used a conditional specification for the generalized linear model and inference based on Bayesian hierarchical modeling. Yasui and Lele (1997) compare and illustrate both marginal and conditional generalized estimating equations for estimation of spatial disease rates using Bayesian methods, and Gotway and Wolfinger (2003) make a similar comparison of spatial prediction methods using penalized quasi-likelihood approaches.

8.4.5 Geostatistical Simulation

For many methods in spatial statistics, Monte Carlo simulation is used for inference (cf. inference methods in Chapters 5, 6, and 7). Simulation is also a powerful tool for the analysis of geostatistical data. Typically, simulation is used here for *uncertainty analysis* in order to generate a distribution of a spatial response from uncertain spatial inputs. The result is an entire probability distribution of values at each spatial location, and thus an ensemble of maps or surfaces, all possible given the data. One of the main differences between geostatistical simulation and other simulation approaches is that geostatistical simulation methods can constrain each simulated surface to pass through the given data points. This is called *conditional simulation*.

There are many different conditional simulation algorithms [see, e.g., Deutsch and Journel (1992), Dowd (1992), and Gotway and Rutherford (1994) for descriptions and comparisons]. One of the most familiar to statisticians is called *LU decomposition*, based on a Cholesky-type decomposition of the covariance matrix between data observed at study locations and data at grid or prediction locations. This covariance matrix can be written as

$$C = \begin{pmatrix} C_{11} & C_{12} \\ C_{21} & C_{22} \end{pmatrix},$$

where C_{11} is the covariance among data at study locations, C_{12} is the covariance between data at study locations and data to be predicted at grid locations, and C_{22} is the covariance among data to be predicted at grid locations. It can be decomposed into a product of a lower triangular matrix and an upper triangular matrix (hence the name *LU decomposition*) as

$$C = \begin{pmatrix} L_{11} & 0 \\ L_{21} & L_{22} \end{pmatrix} \begin{pmatrix} U_{11} & U_{12} \\ 0 & U_{22} \end{pmatrix}$$

(a well-known result from matrix algebra). A conditional Gaussian simulation is obtained by simulating a vector, $\boldsymbol{\epsilon}$, of independent Gaussian random variables with mean 0 and variance 1 and using the data vector $\mathbf{Z}$ in the transformation

$$\begin{pmatrix} L_{ZZ} & 0 \\ L_{21} & L_{22} \end{pmatrix} \begin{pmatrix} L_{11}^{-1} \\ \boldsymbol{\epsilon} \end{pmatrix} = \begin{pmatrix} \mathbf{Z} \\ L_{21}L_{11}^{-1}\mathbf{Z} + L_{22}\boldsymbol{\epsilon} \end{pmatrix}. \qquad (8.34)$$

This transformation induces spatial correlation (specified by C) in the simulated values and also forces them to be equal to the Z values at observed data locations. It is also possible to generate realizations that do not honor the data. More details about this approach as well as other geostatistical simulation algorithms can be found in Deutsch and Journel (1992), Dowd (1992), and Gotway and Rutherford (1994).

8.4.6 Use of Non-Euclidean Distances in Geostatistics

Throughout this chapter we have used Euclidean distance as a basis for measuring spatial autocorrelation. In many applications, particularly those in the environmental sciences, this measure of distance may not be realistic. For example, mountains, irregularly shaped domains, and partitions in a building can present barriers to movement. Although two points on either side of a barrier may be physically close, it may be unrealistic to assume that they are related. Geostatistical analyses can also be done using non-Euclidean distances (e.g., city-block distance) provided that two conditions hold: (1) the distance measure is a valid metric in $\Re^2$ (i.e., it must be nonnegative, symmetric, and satisfy the triangle inequality); and (2) the semivariogram used with this metric must satisfy the properties of a semivariogram (i.e., it must be conditionally negative definite). Using these criteria, Curriero (1996) showed that the exponential semivariogram is valid with city-block distance, but the Gaussian semivariogram is not. This general issue and a proposed alternative using multidimensional scaling is given in Curriero (1996). Rathbun (1998) used these results to evaluate the use of *water distance* (the shortest path between two sites that may be traversed entirely over water) for kriging estuaries.

8.4.7 Spatial Sampling and Network Design

When we have the luxury of choosing the data locations, some thought should go into the *design* of our sampling plan. Olea (1984), Cressie (1993), and Gilbert (1997) review many different spatial sampling plans in the context of different objectives (e.g., estimation of a mean or total, estimation of spatial patterns, detection of hot spots). A systematic sampling plan using a regular grid with a random start was recommended for estimating trends and patterns of spatial variability in fixed (not mobile) populations. A triangular grid is the most efficient for semivariogram estimation and kriging and EPA's Environmental Monitoring and Assessment Program (EMAP) is based on this design [see, e.g., Stevens (1994) for an overview of this program]. Instead of a systematic triangular grid design, Stehman and Overton (1994) suggest a *tessellation-stratified design*, where the strata are defined by the squares or triangles of a regular or triangular grid and the sampling locations are chosen randomly within each stratum. This type of design allows greater variability in distances, including some that are small, and so may allow for better estimation of the semivariogram.

Since all of these sampling plans are probability based, probability sampling theory offers many tools for estimation and inference (e.g., the Horvitz–Thompson estimator and a variety of methods for variance estimation from systematic sampling). Model-based analysis (e.g., regression and kriging) can also be done. Another approach to the construction of spatial sampling plans useful in network design is based on the kriging variance. Since the kriging variance depends only on the spatial locations and not on the data values themselves, prediction errors from kriging can be determined for any particular sampling plan before the sampling is actually performed. We may then choose the sampling plan that minimizes the average (or the maximum) prediction error. Cressie et al. (1990) illustrate this approach. More recently, Bayesian methods have been used to provide a flexible framework for network design (Zidek et al. 2000).

8.5 EXERCISES

8.1 The data in Table 8.3 were collected to assess the suitability of a waste isolation pilot plant (WIPP) in southeastern New Mexico for disposal of transuranic wastes (see, e.g., Gotway 1994). Transmissivity values measuring the rate of water flow through the Culebra aquifer that lies just above the WIPP site were collected from 41 wells.

Table 8.3 WIPP Transmissivity Data[a]

East (km)	North (km)	log(*T*)	East (km)	North (km)	log(*T*)
14.2850	31.1240	−4.6839	7.0330	17.6060	−2.9136
7.4450	29.5230	−3.3692	16.7480	17.3390	−5.6089
16.7400	26.1450	−6.6023	15.3600	16.7980	−6.4842
24.1450	25.8250	−6.5535	21.3860	16.7940	−10.1234
16.7020	21.7380	−4.0191	18.2220	16.7770	−4.9271
13.6130	21.4520	−4.4500	18.3650	15.5740	−4.5057
19.8910	21.2450	−7.0115	11.7210	15.3210	−5.6897
15.6630	20.6910	−4.1296	13.6430	15.1910	−7.0354
9.4040	20.4720	−3.5412	0.0000	15.1380	−2.9685
16.7290	19.9680	−6.9685	15.3990	14.9270	−5.9960
16.7540	19.6230	−6.4913	16.2100	14.4930	−6.5213
15.2830	19.6100	−5.7775	18.7370	13.9570	−6.6361
16.7580	19.2260	−6.1903	16.9450	13.9100	−5.9685
16.7580	19.0970	−6.4003	20.0420	11.8960	−6.7132
16.7620	18.7630	−6.5705	11.1430	11.0920	−2.8125
16.3880	18.6560	−6.1149	25.9940	8.9170	−7.1234
12.1030	18.4200	−3.5571	9.4810	5.9030	−3.2584
16.7150	18.4020	−6.2964	17.0080	4.7050	−3.9019
18.3340	18.3030	−6.8804	17.9720	3.8980	−4.3350
16.4420	18.1280	−6.0290	11.7020	0.0000	−5.0547
15.6700	18.0950	−6.2005			

[a]Data are the UTM coordinates in kilometers measured from a fixed location and the log transmissivity (T) in $\log_{10}(\text{m}^2/\text{s})$.

(a) Estimate the omnidirectional semivariogram and the empirical semivariograms in the east-west and north-south directions. For each, provide the average lag distance, number of pairs, and semivariogram estimate as well as a graph of the empirical semivariograms. Do you see evidence of trend or anisotropy? Discuss.

(b) Repeat your analysis deleting the large negative log(*T*) value of −10.12. What effect does this have on your results?

8.2 Suppose that we have data $Z(\boldsymbol{s}_1), \ldots Z(\boldsymbol{s}_N)$ from an intrinsically stationary process with covariance function $C(\boldsymbol{s}_i - \boldsymbol{s}_j)$. Find the variance of the sample mean, $\overline{Z} = \sum_{i=1}^{N} Z(\boldsymbol{s}_i)/n$. Express this result in terms of the autocorrelation function $\rho(s_i - s_j)$ and compare it to the result you obtain assuming that the data are independent. What implication does this have for survey design based on spatial data?

8.3 Referring to the dioxin case study, Zirschky and Harris (1986) provide the TCDD data. Use ordinary kriging to map the logarithm of the TCDD concentration. How do your conclusions about waste remediation differ from those obtained using lognormal kriging and indicator kriging?

8.4 Using the logarithm of the TCDD concentration values, use different nugget effects, sills, ranges, and search neighborhoods to investigate systematically the effects of your choices on the maps of log(TCDD) concentration and prediction standard errors obtained from ordinary kriging. What conclusions can you draw about the effect of these parameters on the kriged values and standard errors? Do the maps you draw reflect the differences?

8.5 Using the TCDD data, obtain standard error maps for lognormal kriging, indicator kriging, and a probability map from the lognormal kriging using properties of the Gaussian distribution. Discuss the differences in the maps and relate them to the assumptions underlying each method.

8.6 Derive the filtered kriging equations given in equations (8.27).

8.7 Refer to the graveyard data set described in Chapter 5 and given in Table 5.2. Suppose that the affected grave sites are coded as 1's and the nonaffected grave sites are coded as 0's, so that the data set consists of x location, y location, and grave site type. Discuss the implications of using indicator kriging to map the probability of an affected grave site. What assumptions need to be made? How realistic are these?

CHAPTER 9

Linking Spatial Exposure Data to Health Events

...all models are wrong. The practical question is how wrong do they have to be to not be useful.

Box and Draper (1987, p. 74)

In Chapters 4, 5, 6, and 7 we describe and illustrate methods for making inferences about the spatial distribution of health events, observed either at point locations (Chapters 4, 5, and 6) or as aggregated counts, rates, and standardized mortality ratios (Chapters 4 and 7). In Chapter 8 we consider some of the geostatistical methods for assessing the spatial variation in exposure measurements. Through the data breaks and case studies, we show how all of these statistical methods can provide much more substantial conclusions than we could obtain using just visualization and a GIS. There is, however, an alternative approach based on the use of *spatial regression models* that can help us refine our conclusions even more. These models allow us to adjust our analyses and our maps for important covariate information. They also allow us to more explicitly use spatial exposure measurements to help describe the spatial distribution of public health events. In this chapter we integrate much of the knowledge we have acquired thus far and use it to develop several different types of spatial regression models to link spatial exposure data to health events.

In traditional statistics, we frequently assess the effects of exposure on health outcomes through regression analysis. Such analysis can take many forms: Linear, Poisson, and logistic regression are perhaps the most familiar, and we gave an overview of these (for nonspatial data) in Chapter 2. The same ideas can be used in spatial analysis after we adapt them to incorporate our ideas about neighborhood relationships and spatially correlated error terms.

Our goal in this chapter is to quantify the nature of the association between a spatially referenced outcome of interest, $Y(\boldsymbol{s})$, and a set of spatially referenced explanatory variables $x_0(\boldsymbol{s}), x_1(\boldsymbol{s}), \ldots, x_{p-1}(\boldsymbol{s})$. We begin in Section 9.1 with a brief review of multivariate linear regression, assuming that the data follow a multivariate

Applied Spatial Statistics for Public Health Data, by Lance A. Waller and Carol A. Gotway
ISBN 0-471-38771-1

Gaussian distribution and the relationship between $Y(\boldsymbol{s})$ and $x_1(\boldsymbol{s}), \ldots, x_p(\boldsymbol{s})$ can be described adequately by a linear model with independent errors. We present basic results from the theory of maximum likelihood estimation and rely on matrix notation to provide a parsimonious development [see, e.g., Draper and Smith (1998) for an introductory treatment of ordinary least squares regression and relevant matrix notation].

9.1 LINEAR REGRESSION MODELS FOR INDEPENDENT DATA

Many spatial models generalize the basic structure of linear models and we review basic results here to provide a point of reference and comparison for the spatially motivated generalizations to follow. Most of our development in Chapter 8 builds from the assumption of a constant mean [i.e., $E(Y(\boldsymbol{s})) = \mu$]. In this chapter we relax this assumption and allow the mean to depend on a linear combination of covariates using the regression model

$$\mathbf{Y} = X\boldsymbol{\beta} + \boldsymbol{\epsilon}, \tag{9.1}$$

where $\mathbf{Y} = [Y(\boldsymbol{s}_1), Y(\boldsymbol{s}_2), \ldots, Y(\boldsymbol{s}_N)]'$ is the data vector of measurements at locations $\boldsymbol{s}_1, \ldots, \boldsymbol{s}_N$, $\boldsymbol{\beta} = (\beta_0, \beta_1, \ldots, \beta_{p-1})'$ is the vector of regression parameters, and the matrix

$$X = \begin{bmatrix} 1 & x_1(\boldsymbol{s}_1) & \cdots & x_{p-1}(\boldsymbol{s}_1) \\ 1 & x_1(\boldsymbol{s}_2) & \ldots & x_{p-1}(\boldsymbol{s}_2) \\ \vdots & \vdots & \vdots & \vdots \\ 1 & x_1(\boldsymbol{s}_N) & \ldots & x_{p-1}(\boldsymbol{s}_N) \end{bmatrix}$$

contains the covariate values observed at each location. [We assume that $x_0(\boldsymbol{s}) \equiv 1$, so our models fit an intercept.] We assume that the residual (or error) vector $\boldsymbol{\epsilon} = [\epsilon(\boldsymbol{s}_1), \ldots, \epsilon(\boldsymbol{s}_N)]'$ has mean $\mathbf{0}$ and variance–covariance matrix

$$\Sigma = \text{Var}(\mathbf{Y}) = \text{Var}(\boldsymbol{\epsilon}) = \sigma^2 I, \tag{9.2}$$

where I is the $N \times N$ identity matrix. With this variance–covariance matrix [equation (9.2)] we are assuming that the data are uncorrelated. This assumption implies that all of the spatial variation in the data is assumed to be due to the covariates. This is in sharp contrast to most of the development in Chapter 8, where we effectively assume that all of the spatial variation in $\mathbf{Y}$ is due to spatial autocorrelation as quantified by the semivariogram. Our goal in this chapter is a compromise between these two extremes, and we extend the model defined by equations (9.1) and (9.2) in several ways. First, in Section 9.2 we modify $\Sigma = \text{Var}(\mathbf{Y})$ to allow spatially autocorrelated error terms. Our treatment here will be somewhat general, with specific examples utilizing the geostatistical framework in Chapter 8. Second, in Section 9.3 we allow more flexible neighborhood structures for aggregated spatial data, as described in Sections 4.4.1 and 7.4.2. This takes many of the ideas regarding spatial clustering described in Chapters 5, 6, and 7 and puts them into a regression context, so we use not only neighboring information to ascertain clustering of disease cases, but also spatially varying covariate information to provide potential reasons for the clustering. Third, we adapt the models for Poisson and logistic regression in Section 9.4. This allows us to extend traditional public health analytic methods to a spatial setting and to introduce random effects and hierarchical modeling. Finally, we treat random effects and hierarchical models for spatial data in more detail and conclude with an introduction to Bayesian models for disease mapping in Section 9.5.

9.1.1 Estimation and Inference

To quantify associations between $Y(\boldsymbol{s})$ and $x_0(\boldsymbol{s}), x_1(\boldsymbol{s}), \ldots, x_{p-1}(\boldsymbol{s})$ using the linear model defined by equations (9.1) and (9.2), we need to estimate $\boldsymbol{\beta}$. In order to obtain standard errors needed for confidence intervals and significance tests, we also need to estimate σ^2. Since we are assuming that the data follow a multivariate Gaussian distribution [i.e., we assume $\mathbf{Y} \sim MVN(X\boldsymbol{\beta}, \sigma^2 I)$], we could use either *ordinary least squares* or *maximum likelihood methods* to provide these estimates. We concentrate on maximum likelihood here since there is a very rich theory underlying this approach, providing general methods for obtaining standard errors, deriving the asymptotic distributions of the resulting estimators, and constructing hypothesis tests. We use maximum likelihood as a starting point for developing inference for the more complex models in subsequent sections in this chapter. In this section we give an overview of maximum likelihood estimation for the parameters of the linear model defined by equations (9.1) and (9.2). We focus on major points and main results to facilitate a general understanding of how the estimators, confidence intervals, and hypothesis tests operate in order to better motivate their use with more complex models in subsequent sections. Even so, we admittedly omit many important details needed for complete understanding and computation. These can be found in Cox and Hinkley (1974), Graybill (1976), Judge et al. (1985), and Searle et al. (1992). The equations we provide in this section and in Section 9.2 have been synthesized and adapted from all of these references, primarily Judge et al. (1985).

Maximum likelihood (ML) estimators are those estimators that maximize the probability of obtaining the data over the set of possible values of the model parameters. This probability is quantified by the joint probability distribution of the data, given parameter values. Thus, for the linear model defined by equations (9.1) and (9.2), the maximum likelihood estimators of $\boldsymbol{\beta}$ and σ^2 maximize the joint likelihood of the data given by the multivariate Gaussian probability density

$$l(\boldsymbol{\beta}, \sigma^2 | \mathbf{Y}, X) = (2\pi\sigma^2)^{-N/2} \exp\left[-\frac{(\mathbf{Y} - X\boldsymbol{\beta})'(\mathbf{Y} - X\boldsymbol{\beta})}{2\sigma^2}\right],$$

or equivalently, maximize the natural logarithm of the likelihood

$$\mathcal{L} = \ln(l(\boldsymbol{\beta}, \sigma^2 | \mathbf{Y}, X)) = -\frac{N}{2}\ln(2\pi) - \frac{N}{2}\ln(\sigma^2) - \frac{(\mathbf{Y} - X\boldsymbol{\beta})'(\mathbf{Y} - X\boldsymbol{\beta})}{2\sigma^2}. \quad (9.3)$$

The maximum of this function can be obtained analytically using calculus: We take the partial derivatives with respect to $\boldsymbol{\beta}$ and σ^2, set them to zero, and solve the resulting set of equations for the optimal values. This procedure yields

$$\frac{\partial \mathcal{L}}{\partial \boldsymbol{\beta}} = \frac{1}{\sigma^2}(X'\mathbf{Y} - X'X\boldsymbol{\beta}) = 0$$

$$\frac{\partial \mathcal{L}}{\partial \sigma^2} = -\frac{N}{2\sigma^2} + \frac{N}{2\sigma^4}(\mathbf{Y} - X\boldsymbol{\beta})'(\mathbf{Y} - X\boldsymbol{\beta}) = 0.$$

These equations are termed the *score equations*. Solving the first of these equations for $\boldsymbol{\beta}$ gives the maximum likelihood estimator of $\boldsymbol{\beta}$. Since we are assuming that the data follow a Gaussian distribution, the ML estimator of $\boldsymbol{\beta}$ is equivalent to the *ordinary least squares* (OLS) *estimator* of $\boldsymbol{\beta}$ since it also minimizes the residual sum of squares $[(\mathbf{Y} - X\boldsymbol{\beta})'(\mathbf{Y} - X\boldsymbol{\beta})]$. Most regression textbooks (e.g., Draper and Smith 1998) use the least squares approach and for Gaussian data, least squares estimators and maximum likelihood estimators are equivalent. We refer to the maximum likelihood estimators of $\boldsymbol{\beta}$ and σ^2 derived in this section as OLS estimators to distinguish them from other estimators derived under different assumptions in subsequent sections. Thus, solving the first score equation for $\boldsymbol{\beta}$, we obtain the maximum likelihood estimator (and the OLS estimator) of $\boldsymbol{\beta}$ as

$$\hat{\boldsymbol{\beta}}_{\text{OLS}} = (X'X)^{-1}X'\mathbf{Y}. \tag{9.4}$$

Substituting this solution into the second score equation gives the maximum likelihood estimator of σ^2:

$$\hat{\sigma}^2 = \frac{(\mathbf{Y} - X\hat{\boldsymbol{\beta}}_{\text{OLS}})'(\mathbf{Y} - X\hat{\boldsymbol{\beta}}_{\text{OLS}})}{N}.$$

This estimator is biased, so instead, we often use the estimator

$$\hat{\sigma}^2_{\text{OLS}} = \frac{(\mathbf{Y} - X\hat{\boldsymbol{\beta}}_{\text{OLS}})'(\mathbf{Y} - X\hat{\boldsymbol{\beta}}_{\text{OLS}})}{N - p}, \tag{9.5}$$

taking into account the loss in the degrees of freedom associated with estimating $\boldsymbol{\beta}$.

Rather than adjusting the ML estimator of σ^2 for the loss in degrees of freedom, an alternative approach, called *restricted maximum likelihood* (REML), is often used to estimate σ^2. REML uses likelihood methods based on linear combinations of the data that do not involve $\boldsymbol{\beta}$ to estimate σ^2 and is the default estimation procedure in many statistical programs estimating variance components. The restricted likelihood, methods for maximizing it, and the resulting REML estimators are all similar to the corresponding concepts in maximum likelihood theory, and we omit the details here for brevity. Theoretical and computational details of REML can be found in Searle et al. (1992), with additional references provided in Section 9.7.

In order to determine whether solutions to the score equations *maximize* the likelihood function, calculus suggests using what is called *the second derivative test*; that is, we evaluate the second derivatives using the solutions to the score equations (first derivative equations) and assess whether the resulting values are less than zero (for a maximum). In statistics, it is also important to see if there are any values on the edge of the parameter space that give local maxima (e.g., $\sigma^2 = 0$), since it is often difficult (if not impossible) to determine whether an edge value is a true global maximum of the likelihood function. For the models we consider here, these checks have already been done and the details can be found in Cox and Hinkley (1974), Graybill (1976), Judge et al. (1985), and Dobson (1990), and in the other more subject-specific references provided throughout this chapter.

One of the advantages of maximum likelihood estimation is that the resultant estimators have a Gaussian distribution and the theory provides us with a way to derive the associated variance–covariance matrix of the estimators. This is based on the *information matrix*, defined by

$$I(\boldsymbol{\omega}) = -E\left[\frac{\partial^2 \mathcal{L}}{\partial \boldsymbol{\omega}\, \partial \boldsymbol{\omega}'}\right],$$

where $\boldsymbol{\omega} = (\boldsymbol{\beta}', \sigma^2)'$ is a $(p+1) \times (p+1)$ vector containing all the unknown parameters to be estimated. The inverse of the information matrix provides the variance–covariance matrix of the maximum likelihood estimators. For the linear model considered here, this matrix is

$$I(\boldsymbol{\omega})^{-1} = \begin{bmatrix} \sigma^2(X'X)^{-1} & \mathbf{0} \\ \mathbf{0}' & 2\sigma^4/n \end{bmatrix},$$

where $\mathbf{0}$ is a $p \times 1$ vector with all elements equal to 0. Thus, $I(\boldsymbol{\omega})^{-1}$ is a $(p+1) \times (p+1)$ matrix with the (i,j)th element equal to $\mathrm{Cov}(\omega_i, \omega_j)$. For example, in this case, the $(1, 1)$ element is $\mathrm{Var}(\hat{\beta}_0)$, the $(1, 2)$ element is $\mathrm{Cov}(\hat{\beta}_0, \hat{\beta}_1)$, and the $(p, p+1)$ element is $\mathrm{Cov}(\hat{\beta}_p, \hat{\sigma}^2) = 0$.

Thus, the variance–covariance matrix of $\hat{\boldsymbol{\beta}}_{\mathrm{OLS}}$ is $\mathrm{Var}(\hat{\boldsymbol{\beta}}_{\mathrm{OLS}}) = \sigma^2(X'X)^{-1}$, and we estimate it by

$$\widehat{\mathrm{Var}(\hat{\boldsymbol{\beta}}_{\mathrm{OLS}})} = \hat{\sigma}^2_{\mathrm{OLS}}(X'X)^{-1}, \tag{9.6}$$

where $\hat{\sigma}^2_{\mathrm{OLS}}$ is given in equation (9.5). If we denote the diagonal elements of $(X'X)^{-1}$ by v^{kk}, $k = 0, \ldots, p-1$, then the standard error for a single $[\hat{\beta}_{\mathrm{OLS}}]_k$ is

$$\mathrm{s.e.}([\hat{\beta}_{\mathrm{OLS}}]_k) = \hat{\sigma}_{\mathrm{OLS}}\sqrt{v^{kk}}, \tag{9.7}$$

and a $(1-\alpha)\%$ confidence interval for β_k is

$$[\hat{\beta}_{\mathrm{OLS}}]_k \pm (t_{N-p,\alpha/2})\hat{\sigma}_{\mathrm{OLS}}\sqrt{v^{kk}}, \tag{9.8}$$

where $t_{N-p,\alpha/2}$ is the $\alpha/2$ percentage point from a *t*-distribution on $N-p$ degrees of freedom.

In addition to the test of $H_0: \beta_k = 0$ associated with the confidence interval in equation (9.8), we may also test multiparameter hypotheses about $\boldsymbol{\beta}$, estimate standard errors, and obtain confidence intervals for $\hat{\sigma}^2$. Relevant details and examples appear in Rao (1973), Graybill (1976), Judge et al. (1985), and Searle et al. (1992).

9.1.2 Interpretation and Use with Spatial Data

The OLS estimators are unbiased and the associated confidence intervals are correct *only if the model is correctly specified and includes all relevant covariates.* This means we assume that any spatial pattern observed in the outcome **Y** is due entirely to the spatial patterns in the explanatory covariates, X, so we have no residual *spatial* variation. However, if we inadvertently omit an important covariate, estimates of $\boldsymbol{\beta}$ will be biased (see, e.g., Draper and Smith 1998, pp. 235–238), and if this covariate is also one that varies spatially, we will have residual spatial variation. This residual spatial variation will often manifest itself as spatial autocorrelation in the residual process, $\boldsymbol{\epsilon}$. This means that the variance–covariance matrix of the data, Σ, is not $\sigma^2 I$ as we assumed in equation (9.2), but has a more general form whose elements $\text{Cov}(Y(\boldsymbol{s}_i), Y(\boldsymbol{s}_j)) = \text{Cov}(\epsilon_i, \epsilon_j)$ reflect the residual spatial autocorrelation in the data. Thus, the data are no longer independent, but are spatially correlated.

Sometimes, even if we include all relevant covariates, there may still be residual spatial autocorrelation. Some outcomes vary inherently in such a way that the value at any location is strongly related to nearby values, and try as we might, we may never be able to find or measure a suitable covariate or set of covariates to fully describe this complex variation. Examples include the spatial variation in an infectious disease or in a disease with complex environmental risk factors.

Both situations (missing spatially referenced covariates or inherent spatial similarity) result in spatially correlated error terms. Thus, in Section 9.2 we incorporate residual spatial autocorrelation into multiple regression models.

DATA BREAK: Raccoon Rabies in Connecticut We assume that most readers are familiar with the basics of multiple linear regression models with spatially independent errors as outlined above. Nonetheless, the material involves a fair amount of notation and many matrix equations, and we now provide an illustrative application of the approaches to a spatial study of raccoon rabies transmission in Connecticut.

Raccoon rabies has long been endemic in Florida, but it was unknown in the northern states until around the mid-1970s, when a restocking program apparently transported rabid raccoons from Florida to Virginia and West Virginia (see Moore 1999). The data for this data break are Y_i, the month of the first reported case of raccoon rabies for the ith township in Connecticut, u_i, the distance east, in kilometers, from the southwest corner of the state, and v_i, the distance north, in kilometers, from the southwest corner of the state. The goal of our analysis here is to use a particular type of multiple linear regression analysis called *trend surface analysis* to try to determine areas of fast or slow spread of rabid raccoons in order to better understand the speed and direction of transmission in various habitats.

In trend surface analysis, the broad spatial variation in the data is modeled as a linear combination of polynomial functions of the spatial locations. That is, we seek to explain all of the spatial pattern in the data with the (spatially defined) covariates, and do not use spatially correlated errors. A *polynomial trend surface* of degree r is defined by

$$\mu(s) = \sum_{k}\sum_{l}^{0 \le k+l \le r} \beta_{kl} u^k v^l, \qquad s = (u, v)'$$

[consisting of $(r+1)(r+2)/2$ terms]. For example, a quadratic ($r = 2$) trend surface is given by

$$\mu(s) = \beta_{00} + \beta_{10} u + \beta_{01} v + \beta_{20} u^2 + \beta_{11} uv + \beta_{02} v^2.$$

Historically, trend surface analysis has been based on the assumption that any residual variation is spatially uncorrelated, so the trend surface model is equivalent to the regression model given in equation (9.1) with X defined by the u^k and v^l terms in $\mu(s)$ and $\mathrm{Var}(\boldsymbol{\epsilon}) = \sigma^2 I$, as in equation (9.2). The trend surface parameters, $\boldsymbol{\beta}$, can then be estimated using equation (9.4) and a contour map displaying the fitted values $\hat{Y}(s) = \sum_{k}\sum_{l}^{0 \le k+l \le r} \widehat{\beta}_{kl_{\mathrm{OLS}}} u^k v^l$ as a function of u and v depicts the spatial variation in Y.

To determine the order of a trend surface that describes the raccoon rabies data, some appropriate plots can give us a lot of preliminary information. A posting of the data is shown in Figure 9.1, and a three-dimensional scatter diagram is shown in Figure 9.2. From these figures we see that the spread of raccoon rabies moves

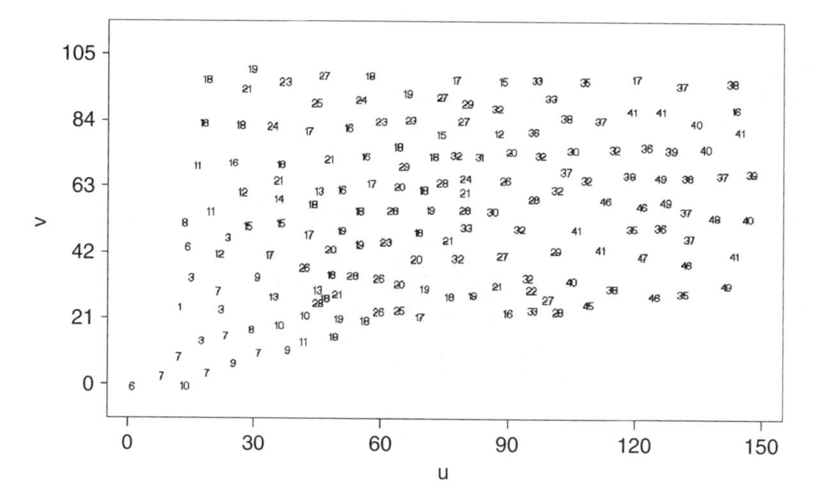

FIG. 9.1 Month of first reported case of raccoon rabies in Connecticut.

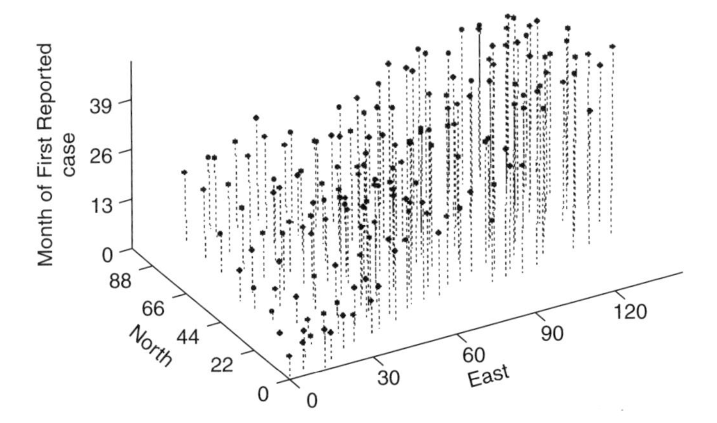

FIG. 9.2 Scatter diagram of raccoon rabies data.

north and east from the southwest corner of the state (entering in the township labeled "1" in Figure 9.1), with the latest occurrence in the southeastern part of the state. We use trend surface analysis to model this spread. From the scatter diagram we can see that there is some curvature to the scatter (this can be seen more clearly by making two-dimensional scatter plots of Y_i vs. u_i and Y_i vs. v_i), so we will fit a second-order trend surface to these data (Figure 9.3). Thus, this trend surface assumes that

$$E[Y] = \beta_0 + \beta_1 u + \beta_2 v + \beta_3 uv + \beta_4 u + \beta_5 v. \tag{9.9}$$

The results are shown in Table 9.1. We could also use stepwise regression to determine the important terms for our regression model. The resulting surface may not be a trend surface per se (since it may not include all of the terms required in the definition of a trend surface function), but instead, would be a response surface model based on just the most important terms in equation (9.9).

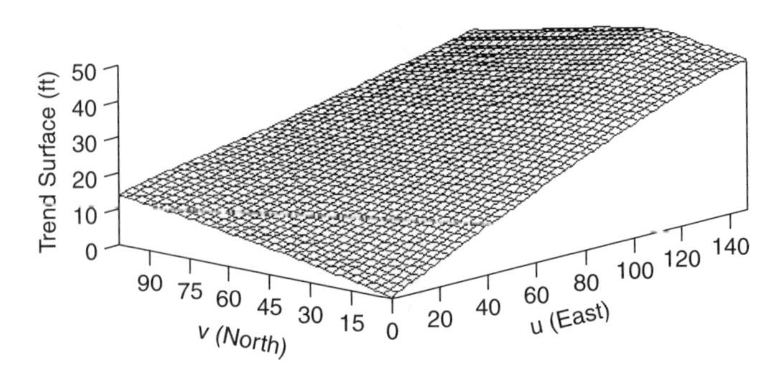

FIG. 9.3 Second-order trend surface fit to the raccoon rabies data.

Table 9.1 Results from Ordinary Least Squares Estimation of Trend Surface Parameters[a]

Order	Effect	$\hat{\beta}$	95% Confidence Interval Lower Bound	95% Confidence Interval Upper Bound
$r = 2$	Intercept	−0.7890		
	u	3.1601	2.1168	4.2035
	v	1.5537	0.0195	3.0880
	uv	−0.2262	−0.3266	−0.1258
	u^2	0.0413	−0.0230	0.1056
	v^2	0.0115	−0.1350	0.1580

[a] Original spatial coordinates (u, v) were divided by 10 so $\hat{\beta}$ and the confidence intervals should be scaled accordingly for interpretation.

To better understand the spread of raccoon rabies, we can determine the direction and magnitude of the most rapid increase in this surface at each location. From vector calculus, this is given by the gradient of $\hat{Y}$, denoted here by $\nabla\hat{Y}(u_0, v_0) = (\partial\hat{Y}/\partial u)_0\vec{i} + (\partial\hat{Y}/\partial v)_0\vec{j}$, where $(\partial\hat{Y}/\partial u)_0$ is the partial derivative of $\hat{Y}$ with respect to u evaluated at (u_0, v_0), $(\partial\hat{Y}/\partial v)_0$ is the partial derivative of $\hat{Y}$ with respect to v evaluated at (u_0, v_0), and $\vec{i}$ and $\vec{j}$ are unit basis vectors [e.g., $\vec{i}$ is the vector from (0,0) to (1,0)]. Thus, for our fitted second-order trend surface,

$$\nabla\hat{Y}(u_0, v_0) = \left(\hat{\beta}_1 + \hat{\beta}_3 v_0 + 2\hat{\beta}_4 u_0\right)\vec{i} + \left(\hat{\beta}_2 + \hat{\beta}_3 u_0 + 2\hat{\beta}_5 v_0\right)\vec{j}.$$

The instantaneous rate of change of $\hat{Y}$ per unit distance in the direction of the gradient is

$$r = \sqrt{(\hat{\beta}_1 + \hat{\beta}_3 v_0 + 2\hat{\beta}_4 u_0)^2 + (\hat{\beta}_2 + \hat{\beta}_3 u_0 + 2\hat{\beta}_5 v_0)^2}.$$

Plotting the direction of most rapid increase in the trend surface as a vector with length r using a *vector plot* shows the spread of raccoon rabies (see Figure 9.4). The initial direction is northeast, but the spread turns southeast about midway across the state. Ecological data important for determining conditions favorable to raccoon habitats and rabies transmission (e.g., location of wooded areas and preferred food and water sources, temperature, and elevation data) might help us better understand the reasons for the transmission pattern of raccoon rabies in Connecticut.

9.2 LINEAR REGRESSION MODELS FOR SPATIALLY AUTOCORRELATED DATA

In previous sections we assumed that all spatial variation in the outcome variable of interest can be completely described by a collection of spatially varying covariates.

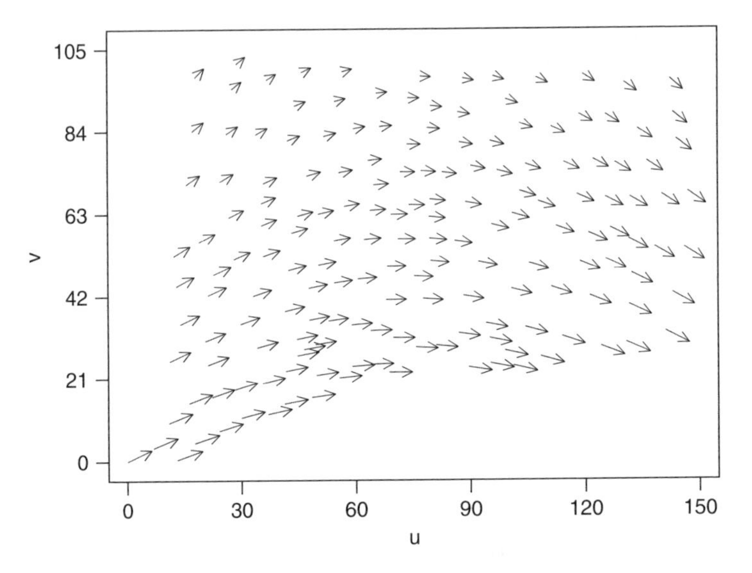

FIG. 9.4 Vector diagram of fitted second-order trend surface.

In this section we relax this assumption. We still assume the same linear relationship between the outcome variable and the covariates [equation (9.1)], but in addition to the spatially varying covariates, we allow the data to be spatially correlated. This means that the variance–covariance matrix of the data becomes

$$\Sigma = \mathrm{Var}(\mathbf{Y}) = \mathrm{Var}(\boldsymbol{\epsilon}), \tag{9.10}$$

where the (i, j)th element of Σ is $\mathrm{Cov}(Y(\boldsymbol{s}_i), Y(\boldsymbol{s}_j))$. The geostatistical models described in Chapter 8 are special cases of this more general linear model obtained by assuming that $X \equiv \mathbf{1}$, where $\mathbf{1}$ is an $n \times 1$ vector whose elements are all equal to 1. In this case, $E[Y(\boldsymbol{s})] = \mu$ for all locations $\boldsymbol{s}$, which is one component of the assumption of second-order stationarity defined in Section 8.1. Thus, the more general linear model allows us to relax the assumptions of stationarity we made in Chapter 8. The term $X\boldsymbol{\beta}$ is often referred to as the *mean structure*, *large-scale variation*, or *trend*, to distinguish this variation from the variation in the residual vector, $\boldsymbol{\epsilon}$, that defines the *small-scale variation* in the data and determines the *stochastic dependence structure* or *residual autocorrelation* in the data. (Note that this usage of the terms *large scale* and *small scale* for broad trends and small details, respectively, is different from the cartographic usages of the terms defined in Chapter 3.) The residual process adjusts the model for any residual spatial variation remaining in the data after accounting for covariate effects.

9.2.1 Estimation and Inference

If Σ is known, we may use maximum likelihood methods to obtain an estimator of $\boldsymbol{\beta}$. It is slightly more general and often easier for computations to assume that

Σ is known up to a constant, that is,

$$\Sigma = \sigma^2 V, \tag{9.11}$$

where σ^2 is an unknown parameter to be estimated and the elements of V reflect the residual spatial correlation [directly generalizing equation (9.2)].

Assuming that $\mathbf{Y} \sim MVN(X\boldsymbol{\beta}, \sigma^2 V)$, the log likelihood is

$$\begin{aligned}\mathcal{L} &= \ln[l(\boldsymbol{\beta}, \sigma^2|\mathbf{Y}, X)] \\ &= -\frac{N}{2}\ln(2\pi) - \frac{N}{2}\ln(\sigma^2) - \frac{1}{2}\ln|V| - \frac{(\mathbf{Y} - X\boldsymbol{\beta})'V^{-1}(\mathbf{Y} - X\boldsymbol{\beta})}{2\sigma^2},\end{aligned} \tag{9.12}$$

where $|V|$ denotes the determinant of V. We use the same approach as for the linear model with uncorrelated residuals (Section 9.1.1) to obtain the maximum likelihood estimators of $\boldsymbol{\beta}$ and σ^2. Thus, the maximum likelihood estimator of $\boldsymbol{\beta}$, also called the *generalized least squares* (GLS) *estimator*, is

$$\hat{\boldsymbol{\beta}}_{\text{GLS}} = (X'V^{-1}X)^{-1}X'V^{-1}\mathbf{Y}, \tag{9.13}$$

and the maximum likelihood estimator of σ^2, adjusted for the loss in degrees of freedom resulting from estimating $\boldsymbol{\beta}$, becomes

$$\hat{\sigma}^2_{\text{GLS}} = \frac{(\mathbf{Y} - X\hat{\boldsymbol{\beta}}_{\text{GLS}})'V^{-1}(\mathbf{Y} - X\hat{\boldsymbol{\beta}}_{\text{GLS}})}{N - p}. \tag{9.14}$$

Of course, Σ is usually not known, and it is difficult to estimate the elements of Σ, since in the spatial setting we have only a single realization. That is, there is no independent replication; we have only a single "subject" with which to work. Even in the case where $\text{Var}(Y(\boldsymbol{s})) = \sigma^2$ (i.e., the diagonal elements of Σ are all equal), there are $N(N-1)/2$ remaining elements to estimate. If $n = 15$, a small sample by most standards, we would have 105 covariance parameters to estimate! One way around this problem is to create a parametric model for the elements of Σ so that the number of parameters in this model is much less than $N(N-1)/2$. However, we cannot use just any model: Since Σ is a variance–covariance matrix, we need to ensure that it satisfies the properties of a variance–covariance matrix (i.e., it must be symmetric and positive definite). Also, since Σ is describing residual spatial variation, we would also like to be able to interpret our estimates in this context. The parametric semivariogram models described in Section 8.2.2 provide a convenient way to meet all of these criteria.

Recall from Section 8.1 that under the assumption of second-order stationarity, the covariances that define the elements of Σ, $\text{Cov}\left(Y(\boldsymbol{s}_i), Y(\boldsymbol{s}_j)\right)$, depend only on the difference between locations $\boldsymbol{s}_i$ and $\boldsymbol{s}_j$, not on the locations themselves. This is quantified by the covariance function, $C(\boldsymbol{s}_i - \boldsymbol{s}_j)$, where $C(\boldsymbol{s}_i - \boldsymbol{s}_j) = \text{Cov}\left(Y(\boldsymbol{s}_i), Y(\boldsymbol{s}_j)\right)$. Also recall from Section 8.2.1 that the covariance function is related to the semivariogram by the relationship

$$C(\boldsymbol{s}_i - \boldsymbol{s}_j) = C(0) - \gamma(\boldsymbol{s}_i - \boldsymbol{s}_j), \tag{9.15}$$

where $C(0) = \mathrm{Var}(Y(\mathbf{s}))$. If the spatial process is isotropic, then $\gamma(\mathbf{s}_i - \mathbf{s}_j)$ is a function only of the distance between locations $\mathbf{s}_i$ and $\mathbf{s}_j$ [i.e., $\gamma(\mathbf{s}_i - \mathbf{s}_j) \equiv \gamma(h)$, where $h = \|\mathbf{s}_i - \mathbf{s}_j\|$]. Thus, from the semivariogram models described and illustrated in Section 8.2.2, we obtain a comparable set of valid models for the covariance function using the relationship in equation (9.15). For example, consider the exponential semivariogram model defined in equation (8.6):

$$\gamma(h; \boldsymbol{\theta}) = \begin{cases} 0, & h = 0 \\ c_0 + c_e[1 - \exp(-h/a_e)], & h > 0, \end{cases}$$

where $\boldsymbol{\theta} = (c_0, c_e, a_e)'$, c_0 is the nugget effect, the sill $c_0 + c_e$ is the variance of $Y(\mathbf{s})$, and the effective range (cf. Section 8.2.2) of autocorrelation is $3a_e$. Using the relationship in equation (9.15), the exponential covariance function is

$$C(h; \boldsymbol{\theta}) = \begin{cases} c_0 + c_e, & h = 0 \\ c_e[\exp(-h/a_e)], & h > 0. \end{cases}$$

Using parametric covariance functions such as this one to describe the matrix elements, Σ becomes a function of $\boldsymbol{\theta}$, denoted here as $\Sigma(\boldsymbol{\theta})$. For example, using the exponential covariance function, the (i, j)th element of $\Sigma(\boldsymbol{\theta})$ is $\mathrm{Cov}(Y(\mathbf{s}_i), Y(\mathbf{s}_j)) = c_e[\exp(-\|\mathbf{s}_i - \mathbf{s}_j\|/a_e)]$. Thus, $\Sigma(\boldsymbol{\theta})$ depends on at most three parameters, c_0, c_e, and a_e, that we estimate from the data. Any of the semivariogram models and the rules for creating more complex semivariogram models given in Section 8.2.2 provide models for the covariance function and $\Sigma(\boldsymbol{\theta})$.

In Sections 8.2.3 and 8.2.4 we describe and illustrate how to estimate the semivariogram from the data and fit parametric models to the empirical semivariogram to ensure a valid semivariogram function. However, in the general linear model where $\mu(\mathbf{s}) = \mathbf{x}(\mathbf{s})'\boldsymbol{\beta} \neq \mu$ (i.e., the mean is not constant but depends on the spatial locations through the covariates) and the residuals are spatially correlated, estimation of the semivariogram is more difficult. To see this, consider estimating $\gamma(\cdot)$ using the classical semivariogram estimator given in equation (8.8). Under the model defined by equations (9.1) and (9.10),

$$\begin{aligned} E[(Y(\mathbf{s}_i) - Y(\mathbf{s}_j)]^2 &= \mathrm{Var}(Y(\mathbf{s}_i) - Y(\mathbf{s}_j)) + [\mu(\mathbf{s}_i) - \mu(\mathbf{s}_j)]^2 \\ &= 2\gamma(\mathbf{s}_i - \mathbf{s}_j) + \left\{ \sum_{k=0}^{p} \beta_k [x_k(\mathbf{s}_i) - x_k(\mathbf{s}_j)] \right\}^2, \end{aligned}$$

with $x_0(\mathbf{s}_i) \equiv 1$ for all i (Cressie 1993, p. 165). Thus, when we average pairs of values to estimate the semivariogram at each lag, the empirical semivariogram will no longer estimate the true, theoretical semivariogram. If the covariates are trend surface functions, the trend often manifests itself in practice by an empirical semivariogram that increases rapidly with $\|\mathbf{h}\|$ (often, quadratically). The empirical semivariogram based on the raccoon rabies data described in the data break following Section 9.1 (Figure 9.5) provides a typical example.

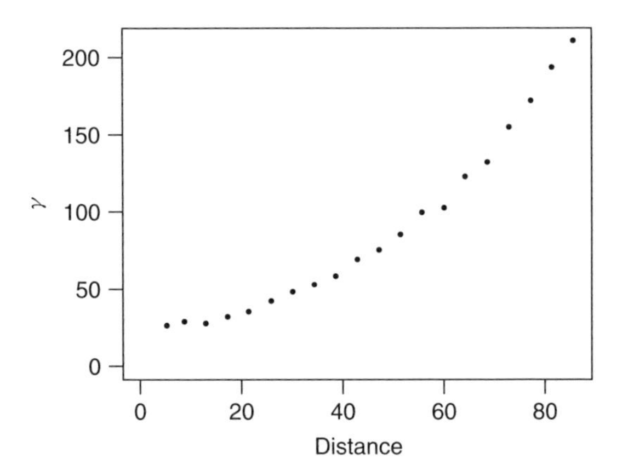

FIG. 9.5 Semivariogram of month of first occurrence of raccoon rabies.

If $\boldsymbol{\beta}$ was known, we could use it to adjust for the bias in the empirical semivariogram estimator. Of course, $\boldsymbol{\beta}$ is not known and to (optimally) estimate it, we need to know $\gamma(\cdot)$! To get us out of this circular argument, we need to estimate $\boldsymbol{\beta}$ and $\gamma(\cdot)$ simultaneously. In the following sections we describe two methods often used to estimate the parameters of a semivariogram model, and equivalently, the parameters in $\Sigma(\boldsymbol{\theta})$, under the general linear model defined by equations (9.1) and (9.10): iteratively reweighted generalized least squares (IRWGLS) and maximum likelihood (ML).

Iteratively Reweighted Generalized Least Squares (IRWGLS) As described in Section 8.2.4, we select a theoretical semivariogram function, $\gamma(h; \boldsymbol{\theta})$, defined up to a vector of parameters $\boldsymbol{\theta}$. To estimate both $\boldsymbol{\theta}$ and $\boldsymbol{\beta}$, we proceed as follows:

1. Obtain a starting estimate of $\boldsymbol{\beta}$, say $\hat{\boldsymbol{\beta}}$.
2. Compute residuals $\boldsymbol{r} = \mathbf{Y} - X\hat{\boldsymbol{\beta}}$.
3. Estimate and model the semivariogram of the residuals using techniques described in Section 8.2. This yields $\gamma(h; \hat{\boldsymbol{\theta}})$ and, correspondingly, $\Sigma(\hat{\boldsymbol{\theta}})$.
4. Obtain a new estimate of $\boldsymbol{\beta}$ using $\hat{\boldsymbol{\beta}} = \hat{\boldsymbol{\beta}}_{\text{GLS}} = (\mathbf{X}'\Sigma(\hat{\boldsymbol{\theta}})^{-1}\mathbf{X})^{-1}\mathbf{X}'\Sigma(\hat{\boldsymbol{\theta}})^{-1}\mathbf{Y}$.
5. Repeat steps 2–4 until the change in estimates of $\boldsymbol{\beta}$ and $\boldsymbol{\theta}$ are "small" (e.g., $<10^{-5}$).

Cressie (1993) shows that the semivariogram estimators based on the residuals $\mathbf{Y} - X\hat{\boldsymbol{\beta}}$ (step 3 above) are biased and discusses some consequences of this bias. He suggests that if the semivariogram parameters are estimated by weighted nonlinear least squares as described in Section 8.2.4, the effect of the bias should be small. Likelihood-based techniques, described below, offer another alternative.

IRWGLS gives an estimator of $\boldsymbol{\beta}$ often referred to as an *estimated generalized least squares* (EGLS) *estimator*, $\hat{\boldsymbol{\beta}}_{\text{EGLS}}$. Thus, if we denote the estimator of $\boldsymbol{\theta}$

obtained from IRWGLS by $\hat{\boldsymbol{\theta}}_{\text{EGLS}}$, the EGLS estimator of $\boldsymbol{\beta}$ is

$$\hat{\boldsymbol{\beta}}_{\text{EGLS}} = [X'\Sigma(\hat{\boldsymbol{\theta}}_{\text{EGLS}})^{-1}X]^{-1}X'\Sigma(\hat{\boldsymbol{\theta}}_{\text{EGLS}})^{-1}\mathbf{Y}. \tag{9.16}$$

Generalizing equation (9.6), an estimator of the variance of $\hat{\boldsymbol{\beta}}_{\text{EGLS}}$ is

$$\widehat{\text{Var}(\hat{\boldsymbol{\beta}}_{\text{EGLS}})} = [X'\Sigma(\hat{\boldsymbol{\theta}}_{\text{EGLS}})^{-1}X]^{-1}. \tag{9.17}$$

If we denote the diagonal elements of $[X'\Sigma(\hat{\boldsymbol{\theta}}_{\text{EGLS}})^{-1}X]^{-1}$ by s^{kk}, the standard error for a single $[\hat{\boldsymbol{\beta}}_{\text{EGLS}}]_k$ in $\boldsymbol{\beta}$ is $\sqrt{s^{kk}}$, and a $(1-\alpha)\%$ confidence interval for β_k is

$$[\hat{\boldsymbol{\beta}}_{\text{EGLS}}]_k \pm (t_{N-p,\alpha/2})\sqrt{s^{kk}}, \tag{9.18}$$

where $t_{N-p,\alpha/2}$ is the $\alpha/2$ percentage point from a t-distribution on $N-p$ degrees of freedom. The theoretical properties of the EGLS estimators are discussed in Judge et al. (1985, pp. 175–177).

Likelihood Methods The procedure described in Section 9.1.1 also provides maximum likelihood estimators of $\boldsymbol{\beta}$ and $\boldsymbol{\theta}$ (Mardia and Marshall 1984). The log likelihood is now

$$\mathcal{L} = \ln[l(\boldsymbol{\beta}, \boldsymbol{\theta}|\mathbf{Y}, X)] = -\frac{N}{2}\ln(2\pi) - \frac{1}{2}\ln|\Sigma| - (\mathbf{Y} - X\boldsymbol{\beta})'\Sigma^{-1}(\mathbf{Y} - X\boldsymbol{\beta}), \tag{9.19}$$

and we assume that $\Sigma \equiv \Sigma(\boldsymbol{\theta})$. Unfortunately, the score equations for $\boldsymbol{\theta}$ do not lead to a closed-form solution for $\boldsymbol{\theta}$. Thus, a common practice is to maximize the *concentrated log likelihood*, obtained from substituting the solution to the score equation for $\boldsymbol{\beta}$ [equation (9.13) with $V = \Sigma(\boldsymbol{\theta})$] into the log likelihood in equation (9.19). The concentrated log likelihood then depends only on $\boldsymbol{\theta}$, and ignoring the constant $(N/2)\ln(2\pi)$ is

$$\mathcal{L}^*(\boldsymbol{\theta}) = -\frac{N}{2}\ln\left[n^{-1}e(\boldsymbol{\theta})'\Sigma(\boldsymbol{\theta})^{-1}e(\boldsymbol{\theta})\right] - \frac{1}{2}\ln|\Sigma(\boldsymbol{\theta})| - \frac{N}{2},$$

where $e(\boldsymbol{\theta}) = \mathbf{Y} - X[X'\Sigma(\boldsymbol{\theta})^{-1}X]^{-1}X'\Sigma(\boldsymbol{\theta})^{-1}\mathbf{Y}$ (the observed values minus the model's predicted values). Maximizing $\mathcal{L}^*$ is equivalent to minimizing

$$\mathcal{Q}(\boldsymbol{\theta}) = N\ \ln[e(\boldsymbol{\theta})'\Sigma(\boldsymbol{\theta})^{-1}e(\boldsymbol{\theta})] + \ln|\Sigma(\boldsymbol{\theta})|. \tag{9.20}$$

There are many algorithms for finding $\boldsymbol{\theta}$ that minimize equation (9.20), and the Newton–Raphson algorithm is perhaps the best known. Most textbooks on nonlinear regression (e.g., Seber and Wild 1989) provide a description of this algorithm and other nonlinear optimization techniques. Most implementations involve a grid search procedure over the range of possible values of $\boldsymbol{\theta}$ evaluating equation (9.20) systematically over a specified range of values and finding the value of $\boldsymbol{\theta}$ producing the minimum value of $\mathcal{Q}(\boldsymbol{\theta})$. More sophisticated algorithms make this search procedure more efficient (and hopefully, faster!), and seek to avoid convergence to a local rather than a global minimum. In practice, we often combine such approaches with additional algorithms to avoid repeated inversion of large unstructured matrices (Mardia and Marshall 1984; Zimmerman 1989).

Given the maximum likelihood estimator of $\boldsymbol{\theta}$, denoted $\tilde{\boldsymbol{\theta}}$, the maximum likelihood estimator of $\boldsymbol{\beta}$ is

$$\tilde{\boldsymbol{\beta}} = [X'\Sigma(\tilde{\boldsymbol{\theta}})^{-1}X)^{-1}X'\Sigma(\tilde{\boldsymbol{\theta}}]^{-1}\mathbf{Y}. \tag{9.21}$$

The asymptotic standard errors of the maximum likelihood estimators derive from the inverse of the information matrix using an approach analogous to that described in Section 9.1.1. In this case, the inverse of the information matrix for $\boldsymbol{\omega} = (\boldsymbol{\beta}', \boldsymbol{\theta}')'$ is (see Breusch 1980; Judge et al. 1985, p. 182)

$$I(\boldsymbol{\omega})^{-1} = \begin{bmatrix} (X'\Sigma(\boldsymbol{\theta})^{-1}X) & \emptyset \\ \emptyset' & \frac{1}{2}\Delta'(\Sigma(\boldsymbol{\theta})^{-1} \bigotimes \Sigma(\boldsymbol{\theta})^{-1})\Delta \end{bmatrix}^{-1}, \tag{9.22}$$

where the matrix $\emptyset$ denotes a $p \times g$ matrix with all elements equal to 0, and $\Delta = \Delta(\boldsymbol{\theta}) = \partial(\text{vec}(\Sigma(\boldsymbol{\theta})))/\partial\boldsymbol{\theta}'$ is an $N^2 \times g$ matrix, where g is the number of elements in $\boldsymbol{\theta}$ that contain the partial derivatives of each element of $\Sigma(\boldsymbol{\theta})$ with respect to each element in $\boldsymbol{\theta}$. The matrix operator vec$(\cdot)$ stacks the columns of a matrix into a single vector, so vec$(\Sigma(\boldsymbol{\theta}))$ is an $N^2 \times 1$ vector. The symbol $\bigotimes$ denotes the matrix direct product multiplying each element in the first matrix by every element in the second matrix producing an $N^2 \times N^2$ matrix.

Although the notation used to define the elements of $I(\boldsymbol{\omega})$ is involved and, in practice, we often leave its computation and inversion to the computer, the variance–covariance matrix of $\tilde{\boldsymbol{\beta}}$ takes the (by now familiar) form

$$\text{Var}(\tilde{\boldsymbol{\beta}}) = [X'\Sigma(\boldsymbol{\theta})^{-1}X]^{-1},$$

estimated via

$$\widehat{\text{Var}}(\tilde{\boldsymbol{\beta}}) = [X'\Sigma(\tilde{\boldsymbol{\theta}})^{-1}X]^{-1}. \tag{9.23}$$

Paralleling previous development, we use $\tilde{v}^{kk}$ to denote the diagonal elements of $[X'\Sigma(\tilde{\boldsymbol{\theta}})X]^{-1}$, so that the standard error for a single $\tilde{\beta}_k$ in $\boldsymbol{\beta}$ can be written as $\sqrt{\tilde{v}^{kk}}$, with a $(1-\alpha)\%$ confidence interval for β_k defined by

$$\tilde{\beta}_k \pm (t_{N-p,\alpha/2})\sqrt{\tilde{v}^{kk}}, \tag{9.24}$$

where $t_{N-p,\alpha/2}$ is the $\alpha/2$ percentage point from a t-distribution on $N-p$ degrees of freedom.

Since maximum likelihood estimators are asymptotically Gaussian, we obtain approximate confidence intervals or associated hypothesis tests for the elements of $\boldsymbol{\theta}$ using

$$\tilde{\theta}_\ell \pm (z_{\alpha/2})\sqrt{\widehat{\text{Var}(\tilde{\theta}_\ell)}}, \tag{9.25}$$

where $\text{Var}(\tilde{\theta}_\ell)$ derives from the inverse of the information matrix, substituting ML estimates for any unknown parameters.

Finally, as discussed in Section 8.2.4, likelihood methods allow us to choose between competing models through the use of likelihood ratio tests of hypotheses about θ_ℓ to see whether a subset of the covariance parameters (θ_ℓs) fits the data as well as the full set. Consider comparing two models of the same form and with the same set of covariates, one based on parameters $\boldsymbol{\theta}_1$ and a larger model based on $\boldsymbol{\theta}_2$, with $\dim(\boldsymbol{\theta}_2) > \dim(\boldsymbol{\theta}_1)$ (i.e., $\boldsymbol{\theta}_1$ is obtained by setting some parameters in $\boldsymbol{\theta}_2$ equal to zero). Then a test of $H_0: \boldsymbol{\theta} = \boldsymbol{\theta}_1$ against the alternative $H_1: \boldsymbol{\theta} = \boldsymbol{\theta}_2$ can be done by comparing

$$2[\mathcal{L}(\boldsymbol{\beta}, \boldsymbol{\theta}_2) - \mathcal{L}(\boldsymbol{\beta}, \boldsymbol{\theta}_1)] \tag{9.26}$$

to a χ^2 with $\dim(\boldsymbol{\theta}_2) - \dim(\boldsymbol{\theta}_1)$ degrees of freedom.

To compare two models that are not nested, we can use Akaike's information criterion (AIC), a penalized-log-likelihood ratio defined by

$$\text{AIC}(\boldsymbol{\beta}, \boldsymbol{\theta}) = \mathcal{L}(\boldsymbol{\beta}, \boldsymbol{\theta}) + 2(p + g), \tag{9.27}$$

where $p + g$ is the number of parameters in the model (Section 8.2.4). We prefer the model with the smallest AIC value.

9.2.2 Interpretation and Use with Spatial Data

In spatial regression, the decomposition of the data into the sum of covariate information and residuals must be done with great thought. Suppose that we left out an important spatially varying covariate (say, x_{p+1}) when we defined X. We might expect residuals from our model to reflect the spatial autocorrelation of the missing variable. By allowing correlated errors, $\boldsymbol{\epsilon}$ effectively "mops up" the excess residual correlation induced by omitting x_{p+1}, and the model omitting x_{p+1} may have overall fit comparable to that of the model including x_{p+1}. So we could have two competing models defined by parameters $(\boldsymbol{\beta}_1, \boldsymbol{\epsilon}_1)$ and $(\boldsymbol{\beta}_2, \boldsymbol{\epsilon}_2)$ with comparable fit. If $X_1\boldsymbol{\beta}_1 \neq X_2\boldsymbol{\beta}_2$, the interpretations in the two models could be *very* different, although both models are valid representations of the spatial variation in the data. In short, for spatial analysis we have to give even greater care to the interpretation of the regression parameters in the models we develop than we would with traditional nonspatial models.

Even if we identify our model with care, there is no guarantee that the statistical estimation algorithms accurately differentiate between what we call the large-scale covariate effects and what we call the small-scale residual autocorrelation parameters, even if a fitting algorithm "converges." The ability to separate these components depends on the data: If covariate effects are strong or the data are not extremely variable, statistical separation of these components usually occurs reliably. However, when the data include a lot of variation and covariate effects are weak, separation of these components is more difficult and the results of the statistical estimation algorithms may be suspect. Careful and varied choices of starting values and thoughtful interpretation of parameter estimates are crucial when fitting the spatial regression models using the iterative approaches outlined above.

9.2.3 Predicting New Observations: Universal Kriging

In addition to providing inferences regarding model parameters, another goal of regression analysis is to use the fitted model to provide predictions of and related inferences for new observations. The same is often true in spatial statistics. We discussed the prediction of new observations in a spatial setting (called *kriging*) in Section 8.3.2. However, in Section 8.3.2 we assumed that the mean was constant [i.e., $E(\mathbf{Y}) = \mu$] and used the semivariogram of the data to develop a spatial prediction technique called *ordinary kriging*. In this section we develop a predictor of $Y(\boldsymbol{s}_0)$, the outcome variable at a new, unobserved location $\boldsymbol{s}_0$, assuming the general linear regression model with autocorrelated errors discussed in Section 9.2. This predictor is known as the *universal kriging predictor*. To parallel the development in Section 8.3.2, we derive the universal kriging predictor in terms of a semivariogram and then show how it can be expressed in terms of a covariance function.

We assume the general linear regression model of equation (9.1) and assume that the residual process has semivariogram $\frac{1}{2}\text{Var}[\epsilon(\boldsymbol{s}_i) - \epsilon(\boldsymbol{s}_j)] = \gamma(\boldsymbol{s}_i - \boldsymbol{s}_j)$. As in 8.3.2, we develop the best linear unbiased predictor (BLUP), following the ideas and notation in Cressie (1993). We consider linear predictors of the form $\hat{Y}(\boldsymbol{s}_0) = \sum_{i=1}^{N} \lambda_i Y(\boldsymbol{s}_i)$, and derive the weights, λ_i, by minimizing the mean-squared prediction error subject to the unbiasedness condition $E[\hat{Y}(\boldsymbol{s}_0)] = \boldsymbol{x}(\boldsymbol{s}_0)'\boldsymbol{\beta}$ for all $\boldsymbol{\beta}$, where the vector of covariates at location $\boldsymbol{s}_0$ is $\boldsymbol{x}(\boldsymbol{s}_0) = [1, x_1(\boldsymbol{s}_0), \ldots, x_{p-1}(\boldsymbol{s}_0)]'$. This condition implies that $\boldsymbol{\lambda}'X = \boldsymbol{x}'(\boldsymbol{s}_0)$, so instead of a single unbiasedness constraint, we need p constraints

$$\sum_{i=1}^{N} \lambda_i = 1, \sum_{i=1}^{N} \lambda_i x_1(\boldsymbol{s}_i) = x_1(\boldsymbol{s}_0), \ldots, \sum_{i=1}^{N} \lambda_i x_{p-1}(\boldsymbol{s}_i) = x_{p-1}(\boldsymbol{s}_0).$$

To find the optimal predictor, we follow the ideas in Section 8.3.2 and minimize the mean-squared prediction error (MSPE), $E\{[\hat{Y}(\boldsymbol{s}_0) - Y(\boldsymbol{s}_0)]^2\}$, subject to $\boldsymbol{\lambda}'X = \boldsymbol{x}'(\boldsymbol{s}_0)$, that is, minimize

$$E\left\{\left[\sum_{i=1}^{N} \lambda_i Y(\boldsymbol{s}_i) - Y(\boldsymbol{s}_0)\right]^2\right\} - 2\sum_{j=0}^{p-1} m_j \left\{\sum_{i=1}^{N} \lambda_i x_j(\boldsymbol{s}_i) - x_j(\boldsymbol{s}_0)\right\} \tag{9.28}$$

[where $x_0(\mathbf{s}) = 1$] with respect to $\lambda_1, \ldots, \lambda_N$, and the p Lagrange multipliers $m_0, \ldots, m_{p-1}$. Expanding terms, we obtain

$$\begin{aligned}\left[\sum_{i=1}^{N} \lambda_i Y(\mathbf{s}_i) - Y(\mathbf{s}_0)\right]^2 &= \left[\boldsymbol{\lambda}' X\boldsymbol{\beta} + \sum_{i=1}^{N} \lambda_i \epsilon(\mathbf{s}_i) - \mathbf{x}'(\mathbf{s}_0)\boldsymbol{\beta} - \epsilon(\mathbf{s}_0)\right]^2 \\ &= \left[\sum_{i=1}^{N} \lambda_i \epsilon(\mathbf{s}_i) - \epsilon(\mathbf{s}_0)\right]^2 \\ &= -\sum_{i=1}^{N}\sum_{j=1}^{N} \lambda_i\lambda_j[\epsilon(\mathbf{s}_i) - \epsilon(\mathbf{s}_j)]^2/2 \\ &\quad + 2\sum_{i=1}^{N} \lambda_i[\epsilon(\mathbf{s}_0) - \epsilon(\mathbf{s}_i)]^2/2.\end{aligned}$$

Taking expectations (9.28) becomes

$$\begin{aligned}-\sum_{i=1}^{N}\sum_{j=1}^{N} \lambda_i\lambda_j\gamma(\mathbf{s}_i - \mathbf{s}_j) + 2\sum_{i=1}^{N} \lambda_i\gamma(\mathbf{s}_0 - \mathbf{s}_i) \\ - 2\sum_{j=0}^{p-1} m_j\left[\sum_{i=1}^{N} \lambda_i x_j(\mathbf{s}_i) - x_j(\mathbf{s}_0)\right].\end{aligned}$$

Differentiating this expression with respect to $\lambda_1, \ldots, \lambda_N, m_0, \ldots, m_{p-1}$ in turn and setting the derivatives equal to zero gives the system of *universal kriging equations*

$$\boldsymbol{\lambda}_{ug} = \Gamma_u^{-1}\boldsymbol{\gamma}_u, \tag{9.29}$$

where

$$\begin{aligned}\boldsymbol{\lambda}_{ug} &= (\lambda_1, \ldots, \lambda_N, m_0, \ldots, m_{p-1})' \\ \boldsymbol{\gamma}_u &= [\gamma(\mathbf{s}_0 - s_1), \ldots, \gamma(\mathbf{s}_0 - \mathbf{s}_N), 1, x_1(\mathbf{s}_0), \ldots, x_{p-1}(\mathbf{s}_0)]'\end{aligned}$$

and

$$\Gamma_u = \begin{cases}\gamma(\mathbf{s}_i - \mathbf{s}_j), & i = 1, \ldots, N;\ j = 1, \ldots, N \\ x_{j-1-N}(\mathbf{s}_i), & i = 1, \ldots, N;\ j = N+1, \ldots, N+p \\ 0, & i = N+1, \ldots, N+p; \\ & j = N+1, \ldots, N+p\end{cases}$$

[with $x_0(\boldsymbol{s}) \equiv 1$]. Thus, the *universal kriging predictor* is

$$\hat{Y}(\boldsymbol{s}_0)_{\text{UK}} = \sum_{i=1}^{N} \lambda_i Y(\boldsymbol{s}_i), \tag{9.30}$$

where the weights $\{\lambda_i\}$ satisfy equations (9.29).

The optimal universal kriging weights also give the minimized MSPE (kriging variance):

$$\begin{aligned}\sigma_k^2(\boldsymbol{s}_0) &= \boldsymbol{\lambda}_{ug}'\boldsymbol{\gamma}_u \\ &= 2\sum_{i=1}^{N} \lambda_i \gamma(\boldsymbol{s}_0 - \boldsymbol{s}_i) - \sum_{i=1}^{N}\sum_{j=1}^{N} \lambda_i\lambda_j\gamma(\boldsymbol{s}_i - \boldsymbol{s}_j).\end{aligned}$$

We can also write the universal kriging equations using general covariance terms:

$$\boldsymbol{\lambda}_u = \Sigma_u^{-1}\mathbf{c}_u, \tag{9.31}$$

where

$$\begin{aligned}\boldsymbol{\lambda}_u &= (\lambda_1, \ldots, \lambda_N, -m_0, \ldots, -m_{p-1})' \\ \mathbf{c}_u &= [\mathbf{c}', 1, x_1(\boldsymbol{s}_0), \ldots, x_{p-1}(\boldsymbol{s}_0)]' \\ \mathbf{c} &= [\text{Cov}(Y(\boldsymbol{s}_0), Y(\boldsymbol{s}_1)), \text{Cov}(Y(\boldsymbol{s}_0), Y(\boldsymbol{s}_2)), \ldots, \text{Cov}(Y(\boldsymbol{s}_0), Y(\boldsymbol{s}_N))]'\end{aligned}$$

and [with $x_0(\boldsymbol{s}) \equiv 1$]

$$\Sigma_u = \begin{cases} \text{Cov}[Y(\boldsymbol{s}_i), Y(\boldsymbol{s}_j)], & i = 1, \ldots, N;\ j = 1, \ldots, N \\ x_{j-1-N}(\boldsymbol{s}_i), & i = 1, \ldots, N;\ j = N+1, \ldots, N+p \\ 0, & i = N+1, \ldots, N+p; \\ & j = N+1, \ldots, N+p. \end{cases}$$

Then, the universal kriging predictor is given in equation (9.30), where the weights $\{\lambda_i\}$ satisfy equations (9.31) and the kriging variance is

$$\sigma_k^2(\boldsymbol{s}_0) = C(\mathbf{0}) - 2\sum_{i=1}^{N} \lambda_i \text{Cov}[Y(\boldsymbol{s}_0), Y(\boldsymbol{s}_i)] + \sum_{i=1}^{N}\sum_{j=1}^{N} \lambda_i\lambda_j \text{Cov}[Y(\boldsymbol{s}_i), Y(\boldsymbol{s}_j)].$$

Developing the universal kriging predictor using covariance terms allows us to use it for prediction with the general linear regression model with autocorrelated errors, specified by the mean function in equation (9.1) and the general variance–covariance matrix Σ defined in equation (9.10). In practice, we assume second-order stationarity so that $\text{Cov}[Y(\boldsymbol{s}_i), Y(\boldsymbol{s}_j)] = C(\boldsymbol{s}_i - \boldsymbol{s}_j)$, and model Σ using parametric functions as described in Section 9.2.1.

Since many geostatistical software packages do not implement universal kriging, it is tempting to try to bypass the universal equations [equations (9.29) and (9.31)] by using ordinary kriging with *detrended data*. The idea is to remove the large-scale mean structure, $X\boldsymbol{\beta}$, and cast the prediction problem into one based on a constant mean that can be handled with ordinary kriging. In this approach, detrending is done by using either ordinary least squares or estimated generalized least squares to estimate $\boldsymbol{\beta}$, and then obtaining the residuals from the fitted model as $\hat{\boldsymbol{\epsilon}} = \mathbf{Y} - X\hat{\boldsymbol{\beta}}$. The residuals have expectation 0, so we can use ordinary kriging (Section 8.3.2) to predict the residual at a new location $\boldsymbol{s}_0$, thus obtaining $\hat{\epsilon}(\boldsymbol{s}_0)_{\text{OK}}$. We can then add the trend or covariates observed at this location, $\boldsymbol{x}(\boldsymbol{s}_0)$, to the kriged residual. Thus, our predicted value of $Y(\boldsymbol{s}_0)$ is $\hat{Y}(\boldsymbol{s}_0) = \boldsymbol{x}'(\boldsymbol{s}_0)\hat{\boldsymbol{\beta}} + \hat{\epsilon}(\boldsymbol{s}_0)_{\text{OK}}$. This approach will give us the same predictions as universal kriging (if the semivariogram or covariance function used in ordinary kriging with model residuals is used in universal kriging and if $\boldsymbol{\beta}$ is estimated using GLS or EGLS and not OLS). However, the prediction errors obtained from the kriging variance will be incorrect for the predictions based on detrended data. The reason for this is somewhat intuitive: The kriging variance from kriging the detrended data does not reflect the uncertainty associated with estimating $\boldsymbol{\beta}$. This reason is also somewhat counterintuitive, since universal kriging does not require estimation of $\boldsymbol{\beta}$. However, if we explicitly solve the universal kriging equations for $\boldsymbol{\lambda}$, the dependence of the UK predictor on $\hat{\boldsymbol{\beta}}_{\text{GLS}}$ and the UK variance on $\text{Var}(\hat{\boldsymbol{\beta}}_{\text{GLS}})$ become clear (see Gotway and Cressie 1993; Cressie 1993, pp. 154, 173). Thus, the kriging variance from universal kriging accounts for the uncertainty in estimating $\boldsymbol{\beta}$, whereas kriging with detrended data does not, and consequently, the prediction errors from kriging detrended data are too low.

By allowing covariate effects, we often simplify the spatial correlation structure required for prediction since many times any anisotropy, nonstationarity, or even spatial correlation in the outcome variable may be due to spatial patterns in relevant covariate effects ignored in the prediction models in Chapter 8. For example, in the model in Section 9.1, the covariates completely describe the spatial variation in the outcome, yielding independent errors and making spatial autocorrelation adjustments irrelevant. In such cases, $\gamma(\boldsymbol{s}_i - \boldsymbol{s}_j)$ represents only a pure nugget effect (i.e., no spatial autocorrelation) and $\Sigma = \sigma^2 I$ [equation (9.2)]. Hence, universal kriging reduces to the traditional prediction with multiple linear regression models. In other applications, directional variation in the outcome process (suggesting anisotropic semivariograms for the outcome variable) may be due entirely to covariate effects. Then, the residual spatial variation characterized by $\gamma(\boldsymbol{s}_i - \boldsymbol{s}_j)$ or Σ exhibits only isotropic spatial variation [see, e.g., Cressie (1993, Section 4.1) and Gotway and Hergert (1997) for some comparative illustrations]. When obtaining point predictions, it matters little if we model the spatial variation entirely through the covariates, entirely as small-scale variation characterized by the semivariogram or Σ, or through some combination of covariates and residual autocorrelation. However, our choice of covariates to include in the model affects both the interpretation of our model and the magnitude of the prediction standard errors, so, as above, it is important to choose our model carefully and rely on a scientific understanding of the spatial process we are studying to help us specify our model.

DATA BREAK: New York Leukemia Data In many public health studies, we would like to use specific covariates to explore associations with the outcome of interest and to adjust our maps for potentially important demographic risk factors. We turn now to a linear regression analysis (with spatially correlated errors) of the New York leukemia data introduced in the data break following Section 4.4.5.

Data Reminder, Assumptions, and Analysis Goals We consider the census tract-level leukemia incidence data introduced earlier covering an eight-county region of upstate New York. As an exposure covariate, we use the inverse distance between each census tract centroid to the nearest of the inactive hazardous waste sites containing trichloroethylene (TCE) (introduced following Section 7.6.5). The use of distance as surrogate for exposure admittedly involves several assumptions. First, we assume that exposure decreases monotonically with the distance from each waste site. Second, we assume that all people residing within a given census tract receive the same exposure. Third, we ignore the amount of TCE reported at each site and treat all sites as sources of equivalent exposure. Finally, we assume that the inverse distance to the *nearest* site represents the only relevant source of TCE exposure. Based on these fairly restrictive simplifying assumptions, we should view all analyses in this chapter as attempts to assess association between leukemia incidence and proximity to locations of sites reporting TCE, not as assessments of associations between leukemia incidence and TCE exposure itself. However, individual exposure is difficult and costly to measure, so these assumptions allow us a fairly fast preliminary indication of elevated leukemia risk that may be associated TCE exposure.

Scrutinizing Model Assumptions Our intent is to use linear regression to model the relationship between the leukemia rate associated with each tract and the inverse distance to the nearest TCE waste site. In using linear regression, we make several rather important assumptions:

1. The linear model with the specified covariates given in equation (9.1) adequately describes the variation in our outcome variable of interest.
2. The error terms, $\epsilon(\boldsymbol{s}_i)$ have zero mean.
3. The data have a constant variance, σ^2.
4. The data are uncorrelated (OLS) or have a specified parametric covariance structure (GLS).
5. The data are multivariate Gaussian.

Diagnostic plots of residuals $\boldsymbol{e} = \mathbf{Y} - X\hat{\boldsymbol{\beta}}$ versus the fitted values $X\hat{\boldsymbol{\beta}}$, residuals versus each covariate, and normal probability plots based on the residuals can be very helpful in assessing model adequacy even when the outcome variable and the covariates are spatially varying [see, e.g., Draper and Smith (1998) for a detailed description and illustration of common methods for residual analysis]. In addition to the traditional methods for residual analysis, a map of the residuals, plots of the residuals versus each spatial coordinate, the empirical semivariogram of the residuals, and maps of local indicators of spatial association based on residuals can be useful in assessing whether there is any remaining spatial variability not accounted for explicitly in the model. If the residuals do show spatial structure, the models described in subsequent sections can be used to account for this spatial variability.

Assumption 5 is necessary if we want to use Gaussian-based likelihood methods for estimation. If we do not want to use likelihood methods, but instead, want to rely on least-squares estimation, we will also need to assume that certain "regularity conditions" are satisfied, so our estimators have nice asymptotic properties and we can construct confidence intervals and make hypothesis tests. In practice, assumption 5 is almost the least of our worries: Linear regression analysis is relatively robust to departures from normality, and even when the data are nonnormal, data transformations, commonly discussed in the literature in most disciplines, can often be used to achieve (or adequately approximate) the desired normality, as illustrated below.

Violations in assumption 3 can have especially severe consequences on statistical inference since standard errors, confidence intervals, and hypothesis tests for the covariate effects (i.e., for the $\hat{\beta}_k$) can be incorrect if this assumption is violated. Assumption 3 is also worth a bit more discussion here since disease counts and rates often violate this assumption in a rather complex way that has not been addressed adequately in the literature.

Referring back to our discussion in Chapter 7, suppose that the number of cases of a particular disease within a region i, Y_i, follows a Poisson distribution under the constant risk assumption. Hence, $E(Y_i) = rn_i$, where n_i is the population size at risk within region i and r is the assumed constant risk of disease. This in turn implies that $\text{Var}(Y_i) = rn_i$, since with the Poisson distribution, $E(Y_i) = \text{Var}(Y_i)$. Thus, when working with disease counts and rates, assumption 3 above is violated in two ways: The variance of the data depends on the mean, and the variance is not constant, but rather, depends on the population sizes that can be very different from region to region. Consequently, we really need to fix two problems: a mean–variance relationship that is usually inherent in discrete data, and heteroscedasticity resulting from the differing population sizes.

A *variance-stabilizing* transformation can be used to remove the dependence of the mean on the variance, and often, an intelligent choice of transformation will fix (or at least improve) nonnormality (violation of assumption 5), nonlinearity (violation of assumption 1), and the mean–variance relationship (violation of assumption 3). There is a wide literature on such transformations, including the well-known families of Box–Cox and power transformations (cf. Carroll and Ruppert 1988; Draper and Smith 1998, Chapter 13; Griffith and Layne 1999, Chapter 2). However, it is rare for any of these transformations to remove heteroscedasticity.

If heteroscedasticity is the only remaining issue following transformation, one solution is to perform a *weighted analysis* (e.g., weighted least squares), where the weights are inversely proportional to the differing variances. Transforming the outcome variable using a variance-stabilizing transformation, and weighting traditional multiple linear regression analysis together provide a widely applied approach for addressing violations in assumption 3.

As we shall see in the rest of this data break, addressing assumptions 1–5 to allow linear modeling of public health data often requires a series of less-than-elegant gyrations and data transformations. However, such analyses remain common in the literature, due primarily to available software and decades of statistical work on methods for assessing departures from these assumptions and making the appropriate corrections. An alternative solution is to use the generalized linear models described in Sections 9.4 and 9.5 that more directly embrace the characteristics of discrete data at the expense of computational simplicity.

Transformations As we mentioned above, the outcome counts, particularly for a rare disease, usually do not follow a Gaussian distribution or even a symmetric distribution (the former a necessary assumption for inference with the maximum likelihood regression methods in Sections 9.1 and 9.2, and the latter for ordinary least squares). Observed incidence proportions (rates) may follow a Gaussian distribution more closely than do counts, but often will not, particularly for very rare outcomes. Second, there is almost always a relationship between the variability in the counts or rates and their expected values (means), violating the Gaussian assumption of independence between regional means and variances.

Functional transformations of the data provide a time-honored approach to addressing these problems in the regression setting where the transformed data better meet the key model assumptions described in Section 9.2.4. The advantages of trying to adapt the analytical methods discussed in Sections 9.1 and 9.2 to spatial counts or rates include the use of widely available software for linear regression and the existence of a broad class of model diagnostics based on residual analysis. The main disadvantage of using linear regression methods with rates or counts lies with the violation of several key model assumptions and the subsequent need to transform the data: it is often difficult to find a suitable transformation addressing all problems simultaneously. Furthermore, unbiased estimation back-transformed to the original scale of measurement is usually impossible. Additional discussion regarding (spatial) regression analysis of regional count data appears in Pocock et al. (1981, 1982), Cook and Pocock (1983), Cressie and Chan (1989), Cressie and Read (1989), Richardson et al. (1992), and Griffith and Layne (1999).

We begin by addressing our first challenge, the need for the outcome data to meet the assumptions of OLS [i.e., the need for the transformed data to be Gaussian (or at least have a relatively symmetric distribution) and to have the variance of the transformed data be independent of the mean]. Note that neither the leukemia counts, Y_i, nor the corresponding proportions, $p_i = Y_i/n_i$, satisfy these assumptions.

Theoretically, we may expect the counts, $Y_i, i = 1, \ldots, N$, to follow binomial distributions since each is bounded above by n_i. However, for large n_i and small p_i their distributions may be approximated adequately by Poisson distributions. Using a Poisson distribution instead of a binomial has the advantage that the square root transformation serves as a variance stabilizing transformation for the Poisson distribution, offering more straightforward implementation and interpretation than the variance stabilizing transformation for the binomial distribution (the arcsine transformation; cf. Draper and Smith 1998, pp. 292–294). However, discussion and analysis in Cressie (1993, pp. 395–396) suggest that the presence of spatial autocorrelation may require a stronger transformation. In his analysis of sudden infant death syndrome (SIDS) data, Cressie (1993, p. 395) suggests three potential transformations. One of these is particularly useful here since it helps to discriminate among the tracts with $Y_i \leq 1$ but with different population sizes:

$$Z_i = \log\left(\frac{1000(Y_i + 1)}{n_i}\right).$$

The effect of this transformation on the data is quite nice, taking a very skewed distribution (Figure 9.6) and transforming it into one that is reasonably symmetric, with a mean value of -0.21 and a median value of -0.28 (Figure 9.7).

Figure 9.7 reveals three rather large observations in the transformed data: 4.71, 2.64, and 2.31. These correspond to tracts with observed leukemia counts of 0, 1, and 0 cases, and associated population counts of 9, 143, and 99 people, respectively. Such extreme observations could affect the results of linear regression analysis, and we briefly take a closer look at these observations.

These three observations provide excellent examples of the small-number problem, having both a very small number of cases and very small population sizes. This is one of the main arguments for spatial smoothing (cf. Section 4.4), but if we smooth the incidence proportions (rates) prior to regression analysis we might also smooth away any effect of the proximity of the TCE locations on the risk of leukemia. We could proceed with linear regression and use the traditional

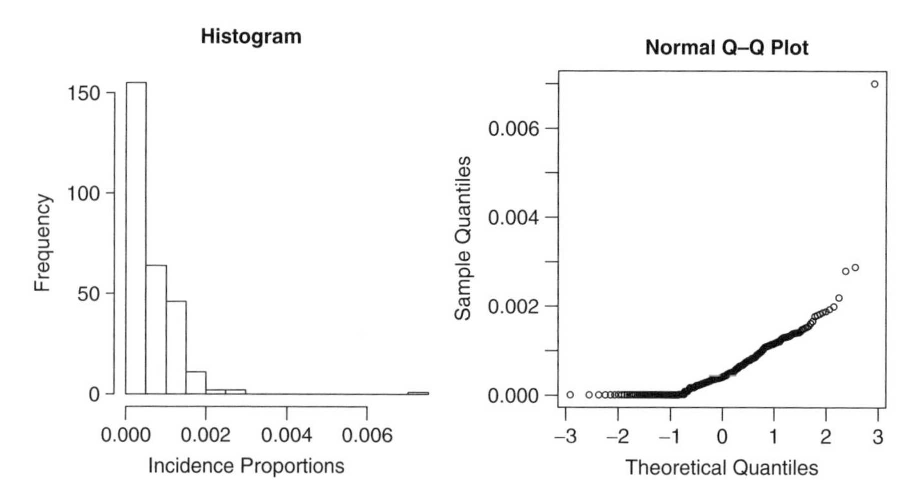

FIG. 9.6 Histogram and QQ plot of incidence proportions for the New York leukemia data.

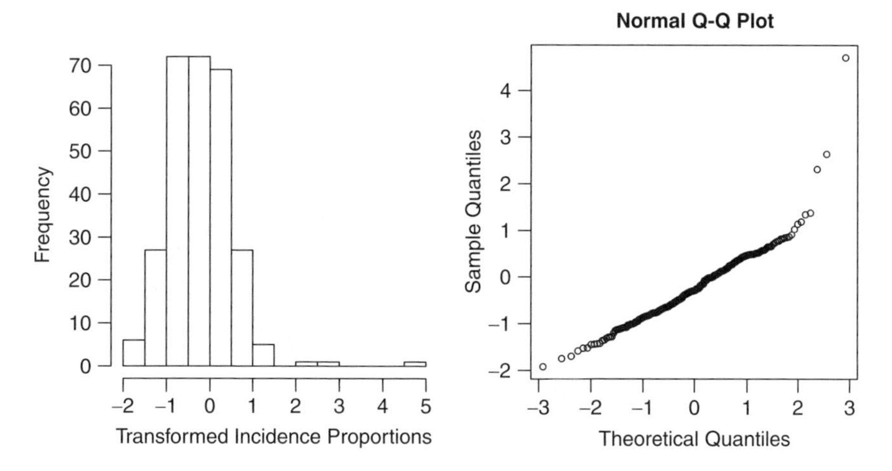

FIG. 9.7 Histogram and QQ plot of the transformed New York leukemia data.

influence diagnostics to help us decide how to treat these observations. However, these diagnostics must be used with caution with spatial data since many of the distributions and test statistics used to measure the potential influence of any one observation on model results can be distorted by residual spatial autocorrelation (cf. Haining 1995). Instead, since our goal is a spatial analysis, we first examine the locations of these observations before we decide what, if anything, we are going to about them. Doing so leads to an interesting revelation: the outlying (transformed) observations occur in adjacent tracts within the city of Syracuse at the southeast end of Lake Onondaga (Figure 9.8). The tracts are bounded by two interstate highways and the lake and have experienced steady emigration from the 1970s to the 1990s as the area became more industrial and commercial. In fact, the three tracts were merged to one in the 1990 U.S. Census, due primarily to their low population sizes. For this analysis, since the potential spatial information contained within these tracts could be important, we leave these observations "as is" in all of our analyses. Analyses without these observations are left as exercises.

Mean–Variance Relationship and Heteroscedasticity While the distribution of the transformed data, Z_i, is fairly Gaussian, we need to determine if the transformation has removed the dependence between the mean and the variance. Such an assessment is rather problematic in this case since both the mean and the variance depend on the population sizes, n_i.

To assess whether or not our transformation removes mean–variance dependence, we follow a procedure suggested by Cressie (1993, p. 395) and partition the tracts into "similarly sized" subsets, each with roughly equal n_i values. Specifically, we split the tracts into seven groups, corresponding to groups of tracts with population sizes between 0 and 999, 1000–1999, 2000–2999, ... , 6000+ people. For each group, we compute the interquartile range of the Z_i, IQ_Z, and then plot $\text{IQ}_Z^2/\text{avg}\{1/n_i\}$ against the median of the Z_i's in each group, where $\text{avg}\{1/n_i\}$

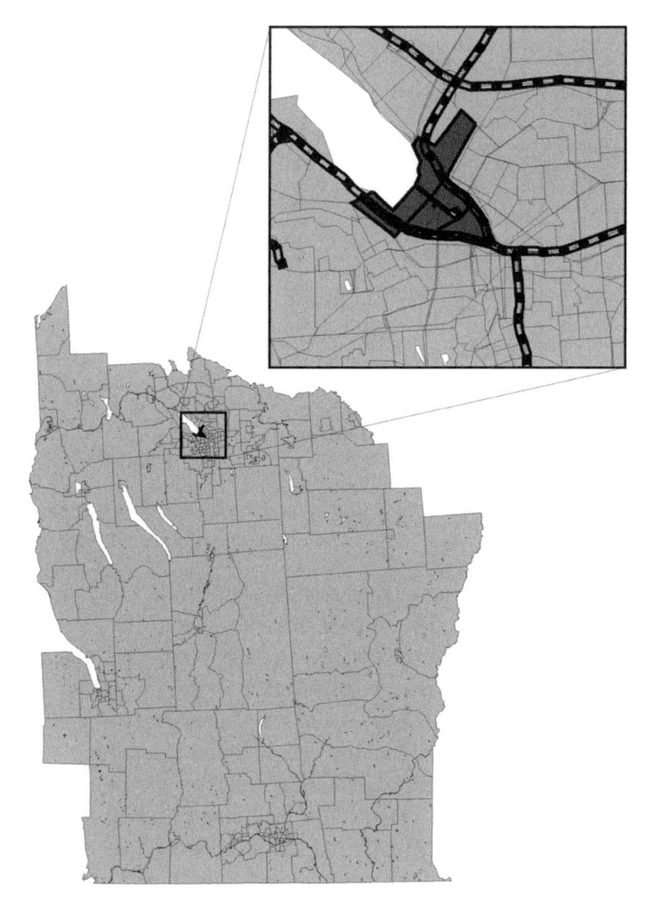

FIG. 9.8 Locations of the tracts containing the three largest values of Z_i (dark gray regions in inset). White area in inset represents Lake Onondaga and black dashed lines represent interstate highways.

is the average (sample mean) of the $1/n_i$ within each group. For each group, IQ_Z^2 provides a resistant (to extreme observations) estimate of $\text{Var}(Z_i)$ and since $\text{Var}(Z_i) \propto 1/n_i$, $\text{IQ}_Z^2/\text{avg}\{1/n_i\}$ should not depend on the n_i, but any dependence on the mean (estimated with the sample median from each group) will remain. Plotting $\text{IQ}_Z^2/\text{avg}\{1/n_i\}$ against the median of the Z_i's in each subset provides a diagnostic plot indicating what relationship, if any, the variance of the Z_i (adjusted for the n_i) has with the mean of the Z_i.

To illustrate the approach, consider the relationship resulting when we use the untransformed proportions, p_i. The relationship depicted in the top plot of Figure 9.9 shows a roughly linear relationship, as may be expected for a Poisson variable. Following transformation to Z_i, a substantial portion of the linear dependence of the variance on the mean has been removed (or least reduced), as shown in the bottom plot of Figure 9.9. Although some dependence between the mean and variance may remain, it appears less pronounced in the Z_i than for the original

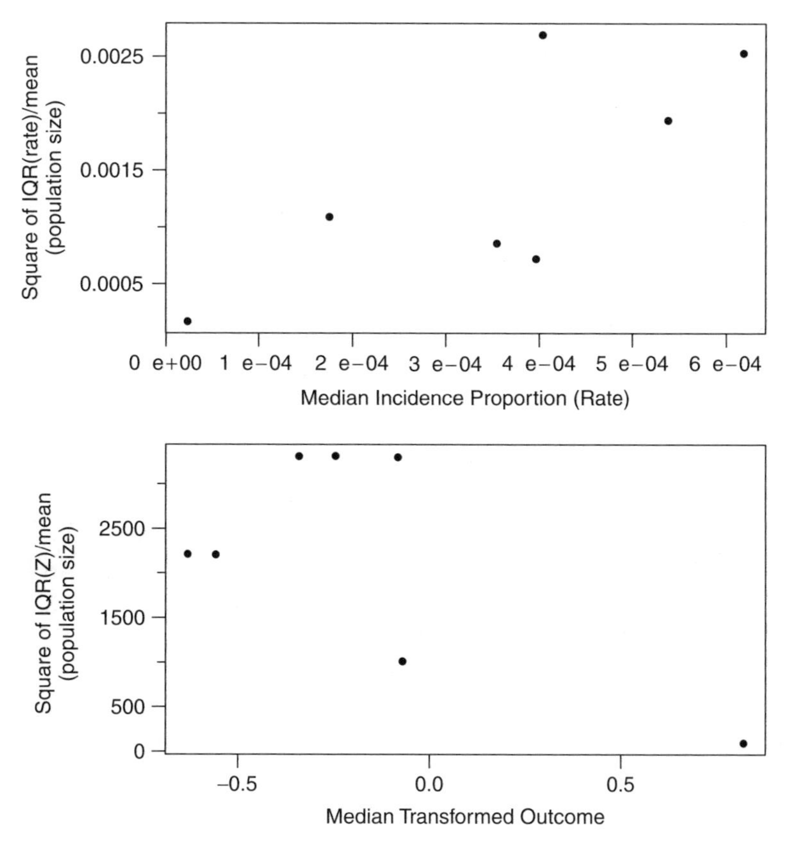

FIG. 9.9 Estimated variance–mean relationship for the incidence proportions (rates), p_i (top), and the transformed outcome Z_i (bottom).

$p_i, i = 1, \ldots, N$, and the Z_i appear to meet linear model assumptions better than do the p_i.

Selecting an appropriate transformation is as much art as science. In practice, we usually consider, compare, and contrast several transformations to arrive at the final transformation. Griffith and Layne (1999, Section 2.2) give a detailed discussion of transformations and provide several examples illustrating their use and evaluation with many different types of spatial data.

Covariates and Transformations In using linear regression analysis, we assume the relationship between the outcome (the transformed proportions, Z) and the potential exposure (the inverse distance between each census tract centroid and the nearest TCE waste site, IDIST) is in fact linear. A scatterplot of the relationship between these two variables (Figure 9.10, upper left) shows a very skewed exposure distribution where the slope of the regression line may be strongly influenced by the five highest exposure values, and the constant variance assumption is questionable. Thus, we chose to transform this variable using $X_1 = \log(100 \times \text{IDIST})$. (The

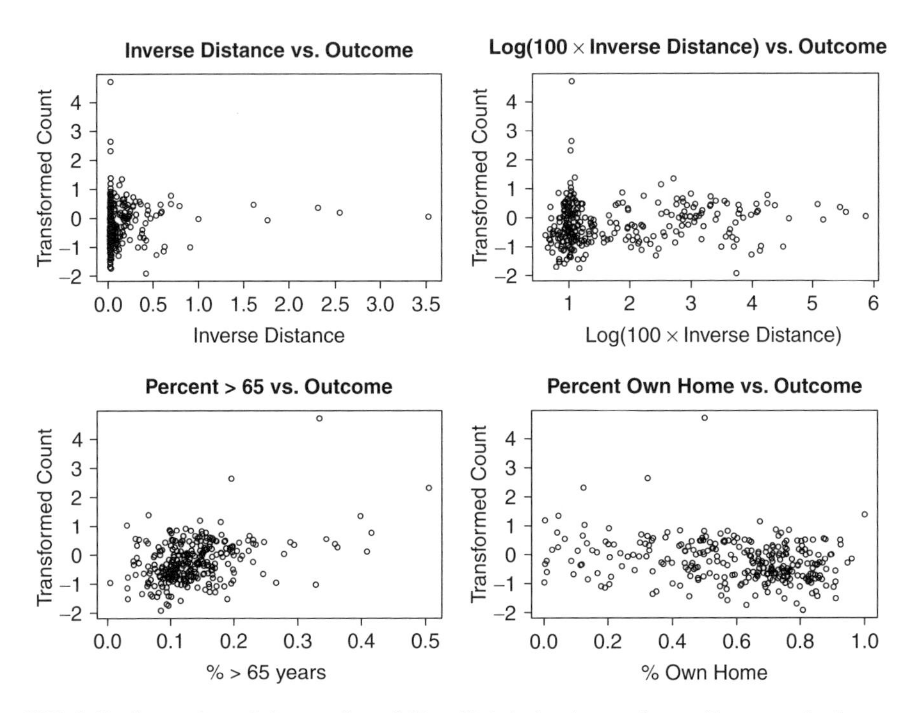

FIG. 9.10 Scatterplots of the transformed New York leukemia prevalence, Z_i, versus the inverse distance to the nearest TCE site IDIST (upper left), Z_i versus log(100 × IDIST) (upper right), Z_i versus the percent in tract i aged over 65 years (lower left), and Z_i versus the percent in tract i that own their own home (lower right).

constant multiplier of 100 is used for convenience to make the values positive.) The scatterplot of this relationship in Figure 9.10 suggests a pattern less driven by high exposure values than the nontransformed exposure and a pattern better meeting the assumption of constant variance (with the possible exception of the three outliers discussed previously).

Any relationship between outcome and our surrogate measure of exposure may be confounded by demographic variables that also potentially affect leukemia rates. For instance, the risk of leukemia increases with age so we expect tracts containing a higher proportion of older people to have a higher incidence of leukemia, regardless of proximity to TCE sites. In addition, measures of socioeconomic status are also of interest in the analysis of health outcomes. For illustration, we include two Census-based variables in our analysis, X_2 = the percentage of residents over 65 years of age, and X_3 = the percentage of the population that own their own home. This latter variable serves as a surrogate for income. Scatterplots of our transformed outcome (Z) and each of these variables appear in the bottom row of Figure 9.10 and the data themselves appear in Table 9.15 at the end of the chapter. In the scatterplots, we see a fairly linear upward trend in Z with increasing percentages over 65 years and perhaps a slight linear decrease in Z with increasing percentages of residences owning homes. We note that this analysis does not fully capture all possible covariates, but rather serves as a general illustration of the modeling techniques described above.

Linear Regression Assuming Independent Errors We are now ready to fit models. To begin, we consider a linear regression model of the form

$$Z_i = \beta_0 + \beta_1 X_{1i} + \beta_2 X_{2i} + \beta_3 X_{3i} + \epsilon_i,$$

where X_{ji} denotes the value of covariate X_j associated with region (tract) i. As a point of comparison, we begin with ordinary least squares (or the equivalent maximum likelihood procedures discussed in Section 9.1.1) to estimate the unknown parameters (the β's) and assess the potential significance of our explanatory variables (the X's) on our transformed outcome.

As we do so, there is one important issue remaining. Recall that in using linear regression models with independent errors (Section 9.1) we assume the variance–covariance matrix of the data is $\sigma^2 I$, i.e., we assume that the data are uncorrelated with constant variance. However, from our earlier discussion we know that the data do not have constant variance. Even though our transformation removed (or at least reduced) dependence on the mean, it did not necessarily remove the heteroscedasticity arising from the differing population sizes since the variance of Z_i is still dependent on the population size n_i. The usual statistical remedy is to perform a *weighted* analysis, where the weights are inversely proportional to the variances. In this case, weighting inversely proportional to $1/n_i$ means that our weights will be n_i. Thus, in performing a weighted analysis, we assume that the variance–covariance matrix of the data is $V = \sigma^2 \text{diag}[1/n_i] \equiv \sigma^2 D$, where $D = \text{diag}[1/n_i]$ is a diagonal matrix with elements $1/n_i$, and use generalized least squares (Section 9.2.1) to estimate the regression parameters. In the statistical literature, this is known as *weighted least squares* and we obtain our estimated parameters via

$$\hat{\boldsymbol{\beta}}_{\text{WLS}} = (X'D^{-1}X)^{-1}X'D^{-1}\mathbf{Z}.$$

Many software packages for linear regression analysis allow the use of a weight variable, but they often differ on how the weights must be specified. Some programs weight inversely proportional to the variable specified (e.g., $1/n_i$ is provided as the weight variable, and the program computes D^{-1}, so weights n_i are actually used), while others assume that the weights themselves are specified (so the program expects that the elements of D^{-1}, the n_i, are specified). Improper weighting can have a disastrous effect on results and conclusions, so it is important to understand what any particular software program actually does. Traditional linear regression software can also be tricked into performing a weighted analysis by regressing $n_i^{1/2} Z_i$ on $n_i^{1/2}$, $n_i^{1/2} X_1$, $n_i^{1/2} X_2$, and $n_i^{1/2} X_3$. Pocock et al. (1981) give a more sophisticated model for weighting in regression analyses of regional health counts and proportions, but for simplicity we will use WLS.

We fit the regression model using both OLS and WLS for comparison. The results, presented in Tables 9.2 and 9.3, respectively, are based on partial sums of squares, where every variable is adjusted for every other variable and not on

Table 9.2 Results of Ordinary Least Squares Linear Regression Applied to the (Transformed) New York Leukemia Data

Parameter	Estimate	Std. Error	t-Value	p-Value
$\hat{\beta}_0$ (intercept)	−0.5173	0.1586	−3.26	0.0012
$\hat{\beta}_1$ (TCE)	0.0488	0.0351	1.39	0.1648
$\hat{\beta}_2$ (% age > 65)	3.9509	0.6055	6.53	<0.0001
$\hat{\beta}_3$ (% own home)	−0.5600	0.1703	−3.29	0.0011
$\hat{\sigma}^2$	0.4318	277 df		
$R^2 = 0.1932$	AIC = 567.5[a]			

[a]Based on maximum likelihood fitting.

Table 9.3 Results of Weighted Least Squares Linear Regression Applied to the (Transformed) New York Leukemia Data

Parameter	Estimate	Std. Error	t-Value	p-Value
$\hat{\beta}_0$ (intercept)	−0.7784	0.1412	−5.51	<0.0001
$\hat{\beta}_1$ (TCE)	0.0763	0.0273	2.79	0.0056
$\hat{\beta}_2$ (% age > 65)	3.8566	0.5713	6.75	<0.0001
$\hat{\beta}_3$ (% own home)	−0.3987	0.1531	−2.60	0.0097
$\hat{\sigma}^2$	1121.94	277 df		
$R^2 = 0.1977$	AIC = 513.5[a]			

[a]Based on maximum likelihood fitting.

sequential sums of squares, where inference for each variable depends on the order in which variables enter the model (cf. Draper and Smith 1998, pp. 151–153).

Referring to Table 9.2, we see that in the OLS analysis, the two census variables are significant, but our surrogate exposure is not. In the weighted analysis (Table 9.3), all covariates are associated significantly with the outcome. Weighting has little effect on model fit (as measured by R^2), but it does have a large impact on some of the parameter estimates and their standard errors. The impact of weighting is most pronounced in the estimate of the effect of our surrogate exposure variable X_1, nearly doubling the parameter estimate and indicating a statistically significant effect (after accounting for the impact of the other covariates). The change indicates the impact of the heterogeneity in population sizes even after transformation, due primarily to lessening the impact of the three outliers (all from counts with small population sizes) on the estimated slope associated with the exposure surrogate.

Figure 9.11 maps the outcome variables predicted (transformed) Z_i. In general, we find higher predictions in the cities and towns, and an interesting set of low

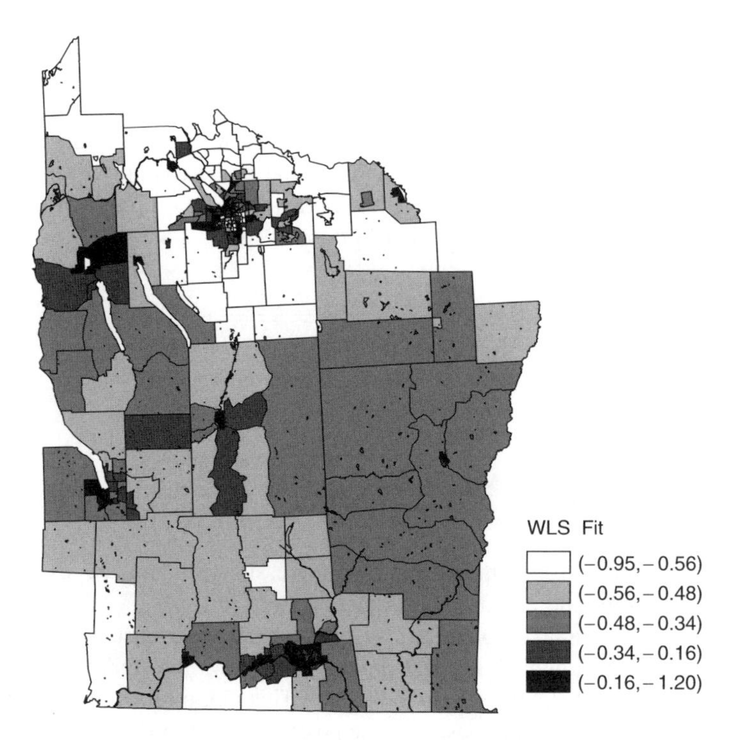

FIG. 9.11 Map of fitted transformed outcomes (Z_i) based on the weighted least squares linear regression model defined in Table 9.3.

predicted values in a ring surrounding Syracuse. There is some suggestion of spatial autocorrelation in the fitted values, as high values tend to occur near other high values and low values near other low values. To this point, we have not used spatial correlation in our models, so this visual tendency is induced entirely by spatial patterns in the covariate values.

Residual Analysis To assess the fit of the model, we consider the vector of residuals from our regression defined by

$$\boldsymbol{e} = \mathbf{Z} - X\hat{\boldsymbol{\beta}}_{\mathrm{WLS}}.$$

The variance–covariance matrix of this residual vector is

$$\mathrm{Var}(\boldsymbol{e}) = \sigma^2(I - H)D,$$

where $H = X(X'D^{-1}X)^{-1}X'D^{-1}$. Since D is a diagonal matrix, the variance of the ith residual is

$$\mathrm{Var}(e_i) = \frac{\sigma^2}{n_i}(1 - h_{ii}),$$

where h_{ii} is the (i, i)th element of H. Consequently, the residuals have different variances and these depend on the n_i even though we used a weighted regression to estimate $\boldsymbol{\beta}$. It is a good idea to take this inequality of variance into account in residual analysis. In our case, it is even more important to do so to make sure that any patterns in the residuals reflect lack of fit and are not simply due to patterns in the different population sizes. Thus, we use *studentized residuals*, residuals that are each divided by their estimated standard error:

$$e_i^s = \frac{e_i}{\sqrt{\widehat{\text{Var}}(e_i)}} = \frac{e_i\sqrt{n_i}}{\sqrt{\hat{\sigma}^2_{\text{WLS}}(1 - h_{ii})}}, \tag{9.32}$$

where

$$\hat{\sigma}^2_{\text{WLS}} = \frac{(\mathbf{Z} - X\hat{\boldsymbol{\beta}}_{\text{WLS}})' D^{-1}(\mathbf{Z} - X\hat{\boldsymbol{\beta}}_{\text{WLS}})}{N - p}$$

is the mean-squared error from the weighted regression. Studentized residuals have expected value zero and a constant variance $\text{Var}(e_i^s) = 1$.

The plot of the residuals against the fitted values provides a standard diagnostic tool in linear regression analysis, and Figure 9.12 shows the studentized residuals plotted against the fitted values from the model. This plot offers no strong evidence of violation of model assumptions, with the possible exception of a particularly low negative residual value, occurring just to the west of Binghamton. In this tract the

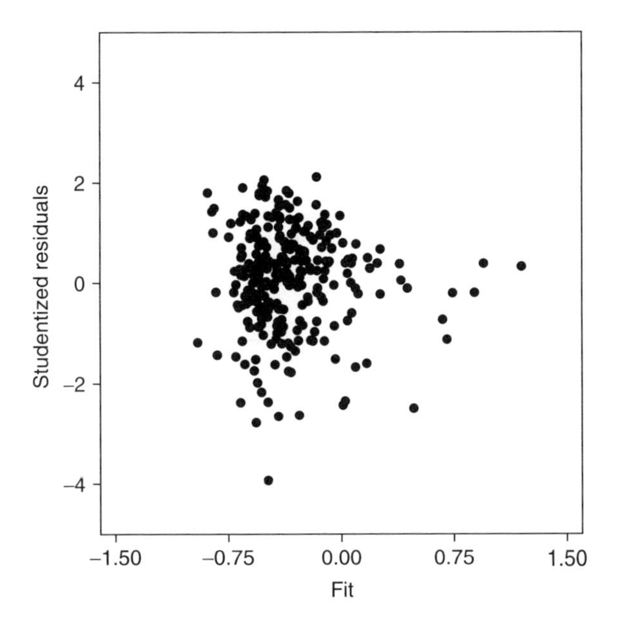

FIG. 9.12 Studentized residuals vs. fitted values from WLS regression (no spatial correlation).

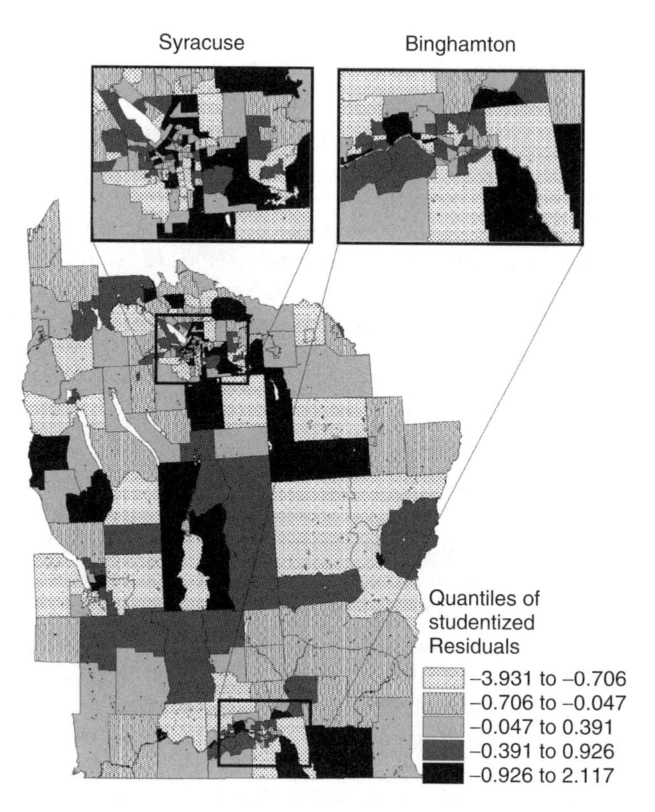

FIG. 9.13 Choropleth map of studentized residuals from weighted least squares (WLS) regression. Positive studentized residuals appear in gray-scale, negative studentized residuals as dots.

fitted value (based on covariate values) is much higher than the incidence proportion observed.

To assess the fit spatially, we first consider a choropleth map of the studentized residuals (Figure 9.13). The figure illustrates locations of positive (gray-scale) and negative (dot-pattern) studentized residuals, with insets showing patterns in the cities of Syracuse and Binghamton. We see the slight suggestion of a concentration of positive residuals (indicating an area underfit by the model) through the middle of the study area. The highest positive residuals appear in many of the cities and towns but often do not display a strong spatial pattern (e.g., within the city of Syracuse we find high residuals occurring in tracts adjacent to tracts with very low residuals). However, for geographically larger tracts, we tend to find positive (negative) residuals in tracts adjacent to other tracts with positive (negative) residuals, suggesting positive spatial autocorrelation. We turn next to numerical summaries to assess the level and significance of any residual spatial correlation.

Assessing Residual Spatial Autocorrelation The studentized residuals estimate a scaled version of the ϵ_i, the true errors associated with our regression model.

Thus, we can investigate the possibility that our errors are spatially autocorrelated. Analysis of residual correlation is complicated by the fact that the sample residuals (the e_i) are correlated even when the true error terms (the ϵ_i) are independent (cf. Draper and Smith 1998, p. 206). We examine this in more detail below, but stress here that much of the literature on spatial regression (and the remainder of our analyses here) build on heuristic assessments of spatial correlation in the sample residuals. The two most common approaches in applications are: (1) explore the semivariogram (or correlogram) of the residuals, or (2) summarize correlation through indexes of spatial autocorrelation (cf. Sections 7.4 and 7.5). In this data break, we assess residual spatial correlation using the geostatistical methods discussed in Section 8.2, deferring assessments via indexes of autocorrelation to the data break following Section 9.3.3.

The studentized residuals should have roughly a constant mean (0) and a constant variance (1), and their distribution should be approximately Gaussian. We found little in the residual analysis above to indicate gross departures from these characteristics for the transformed data. Thus, the studentized residuals should approximately satisfy the assumption of intrinsic stationarity discussed in Section 8.2, and we can use them to estimate the semivariogram of the regression error term, basing distance calculations on distances between the tract centroids. As discussed in Section 9.2.1, this semivariogram is biased and in this case, where we are working with proportions, the covariances of the errors still depend on the n_i. Again, the goal is not perfection (i.e., finding *the* right model) but a substantial improvement over methods that do not adjust for covariates, unequal population sizes, or spatial correlation.

The empirical semivariogram of the studentized residuals appears in Figure 9.14. We notice immediately the fairly large relative nugget effect, reflecting one of our conclusions based on the insets in Figure 9.13: For small tracts that are very close

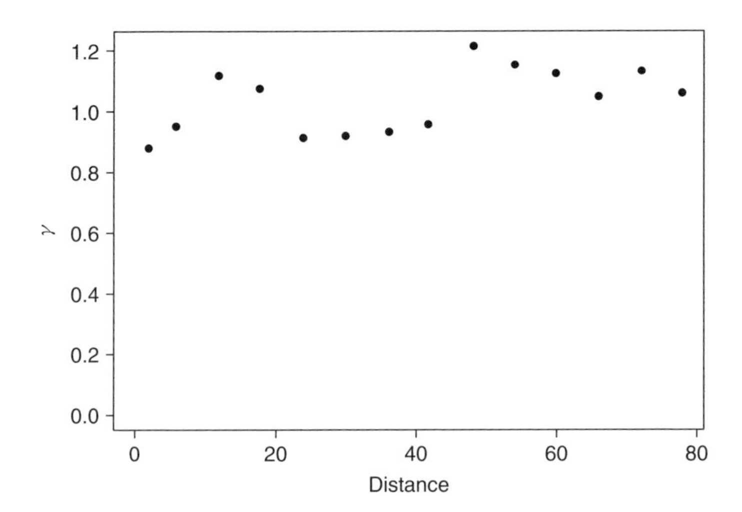

FIG. 9.14 Empirical semivariogram of studentized residuals from WLS regression.

together (e.g., in Syracuse) there are high residuals occurring in tracts adjacent to tracts with very low residuals. The empirical semivariogram appears to then increase up until a distance of about 18 km (roughly the width of the metropolitan area of Syracuse), suggesting that tracts separated by distances less than 18 km tend to have similar values (cf. Figure 9.13). Beyond this distance, there is a drop in the empirical semivariogram, perhaps indicating some negative spatial autocorrelation between rural tracts and those in the major urban areas, and then it eventually levels off to a sill. The empirical semivariogram seems to exhibit an overall cyclical pattern, but it is not clear whether this is real, due to noise in residual process (including that induced by our three outliers), or perhaps induced artificially by the spatial distribution of the tract centroids. Interestingly, Cressie (1993, p. 544) notes a similar oscillatory pattern in empirical semivariograms of residuals from a spatial regression of health data and attributes the pattern to the relative location of outliers in the data.

To investigate the effect of any potential spatial correlation among the studentized residuals on the fit of our model, we next use a linear regression model that has the same form as the one we used earlier:

$$Z_i = \beta_0 + \beta_1 X_1 + \beta_2 X_2 + \beta_3 X_3 + \epsilon_i,$$

but instead of assuming that the errors are uncorrelated, we apply the ideas in Section 9.2.1 and assume that they have a variance–covariance matrix $\Sigma(\boldsymbol{\theta})$. We use a semivariogram model to describe the elements of $\Sigma(\boldsymbol{\theta})$ as a function of nugget (c_0), partial sill (c_s), and range (a) parameters in $\boldsymbol{\theta} = (c_0, c_s, a)'$. To complete our regression model specification, we need to choose a functional form for the semivariogram model. We use the empirical semivariogram of the studentized residuals to infer the shape of this model and choose a spherical semivariogram to model this shape. Thus, our model is now specified completely, up to the unknown values of the parameters $\boldsymbol{\beta}$ and $\boldsymbol{\theta}$.

To estimate these unknown parameters, we use maximum likelihood fitting of the linear regression model with correlated errors described in Section 9.2.1. Since we are now estimating both covariate effects (related to the mean of the outcome) and covariance parameters (related to the variance–covariance matrix of the outcome), we shift focus from least squares to maximum likelihood estimation (recalling that weighted and generalized least-squares estimation assume a fixed and known variance–covariance function).

More specifically, we chose a grid of values around a range of 15 km for the range parameter a. Since we use the studentized residuals, the values for the nugget and partial sill have been scaled so that the overall variance is 1.0. To scale these back to the data, we express the nugget and partial sill as percentages of the total variance estimated from the OLS regression, $\hat{\sigma}^2 = 0.4318$. From the empirical semivariogram of the studentized residuals, the nugget effect appears to be about 80% of the total sill, so we use a grid search around the values of $0.80 \times 0.4318 = 0.35$ for the nugget effect, and $0.20 \times 0.4318 = 0.09$ for the partial sill. The resulting estimates appear in Table 9.4. Note that with residual

Table 9.4 Results of Unweighted Regression with Spatially Correlated Errors

Parameter	Estimate	Std. Error	F-Value	p-Value
$\hat{\beta}_0$ (intercept)	−0.7222	0.1972	13.40	<0.0001
$\hat{\beta}_1$ (TCE)	0.0826	0.0434	3.63	0.0576
$\hat{\beta}_2$ (% age > 65)	3.7093	0.6188	35.93	<0.0001
$\hat{\beta}_3$ (% own home)	−0.3245	0.2044	2.52	0.1136
$\hat{c}_0 = 0.3740$	$\hat{c}_s = 0.0558$	$\hat{a} = 6.93$		
AIC = 565.6[a]	277 df			

[a]Based on maximum likelihood fitting.

correlation, R^2 is no longer a valid measure of model fit, but the AIC suggests a slightly better fit than the model with no residual correlation. Comparing results from Tables 9.2 and 9.4, we see that accounting for spatial correlation substantially affects our conclusions about the effects of TCE concentration and income on the risk of leukemia.

Although these results account for the spatial autocorrelation in the data, they do not account for heteroscedasticity that results from the unequal population sizes in each tract. Although we used the studentized residuals (that do use the n_i to account for this heteroscedasticity) to infer the shape of the underlying correlation structure in the regression error term, this is not enough to account for the heteroscedasticity in our data. As before, we must also explicitly adjust for this heteroscedasticity in our model. Thus, we also weight our regression with spatially correlated errors in the same way that we weighted our regression with uncorrelated errors. Our variance–covariance term is now modeled as

$$\text{Var}(\mathbf{Z}) = D^{1/2}\Sigma(\boldsymbol{\theta})D^{1/2},$$

instead of $\Sigma(\boldsymbol{\theta})$, as in the previous analysis. The results from this weighted regression with spatially correlated errors appear in Table 9.5. Weighting induces subtle changes in the estimates of the covariate effects and their standard errors and places the nugget and sill estimates on different scales. The primary difference concerns the estimated standard errors of the estimates of $\boldsymbol{\beta}$, affecting the significance level observed for the covariates. As in the independent error case, the exposure surrogate is significant in the weighted analysis but not in the unweighted analysis, again influenced by heteroscedasticity induced by the three outlying variables.

Figure 9.15 presents a choropleth map of the fitted values (predicted outcomes) based on the model with spatially correlated errors. Since the overall model fit (as measured by AIC) is not improved by inclusion of the spatial error terms, we would not expect drastic differences in predicted values with the addition of the correlation term, but some subtle differences are apparent. Comparing this map

Table 9.5 Results of Weighted Regression with Spatially Dependent Errors

Parameter	Estimate	Std. Error	F-Value	p-Value
$\hat{\beta}_0$ (intercept)	−0.9161	0.1648	30.91	<0.0001
$\hat{\beta}_1$ (TCE)	0.0956	0.0322	8.85	0.0032
$\hat{\beta}_2$ (% age > 65)	3.5763	0.5920	36.49	<0.0001
$\hat{\beta}_3$ (% own home)	−0.2285	0.1761	1.68	<0.1956
$\hat{c}_0 = 997.65$	$\hat{c}_s = 127.12$	$\hat{a} = 6.86$		
AIC = 514.7[a]	277 df			

[a]Based on maximum likelihood fitting.

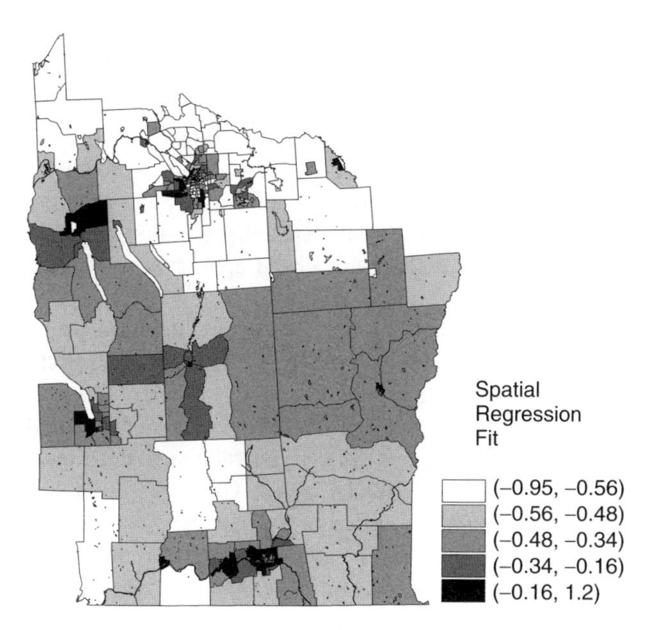

FIG. 9.15 Map of fitted transformed outcomes (Z) based on the weighted regression with spatially correlated errors.

to the map of WLS fitted values (no spatial correlation, Figure 9.11) we observe greater spatial smoothing of fitted values, most notably in the expanded region of very low fitted values surrounding Syracuse.

In summary, in this section we describe and illustrate how the traditional linear regression model can be adapted for spatial analysis. Using a weighted analysis that accounts for population heterogeneity and incorporating spatial correlation not explained by the covariates can both be crucial for obtaining valid conclusions. The general linear regression model that incorporates geostatistical methods for modeling spatial autocorrelation in the data provides one approach to doing this, but another class of linear regression models, which allows the use of the more flexible spatial proximity measures, offers an interesting alternative. These models are described in the next section.

9.3 SPATIAL AUTOREGRESSIVE MODELS

Once we define the covariates we want to include in our regression model, we complete our specification of a spatial regression model by specifying the elements of the variance–covariance matrix Σ. In the preceding section we specified this variance–covariance matrix directly using parametric functions of distance. However, with regional data, this approach will limit our measure of spatial proximity to the distances among points assumed to represent each region (e.g., intercentroid distances). In the case of counts, rates, and proportions from a fixed set of administrative regions, we often require only inference for the given set of regions, and the full generality afforded by geostatistical methods (e.g., observations occurring at *any* location) expressed in the models of Chapter 8 and Section 9.2 may not make sense. For example, do we really wish to model the number of incident cases occurring within some hypothetical region centered between two adjacent counties? To restrict inference to a given set of regions and to build spatial models *for these regions*, we make use of the spatial proximity measures described in Sections 4.4.1 and 7.4.2 and discuss associated approaches to specifying residual spatial autocorrelation.

We consider a structure mirroring the time-series literature which makes wide use of *autoregressive* models wherein we regress the current observation on observed values of all or, more commonly, a subset of other observations. In time series, the "other" observations occur in the recent past; in the spatial setting, they occur nearby. Just as the term *autocorrelation* reflects self-correlation, the term *autoregressive* reflects self-regression. Through such regressions, we incorporate spatial similarity by treating observations of the outcome variable at other locations as additional covariates in the model with associated parameters defining spatial association, rather than building an explicit parametric model of the covariance function of the error terms. The autoregressive model induces a particular covariance structure for the joint distribution of variables, but we typically do not fit the covariance directly. Instead, the autoregressive model itself defines this covariance for us.

In the spatial setting, we lose the ordering (past before present) inherent in a time series, somewhat complicating development and application of spatially autoregressive models. We describe two general classes of spatial autoregressive models and their associated covariance structures in subsequent sections. We retain the general multiple linear regression focus of Sections 9.1 and 9.2, expanding the framework to address Gaussian outcomes from a regional setting. In developing the material for these sections, we synthesize important contributions originally provided in Cliff and Ord (1981), Haining (1990), and Cressie (1993).

9.3.1 Simultaneous Autoregressive Models

We begin by applying the idea of spatial autoregression to the vector of residual errors, $\boldsymbol{\epsilon}$, in the linear regression specification depicted in equation (9.1). That is, we regress $\epsilon(\boldsymbol{s}_i)$ on all the other residual terms, giving

$$\epsilon(\boldsymbol{s}_i) = \sum_{j=1}^{N} b_{ij}\epsilon(\boldsymbol{s}_j) + \upsilon(\boldsymbol{s}_i), \tag{9.33}$$

with $b_{ii} = 0$ [so we don't regress $\epsilon(\boldsymbol{s}_i)$ on itself] and assume that the residual errors ("residual residuals"!) from this regression, $\upsilon(\boldsymbol{s}_i), i = 1, \ldots, N$, have mean zero and a diagonal variance–covariance matrix $\Sigma_\upsilon = \text{diag}[\sigma_1^2, \ldots, \sigma_n^2]$. The terms $\{b_{ij}\}$ represent *spatial dependence parameters* since they measure the contribution of the "other" observations [i.e., $\{\epsilon(\boldsymbol{s}_j), j \neq i\}$] to the variation of $\epsilon(\boldsymbol{s}_i)$. Thus our linear regression model, $Y(\boldsymbol{s}_i) = \boldsymbol{x}(\boldsymbol{s}_i)'\boldsymbol{\beta} + \epsilon(\boldsymbol{s}_i)$, where $\boldsymbol{x}(\boldsymbol{s}_i)' = (1, x_1(\boldsymbol{s}_i), \ldots, x_{p-1}(\boldsymbol{s}_i))$, becomes

$$Y(\boldsymbol{s}_i) = \boldsymbol{x}(\boldsymbol{s}_i)'\boldsymbol{\beta} + \sum_{j=1}^{N} b_{ij}\epsilon(\boldsymbol{s}_j) + \upsilon(\boldsymbol{s}_i).$$

If all the b_{ij} are zero, there is no autoregression and the model reduces to the traditional linear regression model with independent errors.

Using the relationship $\epsilon(\boldsymbol{s}_j) = Y(\boldsymbol{s}_j) - \boldsymbol{x}(\boldsymbol{s}_j)'\boldsymbol{\beta}$ from our original linear regression model [equation (9.1)], we obtain

$$Y(\boldsymbol{s}_i) = \boldsymbol{x}(\boldsymbol{s}_i)'\boldsymbol{\beta} + \sum_{j=1}^{N} b_{ij}[Y(\boldsymbol{s}_j) - \boldsymbol{x}(\boldsymbol{s}_j)'\boldsymbol{\beta}] + \upsilon(\boldsymbol{s}_i), \quad i = 1, 2, \ldots, N. \tag{9.34}$$

This model allows us to assess the degree of spatial dependence in the data through the inclusion of the term $\sum_{j=1} b_{ij}(Y_j - \boldsymbol{x}(\boldsymbol{s}_j)'\boldsymbol{\beta})$ (a weighted sum of the deviation of the jth observation from its modeled mean value) while controlling for covariate effects within region i. Conversely, the formulation also allows us to measure covariate effects while controlling for spatial dependence. We express the model in matrix form as

$$(I - B)(\mathbf{Y} - X\boldsymbol{\beta}) = \boldsymbol{\upsilon}, \tag{9.35}$$

where the $N \times N$ matrix B contains the spatial dependence parameters, b_{ij}, and $b_{ii} = 0$ for all i. From this, we can derive the variance–covariance matrix of $\mathbf{Y}$ as

$$\Sigma_Y = \text{Var}(\mathbf{Y}) = (I - B)^{-1}\Sigma_\upsilon(I - B')^{-1}, \tag{9.36}$$

assuming that $(I - B)^{-1}$ exists. Thus, the autoregression induces a particular model for the general covariance structure (Σ_Y) of the data $\mathbf{Y}$ that is defined by the parameters b_{ij}.

The model given in equation (9.34) [and equivalently, in equation (9.35)] was introduced by Whittle (1954) and often appears in the literature as the *simultaneous autoregressive* (SAR) *model*, where the adjective *simultaneous* describes the simultaneous application of equation (9.34) to each data location and distinguishes this type of spatial model from the class of *conditional* autoregressive models defined in Section 9.3.2.

Spatial Dependence and Covariance Matrices The relationship between matrices B and Σ_Y merits some special attention. We note that Σ_Y relates to the *inverse* of the matrix of spatial dependence parameters, so the link between particular values of B and corresponding values of Σ_Y is not immediately obvious and may, in fact, be somewhat counterintuitive. For example, spatial dependence parameters that decrease monotonically with distance do not necessarily correspond to spatial covariances that decrease monotonically with distance. Although the correspondence between B and Σ_Y appears mathematically throughout the spatial autoregressive literature, in practice, we often find similar decreasing functions of distance (e.g., an exponentially decaying function of intercentroid distance) used to define elements of B for an autoregressive analysis or Σ_Y for a generalized least squares analysis. Griffith (1996) performs an empirical examination of similar parametric families of autoregressive parameters and covariances on a set of regular regions, but the matrix inversion linking B and Σ_Y often makes general conclusions impossible.

Clearly, the matrix of spatial dependence parameters, B, plays an important role in SAR models. To make progress with estimation and inference, we will need to reduce the number of spatial dependence parameters through the use of a parametric model for the $\{b_{ij}\}$ and, for interpretation, we would like to relate them to the ideas of proximity and autocorrelation that we described previously. One way to do this is to take $B = \rho W$, where W is one of the spatial proximity measures discussed in Sections 4.4.1 and 7.4.2. In this case, the SAR model can be written as

$$Y(\mathbf{s}_i) = \boldsymbol{x}(\mathbf{s}_i)'\boldsymbol{\beta} + \rho \sum_{j \in \mathcal{N}_i} w_{ij} \left[Y(\mathbf{s}_j) - \boldsymbol{x}(\mathbf{s}_j)'\boldsymbol{\beta}\right] + \upsilon(\mathbf{s}_i), \qquad i = 1, 2, \ldots, N,$$

where N denotes the number of regions and $\mathcal{N}_i$ denotes the neighborhood set of the ith region [i.e., $\mathcal{N}_i = \{j : j \text{ is a neighbor of } i\}$], as defined in Section 4.4.1. This model derives from the autoregressive structure

$$\begin{aligned} \mathbf{Y} &= X\boldsymbol{\beta} + \boldsymbol{\epsilon} \\ \boldsymbol{\epsilon} &= \rho W \boldsymbol{\epsilon} + \boldsymbol{\upsilon}, \end{aligned} \tag{9.37}$$

where $B = \rho W$. We can manipulate this model in a variety of ways, and it is often intuitive to write the model as

$$\mathbf{Y} = X\boldsymbol{\beta} + (I - \rho W)^{-1}\boldsymbol{\upsilon} \tag{9.38}$$

$$= X\boldsymbol{\beta} - \rho W X\boldsymbol{\beta} + \rho W \mathbf{Y} + \boldsymbol{\upsilon}. \tag{9.39}$$

From equation (9.38) we can see how the autoregression induces spatial autocorrelation in the linear regression model through the term $(I - \rho W)^{-1}\boldsymbol{\upsilon}$. From equation (9.39) we obtain a better appreciation for what this means in terms of a linear regression model with uncorrelated errors: We now have two additional terms in the regression model: $\rho WX\boldsymbol{\beta}$ and $\rho W\mathbf{Y}$. These terms reflect *spatially lagged variables*. If we include $\rho WX\boldsymbol{\beta}$, the covariates are spatially lagged (i.e., covariate values nearby affect the outcome in region i), and if we include $\rho W\mathbf{Y}$, the outcome variable is spatially lagged (i.e., observed outcomes nearby impact the outcome in region i). Thus, in a SAR, both the covariates and the outcome variable are spatially lagged. Econometricians, seeking to develop spatial models that are direct analogues of time-series models, develop spatial models, including either the lagged variables $\rho WX\boldsymbol{\beta}$ *or* $\rho W\mathbf{Y}$ (see Anselin 1988, (1990), (1993)). Often, such models are difficult to motivate in purely spatial applications (they are more useful in space–time applications) and we defer details of such models to the spatial econometric references above.

For a well-defined model, we require $(I - \rho W)$ to be nonsingular (invertible). This restriction imposes conditions on W and also on ρ, best summarized through the eigenvalues of the matrix W. If $\vartheta_{\max}$ and $\vartheta_{\min}$ are the largest and smallest eigenvalues of W, and if $\vartheta_{\min} < 0$ and $\vartheta_{\max} > 0$, then $1/\vartheta_{\min} < \rho < 1/\vartheta_{\max}$ (Haining 1990, p. 82). For a large set of identical square regions, these extreme eigenvalues approach -4 and 4, respectively, as the number of regions increases, implying that $|\rho| < 0.25$, but actual constraints on ρ should be checked by computing the eigenvalues of W, especially when the sites are located on a set of irregularly shaped regions. Often, the row sums of W are standardized to 1 by dividing each entry in W by its row sum, $\sum_j w_{ij}$. Then, $\vartheta_{\max} = 1$ and $\vartheta_{\min} \leq -1$, so $\rho < 1$ but may be less than -1 (see Haining 1990, Section 3.2.2).

Estimating the Parameters in SAR Models Suppose that the data are multivariate Gaussian with the general SAR model defined in equations (9.35) and (9.36) [i.e., the data are multivariate Gaussian with mean $X\boldsymbol{\beta}$ and variance covariance matrix given in equation (9.36)]. Following the ideas in Section 9.2.1, we reparameterize the diagonal matrix Σ_υ as $\Sigma_\upsilon = \sigma^2 V_\upsilon$, so the variance–covariance matrix of a SAR can be written as

$$\Sigma_{\text{SAR}} = \sigma^2 (I - B)^{-1} V_\upsilon (I - B')^{-1} = \sigma^2 V_{\text{SAR}}(\boldsymbol{\theta}), \tag{9.40}$$

where $\boldsymbol{\theta}$ is a vector containing the spatial dependence parameters b_{ij} and the parameters of V_υ. This is exactly the form of the variance–covariance matrix in equation (9.11) of Section 9.2.1. Thus, if $V_{\text{SAR}}(\boldsymbol{\theta})$ is known, the results from maximum likelihood estimation and inference for the general linear model with autocorrelated errors, described in Section 9.2.1, apply directly to estimation and inference with a SAR model, replacing $V(\boldsymbol{\theta})$ in equation (9.11) with $V_{\text{SAR}}(\boldsymbol{\theta})$ defined in equation (9.40). In practice, of course, $V_{\text{SAR}}(\boldsymbol{\theta})$ is not known and we estimate $\boldsymbol{\theta}$ using methods analogous to those described in Section 9.2.1. Specifically, we estimate $\boldsymbol{\theta}$ by $\tilde{\boldsymbol{\theta}}$ obtained by minimizing $\mathcal{Q}(\boldsymbol{\theta})$ in equation (9.20) with $\Sigma(\boldsymbol{\theta})$ replaced with $V_{\text{SAR}}(\boldsymbol{\theta})$.

Given $\tilde{\boldsymbol{\theta}}$, we estimate $\boldsymbol{\beta}$ using equation (9.13) with V replaced by $V_{\text{SAR}}(\tilde{\boldsymbol{\theta}})$, and we estimate σ^2 using equation (9.14), again with V replaced by $V_{\text{SAR}}(\tilde{\boldsymbol{\theta}})$. We obtain the standard errors of these parameter estimates from the information matrix as discussed in Sections 9.1.1 and 9.2.1.

In this general development, many model parameters are contained in the vector $\boldsymbol{\theta}$, and thus minimizing $\mathcal{Q}(\boldsymbol{\theta})$ may be difficult or impossible. Thus, in practice, we usually assume that the parameters in V_{υ} are known (e.g., the (i,i)th element is equal to 1 or equal to $1/n_i$ to account for differing population sizes). Such assumptions still may not be enough allow minimization of $\mathcal{Q}$, so we also often parameterize B as a parametric function of a spatial proximity matrix W. For example, if we take $B = \rho W$ and $V_{\upsilon} = \sigma^2 I$, the only unknown parameter is ρ. In this case, minimizing $\mathcal{Q}(\rho)$ with respect to ρ is typically straightforward and the information matrix has a much simpler form (Ord 1975; Cliff and Ord 1981, p. 242):

$$I(\boldsymbol{\beta}, \sigma^2, \rho) = \begin{bmatrix} \sigma^{-2}[X'A(\rho)^{-1}X] & \mathbf{0} & \mathbf{0} \\ \mathbf{0}' & \frac{N}{2}\sigma^{-4} & \sigma^{-2}\text{tr}(G) \\ \mathbf{0}' & \sigma^{-2}\text{tr}(G) & \sigma^{-2}[\alpha + \text{tr}(G'G)] \end{bmatrix}, \tag{9.41}$$

where $A(\rho) = (I - \rho W)^{-1}(I - \rho W')^{-1}$, $G = W(I - \rho W)^{-1}$, $\text{tr}(\cdot)$ denotes the trace function (summation of the diagonal elements of a matrix), and $\alpha = \sum[\vartheta_i^2/(1 - \rho\vartheta_i)^2]$, where ϑ_i are the eigenvalues of W. Again, we see that the matrix of spatial dependence parameters $B = \rho W$ affects results through its eigenvalues.

The information matrix in equation (9.41) looks similar to those associated with least squares techniques [cf. Section 9.1.1 for OLS and equation (9.22) for GLS], which makes us wonder why we can't simply use least squares to estimate all the parameters in a SAR model. If ρ is known or specified, we can. The ML estimators of $\boldsymbol{\beta}$ and σ^2 for the SAR are equivalent to their generalized least squares estimators. However, if ρ is not known, the least squares estimator of ρ is inconsistent (Whittle 1954; Haining 1990, p. 130).

Testing Residual SAR Dependence The one-parameter SAR model described above (with $B = \rho W$ and $V_{\upsilon} = \sigma^2 I$) is by far the most prevalent SAR model used in practice. One of its most common uses is to provide an alternative model for a test of residual spatial autocorrelation in OLS residuals. That is, we consider the following two models, a traditional linear regression model with independent errors and the one-parameter SAR model:

$$\mathbf{Y} = \begin{cases} X\boldsymbol{\beta} + \boldsymbol{\epsilon}, & \Sigma_Y = \sigma^2 I \quad (9.42) \\ X\boldsymbol{\beta} + (I - \rho W)^{-1}\boldsymbol{\upsilon}, & \Sigma_Y = \sigma^2(I - \rho W)^{-1}(I - \rho W')^{-1}. \quad (9.43) \end{cases}$$

Setting $\rho = 0$ in the SAR model [equation (9.43)], we obtain the traditional linear regression model with independent errors [equation (9.42)]. This nesting of the two models, together with a traditional null model for which estimation is rather straightforward (i.e., OLS), provide several approaches for constructing tests of $H_0: \rho = 0$ vs. $H_1: \rho \neq 0$ (or a corresponding one-sided alternative). We review some of these briefly here.

Moran's I with OLS Residuals The residuals from ordinary least squares or maximum likelihood fitting of the model in equation (9.42) are

$$e = \mathbf{Y} - X\hat{\boldsymbol{\beta}}_{\mathrm{OLS}},$$

where

$$\hat{\boldsymbol{\beta}}_{\mathrm{OLS}} = (X'X)^{-1}X'\mathbf{Y}.$$

As we saw in Section 9.2.3, it is natural to use residuals from fitting a model with uncorrelated errors to assess whether there is any residual spatial autocorrelation in the data after accounting for covariate effects. Instead of the residual semivariogram, we use a variant of Moran's I statistic with these residuals. Specifically, we replace the overall mean in Moran's I [given in equation (7.8)] with the model's predicted value $\hat{\mathbf{Y}} = X\hat{\boldsymbol{\beta}}$, yielding

$$\begin{aligned} I_{\mathrm{res}} &= \frac{1}{(1/N)\sum_{i=1}^{N}\left(Y_i - \hat{Y}_i\right)^2}\left[\frac{\sum_{i=1}^{N}\sum_{j=1}^{N} w_{ij}(Y_i - \hat{Y}_i)(Y_j - \hat{Y}_j)}{\sum_{i=1}^{N}\sum_{j=1}^{N} w_{ij}}\right] \\ &= \frac{N}{\sum_{i=1}^{N}\sum_{j=1}^{N} w_{ij}}\left[\frac{\sum_{i=1}^{N}\sum_{j=1}^{N} w_{ij}(Y_i - \hat{Y}_i)(Y_j - \hat{Y}_j)}{\sum_{i=1}^{N}\left(Y_i - \hat{Y}_i\right)^2}\right] \\ &= \frac{N}{\sum_{i=1}^{N}\sum_{j=1}^{N} w_{ij}}\frac{e'We}{e'e} \end{aligned} \tag{9.44}$$

(cf. Cliff and Ord 1981, Chapter 8; Haining 1990, p. 146).

As in Chapters 6 and 7, it is critically important to consider what null and alternative hypotheses are of interest when applying a specific test statistic, in this case I_{res}. To begin, a null hypothesis based on randomization (cf. Section 7.4) is no longer appropriate here, even with stationary Gaussian residuals (cf. Cliff and Ord 1981, p. 200; Anselin and Rey 1991). Recall from Section 7.4 that under the randomization assumption, each data value is equally likely to be observed at any location. This assumption is not satisfied with sample residuals since they are correlated, even in the absence of residual spatial autocorrelation.

If we assume that the error terms follow a multivariate Gaussian distribution, Cliff and Ord (1981, pp. 202–203) show that under the null hypothesis of independent error terms, I_{res} asymptotically (N going to infinity) follows a Gaussian distribution with mean

$$E(I_{\text{res}}) = \frac{N}{(N-p)\sum_{i=1}^{N}\sum_{j=1}^{N} w_{ij}} \text{tr}(I - HW)$$
$$= -\frac{N}{(N-p)\sum_{i=1}^{N}\sum_{j=1}^{N} w_{ij}} \text{tr}\left[(X'X)^{-1}X'WX\right], \quad (9.45)$$

where tr(·) again denotes the trace function, and $H = X(X'X)^{-1}X'$ (called the "hat" matrix of regression). Cliff and Ord (1981, pp. 202–203) also derive the asymptotic variance of I_{res} as

$$\text{Var}(I_{\text{res}}) = \frac{N^2}{(\text{Sum}_0)^2(N-p)(N-p+2)}$$
$$\times \left\{\text{Sum}_1 + 2\text{tr}\left[G^2\right] - \text{tr}(F) - \frac{2[\text{tr}(G)]^2}{N-p}\right\}, \quad (9.46)$$

where

$$\text{Sum}_0 = \sum_{i=1}^{N}\sum_{j=1}^{N} w_{ij}$$
$$\text{Sum}_1 = \frac{1}{2}\sum_{i=1}^{N}\sum_{j=1}^{N}(w_{ij} + w_{ji})^2$$
$$F = (X'X)^{-1}X'(W + W')^2 X$$
$$G = (X'X)^{-1}X'WX.$$

Based on the asymptotic results in equations (9.45) and (9.46), we obtain an approximate test of the null hypothesis of independent observations by comparing the observed value of

$$z = \frac{I_{\text{res}} - E(I_{\text{res}})}{\sqrt{\text{Var}(I_{\text{res}})}} \quad (9.47)$$

to the appropriate percentage point of the standard normal distribution.

The asymptotic results of Cliff and Ord (1981) derive from results assuming constant variance for the OLS residuals, a situation that may not hold in practice. Even so, Cliff and Ord (1981, Section 2.4) and Haining (1990, p. 147) report the approximation works well in practice and in simulation studies for as few as $N = 10$ regions. An important exception occurs when the W matrix is very sparse (i.e., most regions have very few neighbors) and asymptotic normality no longer holds (cf. Cliff and Ord 1981, p. 50).

Using Moran's I with OLS residuals to test for residual spatial autocorrelation has several advantages. First, obtaining OLS residuals is fairly straightforward and can be done by most statistical software packages. Second, since we do not have to estimate our alternative (SAR) model to make the test, we avoid the need to obtain the more computationally intensive maximum likelihood estimates for the SAR model. Finally, I_{res} has several nice statistical properties [e.g., it is locally best invariant against SAR alternatives and even a uniformly most powerful invariant test for particular SAR models (King 1981; Tiefelsdorf 2000)]. The main practical disadvantage in applying the normal approximation of Cliff and Ord (1981) is that it requires several assumptions that may not be satisfied in practice. OLS residuals are correlated and have different variances, even when the original data are i.i.d. In public health applications where we are working with counts, rates, and proportions, OLS residuals are even more suspect since their variances depend on the population sizes, even after transformation. As we show in the next data break, using Moran's I with studentized residuals from weighted least squares may offer a feasible alternative, although little is known about the statistical properties of the resulting statistic.

Finally, it is important to state that I_{res} also has power against other (non-SAR) alternatives and may not distinguish between competing types of residual spatial correlation (Anselin and Rey 1991). Furthermore, McMillen (2003) illustrates that Moran's I cannot distinguish between residual spatial autocorrelation and local model misspecification, a point raised in Section 7.7. That is, Moran's I is *sensitive* to departures from standard model assumptions (under the usual i.i.d. Gaussian assumptions) but is not *specific* to exactly what sort of departure is driving any unusual observed pattern.

Wald Test Since maximum likelihood estimators are asymptotically Gaussian, an approximate confidence interval for ρ is

$$\hat{\rho} \pm (z_{\alpha/2})\sqrt{\widehat{\text{Var}(\hat{\rho})}}, \tag{9.48}$$

where $\widehat{\text{Var}(\hat{\rho})}$ is obtained from the inverse of the information matrix, substituting ML estimates for any unknown parameters. A Wald test of $H_0\colon \rho = 0$ is made by comparing

$$z = \hat{\rho}/\sqrt{\widehat{\text{Var}(\hat{\rho})}}$$

to a standard normal distribution. Wald tests can also be used easily to test hypotheses about $\boldsymbol{\beta}$ and ρ simultaneously. The main advantage of Wald tests is their flexibility once the alternative model is fit. The main disadvantage lies in having to fit the alternative model by maximum likelihood. Also, with small data sets, Wald tests tend to have an inflated type I error rate (i.e., they tend to reject the null hypothesis too often with small data sets).

Likelihood Ratio Test We introduced likelihood ratio tests in Chapters 6 and 7 and again in Section 8.2.4. The same idea applies here. In this case we are comparing our alternative model in equation (9.43) with parameters $\boldsymbol{\theta}_2 = (\boldsymbol{\beta}', \sigma^2, \rho)'$

to our null model defined by equation (9.42) with parameters $\boldsymbol{\theta}_1 = (\boldsymbol{\beta}', \sigma^2)'$, with $\dim(\boldsymbol{\theta}_2) - \dim(\boldsymbol{\theta}_1) = 1$. A test of $H_0\colon \boldsymbol{\theta} = \boldsymbol{\theta}_1$ against the alternative $H_1 : \boldsymbol{\theta} = \boldsymbol{\theta}_2$ is also a test of $H_0\colon \rho = 0$ vs. $H_1 : \rho \neq 0$, and it can be done by comparing

$$2(\mathcal{L}(\boldsymbol{\beta}, \sigma^2, \rho) - \mathcal{L}(\boldsymbol{\beta}, \sigma^2, 0)) \tag{9.49}$$

to a χ^2 distribution with one degree of freedom.

The main advantage of this test is the beautiful theory underlying maximum likelihood estimation and inference. It also has the advantage that more complex models can be considered if their likelihoods can be obtained. The main disadvantage is the amount of computation required to fit both the null and the alternative models. Also, the χ^2 distribution can be a poor approximation to the distribution of the likelihood ratio for small data sets.

Concluding Remarks All tests here are asymptotic [i.e., they give approximately valid inference only for large N (number of regions in the study area)]. How large is large enough depends on several factors, including the particular structure of the spatial weight matrix W. If the accuracy of the normal approximation is in question, we may use Monte Carlo hypothesis tests, provided that we simulate the original data from the null model of no independence and a fixed set of covariates. However, this approach often will be labor intensive since we must fit a regression model for each simulation (e.g., 999 or more regressions!). As an alternative to Monte Carlo tests, Tiefelsdorf and Boots (1995, 1996), Hepple (1998), Tiefelsdorf (1998, 2000), and Hill (2002) explore other computational approaches for obtaining the exact distribution of Moran's I as applied to OLS residuals from a particular set of zones with a particular spatial weight matrix.

In addition, all tests described here are applied to OLS residuals. Development of appropriate tests of spatial autocorrelation in error terms of SAR models (or any other spatial model for that matter) remains an open area of research, despite an early call for such work by Cliff and Ord (1981, p. 240).

9.3.2 Conditional Autoregressive Models

In Sections 9.2 and 9.3.1 we present models of the *joint* probability distribution $f[Y(\boldsymbol{s}_1), \ldots, Y(\boldsymbol{s}_n)]$ with spatial association incorporated through the variance–covariance matrix $\Sigma = \text{Var}(\mathbf{Y})$. In some applications, we may find it more intuitive to specify models for the set of *conditional* probability distributions of each observation, $Y(\boldsymbol{s}_i)$, given the observed values of all of the other observations. That is, we model $f[Y(\boldsymbol{s}_i)|\mathbf{Y}_{-i}]$, where $\mathbf{Y}_{-i}$ denotes the vector of all observations except $Y(\boldsymbol{s}_i)$, and we do this for each observation in turn.

As with the SAR models in Section 9.3.1, we may simplify the situation by assuming that $Y(\boldsymbol{s}_i)$ depends only on a set of *neighbors* [i.e., $Y(\boldsymbol{s}_i)$ depends on $Y(\boldsymbol{s}_j)$ only if location $\boldsymbol{s}_j$ is in the neighborhood set, $\mathcal{N}_i$, of $\boldsymbol{s}_i$]. If we assume that each conditional distribution is Gaussian, we need only specify the conditional mean and conditional variance of each observation in order to complete our model.

More formally, we define a *conditional autoregressive* (CAR) *model* by specifying the conditional mean and variance:

$$E[Y(\boldsymbol{s}_i)|\mathbf{Y}_{-i}] = \boldsymbol{x}(\boldsymbol{s}_i)'\boldsymbol{\beta} + \sum_{j=1}^{N} c_{ij}[Y(\boldsymbol{s}_j) - \boldsymbol{x}(\boldsymbol{s}_i)'\boldsymbol{\beta}], \tag{9.50}$$

$$\text{Var}[Y(\boldsymbol{s}_i)|\mathbf{Y}_{-i}] = \sigma_i^2, \qquad i = 1, \ldots, N, \tag{9.51}$$

where the c_{ij} denote spatial dependence parameters (we use a different notation to distinguish spatial dependence parameters in CAR models from those in SAR models). The c_{ij} are nonzero only if $\boldsymbol{s}_j \in \mathcal{N}_i$. By convention, we set $c_{ii} = 0$ since we do not want to regress any observed value on itself, so as a consequence, no region is a neighbor to itself. (As an aside, this "a region can't be its own neighbor" convention, which makes intuitive sense for autoregressions, often carries over to the indexes of spatial autocorrelation introduced in Section 7.4, resulting in tests of correlation that entirely ignore issues of goodness of fit, as noted in Section 7.6.3.)

To illustrate how a set of conditional distributions, each defined over a set of spatial neighbors, might define a joint distribution with positive spatial autocorrelation, consider a classroom with seats arranged in rows and columns. Students occupy each seat, and each student receives a piece of paper with a number on it. The instructor tells the class that each student's number represents a measurement from a smoothly varying spatial process (e.g., temperature) measured at that student's seat's location. The instructor asks students to raise a hand to a height corresponding to their individual measurements. As the instructor glances at the course notes, each student quickly glances at the height of the hands displayed by her or his neighboring students. Each student adjusts the height of her or his hand to be closer to the perceived neighboring measurements. In this example, each student considers the conditional probability of her or his own measurement, compared to the associated neighboring measurements. Taken together, the set of conditional distributions induces a joint distribution of measurements with positive spatial autocorrelation.

More formally, a mathematical result known as the *Hammersley–Clifford theorem* [first proved in Besag (1974)] describes the conditions necessary for a set of conditional distributions to define a valid joint distribution. Whereas deriving Gaussian conditional distributions from a multivariate Gaussian (joint) distribution follows standard results in multivariate distribution theory, the conditions needed for a set of conditional distributions to define a valid joint distribution are less straightforward (Besag and Kooperberg 1995; Arnold et al. 1999). A set of conditional distributions defined over spatial neighborhoods and meeting these conditions defines a *Markov random field*, where each observation (given the other observations) depends only on values at neighboring locations.

A full treatment of the Hammersley–Clifford theorem and its related conditions falls beyond our scope, and we defer to Besag (1974) and Cressie (1993, Chapter 6) for technical details. For our Gaussian modeling needs, the conditions required by the Hammersley–Clifford theorem are not too restrictive and Besag (1974) shows (see also Cliff and Ord 1981, p. 180) that the set of Gaussian conditional distributions with conditional means and variances defined by equations (9.50) and (9.51) generates a valid joint multivariate Gaussian distribution with mean $X\boldsymbol{\beta}$ and variance

$$\Sigma_Y = (I - C)^{-1}\Sigma_c, \tag{9.52}$$

where $\Sigma_c = \text{diag}[\sigma_1^2, \ldots, \sigma_n^2]$. To ensure that this variance–covariance matrix is symmetric, we have to impose the constraints

$$\sigma_j^2 c_{ij} = \sigma_i^2 c_{ji}. \tag{9.53}$$

Just as in Section 9.3.1, the link between particular values of C and corresponding values of Σ_Y is not immediately obvious and may, in fact, be somewhat counterintuitive. Again, for example, spatial dependence parameters that decrease monotonically with distance do not necessarily correspond to spatial covariances that decrease monotonically with distance.

In summary, CAR models provide us with yet another model for the general Σ in equation (9.10), including parameters to measure residual spatial autocorrelation. We now consider some particular CAR models in order to better understand how they model spatial dependence in our data.

Relationship to SARs If we set $\Sigma_c = \sigma^2 I$ and if in the development of the SAR models, we set $\Sigma_\upsilon = \sigma^2 I$, then comparing the variances in equations (9.36) and (9.52), we see that any SAR model with spatial dependence matrix B can be expressed as a CAR model with spatial dependence matrix $C = B + B' - BB'$. Any CAR model can also be expressed as a SAR model, but the relationships between B and C are somewhat contrived (see Haining 1990, p. 89), and the neighborhood structure of the two models may not be the same (Cressie 1993, p. 409).

Estimation and Inference with CAR Models Using results from Besag (1974), the joint distribution of data specified with a CAR model is multivariate Gaussian with mean $X\boldsymbol{\beta}$ and variance–covariance matrix given in equation (9.52). Following the ideas in Section 9.2, we reparameterize the diagonal matrix Σ_c as $\Sigma_c = \sigma^2 V_c$, so the variance–covariance matrix of a CAR can be written as

$$\Sigma_{\text{CAR}} = \sigma^2 (I - C)^{-1} V_c = \sigma^2 V_{\text{CAR}}(\boldsymbol{\theta}), \tag{9.54}$$

where $\boldsymbol{\theta}$ is a vector containing all the spatial dependence parameters c_{ij}, and the parameters of V_c. This is exactly the form of the variance–covariance matrix in equation (9.11) of Section 9.2.1. Thus, if $V_{\text{CAR}}(\boldsymbol{\theta})$ is known, the results from maximum likelihood estimation and inference for the general linear model with autocorrelated errors, described in Section 9.2.1, apply directly to estimation and inference with a CAR model, replacing $V(\boldsymbol{\theta})$ in equation (9.11) with $V_{\mathrm{CAR}}(\boldsymbol{\theta})$ defined in equation (9.54), just as we did with the SAR model in Section 9.3.1. In practice, of course, $V_{\mathrm{CAR}}(\boldsymbol{\theta})$ is not known and we estimate $\boldsymbol{\theta}$ using methods analogous to those described in Section 9.2.1. Specifically, we estimate $\boldsymbol{\theta}$ by $\tilde{\boldsymbol{\theta}}$ obtained by minimizing $\mathcal{Q}(\boldsymbol{\theta})$ in equation (9.20) with $\Sigma(\boldsymbol{\theta})$ replaced with $V_{\mathrm{CAR}}(\boldsymbol{\theta})$. Given $\tilde{\boldsymbol{\theta}}$, we estimate $\boldsymbol{\beta}$ using equation (9.13) with V replaced by $V_{\mathrm{CAR}}(\tilde{\boldsymbol{\theta}})$ and we estimate σ^2 using equation (9.14), again with V replaced by $V_{\mathrm{CAR}}(\tilde{\boldsymbol{\theta}})$. We obtain the standard errors of these parameter estimates from the information matrix as discussed in Sections 9.1.1, 9.2.1, and 9.3.1.

As with estimation in the SAR models described in Section 9.3.1, there are many parameters in $\boldsymbol{\theta}$, and thus minimizing $\mathcal{Q}(\boldsymbol{\theta})$ is often difficult or impossible. Thus, in practice, we usually assume that the parameters in V_c are known [e.g., the (i, i)th element is equal to 1 or equal $1/n_i$ to account for differing populations]. This still may not be enough to allow minimization of $\mathcal{Q}$, so we also parameterize C as a parametric function of a spatial proximity matrix W, as described in Section 9.3.1.

In the case of the one-parameter CAR with $C = \rho W$ and $V_c = \sigma^2 I$, minimizing $\mathcal{Q}(\rho)$ is usually straightforward. In this case, the information matrix reduces to (Cliff and Ord 1981, p. 242)

$$I(\boldsymbol{\beta}, \sigma^2, \rho) = \begin{bmatrix} \sigma^{-2}(X'A(\rho)^{-1}X) & \mathbf{0} & \mathbf{0} \\ \mathbf{0}' & \frac{N}{2}\sigma^{-4} & \frac{1}{2}\sigma^{-2}\mathrm{tr}(G) \\ \mathbf{0}' & \frac{1}{2}\sigma^{-2}\mathrm{tr}(G) & \frac{1}{2}\alpha \end{bmatrix}, \qquad (9.55)$$

a form very similar to equation (9.41), but where $A(\rho) = (I - \rho W)^{-1}$, $G = W(I - \rho W)^{-1}$, and $\alpha = \sum[\vartheta_i^2/(1 - \rho\vartheta_i)^2]$, where ϑ_i are the eigenvalues of W.

The primary difference between CAR and SAR models based on Gaussian data is the different definitions of Σ_Y. In the simplest one-parameter cases, $\Sigma_Y = \sigma^2(I - \rho W)^{-1}$ for a CAR and $\Sigma_Y, = \sigma^2(I - \rho W)^{-1}(I - \rho W')^{-1}$ for a SAR. Thus, the methods for testing $H_0\colon \rho = 0$ vs. $H_1\colon \rho \neq 0$ for the simple CAR model are the same as those discussed in Section 9.3.1.

Unlike the SAR model, least squares estimators of the parameters in CAR models are consistent. Thus, iteratively reweighted generalized least squares (described in Section 9.2.1) can also be used to estimate the parameters of the simple CAR model. In this case, when we obtain the residuals, we estimate ρ using ordinary least squares (Haining 1990, p. 130)

$$\hat{\rho}_{\mathrm{OLS}} = \frac{\boldsymbol{e}'W\boldsymbol{e}}{\boldsymbol{e}'W^2\boldsymbol{e}}$$

[cf. equation (9.44)].

9.3.3 Concluding Remarks on Conditional Autoregressions

Just as with the SAR models introduced in Section 9.3.1, the primary purpose of CAR models is to provide a modeling mechanism to account for residual spatial correlation (i.e., spatial trends not explained by spatial patterns in covariate values). As we illustrated in the data break following Section 9.2.3, residual correlation can bias parameter estimates and their standard errors, leading to incorrect inference regarding the impact of covariates on the outcome value.

Spatial autoregressive models were developed primarily for use with geographically aggregated spatial data, in contrast to the geostatistical models developed for spatially continuous data, where measurements could be taken (at least theoretically) at any location in the study area. Unlike the regression models with spatially autocorrelated data, where universal kriging allows us to predict an outcome variable at an unmeasured location, prediction of new observations is not usually the focus of SAR and CAR modeling. The interpretation of a predicted value located between adjacent areal units is at best unclear (e.g., if we have the disease rate for each state in the continental United States, what does it mean to predict the disease rate at a "location" between Texas and Louisiana?). However, when data are missing, prediction of areal values may be a goal, and in such cases, the universal kriging predictor (Section 9.2.3) can be used, with Σ_Y corresponding to either a SAR or a CAR model.

DATA BREAK: New York Leukemia Data (*cont.*) In this portion of the data break, we consider spatial autoregressive models for the New York leukemia data. Most of the assumptions underlying OLS regression (discussed in Sections 9.1 and 9.2) must be made for these models as well. In particular, we assume that the data follow a multivariate Gaussian distribution with the mean independent of the variance. As we discussed earlier, the incidence proportions do not satisfy these assumptions, but much of the work needed to overcome this difficulty was done in the data break following Section 9.2.3. We continue with our analysis of the transformed proportions, Z_i, and use the same covariates as before. Essentially, we pick up this data break just after fitting the OLS and WLS regression models in the preceding data break (results in Tables 9.2 and 9.3).

Earlier, we assessed whether there was any residual spatial autocorrelation by computing the semivariogram of the residuals. In this data break, we apply the ideas in Sections 7.4 and 7.5 to assess residual autocorrelation. We continue using the binary connectivity matrix with elements $w_{ij} = 1$ if regions i and j share any portion of their borders with one another, to specify the neighborhood structure as we did in the data break following Section 7.4.3.

Assessing Residual Autocorrelation Using Moran's I In Section 9.3.1 we described how Moran's I can be used to test for residual spatial autocorrelation. Based on the traditional OLS residuals from our New York leukemia case study, $\boldsymbol{e} = \mathbf{Y} - X\hat{\boldsymbol{\beta}}_{\text{OLS}}$, we obtain a Moran's I value of $I_{\text{res}} = 0.08309$ [equation (9.44)] that has a variance of 0.0013. The test statistic in equation (9.47) suggests significant residual spatial autocorrelation ($p = 0.0155$). Thus, we fit both a SAR and a CAR model and compare our results to those in the earlier data break.

We first fit a one-parameter SAR model with variance–covariance matrix

$$\Sigma_{\text{SAR}} = \sigma_S^2(I - \rho_S W)^{-1} V_v (I - \rho_S W')^{-1},$$

with $V_v = I$, and then a comparable one parameter CAR model with variance–covariance matrix

$$\Sigma_{\text{CAR}} = \sigma_C^2(I - \rho_C W)^{-1} V_c,$$

with $V_c = I$. We use different subscripts on σ^2 and ρ to indicate that the parameters differ between the two models. Their values need not be similar, although their interpretations are the same. The results appear in Tables 9.6 and 9.7.

Comparing these results we see many similarities. The estimates of the covariate effects are similar, as are the associated standard errors. The main difference lies in the estimate of β_3 corresponding to the percentage who own their own home.

Table 9.6 Results of Unweighted SAR Regression for the New York Leukemia Data

Parameter	Estimate	Std. Error	t-Value	p-Value
$\hat{\beta}_0$ (intercept)	−0.6182	0.1781	−3.47	0.0006
$\hat{\beta}_1$ (TCE)	0.0710	0.0424	1.68	0.0947
$\hat{\beta}_2$ (% age > 65)	3.7542	0.6292	5.97	<0.0001
$\hat{\beta}_3$ (% own home)	−0.4199	0.1927	−2.18	0.0302
$\hat{\sigma}_S^2$	0.4198	276 df		
$\hat{\rho}_S = 0.04049$	AIC = 564.2[a]			

[a]Based on maximum likelihood estimation.

Table 9.7 Results of Unweighted CAR Regression for the New York Leukemia Data

Parameter	Estimate	Std. Error	t-Value	p-Value
$\hat{\beta}_0$ (intercept)	−0.6484	0.1824	−3.55	0.0004
$\hat{\beta}_1$ (TCE)	0.0779	0.0440	1.77	0.0778
$\hat{\beta}_2$ (% age > 65)	3.7038	0.6317	5.86	<0.0001
$\hat{\beta}_3$ (% own home)	−0.3828	0.1970	−1.94	0.0530
$\hat{\sigma}_C^2$	0.4135	276 df		
$\hat{\rho}_C = 0.08412$	AIC = 563.7[a]			

[a]Based on maximum likelihood estimation.

The absolute value of the SAR estimate is larger, indicating a significant effect, whereas the same covariate in the CAR model is not technically statistically significant. Both models indicate no significant effect of our surrogate exposure variable on the incidence of leukemia at $\alpha = 0.05$. Comparing these to the results from OLS regression in Table 9.2, we see how including spatial autocorrelation affects results and conclusions. The AIC criteria are smaller for the SAR and CAR models, indicating that these models have a slightly better fit. The impact of including spatial autocorrelation is most pronounced for our surrogate exposure variable X_1, greatly increasing the parameter estimate. With the SAR and CAR models, this effect is significant at $\alpha = 0.10$ but is not significant with traditional OLS regression at this level. We observe the same tendency using geostatistical methods of incorporating spatial autocorrelation (Table 9.4), where spatial proximity is defined by the intercentroid distances. The estimated regression coefficients from the SAR and CAR models are comparable to those in Table 9.4, with the exception of the estimated effect of X_3, our surrogate income variable.

The estimates of ρ_S and ρ_C are small, even when we interpret them against their plausible range of $(-0.3029, 0.1550)$ defined by the reciprocals of the smallest and largest eigenvalues of W, $\vartheta_{\min} = -3.3012$, and $\vartheta_{\max} = 6.4535$. Since the OLS model can be obtained as a special case of both the SAR and the CAR models by taking $\rho = 0$, we can use a likelihood ratio test to test for the significance of the autocorrelation parameters. For example, the value of $\mathcal{L}(\boldsymbol{\beta}, \boldsymbol{\theta}_1)$ from equation (9.26) for the OLS model with five parameters is -278.75. For the SAR model with six parameters, $\mathcal{L}(\boldsymbol{\beta}, \boldsymbol{\theta}_2) = -276.12$. Thus, our likelihood ratio test statistic is $2[-276.12 - (-278.75)] = 5.3$. Comparing this to a χ^2 distribution on one degree of freedom gives a p-value of 0.0294. An analogous test can be used with the CAR model.

Assessing the effects of important covariate factors is usually the primary goal in most regression analyses. With spatial regression analysis, we might want to go beyond this primary goal to assess whether the leukemia incidence proportions or rates are clustered so that we might identify areas of potentially elevated risk. The test based on I_{res} using Moran's I and the likelihood ratio test of $H_0: \rho = 0$ in SAR and CAR models are tests of overall clustering. However, these are global tests. The local indicators of spatial association described in Section 7.5 provide local measures of spatial similarity that can provide insight into areas with comparatively high or low association with neighboring values. Figure 9.16 shows a map of local Moran's I values, computed from the OLS residuals. Thus, this map represents a local version of I_{res} in equation (9.44) that can also be interpreted as a map of local Moran's I values given by $I_{i,\text{std}}$ in equation (7.12) adjusted for the covariates.

Local I_{res} maps require extra effort in interpretation, and we first describe what values capture our interest and for what reasons. High extreme values reveal tracts where all surrounding tracts have similar values. High values of I_{res} may result from high, medium, or low residual values as long as the neighbors have residuals of similar magnitudes. Therefore, high I_{res} values do not necessarily correspond to high residual values, as we might be tempted to conclude. In fact, comparing Figure 9.16 to the map of studentized residuals (Figure 9.13, which is qualitatively

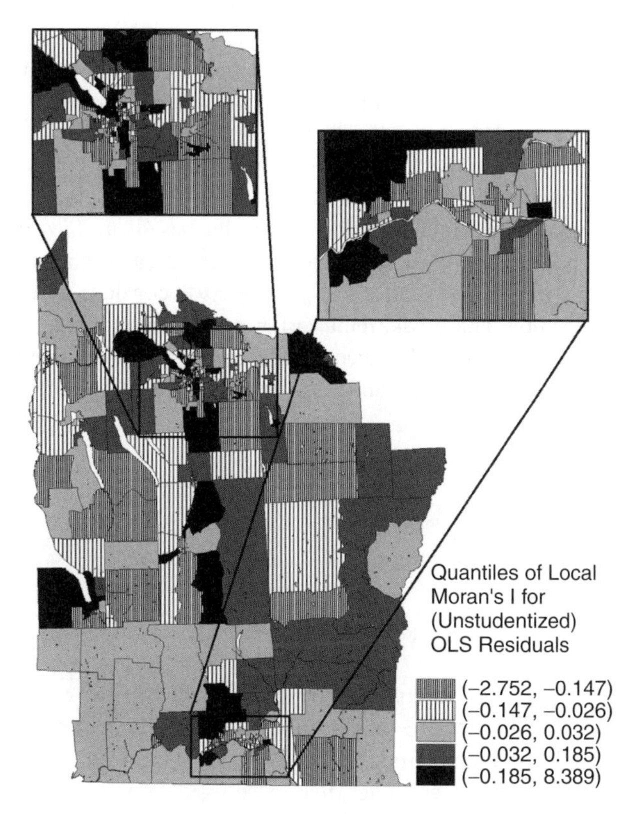

FIG. 9.16 Map of local Moran's I values based on OLS residuals for the New York leukemia data. The map is based on the row-standardized binary connectivity matrix.

similar to the map of OLS residuals, which we do not show), we see that several of the high I_{res} values correspond to clusters of low studentized residual values (where we observe fewer cases than predicted by the model). Low values of I_{res} suggest tracts with residual values very different from those associated with surrounding tracts. These may be high values surrounded by low values, or low values surrounded by high values. Consistent with these interpretations, the three outliers (all high positive residuals and all adjacent to one another) produce three of the five highest observed local values of I_{res}, and a tract neighboring one of the outliers produces the lowest observed local value.

Both extremes of I_{res} values may suggest clusters of interest. A collection of high values of I_{res} suggests an aggregation of regions with similar residuals, thus potentially indicating a spatial pattern in the residuals. A low value of I_{res} suggests a residual that is different from the neighboring residuals, which we might expect if the residuals show no spatial structure, or a local outlier is different from its spatial neighbors. A collection of low values could reflect negative spatial autocorrelation or spatial noise in the residual process (e.g., those near Syracuse, as suggested previously by the high relative nugget effect in the empirical residual semivariogram in Figure 9.14). As a result, the residual LISA map must be interpreted in concert with a map of the residual values. Even so, we must remember that some regions will contain the highest or lowest local values of I_{res}, even for models with independent error terms. The trick is to identify when the extremes are "too extreme," a task complicated by the multiple numbers of correlated statistics encountered in consideration of the set of local statistics (Anselin 1995).

We caution against overinterpretation of results based on I_{res} since the OLS residuals are correlated and have different variances, even when the original data are i.i.d. They are even more suspect in the case we consider here, since as we discussed the preceding data break, their variances depend on the population sizes, n_i, even after transformation. To account for this population heterogeneity, we fit weighted versions of the SAR and CAR models considered previously. Since $\text{Var}(Z_i) \propto 1/n_i$, we take

$$\Sigma_{\text{SAR}} = \sigma^2(I - \rho W)^{-1} V_\upsilon (I - \rho W')^{-1},$$

with $V_\upsilon = \text{diag}[1/n_i]$, and for the CAR we use

$$\Sigma_{\text{CAR}} = \sigma^2(I - \rho W)^{-1} V_c,$$

with $V_c = \text{diag}[1/n_i]$. The results are shown in Tables 9.8 and 9.9.

Comparing these tables, there seems to be little difference between the results from the SAR model and those from the CAR model. All three covariate values are significant at $\alpha = 0.05$. Note, however, that these results do not differ substantially from those obtained using WLS regression with independent errors (Table 9.3). A comparison of the AIC criteria suggests that the WLS regression model fits slightly better than the weighted SAR or weighted CAR, indicating that adjustment for spatial autocorrelation was unnecessary. The nature of the weighted and unweighted results suggests that the residual spatial autocorrelation for the OLS results may be driven by spatial patterns in population size, in particular the collection of the three outliers mapped in Figure 9.8.

Table 9.8 Results of Weighted SAR Regression for the New York Leukemia Data

Parameter	Estimate	Std. Error	t-Value	p-Value
$\hat{\beta}_0$ (intercept)	−0.7971	0.1451	−5.49	<0.0001
$\hat{\beta}_1$ (TCE)	0.0805	0.0285	2.82	0.0051
$\hat{\beta}_2$ (% age > 65)	3.8167	0.5802	6.58	<0.0001
$\hat{\beta}_3$ (% own home)	−0.3808	0.1576	−2.42	0.0164
$\hat{\sigma}^2$	1120.24	276 df		
$\hat{\rho} = 0.009564$	AIC = 515.23			

Table 9.9 Results of Weighted CAR Regression for the New York Leukemia Data

Parameter	Estimate	Std. Error	t-Value	p-Value
$\hat{\beta}_0$ (intercept)	−0.8132	0.1459	−5.57	<0.0001
$\hat{\beta}_1$ (TCE)	0.0812	0.0288	2.82	0.0051
$\hat{\beta}_2$ (% age > 65)	3.7874	0.5819	6.51	<0.0001
$\hat{\beta}_3$ (% own home)	−0.3662	0.1586	−2.31	0.0217
$\hat{\sigma}^2$	1118.9	276 df		
$\hat{\rho} = 0.02242$	AIC = 515.14			

9.3.4 Concluding Remarks on Spatial Autoregressions

In this section we describe and illustrate how the idea of spatial autoregression can be used to adapt the traditional linear regression model for spatial analysis. As in the data break following Section 9.2.3, using a weighted analysis that accounts for population heterogeneity and incorporating spatial correlation not explained by the covariates can both be crucial for obtaining valid conclusions.

Spatial autoregressive models incorporate spatial dependence through the use of spatial proximity measures. As we saw in Chapter 7, these measures provide a flexible modeling tool for geographical data. An alternative approach is provided by geostatistics, where the semivariogram based on inter-centroid distances quantifies the spatial autocorrelation in the data. These two different approaches, and the differences in the results obtained with them, lead us to wonder to what extent the choice of spatial dependence measure has on conclusions. Conceptually, given the differences in the spatial proximity measures, the impact of the choice of spatial proximity measure is likely to be great, as it will result in very different neighborhood structures and thus allow much different interactions among the data.

Griffith (1996) posits several rules of thumb concerning the choice of spatial proximity measure. Although his focus is limited to spatial proximity measures, several of his rules and conclusions apply to modeling spatial dependence in general, whether it be through spatial proximity measures or geostatistical methods. We adapt his rules for our discussion here and interweave some of our own.

1. It is better to use any reasonable method for modeling spatial autocorrelation than to assume that the data are independent.
2. However, the choice of spatial dependence model can greatly affect both the estimates from regression models and their standard errors. Thus, exploratory spatial analysis is important since it can provide valuable information concerning the spatial relationships among the data that can be used to choose a spatial dependence model substantiated by the data. It is also wise to compare results from several different spatial dependence models and to try to understand their differences.

3. Many inferential procedures in spatial statistics are based on asymptotic results which assume that the number of spatial units (points or regions) is large. For inference about the mean with i.i.d data, a sample size of 30 data values is considered a "large" sample. With spatial data, *large* depends on the specific application and the strength and type of the spatial dependence. Our rule of thumb when working with spatial data is based on the idea of effective sample size. If the data are correlated, each data value contains information about other data values, so we have far less information than would be contained in an independent sample of the same size. How much less information? Although this can be calculated, our conservative rule of thumb is that spatial correlation reduces the information contained in a sample of independent data by a factor of 2. Thus, if 30 data values are needed for asymptotic inference with i.i.d data, we would need 60 correlated values for the same inference. However, we stress that this serves only as a loose rule of thumb and may not (probably will not) apply to all spatial data analytic settings.
4. As shown in the data break, accounting for population heterogeneity in geographically aggregated data is very important. Many of the tools for inference with spatial data assume second-order stationarity and thus may give misleading conclusions when applied to data based on units with differing population sizes or with different spatial support.
5. The principle of parsimony is paramount; we should choose the simplest model that both adequately explains the variation in our data and facilitates an interpretation that is consistent with our knowledge about the people, places, and processes we are studying.

Linear models are probably the most widely used regression models in spatial statistics. However, in public health applications, probably the most widely used regression models are the Poisson and the logistic. In the next section we describe how these can be adapted for the analysis of spatial data.

9.4 GENERALIZED LINEAR MODELS

A linear model may not always be the best approach for modeling health events, particularly when the data are counts or rates, or when we are interested in estimating health risk from binary data. In such cases, generalized linear models (GLMs), with Poisson and logistic regression models as special cases, may be more appropriate. A general description of these models (ignoring spatial correlation) appears in Section 2.6.1. In this section we provide more details about GLMs and adapt them for use with spatial data.

9.4.1 Fixed Effects and the Marginal Specification

Instead of assuming the mean response is a linear function of the explanatory covariates as we did with linear regression models in Sections 9.1 and 9.2 [cf.

equation (9.1)], we assume that some function of the mean, called the *link function*, is linearly related to the covariates:

$$g(\boldsymbol{\mu}) = g(E(\mathbf{Y})) = X\boldsymbol{\beta}, \tag{9.56}$$

where $\boldsymbol{\mu}$ is the vector of mean values $(\mu(\boldsymbol{s}_1), \mu(\boldsymbol{s}_2), \ldots, \mu(\boldsymbol{s}_n))'$ of the data vector $\mathbf{Y} = (Y(\boldsymbol{s}_1), Y(\boldsymbol{s}_2), \ldots, Y(\boldsymbol{s}_n))'$. Recall from Section 2.6.1 that there are two common link functions used with public health data. One is the log link function for count data, $g(\mu) = \log(\mu)$, and the other is the logit link function for binary data, $g(\mu) = \log[\mu/(1 - \mu)]$.

To complete our regression model, we have to assume something about the variance of the data. In many of the discrete statistical distributions used to model count or binary data (e.g., Poisson and binomial), the variance of the data depends on the mean. This dependence is included in the specification of a GLM as the *variance function*, $v(\mu)$. With the log link function for count data, $v(\mu) = \mu$, and with the logit link function for binary data, $v(\mu) = \mu(1 - \mu)$. In traditional applications of GLMs (e.g., in the development of Dobson 1990), the data are assumed to be independent, but with heterogeneous variances given by the variance function. Thus, the variance–covariance matrix of the data $\mathbf{Y}$ is

$$\Sigma = \text{Var}(\mathbf{Y}) = \sigma^2 V_{\boldsymbol{\mu}}, \tag{9.57}$$

where $V_{\boldsymbol{\mu}}$ is a $N \times N$ diagonal matrix with the variance function terms on the diagonal, and the parameter σ^2 allows for "inexactness" in the variance-to-mean relationships called *overdispersion* (in many real data situations the variance is greater than the mean, hence the modifier "over"). The variance–covariance matrix defined in equation (9.57) is a generalization of the variance–covariance matrix assumed for linear regression models with uncorrelated residuals [equation (9.2)].

Technically, our use of σ^2 differs slightly from our previous usage in this chapter. In equation (9.57), σ^2 represents a multiplicative increase (or decrease) in the typical variance associated with the distribution of the data, while earlier σ^2 referenced any multiplicative factor shared across the data variances. The distinction is subtle and does not affect our development below, so we maintain the use of σ^2 here to illustrate similarities in estimation routines between the methods outlined below and those of Sections 9.1 and 9.2.

Marginal GLMs with Spatial Correlation Generalized linear models can be used with spatial data if we assume that the data are independent and that any of the systematic spatial variation we observe in the outcome can be accounted for by the covariates (just as with the linear regression model with independent data in Section 9.1). Since we may not always be willing to assume that the data are independent, we need to adapt the GLM models to allow for spatial autocorrelation. We have already done this for the linear regression model in Section 9.2, where we allowed spatially autocorrelated residuals and the more general variance–covariance matrix $\Sigma(\boldsymbol{\theta})$. We extend this idea by modifying $\Sigma(\boldsymbol{\theta})$ to include the variance-to-mean relationships inherent in a GLM specification. Based on the ideas in Wolfinger and O'Connell (1993) and Gotway and Stroup (1997), one such approach is to model the variance–covariance matrix of the data as

$$\text{Var}(\mathbf{Y}) = \Sigma(\boldsymbol{\mu}, \boldsymbol{\theta}) = \sigma^2 V_{\boldsymbol{\mu}}^{1/2} R(\boldsymbol{\theta}) V_{\boldsymbol{\mu}}^{1/2}, \tag{9.58}$$

where $R(\boldsymbol{\theta})$ is a correlation matrix with elements $\rho(\boldsymbol{s}_i - \boldsymbol{s}_j; \boldsymbol{\theta})$, the spatial correlogram defined in Section 8.2.1. The diagonal matrix, $V_{\boldsymbol{\mu}}^{1/2}$, has elements equal to the square root of variance function, $\sqrt{v(\mu)}$. Recall that the correlogram or correlation function is related directly to the covariance function and the semivariogram, so all of the ideas in Section 8.2 apply here. Often, we assume a single parameter for the correlogram (since the sill of a correlogram is 1; i.e., $\boldsymbol{\theta} \equiv a$, the range of spatial autocorrelation). If we wish, we can add a nugget effect by using

$$\text{Var}(\mathbf{Y}) = \sigma_0^2 V_{\boldsymbol{\mu}} + \sigma_1^2 V_{\boldsymbol{\mu}}^{1/2} R(\boldsymbol{\theta}) V_{\boldsymbol{\mu}}^{1/2}.$$

In this case, $\text{Var}(Y(\boldsymbol{s}_i)) = (\sigma_0^2 + \sigma_1^2)v(\mu(\boldsymbol{s}_i))$, and the covariance between any two variables is $\text{Cov}(Y(\boldsymbol{s}_i), Y(\boldsymbol{s}_j)) = \sigma_1^2\sqrt{v(\mu(\boldsymbol{s}_i))v(\mu(\boldsymbol{s}_j))}\rho(\boldsymbol{s}_i - \boldsymbol{s}_j)$.

Example To see how to set up the matrices in a spatial GLM, we consider the spatial arrangement in Figure 8.13. For now, we do not consider the interpolation problem, so we will ignore the point $\boldsymbol{s}_0$. Assume that the data given in this figure (the Z's) are actually covariate values associated with each location. Further assume that count data $Y(\boldsymbol{s}_1), Y(\boldsymbol{s}_2), Y(\boldsymbol{s}_3), Y(\boldsymbol{s}_4), Y(\boldsymbol{s}_5)$ will be observed at spatial locations $\boldsymbol{s}_1, \boldsymbol{s}_2, \boldsymbol{s}_3, \boldsymbol{s}_4, \boldsymbol{s}_5$ in the figure. Since the data are counts, we will use the log link function and specify the mean function in equation (9.56) as

$$\log(E(\mathbf{Y})) = \log(\boldsymbol{\mu}) = \begin{bmatrix} \log(\mu(\boldsymbol{s}_1)) \\ \log(\mu(\boldsymbol{s}_2)) \\ \log(\mu(\boldsymbol{s}_3)) \\ \log(\mu(\boldsymbol{s}_4)) \\ \log(\mu(\boldsymbol{s}_5)) \end{bmatrix} = \begin{bmatrix} 1 & 2 \\ 1 & -3 \\ 1 & 3 \\ 1 & -4 \\ 1 & 2 \end{bmatrix} \begin{bmatrix} \beta_0 \\ \beta_1 \end{bmatrix},$$

and the variance function as $v(\mu)$, so that $V_{\boldsymbol{\mu}}^{1/2}$ in equation (9.58) is

$$V_{\boldsymbol{\mu}}^{1/2} = \begin{bmatrix} \sqrt{\mu(\boldsymbol{s}_1)} & 0 & 0 & 0 & 0 \\ 0 & \sqrt{\mu(\boldsymbol{s}_2)} & 0 & 0 & 0 \\ 0 & 0 & \sqrt{\mu(\boldsymbol{s}_3)} & 0 & 0 \\ 0 & 0 & 0 & \sqrt{\mu(\boldsymbol{s}_4)} & 0 \\ 0 & 0 & 0 & 0 & \sqrt{\mu(\boldsymbol{s}_5)} \end{bmatrix}.$$

By taking the inverse of the link function, we find that $\mu_i = \exp(\beta_0 + \beta_1 Z_i)$, so the vector of expected values and the variance–covariance matrix become

$$E(\mathbf{Y}) = \boldsymbol{\mu} = \begin{bmatrix} \exp(\beta + 2\beta_1) \\ \exp(\beta_0 - 3\beta_1) \\ \exp(\beta_0 + 3\beta_1) \\ \exp(\beta_0 - 4\beta_1) \\ \exp(\beta_0 + 2\beta_1) \end{bmatrix}$$

and

$$V_{\boldsymbol{\mu}}^{1/2} = \begin{bmatrix} \sqrt{e^{\beta+2\beta_1}} & 0 & 0 & 0 & 0 \\ 0 & \sqrt{e^{\beta_0-3\beta_1}} & 0 & 0 & 0 \\ 0 & 0 & \sqrt{e^{\beta_0+3\beta_1}} & 0 & 0 \\ 0 & 0 & 0 & \sqrt{e^{\beta_0-4\beta_1}} & 0 \\ 0 & 0 & 0 & 0 & \sqrt{e^{\beta_0+2\beta_1}} \end{bmatrix},$$

respectively.

Now assume that the spatial correlation function can be specified in terms of one of the semivariogram models given in Section 8.2.2. For illustration, we choose the exponential model so that $\rho(\boldsymbol{s}_i - \boldsymbol{s}_j; \boldsymbol{\theta}) = \exp\{-\|\boldsymbol{s}_i - \boldsymbol{s}_j\|/a\}$. Taking $a = 1$ and using the distances defined in Figure 8.13 gives

$$R = \begin{bmatrix} 1 & 0.37 & 0.24 & 0.13 & 0.24 \\ 0.37 & 1 & 0.37 & 0.13 & 0.11 \\ 0.24 & 0.37 & 1 & 0.33 & 0.14 \\ 0.13 & 0.13 & 0.33 & 1 & 0.16 \\ 0.24 & 0.11 & 0.14 & 0.16 & 1 \end{bmatrix}.$$

Notice that the matrices needed to define the GLM are specified in terms of two unknown parameters, β_0 and β_1. In practical applications, a would also be unknown and we might include an extra parameter, σ^2, to account for overdispersion.

To fit the model, we need to estimate these parameters from the data. However, before detailing estimation techniques for spatial GLMs we present an alternative spatial GLM formulation using conditional (rather than marginal) specification of the model. The marginal and conditional specifications provide different approaches for including spatial correlation, similar in spirit to the simultaneous and conditional autoregressive models presented in Section 9.3 but also unique in perspective, as described in the next section.

9.4.2 Mixed Models and Conditional Specification

In the development in Section 9.4.1, we assume that $\boldsymbol{\beta}$ is a vector of fixed, unknown parameters and we modeled $E(\mathbf{Y})$ as a function of these fixed parameters. The literature refers to this approach as the *marginal* specification since we model the marginal mean, $E(\mathbf{Y})$, as a function of fixed, nonrandom (but unknown) parameters. An alternative specification defines the distribution of each outcome, conditional on an unobserved (latent) spatial process defining the spatial similarity between observations. The conditional approach incorporates this unobserved process through the use of *random effects* within the mean function and models the conditional mean and variance of the outcome as a function of both fixed covariate effects and the random effects deriving from the unobserved spatial process. We describe this approach below.

In our discussion of filtered kriging in Section 8.3.2 we assumed that the data were noisy measurements of an underlying smooth spatial process $S(\boldsymbol{s})$. Here again, we make the same assumption and also assume that $S(\boldsymbol{s})$ is a Gaussian random field with mean 0 at any location and covariance function $\sigma_S^2 \rho_S(\boldsymbol{s}_i - \boldsymbol{s}_j)$. We note that $S(\boldsymbol{s})$ enters the GLM model as part of the linear component (i.e., within the link function) and adds (spatially structured) noise around the mean of the transformed mean of the data $Y(\boldsymbol{s})$. We also note that the Gaussian assumption for $S(\boldsymbol{s})$ is separate from the random component of the GLM, which defines the distribution of error terms associated with each observation (e.g., Poisson or binomial).

More specifically, instead of $E(\mathbf{Y})$, we consider the conditional mean

$$E[Y(\boldsymbol{s})|S(\boldsymbol{s})] \equiv \mu(\boldsymbol{s})$$

and let the link function relate this conditional mean to the explanatory covariates and also to the underlying spatial random field, so that

$$g[\mu(\boldsymbol{s})] = \boldsymbol{x}'(\boldsymbol{s})\boldsymbol{\beta} + S(\boldsymbol{s}). \tag{9.59}$$

We note that equation (9.59) illustrates how the particular value $S(\boldsymbol{s})$ of the random effect at location $\boldsymbol{s}$ enters the linear component of the GLM as an addition to the intercept, so at any location we can consider $S(\boldsymbol{s})$ to represent a *random intercept* (or more accurately, a random addition to the intercept).

Now, instead of trying to predict $S(\boldsymbol{s}_0)$ at an unmeasured location $\boldsymbol{s}_0$, our interest will be estimation of fixed effects given the spatial variation in $S(\boldsymbol{s})$ and smoothing [prediction of $S(\boldsymbol{s})$ and the related mean value of the outcome at the data locations].

To allow the variance to depend on the mean, we assume that the data are conditionally independent (i.e., independent *given* the value of S) with conditional variance

$$\mathrm{Var}[Y(\boldsymbol{s})|S(\boldsymbol{s})] = \sigma^2 v(\mu(\boldsymbol{s})), \tag{9.60}$$

where the function $v(\cdot)$ is the variance function described earlier and σ^2 is an overdispersion parameter. The conditional independence assumptions implies that any spatial correlation among the Y's is due solely to spatial patterns within the random field S. Operationally, conditional independence defers treatment of spatial autocorrelation to the consideration of S (i.e., the key component in the estimation techniques below is the approach for incorporating information regarding S). This type of model specification is known as a *generalized linear mixed model* (GLMM), the term *mixed* indicating the model is composed of both fixed ($\boldsymbol{\beta}$) and random effects ($S(\boldsymbol{s})$).

This conditional specification and the marginal specification given in Section 9.4.1 are different in structure and interpretation. For example, consider $g(\mu) = \log(\mu)$ and $v(\mu) = \mu$, and let $m(\boldsymbol{s}) = \exp[\boldsymbol{x}'(\boldsymbol{s})\boldsymbol{\beta}]$. Standard results from statistical theory reveal that the marginal mean is the mean of the conditional mean and the marginal variance is the sum of the mean conditional variance and the variance of the conditional mean. Using these facts together with the mean and variance relationships of the lognormal distribution (see Section 8.3.2) we define the corresponding marginal moments of the data as

$$E(Y(\boldsymbol{s})) = E_S[E(Y(\boldsymbol{s})|S)] = E_S[m(\boldsymbol{s})\exp(S)] = m(\boldsymbol{s})\exp(\sigma_S^2/2) \quad (9.61)$$

$$\text{Var}(Y(\boldsymbol{s})) = m(\boldsymbol{s})[\sigma^2\exp(\sigma_S^2/2) + m(\boldsymbol{s})\exp(\sigma_S^2)(\exp(\sigma_S^2) - 1)] \quad (9.62)$$

$$\text{Cov}(Y(\boldsymbol{s}_i), Y(\boldsymbol{s}_j)) = m(\boldsymbol{s}_i)m(\boldsymbol{s}_j)\exp(\sigma_S^2)\{\exp[\sigma_S^2\rho(\boldsymbol{s}_i - \boldsymbol{s}_j)] - 1\}, \quad (9.63)$$

where $E_S(\cdot)$ denotes the expectation over S. Note $\text{Var}(Y(\boldsymbol{s})) > E(Y(\boldsymbol{s}))$, even if $\sigma^2 = 1$. Also, both the overdispersion and the autocorrelation induced into data by the latent process, $S(\boldsymbol{s})$, depend on the mean, so the conditional model can be used with nonstationary spatial processes where the mean and variance vary across locations.

As with the marginal spatial GLMs described in Section 9.4.1, the correlation function $\rho_S(\boldsymbol{s}_i - \boldsymbol{s}_j)$ can be modeled as a function of a $q \times 1$ vector of unknown parameters $\boldsymbol{\theta}_S$ that completely characterizes the spatial dependence in the underlying surface [i.e., $\text{corr}(S(\boldsymbol{s}_i), S(\boldsymbol{s}_j)) = \rho_S(\boldsymbol{s}_i - \boldsymbol{s}_j; \boldsymbol{\theta}_S)$]. Thus, to use this model, we need to estimate the parameters for the fixed covariate effects, $\boldsymbol{\beta}$, the variance components, σ_S^2 and σ^2, and the spatial autocorrelation parameters, $\boldsymbol{\theta}_S$.

The spatial GLMM is an example of a *hierarchical model*, or a model defined in stages. At the first stage of the model, we define the distribution of the data given values of the random effects. At the second stage, we define the distribution of the random effects. By combining the first and second stages, we obtain inference about the data, taking into account the distribution of the random effects. We use a similar approach in our discussion of empirical Bayes smoothing in Section 4.4.3. The notion of hierarchical models provides a very convenient framework for spatial GLMs, as we illustrate throughout the remainder of this chapter.

9.4.3 Estimation in Spatial GLMs and GLMMs

The likelihood function plays a central role in the statistical estimation of linear model parameters as illustrated in Sections 9.1 and 9.2. As we move from linear models to GLMs, maximum likelihood estimation still provides an attractive approach for inference, but several factors complicate the direct calculation and maximization of the likelihood function in the spatial GLM and GLMM settings. We briefly outline some of these issues, then define and illustrate a variety of estimation techniques for both marginal and conditional specifications.

Likelihood Complications First, as outlined in McCullagh and Nelder (1989, Chapter 9), we often have less detail in GLMs than in linear models regarding the underlying random mechanism generating the data. For instance, the Gaussian distribution arises as a limiting distribution for a wide variety of statistics due to the central limit theorem, leading to the wide use of Gaussian models across application areas. In contrast, for regionally specified data, we tend to assume a Poisson distribution for counts of events within regions due to the properties of a spatial Poisson process outlined in Chapter 5, but often a binomial distribution is more realistic for counts of events among a fixed regional population size (since the Poisson distribution assigns a small but nonzero probability of observing more events than there are people at risk). Differences between the Poisson and binomial likelihoods are typically small for large population sizes and small individual risks, but such differences still exist.

Although the precise random mechanism may not be clear in GLM applications, we often *do* have clear conceptual models of the mean and variance (and perhaps the range) of possible values. For example, the constant risk hypothesis of Chapter 7 provides a model of the mean number of events within a fixed number of people at risk. Often, particularly when working with discrete data like counts or rates, our conceptual models result in mean–variance relationships and we would like to explicitly include these in our statistical models rather than transform them away. Thus, a second issue arises in that the variance in a GLM (or GLMM) is often a function of the mean, and a Gaussian distribution, by definition, does not allow such functional relationships.

Traditional GLMs allow us to move away from the Gaussian distribution and utilize other distributions that allow mean–variance relationships. However, a final complication arises from spatial dependence. For likelihood-based inference we need to build a *multivariate* distribution. When the data are spatially autocorrelated, we cannot easily build this distribution as a product of marginal likelihoods as we do when the data are independent. Constructing multivariate distributions that allow general spatial dependence structures can be very difficult, and few such distributions (outside the multivariate Gaussian) have been fully evaluated for practical modeling value.

We can bypass this problem by using conditionally specified GLMM models, since these models always assume that conditional on random effects, the data are independent. The conditional independence and hierarchical structure allow us to build a multivariate distribution, although we cannot always be sure of the properties of this distribution. The hierarchical structure of GLMMs further complicates matters if we wish to build a likelihood function encompassing all stages of the model. As noted in Breslow and Clayton (1993), exact inference for first-stage model parameters (e.g., covariate effects) typically requires integration over the distribution of the random effects. This necessary multidimensional integration can often result in numerical instabilities, requiring approximations or more computer-intensive estimation procedures.

There are several ways to avoid all of these problems (although arguably each approach introduces new problems). To address the situation where we can define means and variances, but not necessarily the entire likelihood, Wedderburn (1974) introduced the notion of *quasilikelihood* based on the first two moments of a distribution, and the approach sees wide application for GLMs based on independent data (McCullagh and Nelder 1989, Chapter 9). This leads to an iterative *estimating equation* based on just the first two moments of a distribution that can be used with spatial data. Another solution is based on an initial Taylor series expansion that then allows *pseudolikelihood* methods for spatial inference similar to those described in Section 9.2.1. Finally, Bayesian inference (introduced briefly in Section 4.4.3 and revisited in more detail in Section 9.5) is an attractive alternative since it can avoid the approximations and heuristic arguments inherent in working with "quasi" and "pseudo" likelihood methods and uses simulation to obtain parameter estimates and inferential distributions. As detailed in Section 9.5, the Bayesian approach requires more assumptions and more work in model specification since the distributions for simulations must be derived, but it tends to provide a more complete framework for estimation and inference. We provide several modifications and approximations to likelihood-based inference for GLMs and GLMMs in the sections to follow, then transition to the introduction to Bayesian analysis of spatially correlated regional counts in Section 9.5.

Quasilikelihood Estimation and Generalized Estimating Equations As noted briefly above, quasilikelihood builds inference in terms of the first two moments only rather than the entire joint distribution, but it has many of the familiar properties of a joint likelihood. For example, estimates derive from maximizing the quasilikelihood function using score equations (partial derivatives set equal to zero) and have nice asymptotic properties such as Gaussian distributions. Although developed most fully for independent data, McCullagh and Nelder (1989, Section 9.3) extend quasilikelihood estimation to dependent data, and Gotway and Stroup (1997) phrase the approach in a spatial GLM context, which we summarize here.

To define our GLM, let $\boldsymbol{\mu} = (\mu_1, \ldots, \mu_N)$ denote the vector of mean values for the regional counts $Y(\boldsymbol{s}_1), \ldots, Y(\boldsymbol{s}_N)$ and $g(\boldsymbol{\mu})$ denote the link function, where $g(\boldsymbol{\mu}) = X\boldsymbol{\beta}$. For notational convenience, we denote observation $Y(\boldsymbol{s}_i)$ by Y_i. The quasilikelihood function $Q(\mu_i; Y_i)$ is defined by the relationship

$$\frac{\partial Q(\boldsymbol{\mu}; \mathbf{Y})}{\partial \boldsymbol{\mu}} = V^{-1}(\mathbf{Y} - \boldsymbol{\mu}),$$

where V represents the variance–covariance matrix capturing the spatial correlation, where $\mathbf{Y}$ denotes the vector of observed outcomes. We note that in GLMs, the elements of V are often functions of $\boldsymbol{\mu}$. Differentiating $Q(\boldsymbol{\mu}; \mathbf{Y})$ with respect to each element of $\boldsymbol{\beta}$ yields the set of quasilikelihood score equations

$$\Delta' V^{-1}(\mathbf{Y} - \boldsymbol{\mu}) \overset{\text{set}}{=} \mathbf{0}$$

where Δ denotes the matrix with elements $[\partial\mu_i/\partial\beta_j]$ and $j = 0, \ldots, p$ indexes the parameters in the linear portion of the GLM. Solving the score equations for $\boldsymbol{\beta}$ yields the quasilikelihood estimates of the model parameters.

McCullagh and Nelder (1989, pp. 333–335) note the inverse of the variance–covariance matrix V^{-1} must satisfy several conditions to guarantee a solution to the score equations, some not easily verified in practice. As a result, Wolfinger and O'Connell (1993) and Gotway and Stroup (1997) follow Liang and Zeger (1986) and Zeger and Liang (1986) and limit attention to variance–covariance matrices of the form introduced in equation (9.58):

$$V \equiv \Sigma(\boldsymbol{\mu}, \boldsymbol{\theta}) = V_{\boldsymbol{\mu}}^{1/2} R(\boldsymbol{\theta}) V_{\boldsymbol{\mu}}^{1/2}$$

where R denotes a matrix of correlations among the observations parameterized by the vector $\boldsymbol{\theta}$, and $V_{\boldsymbol{\mu}}^{1/2}$ a diagonal matrix of scale parameters (perhaps including overdispersion). With V now also depending on unknown autocorrelation parameters, the quasilikelihood score equations are known as a *generalized estimating equations*. Liang and Zeger (1986) and Zeger and Liang (1986) show that under mild regularity conditions, these equations generate consistent estimators of $\boldsymbol{\beta}$, even with misspecified correlation matrices. Zeger (1988) shows that the same conditions are met for a single time-series replicate, provided that the covariance function is "well behaved" in the sense that $\Sigma(\boldsymbol{\mu}, \boldsymbol{\theta})$ breaks into independent blocks for large n. This same result holds for spatial data as well (McShane et al. 1997). In the spatial setting, to avoid any distributional assumptions in a completely marginal analysis, Gotway and Stroup (1997) suggest using an iteratively reweighted generalized least-squares (IRWGLS) approach to solve the quasilikelihood/generalized estimating equations for $\boldsymbol{\beta}$ and $\boldsymbol{\theta}$ that is very similar to that described in Section 9.2.1. With $\boldsymbol{\eta} = X\boldsymbol{\beta}$, the matrix Δ can be written as $\Delta = \Psi X$, where $\Psi = \text{diag}[\partial\mu_i/\partial\eta_i]$, and the quasilikelihood/generalized estimating equations can be written as

$$(X'A(\boldsymbol{\theta})X)^{-1}\boldsymbol{\beta} = X'A(\boldsymbol{\theta})\mathbf{Y}^*,$$

where $A(\boldsymbol{\theta}) = \Psi'\Sigma(\boldsymbol{\mu}, \boldsymbol{\theta})^{-1}\Psi$ and $\mathbf{Y}^* = X\boldsymbol{\beta} + \Psi^{-1}(\mathbf{Y} - \boldsymbol{\mu})$. The elements of $R(\boldsymbol{\theta})$ can be estimated via standard geostatistical techniques (e.g., based on the residual semivariogram or correlogram), and then IRWGLS is used to obtain estimates of $\boldsymbol{\beta}$ and $\boldsymbol{\theta}$.

The quasilikelihood approach outlined above provides *marginal* inference regarding covariate effects (i.e., estimates of the average effect of each covariate across the entire study population). Breslow and Clayton (1993), Leroux (2000), and Gotway and Wolfinger (2003) provide additional details and related analytic approaches for GLMs applied to spatial data.

Pseudolikelihood Estimation Instead of quasilikelihood, Wolfinger and O'Connell (1993) suggest an approach termed *pseudolikelihood* (PL) as a flexible and efficient way of estimating the unknown parameters in a generalized linear mixed model (GLMM). (We note that different uses of the term *pseudolikelihood* appear in other statistical estimation contexts; cf. Besag 1975; Gong and Samaniego 1981.)

The pseudolikelihood approach of Wolfinger and O'Connell (1993) differs from the quasilikelihood approach above in that at any step of the iterative process, a function that is a true joint likelihood is used to estimate unknown parameters. In the case we consider here, a pseudolikelihood approach assumes that $\boldsymbol{\beta}$ is known and estimates σ^2 and $\boldsymbol{\theta}$ using ML (as described in Section 9.2.1), and then assumes that $\boldsymbol{\theta}$ is known and estimates $\boldsymbol{\beta}$ using ML and iterating until convergence. We can apply this approach to marginal GLMs as special cases of a GLMM. We concentrate on the PL method here since in Sections 9.1 and 9.2 we have already developed much of the statistical theory we need and PL procedure can be implemented with standard software for random effects modeling or with repeated calls to such software. There are many important theoretical and implementational details associated with the use of these methods (e.g., asymptotic theory, starting values, convergence criteria, etc.) that we do not provide here and defer to the excellent discussions and examples in Green (1987), Breslow and Clayton (1993), and Wolfinger and O'Connell (1993).

The idea behind the pseudolikelihood approach is to linearize the problem so that we can use the approach in Section 9.2 for estimation and inference. This is done using a first-order Taylor series expansion of the link function to give what Wolfinger and O'Connell (1993) call *pseudodata* (similar to the "working" outcome variable in quasilikelihood, $\mathbf{Y}^*$)

$$Y_i^{(p)} = g(\hat{\mu}_i) + g'(\hat{\mu}_i)(Y_i - \hat{\mu}_i), \tag{9.64}$$

where $g'(\hat{\mu}_i)$, is the first derivative of the link function with respect to μ, evaluated at $\hat{\mu}$, and $\hat{\mu}$ is a current estimate of μ. To apply the methods in Section 9.2, we need the mean and variance–covariance matrix of the pseudodata, $\mathbf{Y}^{(p)}$. Conditioning on $\boldsymbol{\beta}$ and $\boldsymbol{S}$, assuming that Var($\mathbf{Y}|\boldsymbol{S}$) has the form of equation (9.58) and using some probabilistic approximations described in Wolfinger and O'Connell (1993), these can be derived in almost the traditional fashion as

$$E(\mathbf{Y}^{(p)}|\boldsymbol{\beta}, \boldsymbol{S}) = X\boldsymbol{\beta} + \boldsymbol{S}$$
$$\text{Var}(\mathbf{Y}^{(p)}|\boldsymbol{\beta}, \boldsymbol{S}) = \Sigma_{\hat{\boldsymbol{\mu}}},$$

with

$$\Sigma_{\hat{\boldsymbol{\mu}}} = \sigma^2 \Delta_{\hat{\boldsymbol{\mu}}} V_{\hat{\boldsymbol{\mu}}}^{1/2} \; R \; V_{\hat{\boldsymbol{\mu}}}^{1/2} \Delta_{\hat{\boldsymbol{\mu}}}.$$

Here $\Delta_{\hat{\boldsymbol{\mu}}}$ is a $N \times N$ diagonal matrix with elements $[\partial g(\mu(\boldsymbol{s}_i))/\partial \mu(\boldsymbol{s}_i)]$ evaluated at $\hat{\boldsymbol{\mu}}$. The marginal moments of the pseudodata are

$$E(\mathbf{Y}^{(p)}) = X\boldsymbol{\beta}$$
$$\text{Var}(\mathbf{Y}^{(p)}) = \Sigma_S + \Sigma_{\hat{\boldsymbol{\mu}}} \equiv \Sigma_{\mathbf{Y}^{(p)}},$$

and Σ_S has (i, j)th element $\sigma_S^2 \rho_S(\boldsymbol{s}_i - \boldsymbol{s}_j)$. This can be considered as a general linear regression model with spatially autocorrelated residuals described in Section 9.2

since the mean (of the pseudodata $\mathbf{Y}^{(p)}$) is linear in $\boldsymbol{\beta}$. Thus, if we are willing to assume that $\Sigma_{\hat{\boldsymbol{\mu}}}$ is known (or at least does not depend on $\boldsymbol{\beta}$) when we want to estimate $\boldsymbol{\beta}$ and that $\boldsymbol{\beta}$ is known when we want to estimate $\boldsymbol{\theta}$, we can maximize the log-likelihood analytically yielding the least squares equations

$$\hat{\boldsymbol{\beta}} = (X'\Sigma_{\mathbf{Y}^{(p)}}^{-1}X)^{-1}X'\Sigma_{\mathbf{Y}^{(p)}}^{-1}\mathbf{Y}^{(p)} \tag{9.65}$$

$$\hat{\mathbf{S}} = \Sigma_S\Sigma_{\mathbf{Y}^{(p)}}^{-1}(\mathbf{Y}^{(p)} - X\hat{\boldsymbol{\beta}}) \tag{9.66}$$

$$\hat{\sigma}^2 = \frac{(\mathbf{Y}^{(p)} - X\hat{\boldsymbol{\beta}})'\Sigma_{\mathbf{Y}^{(p)}}^{-1}(\mathbf{Y}^{(p)} - X\hat{\boldsymbol{\beta}})}{N}. \tag{9.67}$$

However, $\Sigma_{\hat{\boldsymbol{\mu}}}$ does depend on $\boldsymbol{\beta}$, so we iterate as follows:

1. Obtain an initial estimate of $\hat{\boldsymbol{\mu}}$ from the original data. An estimate from the nonspatial generalized linear model often works well.
2. Compute the pseudodata from equation (9.64).
3. Using ML (or REML) with the pseudodata, obtain estimates of the spatial autocorrelation parameters, $\boldsymbol{\theta}$, and σ_S^2 in $\Sigma_{\mathbf{Y}^{(p)}}$ (cf. Section 9.2.1).
4. Use these estimates to compute generalized least squares estimates (which are also the maximum pseudolikelihood estimators) of $\boldsymbol{\beta}$ and σ^2 from equations (9.65) and (9.67) and to predict $\mathbf{S}$ from equation (9.66).
5. Update the estimate of $\boldsymbol{\mu}$ using $\hat{\boldsymbol{\mu}} = g^{-1}(X\hat{\boldsymbol{\beta}} + \hat{\mathbf{S}})$.
6. Repeat these steps until convergence.

Approximate standard errors for the fixed effects derived from

$$\widehat{\text{Var}}(\hat{\boldsymbol{\beta}}) = \hat{\sigma}^2(X'\widehat{\Sigma}_{\mathbf{Y}^{(p)}}^{-1}X)^{-1}$$

using the converged parameter estimates of $\boldsymbol{\theta}$ in $\Sigma_{\mathbf{Y}^{(p)}}$ to define the estimator $\widehat{\Sigma}_{\mathbf{Y}^{(p)}}$. We can construct approximate p-values using t-tests analogous to those described in Section 9.2.1.

We have a choice as to how to model any spatial autocorrelation: through R or through Σ_S. Marginal models let R be a spatial correlation matrix, $R(\boldsymbol{\theta})$, and set $\mathbf{S} = \mathbf{0}$. Conditional models are specified through $\mathbf{S}$ and Σ_S, with spatial dependence incorporated in $\Sigma_S = \sigma_s^2 V(\boldsymbol{\theta}_S)$ and R equal to an identity matrix. Once we have determined which type of model we want to use, we use the iterative approach just described to estimate any unknown parameters ($\sigma^2, \boldsymbol{\beta}, \boldsymbol{\theta}$ for a marginal model and $\sigma^2, \sigma_S^2, \boldsymbol{\beta}, \boldsymbol{\theta}_S$ for a conditional model).

***Example* (cont.)** Continuing with our example in Section 9.4.1, suppose that we fit a marginal model, but this time with an overdispersion parameter, σ^2, and with an unknown range of autocorrelation, a. The vector $\log(\boldsymbol{\mu})$ and the matrix $V_{\boldsymbol{\mu}}^{1/2}$ remain the same. The spatial correlation matrix is now

$$R(a) = \begin{bmatrix} 1 & \exp\left(\frac{-1.0}{a}\right) & \exp\left(\frac{-1.4}{a}\right) & \exp\left(\frac{-2.1}{a}\right) & \exp\left(\frac{-1.4}{a}\right) \\ \exp\left(\frac{-1.0}{a}\right) & 1 & \exp\left(\frac{-1.0}{a}\right) & \exp\left(\frac{-2.1}{a}\right) & \exp\left(\frac{-2.2}{a}\right) \\ \exp\left(\frac{-1.4}{a}\right) & \exp\left(\frac{-1.0}{a}\right) & 1 & \exp\left(\frac{-1.1}{a}\right) & \exp\left(\frac{-2.0}{a}\right) \\ \exp\left(\frac{-2.1}{a}\right) & \exp\left(\frac{-2.1}{a}\right) & \exp\left(\frac{-1.1}{a}\right) & 1 & \exp\left(\frac{-1.8}{a}\right) \\ \exp\left(\frac{-1.4}{a}\right) & \exp\left(\frac{-2.2}{a}\right) & \exp\left(\frac{-2.0}{a}\right) & \exp\left(\frac{-1.8}{a}\right) & 1 \end{bmatrix}.$$

The link function is $g(\mu) = \log(\mu)$, so $g'(\mu) = 1/\mu$, and

$$\Delta_{\boldsymbol{\mu}} = \text{diag}\left\{1/\mu(\boldsymbol{s}_1), 1/\mu(\boldsymbol{s}_2), 1/\mu(\boldsymbol{s}_3), 1/\mu(\boldsymbol{s}_4), 1/\mu(\boldsymbol{s}_5)\right\}.$$

We can also write this matrix as

$$\begin{aligned}\Delta_{\boldsymbol{\beta}} = \text{diag}\,\{&1/\exp(\beta + 2\beta_1), 1/\exp(\beta_0 - 3\beta_1), 1/\exp(\beta_0 + 3\beta_1),\\ &1/\exp(\beta_0 - 4\beta_1), 1/\exp(\beta_0 + 2\beta_1)\},\end{aligned}$$

to emphasize the dependence on $\boldsymbol{\beta}$. The pseudodata are

$$\mathbf{Y}^{(p)} = \begin{bmatrix} 1 & 2 \\ 1 & -3 \\ 1 & 3 \\ 1 & -4 \\ 1 & 2 \end{bmatrix} \begin{bmatrix} \beta_0 \\ \beta_1 \end{bmatrix} + \Delta_{\boldsymbol{\beta}} \left(\begin{bmatrix} Y(\boldsymbol{s}_1) \\ Y(\boldsymbol{s}_2) \\ Y(\boldsymbol{s}_3) \\ Y(\boldsymbol{s}_4) \\ Y(\boldsymbol{s}_5) \end{bmatrix} - \begin{bmatrix} \exp(\beta + 2\beta_1) \\ \exp(\beta_0 - 3\beta_1) \\ \exp(\beta_0 + 3\beta_1) \\ \exp(\beta_0 - 4\beta_1) \\ \exp(\beta_0 + 2\beta_1) \end{bmatrix} \right),$$

and given values for the data $Y(\boldsymbol{s}_1), Y(\boldsymbol{s}_2), \ldots, Y(\boldsymbol{s}_5)$, they depend only on β_0 and β_1. Thus, given an estimate of $\boldsymbol{\mu}$, or equivalently, estimates of β_0 and β_1, the vector of pseudodata $\mathbf{Y}^{(p)}$ is completely determined and plays the role of the data in generalized least-squares fitting with

$$\Sigma_{\mathbf{Y}^{(p)}} = \sigma^2 \Delta_{\boldsymbol{\mu}} V_{\boldsymbol{\mu}}^{1/2} R(a) V_{\boldsymbol{\mu}}^{1/2} \Delta_{\boldsymbol{\mu}},$$

where $\Delta_{\boldsymbol{\mu}}$ and $V_{\boldsymbol{\mu}}$ are evaluated in terms of β_0 and β_1. Thus, the iteration proceeds as follows: Given initial estimates of β_0 and β_1, we compute the means $\mu_i = \exp(\beta_0 + \beta_1 Z_i)$ and then evaluate $\Delta_{\boldsymbol{\mu}}, V_{\boldsymbol{\mu}}^{1/2}$, and $\mathbf{Y}^{(p)}$. Given data $\mathbf{Y}^{(p)}$, we estimate σ^2 and a using ML or REML. Then we substitute these estimates into $\Sigma_{\mathbf{Y}(p)}$ and estimate β_0 and β_1 using generalized least squares and repeat this procedure until convergence.

DATA BREAK: Modeling Lip Cancer Morbidity in Scotland Spatial GLMMs are often used to smooth spatial disease rates, and they provide a nice extension to the empirical Bayes smoothing methods illustrated in Section 4.4.3. In this data break, we use spatial GLMMs to estimate the effect of an exposure variable on lip cancer rates in Scotland and then to smooth the rates, adjusting for this exposure.

As an aside, we originally intended to use the New York leukemia data throughout the data breaks in this chapter to illustrate the differences and the similarities that result from the various modeling approaches. However, the Scottish lip cancer data represent a "classic" data set for regionally specified health data and receives much attention in the literature, so we could not resist including it here. The data permit a nice comparative illustration of many statistical methods spanning a spectrum from traditional Poisson regression through random effects modeling to spatial GLMMs. In addition, the multiple analyses of the lip cancer data appearing in the spatial literature provide interesting cross-references for the results presented here. A GLMM analysis of the New York leukemia data is left as an exercise.

Clayton and Kaldor (1987) report the number of lip cancer cases registered during 1975–1980 in each of 56 districts of Scotland, which we denote Y_i, $i = 1, \ldots N$, $N = 56$. Clayton and Kaldor (1987) also report estimates of the expected number of cases per district, E_i, accounting for the different age distributions in each district. Assuming that the E_i are fixed constants, Clayton and Kaldor (1987) use the standardized morbidity ratio (SMR), $r_i = Y_i/E_i$, as the data for their analyses. We follow Cressie (1993, p. 536) in the use of the term *districts*, since the 56 regions correspond to a collection of political regions defined in 1973 corresponding to 53 districts and three "island authorities." The 1994 Local Government (Scotland) Act redefined the political geography of Scotland, replacing the 53 districts with 32 "council areas," so the districts in this analysis are no longer in use.

Clayton and Bernardinelli (1992) and Breslow and Clayton (1993) also report the percentage of the workforce in each district employed in agriculture, fishing, and forestry (%AFF). These authors note that the original compilers of the data, Kemp et al. (1985), observed spatial variation in this covariate similar to that observed for the lip cancer SMRs. Kemp et al. (1985) suggest that exposure to sunlight, a known risk factor for lip cancer and a frequent occurrence for those engaged in the agriculture, fishing, and forestry professions, might be the reason. We provide these data, as well as the longitude and latitude coordinate of the center of each district, in Table 2.6. Since we consider distance-based covariance functions in our analysis below, we projected the data using the British National Grid (a transverse Mercator projection), so distances are measured in meters. Figures 9.17 and 9.18 show the spatial distributions of the SMRs and the exposure values, respectively.

Recall from the discussion in Section 4.4.3 the concept of an unobserved relative risk for each region, ζ_i, whose spatial distribution we want to depict on a map. We

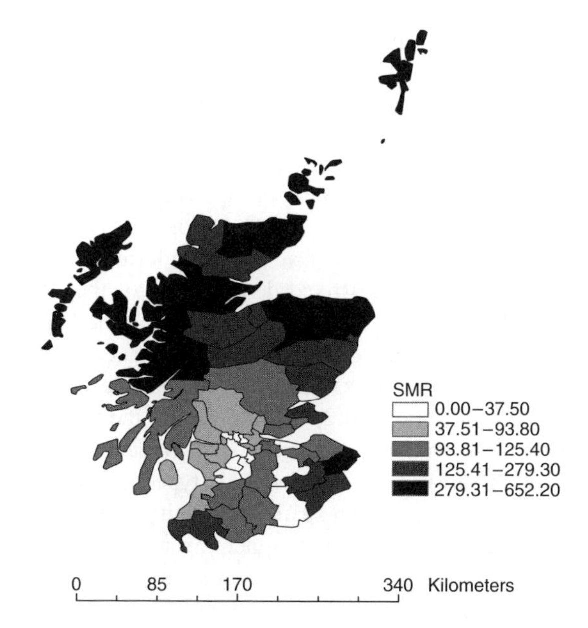

FIG. 9.17 Lip cancer SMRs during 1975–1980 in the 56 districts of Scotland.

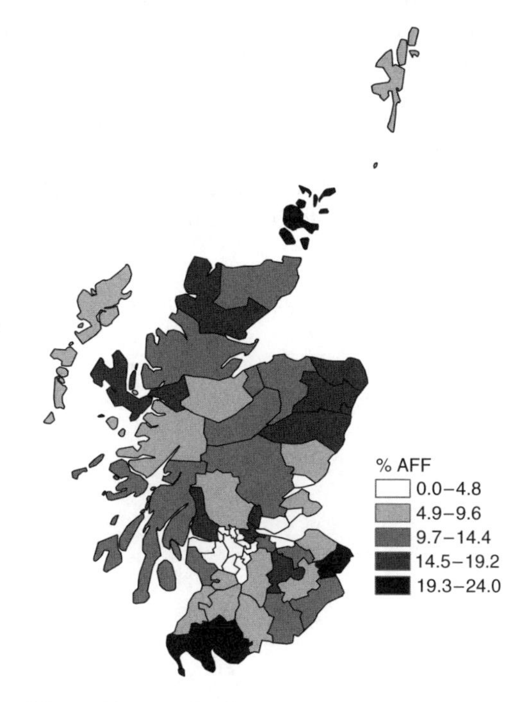

FIG. 9.18 Percentage of the workforce engaged in agriculture, fishing, or forestry during 1975–1980 in the 56 districts of Scotland.

assumed, and we do so again here, conditional on these true but unobserved relative risks, that the disease district in the N districts, $Y_1, \ldots, Y_N$ are independent Poisson random variables with means $\mu_i = E(Y_i|\zeta_i)$ and variances $\text{Var}(Y_i|\zeta_i) = \sigma^2\mu_i$. In contrast to the smoothing methods in Section 4.4.3, in this data break we relate these means to an exposure covariate, x_i =%AFF/10 (we divide the covariate by 10 in order to compare our results more easily with those in the literature). Since the data are Poisson, we choose the link function $g(\mu) = \log(\mu)$, so that $\mu_i = \exp[\log(E_i) + \boldsymbol{x}_i'\boldsymbol{\beta} + \zeta_i]$, where $\boldsymbol{\beta} = (\beta_0, \beta_1)'$. The term $\log(E_i)$ is an *offset* in the model representing the (assumed) fixed denominator of the SMR, allowing us to model the local SMRs based on local counts following the Poisson distribution.

To complete the model specification, we need to make some assumptions about the distribution of the ζ_i (in this example, ζ plays the role of S in the development in Section 9.4.2). As in Section 9.4.2, we assume that the vector of random effects, $\boldsymbol{\xi}$, is $MVN(\mathbf{0}, \Sigma_\zeta(\boldsymbol{\theta}))$, with the elements of $\Sigma_\zeta(\boldsymbol{\theta})$ modeled with a parametric covariance model. If we use a CAR- or SAR-type model for $\boldsymbol{\xi}$, we can model $\Sigma_\zeta(\boldsymbol{\theta}) = \rho W$, where W is a known spatial proximity matrix. Often, W is taken to be the matrix of adjacency weights, and in fact, the adjacencies are given in Clayton and Kaldor (1987). However, to be curious and different, we try to let the data inform on the spatial correlation in the random effects and use the geostatistical methods described in Chapter 8 and Section 9.2.1 and illustrated in Section 9.2.3 to suggest a parametric model for $\Sigma_\zeta(\boldsymbol{\theta})$. We use the word *try* since we know that for our analysis in Section 9.2.3, this can be tricky to do with rates, and the problem is exacerbated when fitting a GLMM since we lose the nice decomposition of variability into large-scale covariate effects and small-scale autocorrelation.

However, we do have this decomposition on the log scale, so we follow the same procedure that we used in Section 9.2.3. We obtain the empirical semivariogram of the studentized residuals from a weighted (by E_i) regression of $\log(r_i + 1)$ on x_i (Figure 9.19) and use this to infer a model for $\Sigma_\zeta(\boldsymbol{\theta})$. Again we see an

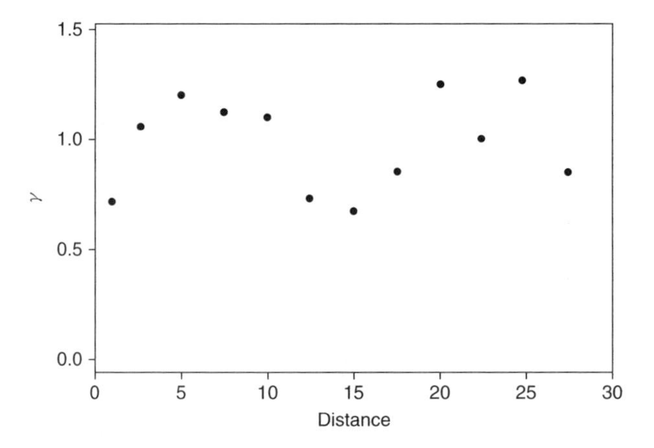

FIG. 9.19 Empirical semivariogram of log(SMR + 1) values for the lip cancer data. Distances are in kilometers.

apparent periodicity in the empirical semivariogram, which seems fairly common when working with health data and is perhaps due to the geographic distribution of the population. Cressie (1993, p. 544) suggests that the apparent negative dependence at distances between 45 and 65 miles (72,000–105,000 meters here) is partly due to districts 4 and 50 being considerably different from their neighboring districts. Either an exponential or a spherical semivariogram model will smooth out the fluctuations and provide a reasonable overall fit to the empirical semivariogram, so we use both as models for $\Sigma_\zeta(\boldsymbol{\theta})$ and compare the results for illustration.

Using traditional likelihood methods for nonspatial GLMs and the methodology described in Section 9.4.3, we fit the following seven models to the lip cancer SMRs:

1. *PR*: traditional (nonspatial) Poisson regression without random effects, not adjusted for overdispersion
2. $PR + OD$: traditional (nonspatial) Poisson regression without random effects, adjusted for overdispersion
3. *GLMMI*: nonspatial Poisson regression with uncorrelated random effects (i.e., with $\Sigma_S = \sigma_S^2 I$), adjusted for overdispersion
4. *GLMME*: the spatial GLMM described above, without adjustment for overdispersion, using an exponential correlation function
5. *GLMMS*: the spatial GLMM described above, without adjustment for overdispersion, using a spherical correlation function
6. $S + OD$: the spatial GLMM described above, with adjustment for overdispersion, using a spherical correlation function
7. *MGLM*: marginal spatial GLM, with adjustment for overdispersion, using a spherical correlation function

We summarize results in Table 9.10. We present the results in a single table to facilitate comparison and discussion, but stress that the entries may have different interpretations depending on the model. We elaborate on this further in the discussion below.

Table 9.10 Results of seven GLMs Fit to the Lip Cancer SMRs[a]

Model	$\hat{\beta}_0$	$\hat{\beta}_1$	$\hat{\sigma}_S^2$	$\hat{\sigma}^2$	$\hat{a}$	p-Value
PR	-0.54 ± 0.07	0.74 ± 0.06	—	—	—	0.0001
PR+OD	-0.54 ± 0.15	0.74 ± 0.13	—	4.92	—	0.0001
GLMMI	-0.43 ± 0.16	0.68 ± 0.14	0.29	1.50	—	0.0001
GLMME	0.44 ± 0.35	0.31 ± 0.12	0.42	—	114.66	0.0155
GLMMS	0.49 ± 0.33	0.30 ± 0.12	0.47	—	256.74	0.0168
S+OD	0.44 ± 0.32	0.33 ± 0.13	0.38	1.38	263.70	0.0125
MGLM	-0.63 ± 0.21	0.70 ± 0.16	—	7.10	53.16	0.0001

[a]The units of the spatial autocorrelation parameter, $\hat{a}$, are in kilometers. The p-value is based on testing $\beta_1 = 0$.

In nonspatial GLMs (PR and PR+OD), it is important to adjust for overdispersion, as it can have a large effect on standard errors. This is clearly illustrated by comparing the results from the PR and PR+OD models: Note that the estimates of β_0 and β_1 are the same, but the associated standard errors are more than twice as large after adjusting for overdispersion. The assumption in the PR model that the variance equals the mean is not valid if there is substantial overdispersion, and thus the standard errors estimated from this model are too low. The impact of including a dispersion parameter in the GLMMs (compare models GLMMS vs. S+OD) is not nearly as great since the conditional models include overdispersion, even without the extra dispersion parameter [cf. equation (9.62)].

The inclusion of independent (nonspatial) random effects in the PR model (model GLMMI) decreases the estimate of β_1 slightly, from 0.74 to 0.68, but adjusts for the overdispersion in the data via the variability in the random effect. The inclusion of spatially correlated random effects (models GLMME, GLMMS, and S+OD) has a substantial impact on the estimate of β_1, essentially reducing it by a factor of 2 (from 0.68 in the GLMMI model to 0.33 in the comparable S+OD model). However, the estimated standard errors for $\hat{\beta}_1$ remain about the same. We observe somewhat different results when fitting the marginal spatial GLM: Including spatial correlation increases the standard errors slightly (from 0.13 in PR+OD to 0.16 in MGLM), but leaves the magnitudes of the estimated β_1 coefficients unchanged.

The results illustrate an important point first made in Section 9.2.2 concerning the interpretation of spatial regression models. All regression models partition the variation in the data into variation that can be attributed to systematic changes in fixed covariates and the remaining random variation. When we are modeling spatial variation with spatially varying covariates, this partitioning is not unique and it can be difficult to decide what part of the spatial variation belongs to the covariates and what part should be treated as residual autocorrelation. The variation that one model attributes to the covariates may be attributed to random variation in another model, and both models could be valid! This is even more difficult with the inclusion of spatially structured random effects, since we now have to partition our variation into three parts instead of two. If the spatial variation in the random effects is related to that in the covariates, some of the covariate effect will be assigned to the random effects. Thus, we have to take great care in interpreting the results from spatial regression models by understanding how the components of our models can affect our interpretation. If the signal in the data is strong, all models should give similar conclusions, even if the particular values parameter estimates and standard errors differ. This seems to be the case with our analyses of the lip cancer rates: All models clearly indicate a significant effect due to occupational exposure as measured by %AFF.

The choice of autocorrelation model has little effect on the results from the spatial GLMMs (recall that the effective range in the exponential model is about $3a$, so the effective range for this model is slightly larger than for the other conditionally specified models). We emphasize that the range of autocorrelation in the conditional models is that of the ζ_i and not that of the data Y_i as with the marginal model, which is why the estimates of a are much different for the two types of models. Although it is not obvious from the correlation function computed using equations (9.63) and (9.62), the strength of the marginal autocorrelation induced by the spatially correlated random effects is probably much smaller than that indicated by the $\hat{a}$. This can be seen theoretically in Zeger (1988) [he assumes that $E(\exp(\zeta)) = 1$, simplifying equations (9.63) and (9.62)] and empirically from results in Gotway and Wolfinger (2003).

How do we know when to use a marginal spatial GLM or a conditional spatial GLMM? The choice between marginal and conditional models is of considerable debate even in nonspatial applications. There are several considerations that may help us choose. The first is the interpretation of the regression parameters. In the marginal model, $\boldsymbol{\beta}$ describes the change in $g(E(\mathbf{Y}))$ with changes in the covariates. Thus, this approach is often referred to as *population averaged*, since it describes the dependence of a population mean on selected covariates. In contrast, when separate random effects are estimated for each "subject" (here, the district), $\boldsymbol{\beta}$ represents covariate effects at the *subject-specific level.* When the subjects are people in a clinical trial, subject-specific inference may be undesirable, but when the subjects are spatial regions, subject-specific inference can be appealing, arguably more appealing than inference with a population-averaged interpretation. A second consideration in the choice between marginal and conditional models is the overall application. In many studies, it may not make sense to assume the existence of unobserved, random, but fairly well-structured variables affecting the response. In other studies, including these variables may provide a much more elegant and direct interpretation than that provided by a marginal model. A third consideration is the overall goal of the analysis. We may not always be interested in estimating covariate effects. For example, we may simply want a smooth map of the rates adjusted for covariates or known confounders. The spatial GLMMs are ideally suited to this since the fitted means, $\hat{\mu}_i = \exp[\log(E_i) + \boldsymbol{x}_i'\hat{\boldsymbol{\beta}} + \hat{\zeta}_i]$, provide the smoothed, adjusted, empirical Bayes estimates of mean counts. Dividing these smoothed mean counts by population sizes provides a smoothed map of local rates, while dividing by the expected counts E_i yields a smoothed map of local SMRs. The smoothed SMR map based on the GLMME model appears in Figure 9.20. Note how the trend in the SMRs is much more apparent after adjusting for the percentage of the workforce engaged in agriculture, fishing, or forestry. The larger rates tend to occur in more rural areas, with the smallest rates near the middle, more urban regions.

Smoothing rates with marginal models is slightly more complicated since we somehow have to adjust for the aggregation effects (this is essentially one interpretation of what the ζ's do). This has not received much attention in the literature, primarily, we think, because theoretical results for inference from a single realization of correlated data are difficult to obtain: Conditioning allows us to assume independence and makes the theory more tractable. We do not we present the details here (see Section 9.7.7 and think about using filtered kriging in a spatial GLM context), but we do provide a smoothed map from a marginal spatial GLM for comparison (Figure 9.21).

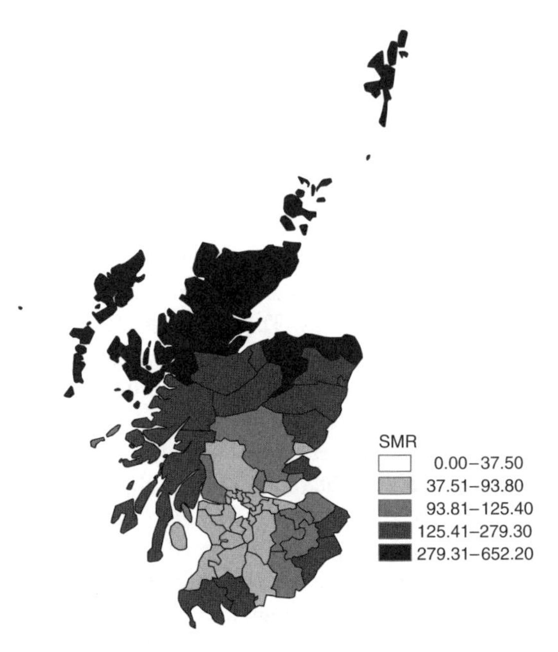

FIG. 9.20 Smoothed lip cancer SMRs using the spatial GLMM described in the text.

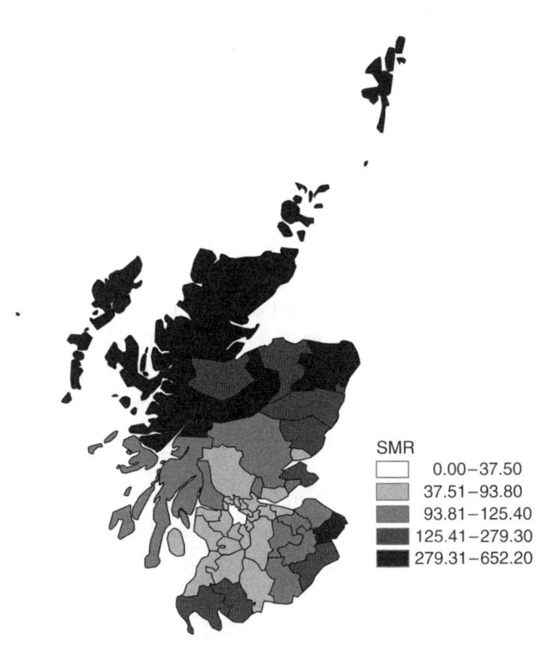

FIG. 9.21 Smoothed lip cancer SMRs using a marginal spatial GLM similar to the one described in the text.

9.4.4 Additional Considerations in Spatial GLMs

The preceding data break illustrates the application of a variety of marginally and conditionally specified GLMs and GLMMs, some incorporating spatial correlation. GLMs and GLMMs model rates, counts, and proportions more directly than the linear regression models of Sections 9.1, 9.2, and 9.3, at the expense of more complicated model formulation and computational implementation and residual diagnostics. These issues, in turn, raise some interesting theoretical and practical issues.

We use geostatistical methods to quantify the spatial autocorrelation in the data primarily to motivate spatial GLMMs as natural extensions to the general linear regression models we describe in Section 9.2. However, we may use the models and the computational procedures described here with a variety of spatial covariance structures, including autoregressive structures similar to those defined in Section 9.3. Breslow and Clayton (1993) provide an example of autoregressive spatial random effects and use a penalized quasilikelihood approach to fit the model to the Scottish lip cancer data.

Theoretically, the distribution of the random effects need not be Gaussian. A Gaussian distribution allows many of the approximations driving the PL approach for fitting GLMMs, but some applications may merit other distributions for the random effects. Changing the random effects distribution sometimes complicates the numerical and computational approaches used to fit GLMMs, but clever choices actually offer advantages over Gaussian assumptions [cf. Lee and Nelder (1996) and associated discussion]. In general, treating the distribution of the random effects as a prior distribution in a Bayesian setting (as introduced with empirical Bayes smoothing approaches in Section 4.4.3) offers additional advantages, which we explore in Section 9.5.

On the practical implementation side, all GLMM parameter estimation algorithms are iterative and require assessment of convergence of the algorithm. Such convergence is often sensitive (sometimes *very* sensitive) to the starting values defined by the user, and robust, general-purpose convergence diagnostics are lacking. In the example above, we implement a parameter search that is sensitive to both the range of possible parameter values and the search increment considered. Agresti et al. (2000) provide a readable overview of GLMMs, including a detailed discussion of the advantages and disadvantages of different computational approaches for GLMM parameter estimation.

Finally, many analyses exploring links between geographically referenced exposures and health outcomes involve data collected on units with different spatial supports (e.g., point measurements of exposure suggesting geostatistical interpolation coupled with outcomes defined by regional counts of a particular health event). Fitting a GLM or GLMM to such *misaligned data* presents considerable analytical and inferential challenges. To illustrate the issue, we now explore an example in detail and in the process incorporate many of the spatial statistical ideas and tools defined throughout the book.

CASE STUDY: Very Low Birth Weights in Georgia Health Care District 9 In many public health studies, particularly those assessing the impacts of the environment on human health, the locations of the exposure data and those of the health data do not coincide. Thus, we cannot apply regression methods, even those in spatial statistics, to such misaligned data. In this case study, we illustrate one approach to overcoming misalignment problems in statistical analysis. Additional approaches are reviewed in Gotway and Young (2002).

In Section 4.2 we used data on very low birth weights to illustrate several different statistical maps useful for the display of spatial data. These data are based on a case–control study of the risk of having a very low birth weight (VLBW) baby, one weighing less than 1500 grams at birth (Rogers et al. 2000). The study area comprised the 25 contiguous counties in Georgia Health Care District 9 (GHCD9) (Figure 4.1). Cases were identified from all live-born, singleton infants born between April 1, 1986 and March 30, 1988. Control selection for this study was based on a pool of potential control subjects derived from a 3% random sample of all live-born infants weighing more than 2499 grams at birth and meeting the same residency and time frame requirements as the case subjects. The addresses of the birth mothers were geocoded to produce 770 georeferenced point locations, 230 of these corresponding to the locations of the VLBW cases, and the remaining 550 corresponding to the controls (Figure 9.22).

One of the hypotheses of the study was that pollution from industrial emissions adversely affected birth weights during this period. Emissions data for 1986–1988 on 32 industrial facilities within GHCD9 were obtained from the Georgia Environmental Protection Division (GAEPD) of the Georgia Department of Natural

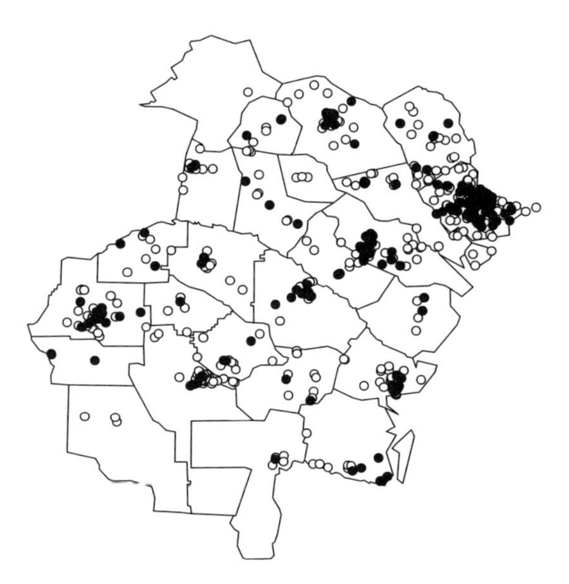

FIG. 9.22 Cases of very low birth weight and controls in Georgia Health Care District 9. Case locations are indicted by filled circles; control locations, by open circles.

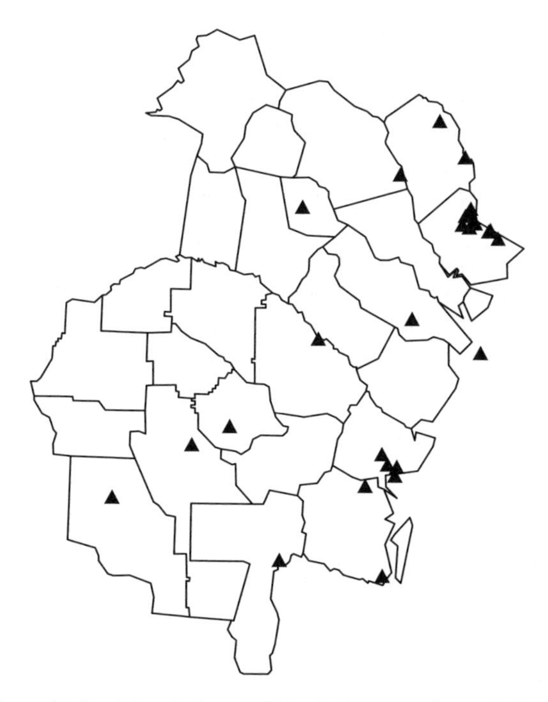

FIG. 9.23 Locations of industrial emissions facilities in GHCD9. The projection used with the map boundary file does not correspond exactly to that used to georeference the facilities, so some locations appear outside the boundary.

Resources (Rogers et al. 2000). These industries produce chemicals, plastics, fertilizers, asphalt, wood, paper, and gypsum and account for almost 95% of the approximately 45,000 tons of total suspended particulate (TSP) emissions in the area per year. The locations of these industrial facilities are shown in Figure 9.23. For each facility, the average annual TSP concentration (in tons) was recorded, and for illustration here, we assume that the emission concentration at each location is proportional to the ground-level concentration. Since particulate matter less than 10μm in diameter, PM_{10}, is often assumed to have the greatest potential impact on human health and accounts for approximately 55% of the TSP concentration (Dockery and Pope 1994), we converted the ground-level TSP concentrations to PM_{10} concentrations and used the PM_{10} concentrations (in $\mu g/m^3$) for our analysis.

In this study, our health outcome of interest, VLBW, is recorded at the residences of the study participants (Figure 9.22), and our exposure of interest, PM_{10}, is measured at the emissions facilities located throughout the region (Figure 9.23). The two sets of locations do not coincide. How can we assess the effect of PM_{10} exposure on the risk of a VLBW baby?

There are several possible answers to this question. One approach is to use a focused test where we consider the exposure locations to be focuses of potentially increased relative risk (see Sections 6.2 and 6.7; Cuzick and Edwards 1990; Diggle 1990; Lawson and Waller 1996; Diggle et al. 2000; Lawson 2001). Another approach is to create a variable that measures the distance from each residence to the nearest emissions facility and then use this variable as a covariate in logistic regression. We used this approach to study the impact of waste exposure on the risk for leukemia. Both of these are feasible approaches, although they would not explicitly use the amount of PM_{10} measured at each location (at least without modification). Another approach, and one that we consider in some detail here, is to use kriging (Chapter 8) to predict the exposure concentration at each residence and then use logistic regression with the estimated exposure as a covariate.

The PM_{10} exposure values range from 1 to 5895 $\mu g/m^3$, with most values below 2000 $\mu g/m^3$. Thus, the distribution of PM_{10} values is very skewed (see Figure 9.24). In such cases (see Section 8.3.2), lognormal kriging may result in better predictions

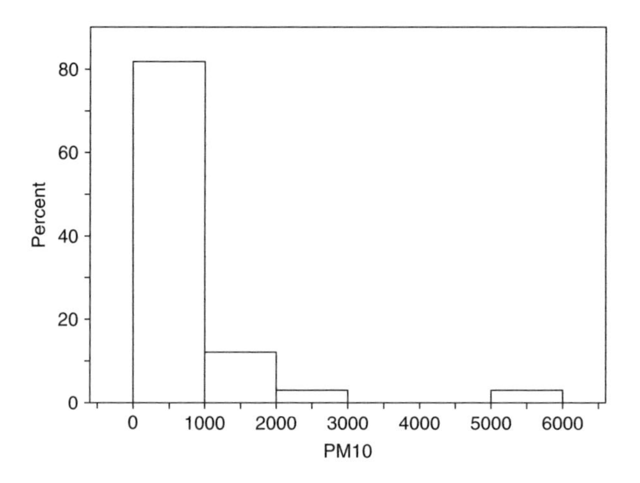

FIG. 9.24 Histogram of PM_{10} values.

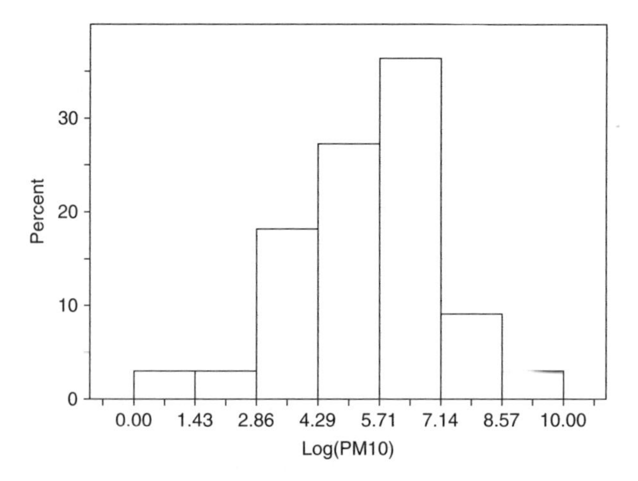

FIG. 9.25 Histogram of $\log(PM_{10})$ values.

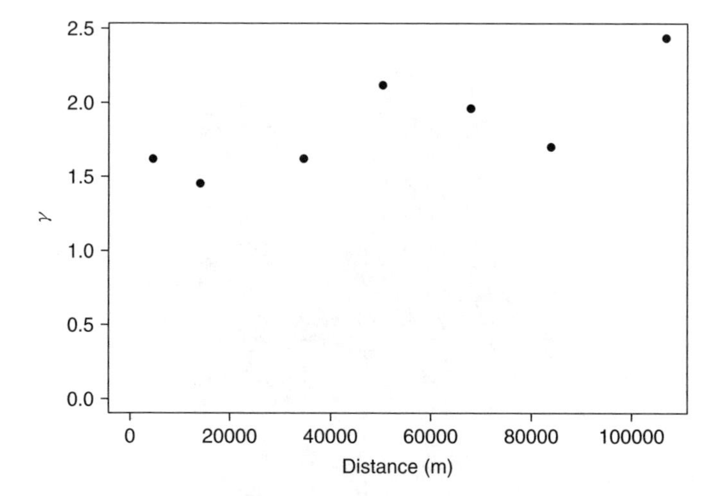

FIG. 9.26 Empirical semivariogram of log(PM_{10}) values. The distances are in meters.

than ordinary kriging, so we should analyze the logarithm of the PM_{10} values. The distribution of this transformed variable is shown in Figure 9.25.

Using these transformed values, we estimated the empirical semivariogram using the methods described in Section 8.2.3 (see Figure 9.26). There is obviously a large nugget effect, and we do not know if this is due to measurement error, lack of information at small distances, or the nature of the spatial variation in the emissions data. We used weighted least squares (Section 8.2.4) to fit a spherical semivariogram model [equation (8.5)] to this empirical semivariogram, and the model fit is shown in Figure 9.27.

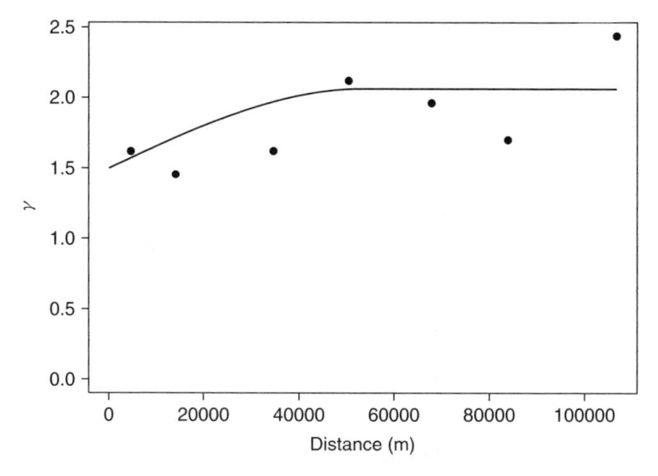

FIG. 9.27 Fit of the spherical semivariogram model to the empirical semivariogram of the log(PM_{10}) values. The estimated parameters are $c_0 = 1.50$, $c_e = 0.56$, and $a_e = 53,385.57$.

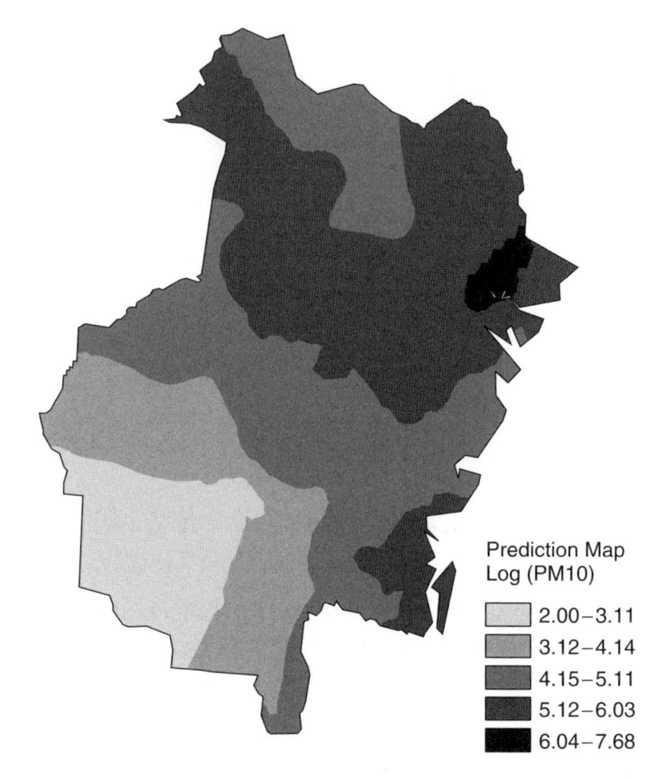

FIG. 9.28 Predicted log(PM_{10}) concentrations in GHCD9 using filtered ordinary kriging.

We used this fitted semivariogram model and filtered ordinary kriging (assuming the nugget effect was 50% measurement error and 50% spatial variation at distances smaller than the smallest distance lag; see Section 8.3.2) to predict the log(PM_{10}) concentrations at the residences of the study participants (the locations shown in Figure 9.22). A contour map of the predicted log(PM_{10}) concentrations is shown in Figure 9.28.

Now that we have a predicted log(PM_{10}) concentration at each of the case and control locations, we can use logistic regression to infer the effect of the predicted log(PM_{10}) concentrations on the risk of VLBW. We first fit a traditional logistic regression model (cf. Section 2.6.2) to the case and control data. Our outcome variable is

$$Y(\mathbf{s}) = \begin{cases} 1 & \text{if location } \mathbf{s} \text{ is a case} \\ 0 & \text{if location } \mathbf{s} \text{ is a control,} \end{cases}$$

and we assume that this variable has a Bernoulli distribution with the probability of a VLBW baby equal to π. We use the logit link function to relate this probability to the log(PM_{10}) concentrations. Following Rogers et al. (2000), we partitioned the predicted log(PM_{10}) concentrations into four categories for ease of interpretation from logistic regression. The categories were defined based on the distribution of the predicted log(PM_{10}) concentrations at only the control locations. Predicted log(PM_{10}) concentrations above the 95th percentile of those at the control locations defined a high exposure group (>6.51μg/m^3). A medium exposure group was delineated by predicted log(PM_{10}) concentrations between the 75th and 95th percentiles of the control concentration distribution (between 6.22 and 6.51 μg/m^3), and a low exposure group was similarly defined using the 50th–75th percentiles (between 5.79 and 6.22 μg/m^3). The reference baseline category for an unexposed group was taken to be any predicted log(PM_{10}) concentration less than the 50th percentile of the predicted exposures at the control locations (i.e., <5.79μg/m^3). Based on these categories for the predicted log(PM_{10}) concentrations, logistic regression was used to estimate the probability of being a case rather than a control as a function of the exposure categories. Thus, our regression model is

$$\log[\pi/(1-\pi)] = \beta_0 + \beta_1 x_1(\boldsymbol{s}) + \beta_2 x_2(\boldsymbol{s}) + \beta_3 x_3(\boldsymbol{s}) + \beta_4 x_4(\boldsymbol{s}), \tag{9.68}$$

where $x_1(\boldsymbol{s})$ is an indicator variable taking the value of 1 if the predicted log(PM_{10}) concentration at location $\boldsymbol{s}$ is a high exposure, $x_2(\boldsymbol{s})$ is an indicator variable taking the value of 1 if the predicted log(PM_{10}) concentration at location $\boldsymbol{s}$ is a medium exposure, and $x_3(\boldsymbol{s})$ and $x_4(\boldsymbol{s})$ are defined similarly, with $x_4(\boldsymbol{s})$ indicating the baseline (no exposure) group, as defined above. The results are summarized in Table 9.11. From this table we can see that the risk of VLBW (as measured by the odds ratio) increases as the predicted log(PM_{10}) concentrations increase. At the highest levels of exposure, this risk is significantly greater than that of the baseline, unexposed group.

To use the spatial generalized linear models described in this section, we need to determine how best to model $\rho(\boldsymbol{s}_i - \boldsymbol{s}_j)$ in equation (9.58) for a marginal spatial GLM, or $\rho_S(\boldsymbol{s}_i - \boldsymbol{s}_j)$, the spatial correlation in $S(\boldsymbol{s})$ of equation (9.59), for a conditional spatial GLMM model. To investigate this, we computed the empirical semivariogram of the Pearson residuals, the raw residuals divided by the square root of the variance function, from the logistic regression [cf. Section 7.4.3 and McCullagh and Nelder (1989, p. 37)]. The resulting empirical semivariogram is shown in Figure 9.29. There seem to be some small periodicities in the semivariogram that may reflect the geographic distribution of the population. Even though

Table 9.11 Results of Logistic Regression of Predicted log(PM_{10}) Exposures on Case–Control Status in GHCD9

Exposure Category	Odds Ratio	95% Confidence Limits
High	2.12	(1.14, 3.93)
Medium	1.79	(1.22, 2.64)
Low	1.09	(0.73, 1.63)

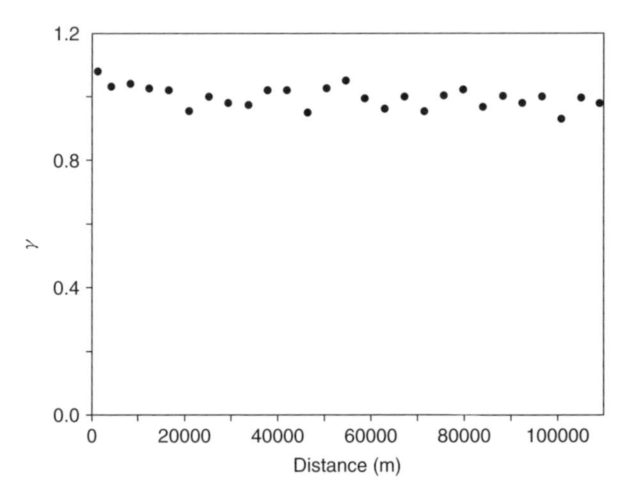

FIG. 9.29 Empirical semivariogram of the case–control data in GHCD9.

the need for hole effect models rarely arises in practice, we considered both a hole effect model and a pure nugget model for this empirical semivariogram. The best-fitting model is the pure nugget model (a straight, horizontal line), indicating the lack of any residual spatial autocorrelation. Thus, adjusting our analyses for small-scale autocorrelation as we did with the earlier data break on lip cancer data seems unnecessary here and we will base our remaining discussion on the use of the traditional logistic regression model described above.

The results from the logistic regression (Table 9.11) are misleading, however, since they are based on predicted exposure concentrations, and the uncertainty associated with these predictions is not incorporated into the logistic regression. If it were, the width of the confidence intervals associated with the odds ratios would undoubtedly increase. We have one measure of the uncertainty in the predicted $\log(PM_{10})$ concentrations: the standard errors associated with the predicted values obtained from filtered ordinary kriging (see Figure 9.30), but how can we incorporate these standard errors into our logistic regression? It is difficult, if not impossible, to derive the effect of this uncertainty analytically on the estimated odds ratios and associated confidence intervals since the amount of uncertainty varies from location to location. Thus, as we have done many times in previous chapters, we turn to Monte Carlo simulation for a more tractable solution.

We touched briefly on geostatistical simulation in Section 8.4.5, and we use these ideas here to generate a Monte Carlo distribution of odds ratios that reflects the uncertainty in the exposure concentrations predicted. Although the details and nuances associated with geostatistical simulation are beyond the scope of this book, the basic idea is simple and we describe it below.

1. We first generate a realization of the exposure distribution at the case and control locations. Since we assumed that the original emissions data were

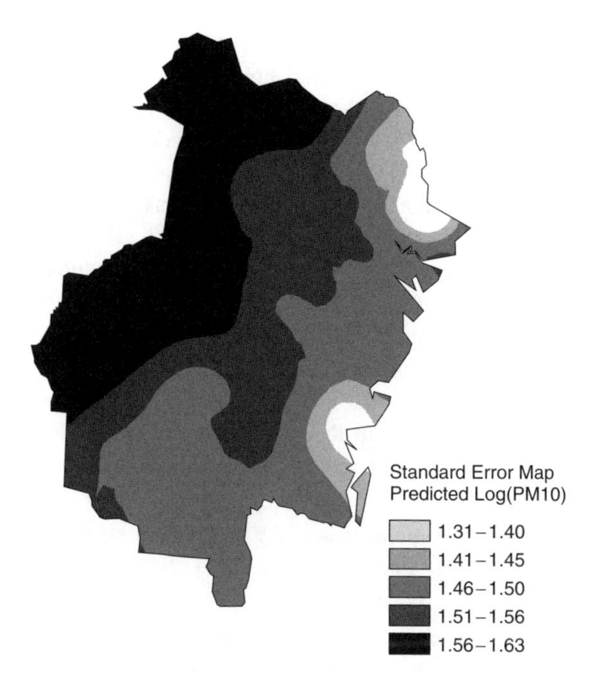

FIG. 9.30 Standard errors of predicted $\log(\text{PM}_{10})$ concentrations in GHCD9.

recorded with error, we use *unconditional simulations* rather than *conditional simulations*, which would force each realization to pass through the original $\log(\text{PM}_{10})$ values [cf. equation (8.34)]. Unconditional realizations can be obtained using an equation similar to equation (8.34) but without the complexity due to the conditioning. Specifically, for the case locations, we first generate a vector $\mathbf{z}_1$ of 230 realizations of an $N(0,1)$ random variable. We induce autocorrelation into this vector using LU decomposition (Section 8.4.5) of $\Sigma_1(\hat{\boldsymbol{\theta}})$, the 230×230 variance–covariance matrix of the unobserved $\log(\text{PM}_{10})$ measurements at the case locations with elements based on the spherical semivariogram (Figure 9.27) using $\hat{\boldsymbol{\theta}} = (c_0 = 1.50, c_e = 0.56, a_e = 53,385.57)'$ and the distances between the 230 residential case locations. Then the LU (or Cholesky) decomposition of $\Sigma_1(\hat{\boldsymbol{\theta}})$ gives $L_1 U_1 = \Sigma_1(\hat{\boldsymbol{\theta}})$, and $L_1\mathbf{z}_1$ has variance–covariance matrix $\text{Var}(L_1\mathbf{z}_1) = L_1\text{Var}(\mathbf{z}_1)L_1' = L_1 L_1' = L_1 U_1 = \Sigma_1(\hat{\boldsymbol{\theta}})$. We assume that the exposure distribution at the control locations has the same spatial variability as the exposure distribution at the case locations, so we apply the same procedure for the control locations and obtain $L_2\mathbf{z}_2$. However, the elements of both $L_1\mathbf{z}_1$ and $L_2\mathbf{z}_2$ have zero expectations (means) and we cannot assume that the mean of the exposure distribution at the case locations is the same as the mean of the exposure distribution at the control locations (if we did make this assumption, we would be assuming that exposure has no effect on risk of a VLBW baby). The mean of the predicted $\log(\text{PM}_{10})$ values for the cases is 5.70 and that for the controls is 5.52, so we will add these means to our simulated vectors for the cases and controls. Thus, for the case locations, our simulated vector is now $\mathbf{P}_1 = \mathbf{5.70} + L_1\mathbf{z}_1$, where **5.70** is a vector with elements all equal to 5.70. Similarly, for the controls, our simulated vector is now $\mathbf{P}_2 = \mathbf{5.52} + L_2\mathbf{z}_2$. To obtain a single realization at both the case and control locations with the desired mean and variance structure, we combine the two vectors into a single realization as $\mathbf{P} = (\mathbf{P}_1', \mathbf{P}_2')'$, a 780×1 vector of autocorrelated values at both the case and control locations. If we repeated this procedure many times (we will, but not yet), each realization $\mathbf{P}_i$ can be used to make a plausible map of predicted $\log(\text{PM}_{10})$ concentrations. The map produced by kriging (Figure 9.28) is an average of these simulated surfaces.

2. For each realization $\mathbf{P}_i$, we fit the logistic regression model described above [equation (9.68)]. The result will be one estimated odds ratio for each realization.
3. Repeat this procedure many times (e.g., 1000). Note that each $\Sigma(\hat{\boldsymbol{\theta}})$ needs to be decomposed only once.

The end result is a *distribution* of odds ratios for each exposure category that reflects the uncertainty in the predicted $\log(\text{PM}_{10})$ measurements. This idea is illustrated in Figure 9.31, where the simulated $\log(\text{PM}_{10})$ surfaces are the realizations, the logistic regression analysis plays the role of a transfer function, and the system response is the odds ratio. We use the mean of the resulting distribution of odds ratios as a point estimate and the 2.5th and 97.5th percentiles of this distribution as an empirical or bootstrap confidence interval. The results of this spatial uncertainty analysis applied to the $\log(\text{PM}_{10})$ and VLBW case–control data described above are presented in Table 9.12. Although the trend of increasing risk with increasing exposure level is still apparent and the estimated odds ratios are similar to those in Table 9.11, the confidence intervals are much wider. Note that at the highest levels of exposure, the risk of VLBW is no longer significantly greater than that of the baseline, unexposed group.

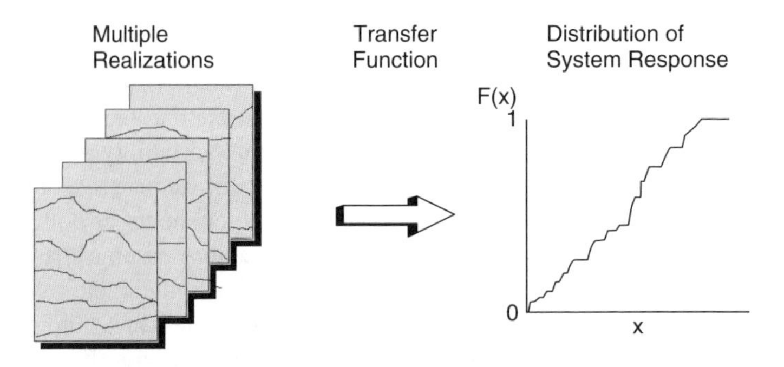

FIG. 9.31 Geostatistical simulation for uncertainty analysis.

Table 9.12 Results of Logistic Regression of Case–Control Indicators on log(PM_{10}) Exposure Categories Obtained Using Geostatistical Simulation of log(PM_{10}) Exposures in GHCD9

Exposure Category	Odds Ratio	95% Confidence Limits
High	2.08	(0.17, 8.99)
Medium	1.48	(0.38, 4.36)
Low	1.26	(0.49, 2.55)

There are other approaches that we could use to predict the log(PM_{10}) concentrations at the residence locations instead of kriging as we have used here. Rogers et al. (2000) used a deterministic atmospheric transport model to predict ground-level exposures as a function of distance between exposure and residence locations, windspeed, and emission stack heights. Regardless of the approach used, it is important to adjust subsequent statistical analyses for the uncertainty in the exposures predicted. Spatial uncertainty analysis, and geostatistical simulation in particular, is a powerful method for making such adjustments.

9.5 BAYESIAN MODELS FOR DISEASE MAPPING

The preceding sections illustrate the structure and application of generalized linear mixed models (GLMMs) as a means of modeling regional counts and rates. The hierarchical structure of spatial GLMMs provides an intuitive structure for spatial model building. We first define the probability structure of the data given the observed covariate values and assuming that the observations are mutually independent. Second, we relax the assumption of independence by inducing spatial correlation through random effects representing unmeasured (or perhaps unmeasurable) effects not otherwise included in our model. The model defined in equation (9.59) incorporates all such effects as a spatially structured random intercept. Although the addition of a random intercept is helpful conceptually, its inclusion often complicates likelihood-based inference, resulting in the quasilikelihood and pseudolikelihood approaches defined above. However, these approaches build from distributional or functional assumptions particular to certain classes of GLMMs (e.g., those with Gaussian random effects) and may not readily apply or be extended to other hierarchically defined GLMMs. In contrast, developments in a very general class of simulation-based algorithms for Bayesian inference allow us to fit very complicated hierarchical models, including those with spatially correlated random effects. Building on the hierarchical structure of GLMMs defined in Section 9.4.2, the brief introduction to Bayesian statistics outlined in Section 4.4.3, and a very brief overview of *Markov chain Monte Carlo* (MCMC) *algorithms*, we conclude the chapter with a Bayesian formulation of GLMMs.

Recall from Section 4.4.3 that in Bayesian statistics we build a probability model linking the distribution of the data to model parameters, and we treat the model parameters as random variables. Contrast this conceptual framework with the classical statistical approach of fixed but unknown model parameters. In a Bayesian setting, we seek inference regarding the probability of unknown model parameters taking on certain values (e.g., given the data and our probability model, what is the probability that the mean is greater than zero?) rather than assessments of the probability of estimates being close to the true (but still unknown) parameter values (e.g., given an estimate of the mean and our probability model, how often would we expect data under this model to generate sample means greater than zero?). The differences in inferential style are sometimes subtle and generate much discussion and debate. For our purposes, the most important notion is that of using the data to define a probability distribution for each of the model parameters, then using these distributions to draw inference.

9.5.1 Hierarchical Structure

More specifically, all Bayesian inference stems from the *posterior distribution*, that is, the conditional distribution of the model parameters given the observed data, denoted for general development by $f(\boldsymbol{\theta}|\mathbf{Y})$, where $\boldsymbol{\theta}$ denotes the vector of model parameters, $\mathbf{Y}$ the data vector, and $f(\cdot)$ represents general notation for any probability density (or mass) function. Using Bayes' theorem, the posterior distribution is proportional to the product of the *likelihood function* (the conditional probability distribution of the data $\mathbf{Y}$ given the parameters $\boldsymbol{\theta}$), denoted $f(\mathbf{Y}|\boldsymbol{\theta})$, and the *prior distribution* of the parameters (the analyst-defined probability distribution of parameters without input from the data), denoted $f(\boldsymbol{\theta})$:

$$f(\boldsymbol{\theta}|\mathbf{Y}) \propto f(\mathbf{Y}|\boldsymbol{\theta})f(\boldsymbol{\theta}), \tag{9.69}$$

where the constant of proportionality, $\int f(\mathbf{Y}|\boldsymbol{\theta})f(\boldsymbol{\theta})$, ensures that the posterior distribution integrates to 1. [We note that our use of $f(\cdot)$ for the posterior, likelihood, and prior densities does not mean that all have the same parametric or functional form.] Carlin and Louis (2000) and Gelman et al. (2004) provide detailed introductions to Bayesian methods and their application in a wide variety of data analysis settings.

Next, we expand the right-hand side of equation (9.69) in light of the GLMMs introduced in Section 9.4.2. In this hierarchical setting we have three types of model parameters:

- A vector of *fixed effects* $\boldsymbol{\beta}$ relating covariates to the expected outcome $\mathbf{Y}$
- A vector of *random effects* $\boldsymbol{\psi}$ typically based on either a Gaussian random field $[S(s)]$ or a multivariate Gaussian distribution with spatial correlation
- A vector of parameters $\boldsymbol{\theta}_{\psi}$ defining the spatial correlations (variance–covariance matrix) of the random effects

The hierarchical structure of the model parameters yields a joint posterior distribution

$$f(\boldsymbol{\theta}_\psi, \boldsymbol{\psi}, \boldsymbol{\beta}|\mathbf{Y}) \propto f(\mathbf{Y}|\boldsymbol{\beta}, \boldsymbol{\psi}) f(\boldsymbol{\psi}|\boldsymbol{\theta}_\psi) f(\boldsymbol{\beta}) f(\boldsymbol{\theta}_\psi). \tag{9.70}$$

The steps between equations (9.69) and (9.70) include the split of the vector of all model parameters [$\boldsymbol{\theta}$ in equation (9.69)] into three components ($\boldsymbol{\beta}$, $\boldsymbol{\psi}$, and $\boldsymbol{\theta}_\psi$), and the specification of the hierarchy of parameters, that is, defining the random effects $\boldsymbol{\psi}$ as dependent on the covariance parameters $\boldsymbol{\theta}_\psi$ (i.e., using the prior distribution $f(\boldsymbol{\psi}|\boldsymbol{\theta}_\psi)$ rather than $f(\boldsymbol{\psi})$), and assuming that the covariance parameters and the fixed effects are random and assigning prior distributions to them. Since the covariance parameters $\boldsymbol{\theta}_\psi$ enter the model at a second level of the hierarchy, we often refer to them as *hyperparameters* and assign a *hyperprior distribution* to them. Finally, we assume statistical independence between the fixed-effects parameters $\boldsymbol{\beta}$ and the hyperparameters $\boldsymbol{\theta}_\psi$, yielding a product of prior distributions for the various categories of model parameters.

As a brief aside and a point of semantics, the term *fixed effects* may seem a bit odd, since a Bayesian analysis treats *all* model parameters as random variables rather than fixed but unknown values. However, in the mixed-models context, we define *fixed effects* as parameters pertaining to all study units (in our example, $\boldsymbol{\beta}$), and *random effects* as parameters that vary between study units and are assumed to be drawn from some common (prior) distribution (in this example, $\boldsymbol{\psi}$). This distinction (every unit experiencing the same effect of a covariate vs. each unit experiencing a unique effect drawn from some overall population distribution of effects) remains a key component of mixed models regardless of the inferential approach.

9.5.2 Estimation and Inference

So how does Bayesian, posterior inference differ from the likelihood (and pseudo-likelihood) inference defined in Section 9.4.2? The key difference involves the prior and hyperprior distributions $f(\boldsymbol{\beta})$ and $f(\boldsymbol{\theta}_\psi)$, which are included in the Bayesian approach but not in the likelihood approximations. To see this, consider the following. A classical development of GLMMs bases inference on the product of the likelihood of the data with the random effects distribution: namely,

$$f(\mathbf{Y}; \boldsymbol{\beta}, \boldsymbol{\psi}) f(\boldsymbol{\psi}; \boldsymbol{\theta}_\psi). \tag{9.71}$$

[We note that traditional likelihood notation replaces the conditioning in equation (9.70) with a semicolon to indicate the classical view of a likelihood as a function of model parameters to be maximized over rather than a conditional probability distribution per se.] Based on equations (9.70) and (9.71), both classical and Bayesian inference proceed in similar ways [e.g., inference regarding the fixed effects $\boldsymbol{\beta}$ results from integrating out (averaging over) the impact of the random effects yielding a marginal likelihood in the classical sense, and a marginal posterior distribution in the Bayesian sense]. Theoretically, inferential differences between the two approaches depend on the impact of the prior and hyperprior distributions for $\boldsymbol{\beta}$ and $\boldsymbol{\theta}_{\psi}$, respectively. If these are broadly defined with wide variances, there will be little difference between the approaches, although the Bayesian approach will incorporate uncertainty in the hyperparameters [reflected in the hyperprior $f(\boldsymbol{\theta}_{\psi})$] that is not included in the classical approach. In practice, implementation of the classical GLMM and Bayesian approaches derives from different numerical approximations and computational algorithms. We present the pseudolikelihood approach for classical inference in Section 9.4.2, and we outline Bayesian computational approaches below.

Building the Hierarchy To illustrate Bayesian inference on one of the most widely applied spatial GLMMs, consider the model proposed by Clayton and Kaldor (1987) and introduced in Sections 4.4.3 and the data break following 9.4.3. Briefly, for each of N regions, we obtain the number of incident cases ($Y_i, i = 1, \ldots, N$) and the number expected based on the population size and structure within region i ($E_i, i = 1, \ldots, N$). We treat the Y_i as random quantities and the E_i as fixed values. Often, the E_i reflect age-standardized values as defined in Section 2.3.

To allow for the possibility of region-specific risk factors in addition to those defining each E_i, Clayton and Kaldor (1987) propose a set of region-specific relative risks $\zeta_i, i = 1, \ldots, N$, and define the first stage of a hierarchical model through equation (4.12):

$$Y_i|\zeta_i \overset{\text{ind}}{\sim} \text{Poisson}(E_i\zeta_i). \tag{9.72}$$

Note that $E[Y_i|\zeta_i] \neq E_i$, since the ζ_i reflect an additional (multiplicative) risk associated with region i not already accounted for in the calculation of E_i.

Recall from Sections 2.3.2 and 4.4.3 that the ratio of observed to expected counts, Y_i/E_i, corresponds to the local *standardized mortality ratio* (SMR_i) and represents the maximum likelihood estimate of the relative risk, ζ_i, experienced by people residing in region i.

We place equation (9.72) in the structure of equation (9.59) through the use of the log link (the canonical link for Poisson data; cf. Section 2.6.1), yielding

$$\log(E[Y_i|\zeta_i]) = \log(E_i) + \log(\zeta_i).$$

If we let $\log(\zeta_i) = \psi_i$, we have a GLMM with offset $\log(E_i)$ and a random intercept ψ_i for each region $i, i = 1, \ldots, N$. We can incorporate fixed and random effects within the relative risk parameter if we include covariates and let

$$\log(\zeta_i) = \boldsymbol{x}_i'\boldsymbol{\beta} + \psi_i \tag{9.73}$$

for $i = 1, \ldots, N$.

Thus, at this stage, our model is

$$Y_i|\boldsymbol{\beta}, \psi_i \overset{\text{ind}}{\sim} \text{Poisson}(E_i \exp(\boldsymbol{x}_i'\boldsymbol{\beta} + \psi_i)), \tag{9.74}$$

which corresponds to the first term in equation (9.70); that is, we have conditionally independent observations with distributions defined by equation (9.74) and parameters $\boldsymbol{\beta}$ and $\boldsymbol{\psi}$ (the vector of ψ_is).

The next step is to specify distributions for the parameters $\boldsymbol{\beta}$ and $\boldsymbol{\psi}$. In our GLMM analysis in the data break following Section 9.4.3, we assume that $\boldsymbol{\beta}$ is fixed and not random, and we assume a multivariate Gaussian distribution for $\boldsymbol{\psi}$. We then (as noted in the preceding section) base inference on

$$f(\mathbf{Y}; \boldsymbol{\beta}, \boldsymbol{\psi}) = f(\mathbf{Y}; \boldsymbol{\beta}, \boldsymbol{\psi}) f(\boldsymbol{\psi}; \boldsymbol{\theta}_{\psi}),$$

where $\boldsymbol{\theta}_{\psi}$ represents parameters of overdispersion or spatial correlation. Both the classical GLMM and Bayesian approaches require specification of the distribution of $\boldsymbol{\psi}$ as a function of $\boldsymbol{\theta}_{\psi}$. However, for the classical GLMM methods, the hierarchy stops here and we iterate between estimates of $\boldsymbol{\beta}$ and $\boldsymbol{\theta}_{\psi}$. A Bayesian hierarchical model is not defined completely until we specify the prior distributions for $\boldsymbol{\beta}$ and $\boldsymbol{\theta}_{\psi}$.

Prior Distributions For the fixed effects $\boldsymbol{\beta}$ (which apply equally to all study units), we typically define a *noninformative prior* such as a uniform or Gaussian distribution with very wide prior variance, since the elements of $\boldsymbol{\beta}$ are typically well estimated by the data. Noninformative priors result in posterior inference very similar to maximum likelihood inference. In the case of a uniform prior distribution, $f(\boldsymbol{\beta})$ is proportional to a constant; hence the posterior distribution is proportional to the likelihood. In this case, the mode of the posterior distribution corresponds to the MLE. Note that for continuous parameters (potentially) taking values anywhere in $[-\infty, \infty]$, the uniform prior distribution is an *improper* distribution (i.e., its probability density function does not integrate to 1). However, when the likelihood is sufficiently well defined, we do obtain a proper posterior distribution. This simple example illustrates that proper posterior distributions are not always associated with proper prior distributions and indicates the need to assess posterior propriety, especially in complex modeling settings.

Bayesian inference differs from the methods described in previous sections in how it incorporates the (spatial) distribution of the random effects $\psi_i, i = 1, \ldots, N$. Before defining a spatially structured prior for $\boldsymbol{\psi}$, we first consider a simpler prior distribution inducing (nonspatial) overdispersion among the Y_i's. Suppose that

$$\psi_i \overset{\text{ind}}{\sim} N(0, v_{\psi}), \qquad i = 1, \ldots, I, \tag{9.75}$$

where v_{ψ} denotes a shared prior variance for the ψ_i (similar to that defined in the method of moments empirical Bayes estimates of Section 4.4.3). With equation (9.75), we assume (prior to collecting or examining the data) each ψ_i is drawn from an underlying Gaussian distribution centered at zero. Under this prior structure, the ψ_i do not depend on location i and are said to be *exchangeable*. The effect of the prior distributions defined in equation (9.75) is to add excess (but not spatially structured) variation to the model in equation (9.73), and hence to the model in equation (9.74).

Even though the prior distributions add spatially unstructured variation, the variation does induce some structure in the model. Each ψ_i represents a value sampled from the same underlying distribution, and the exchangeable prior distribution induces similarity among the observations. In Section 4.4.3 we saw how we can take advantage of this similarity and "borrow strength" across observations to improve estimates of any single estimand. Specifically, we saw that the exchangeable prior distribution defined in equation (9.75) results in posterior estimates of the local relative risks based on weighted averages of the MLE of the local relative risk, Y_i/E_i, and the global relative risk defined across all regions, Y_+/E_+. The weights assigned to the local and global values are functions of the prior variance v_ψ and the variance associated with any particular local SMR. Conceptually, the model smoothes more where local estimates are least stable, precisely where we require more smoothing.

If we estimate the remaining model parameter v_ψ from the data, we obtain empirical Bayes inference, as in Section 4.4.3, but data-based estimates of prior parameters are not entirely in the spirit of Bayesian inference. For *fully Bayes inference*, we complete the hierarchy by defining a *hyperprior distribution* for v_ψ. At higher levels of the hierarchy, we are typically less interested in introducing new structure (particularly because it may not be altogether clear how such structure cascades through the other levels of the hierarchy and eventually affects the posterior distribution). In addition, we often require a *proper hyperprior distribution* (i.e., based on a well-defined density function integrating to 1) to ensure a proper posterior distribution. Therefore, we often choose a proper, *conjugate prior* for v_ψ [i.e., a parametric family of prior distributions yielding a marginal posterior distribution for v_ψ within the same parametric family as the prior; cf. Carlin and Louis (2000, Section 2.2.2) for details]. In our case of a variance parameter for a Gaussian distribution, the inverse gamma distribution (i.e., the reciprocal of v_ψ follows a gamma distribution) provides the conjugate family.

Most applications complete the model at this point, assigning fixed values to the two parameters of the inverse gamma hyperprior. Identifying noninformative choices for these parameters can be tricky since the inverse gamma distribution is defined only for positive values, and zero is a degenerate value. In practice, many analysts assign values corresponding to a very small mean and very large variance as a sort of noninformative hyperprior for v_ψ. However, Kelsall and Wakefield (1999) [in a discussion of Best et al. (1999)] and Gelman et al. (2004, Appendix C) note that even though this definition results in a long, flat upper tail for the prior distribution, it also increases without bound for values very close to zero and may be more informative than is often appreciated. Furthermore, Ghosh et al. (1999) and Sun et al. (1999) define conditions on the inverse gamma parameters to ensure a proper posterior. In practice, some experimentation to assess the sensitivity of inferences to changes in the hyperprior parameters provides valuable insight into the robustness of inference to the choice of these (hyper)parameters.

Defining the prior distribution for $\boldsymbol{\psi}$ offers spatial modeling opportunities. We want to express some sort of spatial pattern among the ψ_i's, perhaps through a parametric correlation model linking pairs ψ_i and ψ_j for $j \neq i$. Also, we want to allow the data to inform on the relative strength and extent (scale) of any correlation through the likelihood, resulting in posterior inference for correlation parameters, and the ψ_i's themselves. We consider two classes of spatially structured prior formulations below.

First, we can follow development in the Scottish lip cancer data break and consider a joint multivariate Gaussian prior distribution for $\boldsymbol{\psi}$ with spatial covariance matrix Σ_ψ, that is,

$$\boldsymbol{\psi} \sim MVN(\mathbf{0}, \Sigma_\psi). \tag{9.76}$$

In this data break we define the elements of Σ_ψ through a parametric semivariogram or correlogram model. A Bayesian hierarchical model is defined in the same way except that we treat the autocorrelation parameters as random and specify prior distributions for them. Diggle et al. (1998) illustrate a Bayesian application of this approach using an isotropic exponential correlation function with parameters governing the rate of decay with distance and controlling the overall smoothness of the prediction. The rate of decay and smoothness parameters are then assigned independent uniform priors.

As an alternative to the joint prior distribution defined in equation (9.76) and as noted in Section 9.4.3, we could consider a conditionally specified prior spatial structure for $\boldsymbol{\psi}$ similar to the conditional autoregressive models introduced in Section 9.3.2. Clayton and Kaldor (1987) propose such *conditionally autoregressive priors* (CAR priors) in an empirical Bayes setting, and Besag et al. (1991) provide the fully Bayes implementation. In addition, Breslow and Clayton (1993) apply CAR priors as random effects distributions within likelihood approximations for GLMMs. The CAR priors see wide use in the area of *disease mapping* or regional smoothing of rates (proportions) of rare events, as discussed in Chapter 4. Clayton and Bernardinelli (1992), Mollié (1996), and Wakefield et al. (2000a) all provide overviews of the application of hierarchical GLMMs with CAR priors to the area of disease mapping.

Due to their widespread use, we consider the CAR disease mapping models in more detail. First, we specify a subset of Gaussian CAR priors defining the prior mean of each ψ_i as a weighted average of the other ψ_j, $j \neq i$,

$$\psi_i | \psi_{j \neq i} \sim N\left(\frac{\sum_{j \neq i} c_{ij} \psi_j}{\sum_{j \neq i} c_{ij}}, \frac{1}{v_{\text{CAR}} \sum_{j \neq i} c_{ij}} \right), \qquad i = 1, \ldots, N. \tag{9.77}$$

Here, the c_{ij}'s denote spatial dependence parameters defining which regions j are neighbors to region i (and quantifying how "neighborly"), and v_{CAR} denotes a hyperparameter related to the conditional variance of ψ_i given the values of the other elements of $\boldsymbol{\psi}$. As with the CAR regression models in Section 9.3.2, we set $c_{ii} = 0$ for all i. Typical applications consider adjacency-based weights where

$c_{ij} = 1$ if region j is adjacent to region i, and $c_{ij} = 0$, otherwise. Other weighting options also appear in the literature (e.g., Best et al. 1999) but are much less widely applied.

For the CAR regression models in Section 9.3.2, we parameterized the covariance matrix induced by the CAR structure, then estimated the covariance parameters (rather than estimating the c_{ij}'s themselves). In applications of Bayesian GLMMs, we often assign fixed values to the c_{ij}'s in equation (9.77) (e.g., based on adjacency within the census geography), with only the hyperparameter v_{CAR} controlling the amount of spatial similarity. We explore reasons for this approach and the links between the joint and conditionally specified prior distributions in Section 9.5.3.

Fitting Bayesian Models: Markov Chain Monte Carlo As noted above, the primary theoretical difference between Bayesian and the likelihood-based approaches to GLMMs involves whether or not one incorporates (Bayesian) or omits (likelihood) the prior distribution for fixed effects and the hyperprior distribution for random effect covariance parameters. The two approaches also differ in the algorithms used to fit the models. In Section 9.4.3 we outlined pseudolikelihood approaches to fitting GLMMs under the classical approach. Although it might seem that the inclusion of prior and hyperprior structures will only complicate calculations, in fact, consideration of the posterior distribution allows application of a fairly general family of simulation-based model-fitting techniques.

We present closed-form empirical Bayes posterior inference for nonspatial random effects in Section 4.4.3. However, when considering spatial prior distributions, analytic calculation of the resulting posterior distribution becomes difficult, due to the dimension of the problem (we have N observations and N random effects in addition to the fixed effects contained in the vector $\boldsymbol{\beta}$) and the inclusion of the spatial structure itself.

Such complications (high-dimensional, complex posterior distributions) hampered the widespread application of Bayesian methods for many years. However, during the 1990s, many statisticians recognized and expanded a class of simulation-based *Markov Chain Monte Carlo* (MCMC) *algorithms* particularly suited to the analysis of hierarchical models, including the spatial models defined here. In this section we provide a brief introduction to the concepts underlying MCMC methods and their connection to the hierarchical spatial GLMMs defined above. Gelfand and Smith (1990), Agresti et al. (2000), Carlin and Louis (2000), and Gelman et al. (2004) provide more detailed development, many examples, and associated references.

A *Markov chain* is a sequence of random variables where the distribution of the next value depends only on the present "state" or value. An example of a Markov chain is the simple *random walk*, where at any point in time we either move one step to the right or to the left with equal probability. Where we go next depends only on where we are right now, not on where we were several steps ago. Under certain conditions, if we "run" a Markov chain (i.e., we generate a long sequence of observed values one at a time), the chain will converge to a *stationary distribution* [i.e., after convergence, the probability of the chain being in any particular "state" (or taking any particular value) at any particular time remains the same]. In other words, after convergence, any sequence of observations from the Markov chain represents a sample from the stationary distribution. Note that each (postconvergence) sequence represents a *correlated sample*, since each new observation still depends on the preceding observation.

In a nutshell, MCMC methods construct (Monte Carlo) simulations generating parameter values from Markov chains having stationary distributions identical (at least theoretically) to the joint posterior distribution of interest. After these Markov chains converge, the simulated values represent a (again, correlated) sample of observations from the posterior distribution. We can often define an MCMC algorithm even when the target posterior distribution is analytically intractable, allowing us to fit complex, highly structured hierarchical models such as the spatial GLMMs considered here.

For illustration of an MCMC algorithm, suppose that we have a model with data vector $\mathbf{Y}$ and three parameters θ_1, θ_2, and θ_3. One of the simplest MCMC algorithms is a *Gibbs sampler*, based on the *full conditional distributions*

$$f(\theta_1|\theta_2, \theta_3, \mathbf{Y})$$
$$f(\theta_2|\theta_1, \theta_3, \mathbf{Y})$$
$$f(\theta_3|\theta_1, \theta_2, \mathbf{Y}).$$

Next, suppose that we have the full conditional distributions and can simulate values from each of the full conditional distributions and we start with values $\theta_1^{(1)}$, $\theta_2^{(1)}$, and $\theta_3^{(1)}$. Then we iterate through the full conditional distributions generating the second value of each parameter from the following distributions:

$$\text{sample } \theta_1^{(2)} \text{ from } f(\theta_1|\theta_2^{(1)}, \theta_3^{(1)}, \mathbf{Y})$$
$$\text{sample } \theta_2^{(2)} \text{ from } f(\theta_2|\theta_1^{(2)}, \theta_3^{(1)}, \mathbf{Y})$$
$$\text{sample } \theta_3^{(2)} \text{ from } f(\theta_3|\theta_1^{(2)}, \theta_2^{(2)}, \mathbf{Y}).$$

As we continue to update the values of $\boldsymbol{\theta}$ sequentially, they will eventually become indistinguishable from samples from the joint posterior distribution $f(\theta_1, \theta_2, \theta_3|\mathbf{Y})$, provided that such a stationary distribution exists (which is the case under fairly mild conditions met by most well-defined models with proper posterior distributions; cf. Gelfand and Smith 1990).

Example. Gelman et al. (2004, pp. 288–289) provide a very simple example illustrating Gibbs sampling, which we repeat here to illustrate the basic idea. Suppose that we have a single observation (Y_1, Y_2) which follows a bivariate Gaussian distribution with unknown mean $\boldsymbol{\theta} = (\theta_1, \theta_2)$, known variances $\text{Var}(Y_1) = \text{Var}(Y_2) = 1$, and a known value for $\text{Cov}(Y_1, Y_2) = \rho$. With a uniform prior on $\boldsymbol{\theta}$, the joint posterior distribution of $\boldsymbol{\theta}$ is multivariate Gaussian with mean (Y_1, Y_2) and variance–covariance matrix with $\text{Var}(\theta_1|\mathbf{Y}) = \text{Var}(\theta_1|\mathbf{Y}) = 1$ and $\text{Cov}(\theta_1, \theta_2|\mathbf{Y}) = \rho$; that is, given values for Y_1 and Y_2,

$$\begin{bmatrix}\theta_1\\ \theta_2\end{bmatrix} \sim MVN\left(\begin{bmatrix}Y_1\\ Y_2\end{bmatrix}, \begin{bmatrix}1 & \rho\\ \rho & 1\end{bmatrix}\right).$$

Standard results from multivariate statistics reveal the full conditional distributions as univariate Gaussian distributions

$$\theta_1|\theta_2, \mathbf{Y} \sim N(Y_1 + \rho(\theta_2 - Y_2), 1 - \rho^2)$$
$$\theta_2|\theta_1, \mathbf{Y} \sim N(Y_2 + \rho(\theta_1 - Y_1), 1 - \rho^2).$$

Since we know both the full joint posterior distribution and the full conditionals in this simple example, we can check how well Gibbs sampling output matches the known full posterior distribution.

To implement a Gibbs sampler, we generate a value from the full conditional distribution of θ_1 given the current value of θ_2 and the data, then generate a value of θ_2 given the current value of θ_1 and the data. We continue to alternate between the full conditionals until we have a sufficient sample of values to estimate the joint posterior density (e.g., using kernel estimates as we did for point patterns in Chapter 5).

Figure 9.32 illustrates the example for $\rho = 0.5$ and $\mathbf{Y} = (0.2655, 0.2742)$. The plot in the upper left-hand corner shows the values and the order of the first 10 updates of θ_1 and θ_2, and so includes 20 points (updating each parameter given the current value of the other). The plot in the upper right-hand corner shows the first 500 updates, revealing that all (but the starting value of (4,0) fall within the elliptical region of the bivariate normal distribution specified. The histograms on the bottom compare the marginal histograms of each parameter (the univariate histograms of each of the parameter samples) to the known marginal Gaussian density functions. Additional illustrative examples of Gibbs sampling appear in Casella and George (1992) and in Gelman et al. (2004, Chapter 11).

Returning to our general description of MCMC algorithms, in some applications we may find that deriving the full conditional distributions may not be possible, or the full conditional distributions may not fall into convenient parametric distributional families. Such cases require more advanced simulation methods typically based on acceptance–rejection sampling, wherein we generate "candidate" values under a more manageable distribution, then accept or reject the candidate value in a manner such that the sample of accepted values follows the desired distribution (cf. Gelman et al. 2004, Chapter 11).

Based on the description of a Gibbs sampler above, the conditional specification of the CAR prior seems almost a "custom fit" to an MCMC algorithm. Indeed, the Hammersley–Clifford theorem detailed in Besag (1974), which defines under what conditions a set of (full) conditional distributions uniquely defines a valid joint distribution, is one of the key results enabling the use of both MCMC and CAR spatial models. However, we cannot directly implement a Gibbs sampler for

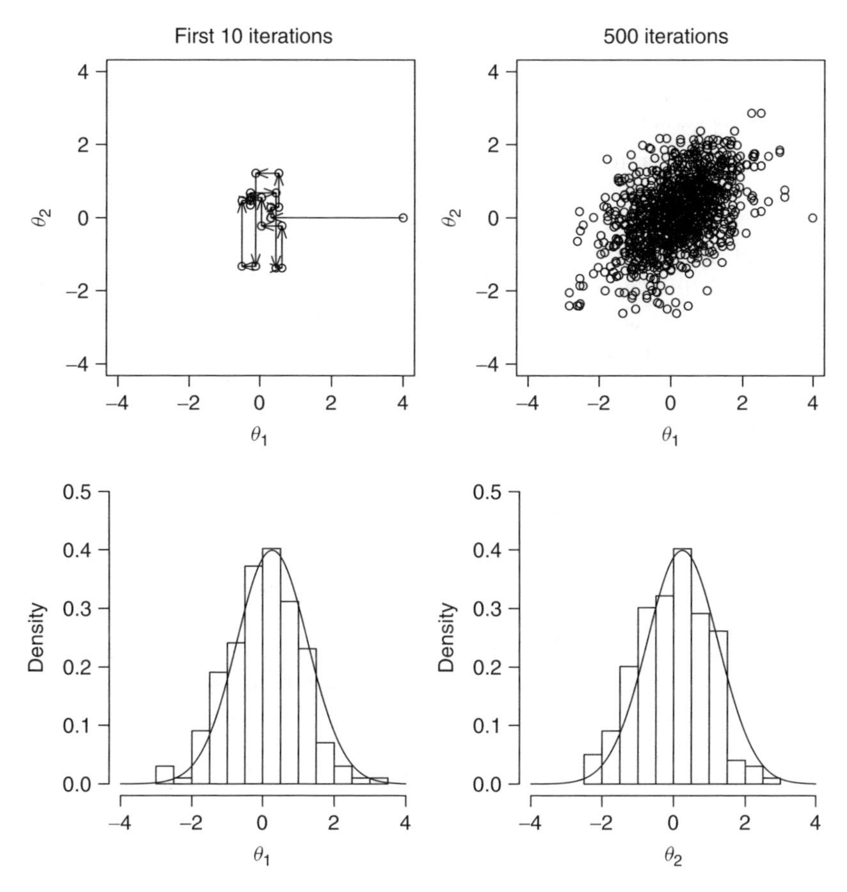

FIG. 9.32 Example of Gibbs sampling for bivariate normal model. The plot on the upper left illustrates the first 10 iterations, the plot on the upper right illustrates the first 500 iterations. The lower plots give histograms of samples of θ_1 and θ_2, compared to the theoretical marginal density functions.

our GLMM since some full conditional distributions are not available in closed form due to the non-CAR parameters (e.g., v_{CAR}) in the model, and we require acceptance–rejection-based sampling. This said, the conditional specification does provide a (relatively) straightforward implementation of MCMC approaches to sample from the joint posterior distribution of all model parameters.

Summaries of the postconvergence MCMC samples provide posterior inference for model parameters. For instance, the sample mean of the (postconvergence) sampled values for a particular model parameter provides an estimate of the marginal posterior mean and a point estimate of the parameter itself. The interval defined by the 2.5th and 97.5th quantiles of the (postconvergence) sampled values for a model parameter provides a 95% interval estimate of the parameter. In the data break following Section 9.4.4 we used a similar idea to provide a summary of a distribution of odds ratios generated using geostatistical simulation and we called this interval a *bootstrap confidence interval*. In Bayesian inference, such an interval is termed a *credible set* to distinguish it from the *confidence interval* of classical statistics. Although similar in spirit, the interpretation of the two intervals is different. A 95% credible set defines an interval having a 0.95 posterior probability of containing the parameter of interest (which is assumed to be a random variable in Bayesian statistics). In contrast, a 95% confidence interval represents an interval such that 95% of intervals constructed similarly from identically distributed and independent data sets would contain the true parameter value (which is assumed to be a fixed but unknown quantity in classical statistics).

The MCMC samples also provide posterior inference for functions of model parameters. For instance, an MCMC implementation of the spatial GLMM with Poisson likelihood and CAR priors provides samples from the posterior distribution of model parameters contained in the vectors $\boldsymbol{\beta}$ and $\boldsymbol{\psi}$. If we define $\boldsymbol{\beta}^{(s)}$ and $\boldsymbol{\psi}^{(s)}$ as the set of simulated values at the sth (postconvergence) iteration of our MCMC algorithm, then

$$\zeta_i^{(s)} = \exp\left(\boldsymbol{x}_i'\boldsymbol{\beta}^{(s)} + \psi_i^{(s)}\right)$$

defines the sth value in a Markov chain having the posterior distribution of ζ_i as its stationary distribution. As with the sampled values of the model parameters themselves, histograms, percentiles, and other summaries provide sampling-based estimates of the posterior distribution for ζ_i for each region i.

Assessing convergence for MCMC algorithms is an active area of statistical interest, particularly for models containing many parameters. Several diagnostics exist, but none are foolproof (Cowles and Carlin 1996). As a result, MCMC algorithms offer an approach to fitting highly complex parametric models but are by no means "automatic" and should be used with care.

9.5.3 Interpretation and Use with Spatial Data

While the hierarchical spatial GLMM defined above contains sensible pieces, they fit together to create a somewhat complicated inferential structure. Although MCMC algorithms offer a means to fit such models, the models are certainly not the most straightforward or basic of hierarchical models, and several features merit further attention.

First, we elaborate on the relationship between the joint and conditional specifications of spatially structured priors. In the discussion of spatial autoregressive models in Section 9.3, we give the joint distribution induced by a conditional autoregression, parameterize the elements of the (induced) covariance matrix, and then estimate these (covariance) parameters from the data. As noted briefly above, most Bayesian implementations of spatial GLMMs based on conditionally specified CAR priors define a (seemingly sensible) set of spatial dependence parameters, $\{c_{ij}\}$, treat these as fixed values, then derive the resulting posterior distributions via MCMC algorithms. However, the connection between the user-defined c_{ij}'s and the resulting (prior or posterior) spatial covariance structure of $\boldsymbol{\psi}$, although theoretically sound, is not altogether transparent. For instance, the connection rarely, if ever, provides a closed-form, functional relationship between the spatial dependence parameters $\{c_{ij}\}$ and the elements of the covariance matrix Σ_ψ for the joint distribution of $\boldsymbol{\psi}$, as we illustrate below.

Besag and Kooperberg (1995) explore the connection between the autoregressive spatial dependence parameters and the spatial covariance matrix in detail, and we highlight several key points here. First, if $\boldsymbol{\psi}$ follows a multivariate Gaussian distribution with covariance $\Sigma_{\boldsymbol{\psi}}$, then the density, $f(\boldsymbol{\psi})$, follows

$$f(\boldsymbol{\psi}) \propto \exp\left(-\frac{1}{2}\boldsymbol{\psi}'\Sigma_\psi^{-1}\boldsymbol{\psi}\right). \tag{9.78}$$

Standard multivariate theory defines the associated conditional distributions as

$$\psi_i|\psi_{j\neq i} \sim N\left(\sum_{j\neq i}\left(\frac{-\Sigma_{\psi,ij}^{-1}}{\Sigma_{\psi,ii}^{-1}}\right)\psi_j, \frac{1}{\Sigma_{\psi,ii}^{-1}}\right), \tag{9.79}$$

where $\Sigma_{\psi,ij}^{-1}$ denotes the (i, j)th element of the Σ_ψ^{-1} matrix. Note that the conditional mean for ψ_i is a weighted sum of ψ_j, $j \neq i$, and the conditional variance is inversely proportional to the diagonal of the inverse of Σ_ψ. Reversing direction and going from a set of user-specified conditional Gaussian distributions to the associated joint distribution is a bit more involved, requiring some constraints on the weights defining the conditional mean and variance to ensure, first, a Gaussian joint distribution, and second, a symmetric and valid covariance matrix Σ_ψ (cf. Besag 1974; Besag and Kooperberg 1995; Arnold et al. 1999).

Note that both the conditional mean and the conditional variance in equation (9.79) depend on elements of the *inverse* of the covariance matrix Σ_ψ. As a result, any MCMC algorithm applied to the joint specification based on updating single elements (or any subset) of $\boldsymbol{\psi}$ based on a full conditional distribution will involve matrix inversion, and we must reinvert whenever we update covariance parameters. This feature suggests that the CAR prior formulation may be more computationally efficient than the joint formulation, since the CAR priors (effectively) limit modeling to the elements of Σ_ψ^{-1}, rather than Σ_ψ, thereby avoiding the potentially costly inversion step.

The preceding paragraph suggests that working directly with the spatial dependence parameters (c_{ij}s) rather than the elements of Σ_ψ has practical advantages for spatial GLMMs, particularly for MCMC implementation. However, much of this book aims to develop models (and intuition) for elements of Σ_ψ rather than for elements of Σ_ψ^{-1}, that is, models of spatial covariance (and correlation), not models of spatial dependence parameters. Also, as noted in Section 9.3.1, the relationship between the dependence parameters (autoregressive weights) and the resulting covariances may not always be intuitive. How, then, do we develop sensible structures for the c_{ij}'s within CAR priors?

To address this issue, we first link the spatial dependence parameters in equation (9.77) with their counterparts in equation (9.79). Doing this, we find that

$$\frac{c_{ij}}{\sum_j c_{ij}} = \frac{-\Sigma^{-1}_{\psi,ij}}{\Sigma^{-1}_{\psi,ii}}$$

and

$$v_{\text{CAR}} \sum_j c_{ij} = \Sigma^{-1}_{\psi,ii}.$$

Therefore, $c_{ij} = \Sigma^{-1}_{\psi,ij}/v_{\text{CAR}}$, and symmetry of Σ_ψ requires symmetry of the spatial dependence parameters, c_{ij}, in the collection of CAR priors defined by equation (9.77).

By limiting attention to CAR priors with symmetric spatial dependence parameters, we restrict attention to a subset of the full class of valid conditionally specified CAR prior distributions, since in general, the weights defining the conditional mean need not be symmetric themselves as long as the diagonal elements of Σ^{-1}_ψ compensate appropriately via

$$\left(\frac{-\Sigma^{-1}_{\psi,ij}}{\Sigma^{-1}_{\psi,ii}}\right)\Sigma^{-1}_{\psi,ii} = \left(\frac{-\Sigma^{-1}_{\psi,ji}}{\Sigma^{-1}_{\psi,jj}}\right)\Sigma^{-1}_{\psi,jj}. \tag{9.80}$$

[Although equation (9.80) may seem trivial, recall that in practice we define the additive weights $\left(-\Sigma^{-1}_{\psi,ij}/\Sigma^{-1}_{\psi,ii}\right)$ and conditional variances $1/\left(\Sigma^{-1}_{\psi,ii}\right)$ without regard to the specific nondiagonal elements of Σ^{-1}_ψ, so verification is important for any proposed conditional structure.] The class of CAR priors defined by equation (9.77) (with associated symmetric c_{ij}'s) includes the widely applied adjacency weights ($c_{ij} = 1$ when regions i and j share a boundary, $c_{ij} = 0$ otherwise), and (symmetric) distance-decay weights such as those considered by Best et al. (1999), and we continue to limit attention to this subset of CAR priors here, for simplicity and to raise some practical issues associated with these particular prior distributions.

Using results in Besag (1974), we find that the set of CAR priors defined in equation (9.77) uniquely defines a corresponding multivariate normal joint distribution

$$\boldsymbol{\psi} \sim MVN(\mathbf{0}, \Sigma_\psi), \tag{9.81}$$

where $\Sigma^{-1}_{\psi,ii} = \sum_j c_{ij}$ and $\Sigma^{-1}_{\psi,ij} = -c_{ij}$. However, for symmetric c_{ij}'s, the sum of any row of the matrix Σ^{-1}_ψ is zero, indicating that Σ^{-1}_ψ is singular (noninvertible), and the corresponding covariance matrix Σ_ψ in equation (9.81) is not well defined. This holds for any symmetric set of spatial dependence parameters c_{ij} (including the adjacency-based c_{ij}'s appearing in many applications). Surprisingly enough, this does not preclude application of the model with such weight matrices (cf. Besag and Kooperberg 1995), but it does prevent easy transition from the spatial dependence parameters to spatial covariances.

A further complication arises by noting that the full class of CAR priors [including those defined by equation (9.77)] falls into the class of *pairwise difference prior distributions* defined by Besag et al. (1995). Such distributions define improper priors since they only define contrasts (differences) between pairs of values $\psi_i - \psi_j$, $j \neq i$. Besag et al. (1995) note that the only source of impropriety for such pairwise difference prior distributions lies in their inability to identify an overall mean value for the elements of $\boldsymbol{\psi}$, since such distributions define the value of each ψ_i relative to the values of the others. In this case, any likelihood function based on data allowing estimation of an overall mean also allows the class of improper pairwise difference priors to generate proper posterior distributions. In practice, we assure this by adding the constraint

$$\sum_{i=1}^{N} \psi_i = 0.$$

This provides a sensible restriction since we do not want the random effects to add to the overall mean value of the outcome, but instead we want the ψ_i to reflect only the spatial similarity between residual values at nearby locations.

As a result of the preceding development, we have a set of conditional prior distributions defined by a sensible set of spatial dependence parameters that do not translate directly into a closed-form model of spatial correlation or covariance. We also have a joint specification that allows direct parametric modeling of the covariance function but is computationally intensive to fit (due to the matrix inversion component). Both induce spatial similarity between observations by borrowing strength from neighboring values. However, the conditionally specified model is much more attractive for practical MCMC implementation. At present, computational demands often win out over direct parameterization of the covariance structure and the literature contains many more examples of CAR priors than the multivariate normal formulation.

DATA BREAK: New York Leukemia Data (*cont.*) To illustrate Bayesian disease mapping models, we turn again to the New York leukemia data set. Our previous modeling efforts revolved around linear models with residual correlation. Meeting the standard assumptions for linear regression required transformations of the outcome and covariates of interest. We now turn toward a hierarchical Poisson regression analysis, very similar to that used in the analysis of the Scotland lip cancer data in Section 9.4. The Poisson model allows us to treat the counts as outcomes without the awkward transformations we utilized earlier in the chapter. In addition, we use similar covariates to those above, but again without transformation.

More specifically, we observe census tract counts $Y_1, \ldots, Y_{281}$ modeled as conditionally independent Poisson random variables with mean

$$Y_i | \zeta_i \overset{\text{ind}}{\sim} \text{Poisson}(E_i \zeta_i)$$

and

$$\log(\zeta_i) = \boldsymbol{x}_i'\boldsymbol{\beta} + \psi_i,$$

where

$$E_i = n_i(Y_+/n_+) = n_i(592/1,057,673),$$

n_i denotes the population size of the ith tract, and $\psi_i, i = 1, \ldots, 281$, denotes tract-specific random effects. We consider three tract-specific covariates: the percent of residents aged greater than 65 years, the percent of residents who own their own home, and a surrogate for exposure to the 11 inactive hazardous waste sites reporting TCE. For illustration we use the natural logarithm of the inverse distance between each tract and the nearest waste site, recalling the precautions in interpretation associated with exposure surrogates noted in the data break following Section 7.6.5.

For the next stage of model specification, we assume uniform prior distributions for the fixed-effect parameters ($\boldsymbol{\beta}$), and consider three different prior specifications for the tract-specific random effects in $\boldsymbol{\psi}$. First, we consider the exchangeable (nonspatial) prior distribution defined in equation (9.75). Next, we assign the spatially structured conditionally autoregressive (CAR) prior defined in equation (9.77). Finally, we consider a model introduced by Besag et al. (1991) that includes a pair of random effects for each tract, one assigned an exchangeable prior, the other assigned a CAR prior. Including both random effects clearly overparameterizes the model (two random intercepts for each observation). The likelihood will only identify the sum of the two parameters for each tract, although the prior distributions allows posterior identifiability (see Besag et al. 1995; Carlin and Louis 2000, p. 263).

To complete the model specification, we assign conjugate inverse-gamma prior distributions to the variance parameters associated with the exchangeable and/or CAR priors. More specifically, we follow discussions in Gelman et al. (2004, Appendix C) and a specific suggestion in Kelsall and Wakefield (1999) and define the hyperpriors

$$\frac{1}{v_\psi} \sim \text{gamma}(0.5, 0.0005)$$

and

$$\frac{1}{v_{\text{CAR}}} \sim \text{gamma}(0.5, 0.0005).$$

We utilize these particular hyperprior distributions primarily for illustration rather than advocate them as any sort of optimal choice. In fact, for the model containing both exchangeable and CAR random effects, the choice is technically not particularly "fair" (in the sense of providing equal prior emphasis on the nonspatial and spatial random effects), due to the marginal nature of the exchangeable effects and the conditional nature of the CAR effects (cf. Bernardinelli et al. 1995b; Best et al. 1999; Carlin and Louis 2000, pp. 263–264).

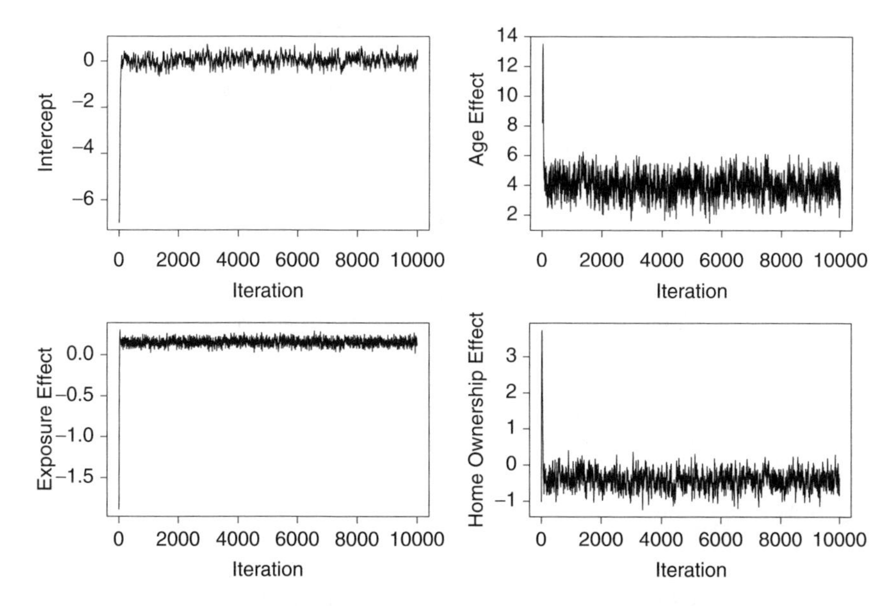

FIG. 9.33 Trace plots of the first 10,000 Markov Chain Monte Carlo (MCMC) updates for the intercept, age effect, exposure effect, and home ownership effect for the hierarchical Poisson regression model with exchangeable random effects.

To fit the model, we implement an MCMC approach using 20,000 updates of each model parameter. Figure 9.33 illustrates a trace of the first 10,000 updates of the fixed effects in $\boldsymbol{\beta} = (\beta_0, \beta_{\text{age}}, \beta_{\text{home}}, \beta_{\text{exposure}})'$. For each parameter, we observe the algorithm move away from the (intentionally distant) starting value and then generate values "wiggling" around within a consistent range of values representing the posterior distribution of each model parameter. Trace plots for the fixed effects based on the CAR and the composite model are similar. Although we do not show any formal diagnostics of convergence, the plots strongly suggest that this is the case. We base inference on iterations 5001 to 20,000 (we do not show the second 10,000 iterations in Figure 9.33), noting that the Markov nature of MCMC algorithms induces correlation within the sequence of simulated values for each parameter so that we are not basing inference on 15,000 independent observations, but rather, on a more modest (but still large) effective sample size for each parameter.

Table 9.13 provides the estimated posterior median and associated 95% credible set for each of the fixed effects and for all three models. In addition, Figure 9.34 provides kernel estimates of the corresponding posterior densities. We note that the particular choice of prior (spatial or not) makes relatively little difference in inference. From the results in Table 9.13, we note a strong age effect (as expected) and a suggestive exposure effect (the posterior density of β_{exposure} primarily covers positive values). In addition, we note that homeownership also has a suggestive negative effect (i.e., the lower the proportion of homeowners in a tract, the higher

Table 9.13 Markov Chain Monte Carlo Results for Hierarchical Poisson Regression of the New York Leukemia Data for Each of Three Models[a]

Priors	Posterior Median	95% Credible Set
	Intercept (β_0)	
Exchangeable	0.034	(−0.335, 0.401)
CAR	0.048	(−0.355, 0.408)
Both	0.049	(−0.368, 0.414)
	% > 65	
Exchangeable	4.034	(2.759, 5.300)
CAR	3.984	(2.736, 5.330)
Both	3.985	(2.708, 5.293)
	Exposure	
Exchangeable	0.153	(0.085, 0.223)
CAR	0.152	(0.066, 0.226)
Both	0.152	(0.069, 0.228)
	% Own Home	
Exchangeable	−0.372	(−0.783, 0.037)
CAR	−0.367	(−0.758, 0.049)
Both	−0.379	(−0.765, 0.072)

[a] Models are identical except for the prior distributions assigned to the random effects. Posterior medians and 95% credible sets are based on 15,000 (postconvergence) iterations.

the incidence of leukemia). While the 95% credible set in Table 9.13 offers one summary, we may also query the simulated values directly and find the proportion of simulated values of β_{home} below zero in iterations 5001 and 20,000 yielding estimates of 0.034, 0.036, and 0.047 for the posterior probability $\Pr(\beta_{\text{home}} < 0|\mathbf{Y})$ from the models with exchangeable, CAR, and both types of random effects, respectively. These results are remarkably consistent with the results from weighted linear regression given in Tables 9.3, 9.5, 9.8, and 9.9.

In addition to inference for the fixed effects, we may also use the MCMC samples to explore patterns in the local standardized mortality/morbidity ratios (SMRs) which incorporate fixed and random effects to provide insight into differences between the modeled expected values and the E_i values (that do not adjust for covariate effects or regional differences). More specifically, we consider inference for

$$\text{SMR}_i = 100 \times \frac{E_i \exp(\boldsymbol{x}_i'\boldsymbol{\beta} + \psi_i)}{E_i} = 100 \times \exp(\boldsymbol{x}_i'\boldsymbol{\beta} + \psi_i),$$

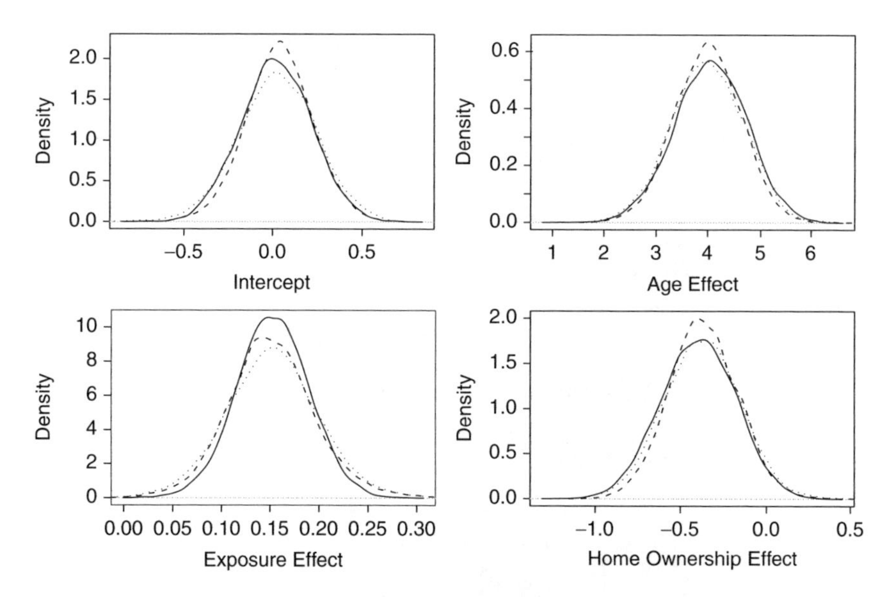

FIG. 9.34 Kernel estimates of the posterior density of the fixed effects in a hierarchical Poisson regression of the New York leukemia data. The three densities correspond to exchangeable (solid line) random effects, conditionally autoregressive (CAR) random effects (dashed line), and both types of random effects (dotted line).

where we multiply by 100 to put the local SMRs on their traditional scale, where $\text{SMR}_i = 100$ indicates the same number observed (or expected under the model, in our case) as expected (as defined by the E_i). The local SMRs are functions of the model parameters. In a likelihood-based setting, obtaining inference for such a function of parameters would require extended calculations or approximations such as the delta method. In our MCMC-based Bayesian analysis, calculating

$$\text{SMR}_i^{(s)} = 100 \times \exp(\boldsymbol{x}_i'\boldsymbol{\beta}^{(s)} + \psi_i^{(s)})$$

for each iteration s of the (postconvergence) MCMC samples [where the superscript (s) denotes the sth simulated value for each parameter], we obtain a sample from the posterior distribution of each of the 281 local SMRs.

Figure 9.35 provides a map of the posterior median value of SMR_i for each tract. We note concentrations of high SMRs in and around the cities and towns of Syracuse (north), Binghamton (south), Cortland (center), Auburn (northwest), and Ithaca (west), perhaps suggesting a need for including an urban–rural effect or some other covariate correlating with occupation that differentiates between urban and rural locations (cf. Ahrens et al. 2001). We note that Figures 9.11 and 9.15 from weighted linear regression showed similar patterns, as did Figure 4.21, based on Poisson probability mapping. It is interesting to note that the three tracts identified as possible outliers in our earlier analyses (identified in Figure 9.8) also exhibit large local SMRs. This provides a nice validation of the approach; we know that these tracts exhibit odd behavior, due primarily to low local population sizes.

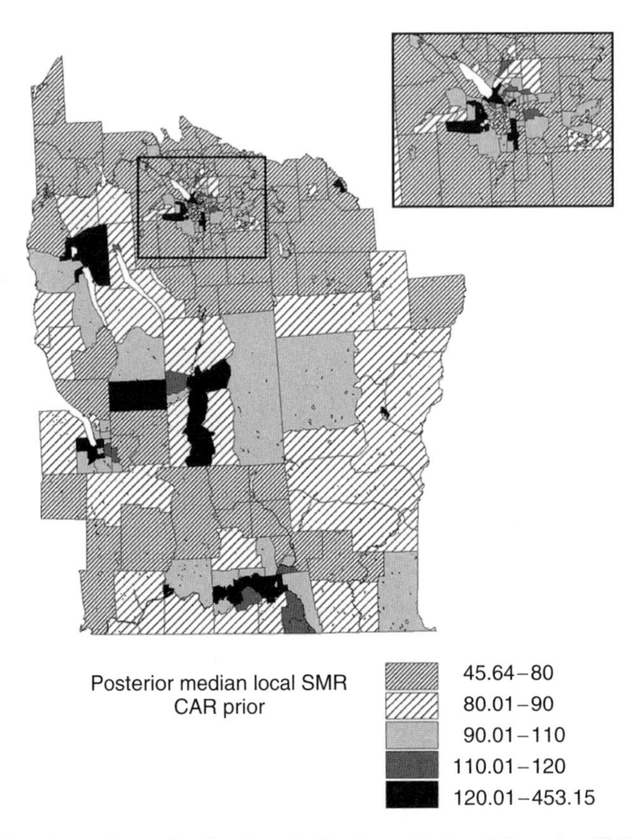

FIG. 9.35 Map of posterior median local standardized mortality/morbidity ratios (SMRs), based on a hierarchical Poisson regression with conditionally autoregressive (CAR) random effects.

Finally, paralleling our calculation of the posterior probability of β_{home} exceeding 0, we can also calculate local posterior probabilities of exceeding particular SMR values. For example, Figure 9.36 maps the local posterior probabilities

$$\Pr(\text{SMR}_i > 150|\mathbf{Y}),$$

(top map) and

$$\Pr(\text{SMR}_i > 200|\mathbf{Y}),$$

estimated as the fraction of MCMC samples exceeding 150 and 200, respectively. These values correspond to model predictions of half again or twice as many cases as expected based on the overall crude proportion Y_+/n_+. As with the map of the local SMRs themselves, we find the tracts with elevated probability of exceeding the cutoff values occurring in the cities and towns of the study area, particularly within Syracuse and Binghamton.

In conclusion, our analyses of the New York leukemia throughout the book provide some suggestion of spatial patterns in the observed counts and proportions,

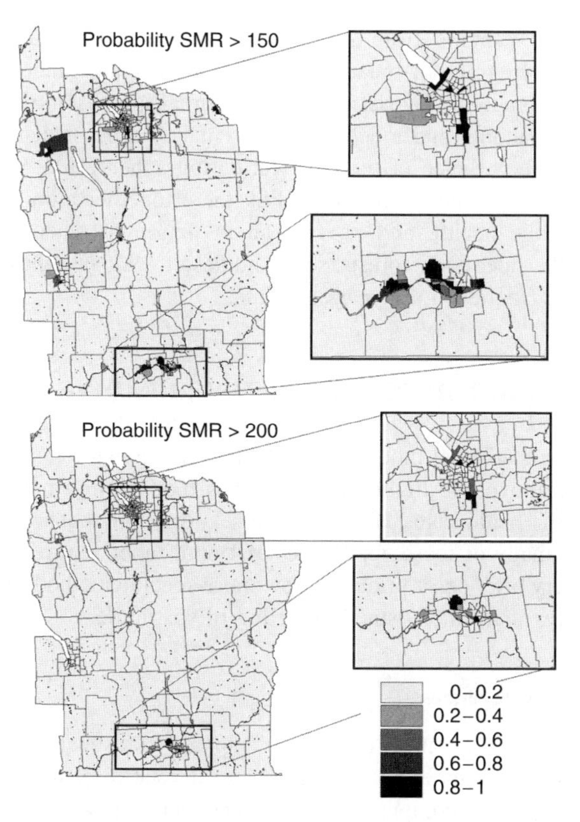

FIG. 9.36 Maps of the posterior probability of the local SMR exceeding 150 (top map and insets) or 200 (bottom map and insets). The insets provide local detail within the cities of Syracuse (north) and Binghamton (south).

but also suggest that many of the spatial patterns are driven by spatially varying covariates (some of which we adjust for in this chapter), a conclusion also proposed by Ahrens et al. (2001). Each analysis addresses different aspects of the data and provides answers to a slightly different set of questions. The underlying "true" picture remains somewhat elusive, but each analysis reveals additional avenues for further investigation. This is often the case in the spatial analysis of public health data, and this chapter in particular illustrates the wide variety of tools and approaches that apply to the myriad of questions surrounding a "simple" map of disease rates.

9.6 PARTING THOUGHTS

We conclude our tour of spatial statistics by noting that we are as much at a beginning point as an end. To stretch a geographic metaphor perhaps a bit too thin, the map of spatial statistics reveals a wide world of applications with the notion of "space" ranging from subatomic particles to the scale of the known universe, crossed by trails of breathtakingly beautiful mathematics linking related applications but sometimes bypassing particular areas of substantive interest. These trails are still expanding and much territory remains to be uncharted ("here there be dragons" in the parlance of the classical cartographers). Our goal has been to send postcards from some scenic areas, link them together around certain spatial questions in public health, and provide an invitation to readers to join in our exploration of the side roads, forests, seas, and deserts. We anticipate many exciting reports from the frontier in the years to come.

9.7 ADDITIONAL TOPICS AND FURTHER READING

The literature on statistical modeling for spatial data is wide ranging and diverse. In the sections above, we highlight approaches that we find most useful for the analysis of public health data. However, we acknowledge that we provide only an introduction to many of these approaches and omit others entirely. In this section we provide a very brief description of a few more specific methods and an overview of the current research in statistical modeling of spatial data.

9.7.1 General References

Readers interested in learning more about spatial statistical modeling can find descriptions and applications in the following references (roughly in the order of increasing mathematical complexity): Bailey and Gatrell (1995), Griffith and Layne (1999), Upton and Fingleton (1985), Haining (1990), Anselin (1988), Lawson (2001), Cressie (1993), Ripley (1981), Banerjee et al. (2003), and Ripley (1988). Each reference has its own special emphasis and tone, and there is much to be learned from each. We have found that some of the best investments in learning about spatial modeling are time, a computer, and a bookcase.

In addition to these general references, we provide brief descriptions and relevant introductory references for several more detailed approaches branching off the basic development in the sections above.

9.7.2 Restricted Maximum Likelihood Estimation

As discussed briefly in Section 9.1.1, *restricted maximum likelihood* (REML) provides an alternative to maximum likelihood estimation (and associated inference) of random effects parameters ($\boldsymbol{\theta}$). There is a large literature on the use of ML and REML for spatial modeling, and this is an area of active research in statistics. The basic theory is fairly straightforward, but the complexities encountered in many practical applications lead to issues and modifications falling beyond our scope here. Mardia and Marshall (1984) provide the basic theory of ML estimation in a spatial setting. Littell et al. (1996) give a nice overview of ML and REML estimation techniques in linear models and some good examples of their use in spatial modeling. Cressie and Lahiri (1996) provide the distributional properties of REML estimators, and Kenward and Roger (1999) provide an overview of related recent theoretical developments.

9.7.3 Residual Analysis with Spatially Correlated Error Terms

Cliff and Ord (1973, 1981), Anselin (1988), Anselin and Rey (1991), and Tiefelsdorf (2000) all describe approaches for exploring spatial autocorrelation in OLS residuals. In the presence of spatially correlated error terms, residual analysis becomes much more complicated. As illustrated in the data breaks above, many of the standard approaches are complicated by the inherent correlation of model residuals, and this problem is further compounded by the spatial correlation already included in fitting the model. Martin (1992) provides one of the earliest discussions on leverage and other diagnostics for the linear regression model with correlated error terms. His ideas were then applied to spatial autoregressive models by Haining (1994). Christensen et al. (1992) and Haslett (1998) extend the "leave one out" ideas of the model diagnostics in ordinary least squares regression to the spatial case based on best linear unbiased prediction.

Unfortunately, in moving from linear regression to GLMs and GLMMs, the picture becomes even more complicated. The current model diagnostics and methods for residual analysis in the case of independent data are often not informative, and with the exception of Jacqmin-Gadda et al. (1997) there has been little work on model diagnostics for the spatial case. There is a need for more general results regarding the properties and behavior of the residuals from the various spatial models outlined above.

9.7.4 Two-Parameter Autoregressive Models

Suppose that we want to allow the spatial dependence to vary with direction. Recall from Section 8.2.5 that this directional spatial dependence is called *anisotropy*. One way to do this is to consider two spatial dependence parameters, one for each direction. For example, if we consider a regular lattice of spatial locations and the first nearest-neighbor structure in a SAR model, we could allow the strength of spatial dependence in the east-west direction to be different from the strength of spatial dependence in the north-south direction and specify that (Whittle 1954)

$$\begin{aligned} Y(u, v) = \rho_1(Y(u+1, v) + Y(u-1, v)) + \rho_2(Y(u, v+1) \\ + Y(u, v-1)) + \upsilon(u, v). \end{aligned}$$

For $(I - B)$ to be invertible, $|\rho_1| + |\rho_2| < 0.5$ (Haining 1990, p. 82). Alternatively, Brandsma and Ketellapper (1979) use two spatial proximity matrices and two spatial dependence parameters to model spatial migration patterns from two different influences. Thus, in the autoregressive framework of equation (9.37), they take $B = \rho_1 W_1 + \rho_2 W_2$. This can easily be extended to consider multiple influences by using $B\rho_1 W_1 + \cdots + \rho_k W_k$, provided that the parameters can be estimated reliably.

Pace and LeSage (2002) consider a sequence of nested nearest-neighbor proximity matrices and use maximum likelihood to select the optimal nearest-neighbor structure. Another approach is to parameterize W directly, so that $W = W(\boldsymbol{\theta})$. For example, we could choose

$$w_{ij} = \begin{cases} d_{ij}^{-\alpha}, & \alpha > 0 \\ 0, & \text{otherwise} \end{cases}$$

so that $\boldsymbol{\theta} \equiv \alpha$, $W(\boldsymbol{\theta}) \equiv W(\alpha)$, the matrix of spatial dependence parameters is $B(\alpha) = W(\alpha)$, and we would then estimate α from the data. Whereas these extensions have focused primarily on SAR models, the same ideas can be used with CAR models. If we need an even more general spatial dependence structure, we could consider the broader geostatistical framework described in Section 9.2, where we drop the use of spatial proximity matrices and autoregression altogether and model Σ directly.

Other than the research described above, very little work has been done on developing multiparameter autoregressive models for practical applications. Although it is simple to conceive of a variety of parametric models for the spatial dependence matrix (B in a SAR model and C in a CAR model), it is necessary to know the theoretical constraints on the specified parameters, and sophisticated computing algorithms may be needed to estimate them.

9.7.5 Non-Gaussian Spatial Autoregressive Models

With the simultaneous approach, there are few alternatives to transformation, primarily because there are few alternatives to the multivariate Gaussian distribution that allow a general variance–covariance matrix. In general, constructing a general multivariate distribution with specified marginals is very difficult, and those distributions that have been developed result in or require constraints on the correlation parameters (see Johnson and Kotz 1969, Chapter 11) that make them unattractive for spatial modeling.

With the conditional approach, in addition to providing the mathematical underpinnings for Gaussian conditional autoregressive models, Besag (1974) also describes non-Gaussian conditional autoregressive models in general. As we mention in Section 9.3.2, the Hammersley–Clifford theorem provides the most general form for a valid joint distribution that can be constructed from a set of specified conditional distributions. This form is quite flexible for Gaussian conditional distributions, but for other distributions, the most general form is much more restrictive, essentially imposing more restrictions on the neighborhood structure than can be used. Thus, Besag (1974) developed a class of models called *auto models* that allow only pairwise dependence between spatial locations and so satisfy the conditions imposed by the Hammersley–Clifford theorem.

The models we describe at length in Section 9.3.2 are often referred to as *auto-Gaussian models*. However, there are other auto models corresponding to other distributions. In particular, the *auto-logistic model* finds application in many fields, including the analysis of plant patterns (Besag 1972; Gumpertz et al. 1997; Huffer and Wu 1998). Besag (1974) also introduces an *auto-Poisson model*, primarily as an example of the care required in developing conditionally specified models, since the constraints on spatial similarity parameters coupled with the small (but nonzero) probability of observing an infinite number of events result in a requirement of negative spatial autocorrelation. Some recent modifications allow positive spatial correlations (Ferrándiz et al. 1995; Kaiser and Cressie 1997), and Kaiser and Cressie (2000) provide additional tools for constructing Markov random fields that allow multiway spatial dependence and a spatial beta process.

9.7.6 Classical/Bayesian GLMMs

For more details regarding comparisons and contrasts between the Bayesian and classical developments, general discussions of Bayesian and classical issues appear in Cox and Hinkley (1974), and particular comments regarding GLMMs and their implementation appear in Breslow and Clayton (1993), Lee and Nelder (1996), and Agresti et al. (2000).

9.7.7 Prediction with GLMs

There are two types of predictions that can be considered with a spatial GLMM. The first is obviously the prediction of random effects. With the pseudolikelihood approach in Section 9.4.3, prediction of random effects is done using equation (9.66). We show in the data break following Section 9.4.3 how these can be used to obtain fitted values and smoothed rates. In the Bayesian setting, prediction of random effects is discussed in Zhang (2002).

However, in many mapping applications, we may also want to predict new observations, just as we did with universal kriging in Section 9.2.3. In this case, for a marginal GLM or with a GLMM using the pseudolikelihood approach in Section 9.4.3, prediction of new observations is very similar to kriging with the GLM mean and variance structure (see Gotway and Stroup 1997; Gotway and Wolfinger 2003). Gotway and Wolfinger (2003) also perform simulations comparing the predictions from a conditionally specified GLMM to those from a marginal GLM. From a Bayesian viewpoint, prediction of new observations in a spatial GLMM is described in Diggle et al. (1998), Christensen and Waagepetersen (2002), and Gelman et al. (2004).

9.7.8 Bayesian Hierarchical Models for Spatial Data

For readers interested in more details regarding Bayesian hierarchical spatial models, key developments appear in Besag (1974), Besag et al. (1991, 1995), Cressie (1993), and Besag and Kooperberg (1995). Detailed descriptions and applications appear in Clayton and Bernardinelli (1992), Mollié (1996), Best et al. (1999), Wakefield et al. (2000a), and Banerjee et al. (2003).

Some of the published extensions of the basic structure include spatiotemporal models (Bernardinelli et al. 1995a; Waller et al. 1997; Knorr-Held and Besag 1998; Xia and Carlin 1998), and models for point process data (Wolpert and Ickstadt 1998). There has also been a great deal published recently regarding the analysis of misaligned data, as mentioned in the case study following Section 9.4.4 (Mugglin et al. 1999, 2000, Best et al. 2000; Gotway and Young 2002). Finally, recent studies allow the covariate effects in equation (9.73) to be random effects and vary (spatially or not) from location to location. This is the concept underlying *geographically weighted regression* as described in Fotheringham et al. (2002) and illustrated in the Bayesian context by Congdon (2003, Chapter 7) and Gelfand et al. (2003).

9.8 EXERCISES

9.1 Fit a fourth-order trend surface to the raccoon rabies data described in Section 9.1.2. (The data are given in Table 9.14.) Use a variable selection routine (e.g., stepwise, or maximizing R^2) to create a response surface based only on the most important terms of this model.

Table 9.14 Connecticut Raccoon Rabies Data[a]

x	y	Month	x	y	Month	x	y	Month
103.02	68.71	37	46.42	28.44	18	118.57	88.25	41
63.44	76.51	18	25.32	91.6	24	47.89	35.93	18
71.1	86.21	19	52.84	35.69	28	20.55	30.59	7
35.41	60.04	14	73.53	80.64	15	97.2	73.99	32
118.71	50.69	34	68.67	22.61	17	37.02	11.93	9
22.75	47.47	3	57.11	64.9	17	21.28	42.25	12
136.23	76.23	40	55.69	73.44	16	27.7	94.77	21
131.83	67.06	38	59.54	84.58	26	122.2	76.69	36
60.68	46.33	23	94.12	35.09	32	89.49	23.9	16
105.41	50.27	41	46.1	99.03	28	107.88	66.1	32
26.24	83.3	18	104.63	75.55	30	79.26	56.69	28
16.12	34.81	3	13.16	0.37	10	95.04	31.28	22
44.68	26.83	28	77.56	41.33	32	73.8	92.47	27
100.77	43.8	29	92.2	50.64	32	82.66	73.53	31
63.94	24.63	25	113.94	31.65	35	86.83	88.88	32
125.5	88.16	41	28.35	18.26	8	99.49	92.12	33
88.21	97.52	27	98.99	28.07	27	30.04	11.01	7
64.89	70.32	29	121	57.98	46	88.8	65.91	26
33.99	83.16	24	65.64	93.66	19	0	0	6
138.2	54.4	48	130.73	30.09	36	75.64	28.99	18
88.25	42.06	27	58.99	34.68	26	127.93	75.82	39
77.2	73.85	32	56.69	99.17	18	47.34	72.61	21
101.05	63.02	32	15.87	70.45	11	144.03	52.38	41

Table 9.14 (*continued*)

x	y	Month	x	y	Month	x	y	Month
86.92	32.57	21	112.52	59.77	46	131.46	39.68	46
131.41	56.46	27	35.96	70.73	18	104.35	34.03	40
80.91	29.49	19	90.22	75.13	20	114.63	75.96	32
95.64	60.18	28	68.3	49.49	18	42.47	48.58	17
75.27	47.06	21	79.58	50.91	33	48.44	16.19	18
34.26	28.9	13	121.23	41.97	47	35.41	65.68	21
47.75	44.03	20	69.35	62.79	18	11.1	9.72	7
13.12	44.49	6	51.79	82.66	16	59.03	24.08	26
124.08	29.17	46	19.04	55.73	11	73.94	65.28	28
29.81	34.91	9	36.92	97.1	21	63.9	31.42	19
28.94	101.14	19	63.94	33.16	20	142.93	42.66	41
17.75	4.59	7	125.45	51.28	36	108.34	26.56	45
101.28	24.26	28	49.58	21.83	19	41.56	38.16	26
140.13	67.7	37	63.9	63.8	20	50.27	62.93	16
133.89	84.49	40	85.91	56.1	30	132.19	47.61	37
54.35	45.36	19	143.16	88.57	16	21.15	24.54	3
11.33	25.46	1	79.12	62.2	24	28.07	51.42	15
111.19	44.22	41	18.26	97.79	18	125.41	67.06	49
44.58	31.05	13	17.48	83.99	18	41.65	22.84	10
12.48	52.2	8	66.46	98.02	23	96.19	98.02	33
87.2	81.14	12	33.21	42.06	17	62.29	56.42	28
126.64	59.26	49	107.43	97.61	35	6.97	3.35	7
147.06	68.44	39	141.05	32.84	49	41.28	14.54	11
77.06	97.93	17	44.91	62.43	13	142.38	97.15	38
103.02	85.96	38	42.38	81.6	17	35.64	19.82	10
119.63	98.39	38	95.36	81.46	36	146.05	54.22	40
67.98	41.05	20	24.5	71.19	16	26.79	62.06	12
50.27	49.86	19	43.3	58.12	18	71.79	73.57	18
55.64	21.19	18	95.27	24.86	33	22.25	16.33	7
24.13	7.71	9	79.4	66.65	24	111.28	85	37
16.38	14.77	3	44.26	90.45	25	118.02	67.79	38
78.8	84.81	27	79.63	90.45	29	54.35	56.14	18
49.36	29.68	21	35.92	52.15	15	130.36	96.33	37

[a] x and y denote the coordinates of each township's centroid from the southwesternmost township centroid, and "month" denotes the number of months until first appearance.

9.2 Fit a second-order trend surface to the raccoon rabies data. Calculate an empirical semivariogram based on the residuals from your model. Are the residuals spatially autocorrelated? Use iteratively reweighted least squares or maximum likelihood to fit the same trend surface function with residual spatial autocorrelation. How does the fit compare to the model assuming independent errors?

9.3 Assess the adequacy of the transformation used in the New York leukemia data break and the impact of excluding the three highest transformed incidence proportions on the analysis. The data are provided in Table 9.15. How does excluding these potential outliers affect the residual spatial autocorrelation? How does excluding these potential outliers affect the regression results and the conclusions obtained from them? Is weighting still necessary?

Table 9.15 Covariate Data for the New York Leukemia Analysis[a]

x	y	Exposure	% Own Home	% Over 65
4.069	−67.353	0.237	0.328	0.147
4.639	−66.862	0.209	0.427	0.235
5.709	−66.978	0.171	0.338	0.138
7.614	−65.996	0.141	0.462	0.119
7.316	−67.318	0.158	0.192	0.142
8.559	−66.934	0.173	0.365	0.141
9.207	−67.179	0.191	0.666	0.231
10.180	−66.879	0.198	0.667	0.279
8.698	−68.307	0.215	0.459	0.172
7.405	−68.078	0.173	0.166	0.179
7.335	−68.351	0.176	0.065	0.344
6.644	−67.644	0.150	0.045	0.398
5.556	−67.778	0.175	0.121	0.225
5.403	−68.525	0.175	0.319	0.166
3.892	−68.166	0.241	0.693	0.194
4.320	−69.593	0.197	0.713	0.188
6.726	−69.763	0.180	0.523	0.165
8.341	−68.803	0.218	0.485	0.125
4.319	−40.067	0.036	0.745	0.124
5.888	−48.612	0.051	0.808	0.110
−3.922	−39.102	0.036	0.756	0.113
−3.473	−53.637	0.072	0.823	0.093
−4.243	−57.960	0.103	0.829	0.104
10.472	−59.754	0.084	0.840	0.102
10.429	−60.770	0.091	0.869	0.144
6.029	−60.332	0.108	0.748	0.121
9.294	−63.504	0.117	0.840	0.167
15.301	−57.990	0.071	0.846	0.107
28.533	−59.213	0.048	0.768	0.114
44.542	−71.661	0.032	0.514	0.143
26.200	−70.753	0.072	0.712	0.100
14.651	−70.153	0.329	0.697	0.111
13.633	−73.304	0.471	0.817	0.105
5.520	−71.256	0.155	0.867	0.100
6.220	−64.636	0.146	0.691	0.197
2.294	−63.134	0.211	0.877	0.122
−1.307	−65.936	0.584	0.803	0.130
−3.056	−67.421	0.698	0.488	0.171
−3.228	−66.656	0.629	0.834	0.196

Table 9.15 (*continued*)

x	y	Exposure	% Own Home	% Over 65
−3.376	−66.134	0.535	0.668	0.152
−7.735	−68.314	0.300	0.644	0.147
−6.265	−66.089	0.42	0.809	0.085
−4.848	−67.158	1.611	0.558	0.185
−4.788	−67.943	2.314	0.218	0.134
−6.278	−68.079	0.538	0.350	0.162
−5.496	−68.645	0.699	0.384	0.156
3.106	−65.587	0.276	0.645	0.248
2.420	−66.551	0.379	0.243	0.166
2.739	−67.014	0.347	0.339	0.142
2.646	−67.673	0.354	0.696	0.247
1.476	−65.563	0.436	0.562	0.289
0.728	−69.439	0.415	0.593	0.109
−4.198	−69.329	0.588	0.815	0.157
−7.078	−71.146	0.229	0.830	0.127
−2.693	−75.291	0.127	0.880	0.091
−50.243	36.814	0.077	0.537	0.032
−48.713	54.252	0.033	0.759	0.091
−44.846	48.834	0.041	0.538	0.105
−51.984	50.333	0.038	0.684	0.103
−54.284	36.220	0.071	0.776	0.102
−48.719	35.411	0.089	0.799	0.127
−45.506	26.448	0.436	0.645	0.205
−44.249	23.500	0.395	0.832	0.166
−46.511	26.100	0.598	0.526	0.187
−47.855	24.276	0.791	0.299	0.208
−53.546	21.137	0.130	0.721	0.159
−46.274	24.648	2.548	0.535	0.155
−55.482	9.899	0.059	0.591	0.116
−45.278	11.980	0.080	0.691	0.127
−32.888	8.954	0.048	0.593	0.130
−30.870	−2.614	0.085	0.712	0.130
−41.620	−4.037	0.065	0.722	0.099
−51.202	−0.781	0.040	0.558	0.119
42.713	−2.720	0.030	0.665	0.140
21.226	−11.684	0.075	0.615	0.123
38.318	−20.559	0.031	0.449	0.161
38.701	−19.448	0.031	0.495	0.223
46.626	−14.208	0.026	0.710	0.150
37.769	−23.729	0.030	0.716	0.152
21.514	−28.348	0.039	0.640	0.138
32.135	−41.099	0.027	0.665	0.127
31.607	−49.284	0.034	0.670	0.132
1.862	−16.601	0.076	0.679	0.123
−10.903	−0.588	0.059	0.736	0.110

(*continued overleaf*)

Table 9.15 (*continued*)

x	y	Exposure	% Own Home	% Over 65
−17.986	−1.508	0.072	0.713	0.106
−18.630	−12.635	0.362	0.639	0.107
−18.906	−11.309	0.246	0.438	0.152
−15.730	−12.060	0.214	0.278	0.200
−12.310	−10.786	0.123	0.672	0.179
−6.136	−23.354	0.066	0.624	0.102
−15.148	−16.950	0.238	0.455	0.133
−19.260	−13.129	0.444	0.607	0.081
−18.944	−22.815	0.134	0.757	0.103
26.365	41.438	0.020	0.459	0.065
27.552	40.655	0.020	0.533	0.357
26.373	41.236	0.020	0.734	0.136
18.846	45.413	0.019	0.687	0.117
18.898	41.544	0.021	0.568	0.155
7.169	48.289	0.018	0.775	0.098
10.795	38.083	0.023	0.847	0.092
8.497	38.279	0.023	0.748	0.111
10.823	24.177	0.033	0.562	0.147
11.161	23.461	0.034	0.791	0.119
23.025	31.970	0.025	0.767	0.088
24.096	19.087	0.035	0.551	0.097
16.640	8.843	0.061	0.574	0.118
36.296	13.316	0.030	0.472	0.086
39.356	14.481	0.028	0.684	0.153
53.509	10.264	0.021	0.707	0.132
−15.326	40.508	0.028	0.500	0.333
−13.793	41.011	0.027	0.421	0.148
−12.939	41.735	0.026	0.710	0.199
−12.226	41.264	0.026	0.701	0.213
−13.906	40.029	0.028	0.201	0.116
−13.351	40.456	0.027	0.296	0.182
−12.758	40.442	0.027	0.441	0.170
−12.147	40.364	0.026	0.504	0.146
−11.244	40.312	0.026	0.648	0.158
−9.848	40.709	0.025	0.336	0.186
−14.694	39.499	0.028	0.323	0.196
−13.917	39.117	0.028	0.124	0.505
−13.303	39.395	0.027	0.114	0.106
−12.970	39.858	0.027	0.315	0.162
−12.276	39.573	0.027	0.322	0.120
−12.173	38.934	0.027	0.044	0.361
−11.109	39.123	0.026	0.423	0.132
−10.519	39.400	0.026	0.570	0.153
−9.809	39.762	0.025	0.548	0.161
−8.752	39.839	0.024	0.658	0.178

Table 9.15 (*continued*)

x	y	Exposure	% Own Home	% Over 65
−16.723	38.980	0.030	0.465	0.155
−15.217	38.544	0.029	0.303	0.180
−14.159	38.501	0.028	0.203	0.124
−12.996	38.885	0.027	0.085	0.150
−11.893	38.702	0.027	0.209	0.084
−16.457	38.264	0.030	0.378	0.162
−16.375	37.649	0.030	0.562	0.167
−15.444	38.028	0.029	0.384	0.149
−14.124	37.801	0.028	0.151	0.133
−13.363	38.134	0.028	0.003	0.147
−12.743	37.939	0.027	0.003	0.109
−12.224	38.122	0.027	0.008	0.041
−11.479	37.992	0.027	0.118	0.042
−10.724	37.938	0.026	0.205	0.047
−9.753	38.180	0.025	0.438	0.083
−8.704	38.332	0.025	0.479	0.088
−15.727	37.105	0.030	1.000	0.066
−15.397	36.783	0.030	0.371	0.144
−14.469	36.803	0.029	0.167	0.058
−13.954	37.319	0.028	0.137	0.069
−13.265	36.954	0.028	0.127	0.031
−12.722	36.979	0.028	0.025	0.087
−12.024	37.260	0.027	0.008	0.107
−11.158	36.577	0.027	0.326	0.047
−10.470	36.651	0.026	0.452	0.079
−8.878	37.115	0.025	0.750	0.231
−16.433	35.815	0.031	0.896	0.172
−15.426	35.799	0.030	0.741	0.138
−14.754	35.563	0.030	0.689	0.094
−13.920	35.189	0.029	0.473	0.084
−13.832	36.218	0.029	0.282	0.068
−12.852	36.222	0.028	0.178	0.087
−12.634	35.421	0.028	0.338	0.069
−11.764	34.930	0.027	0.204	0.328
−10.617	35.288	0.027	0.796	0.194
−10.592	34.676	0.027	0.001	0.004
−14.111	34.358	0.029	0.498	0.099
−13.321	34.785	0.029	0.485	0.062
−12.558	34.582	0.028	0.423	0.063
−13.447	32.917	0.029	0.678	0.170
−12.469	33.387	0.028	0.439	0.409
−11.562	32.740	0.028	0.041	0.416
−12.506	31.784	0.029	0.880	0.185
−4.891	53.764	0.020	0.792	0.110
−10.943	56.410	0.021	0.682	0.106

(*continued overleaf*)

Table 9.15 *(continued)*

x	y	Exposure	% Own Home	% Over 65
−9.834	51.064	0.022	0.789	0.094
−4.197	49.537	0.020	0.746	0.075
−9.488	49.009	0.022	0.909	0.065
−9.754	47.072	0.023	0.658	0.072
−10.954	47.897	0.023	0.662	0.121
−12.085	47.577	0.024	0.625	0.141
−13.100	46.879	0.025	0.903	0.143
−15.175	47.155	0.026	0.515	0.093
−13.057	48.404	0.024	0.730	0.097
−18.973	48.402	0.027	0.837	0.055
−18.418	47.007	0.028	0.093	0.045
−21.552	51.780	0.027	0.825	0.097
−20.175	53.142	0.026	0.873	0.044
−18.852	50.853	0.026	0.859	0.050
−12.434	51.045	0.023	0.910	0.032
−18.052	54.741	0.024	0.752	0.085
−24.874	54.020	0.027	0.601	0.166
−30.753	53.944	0.030	0.854	0.075
−22.711	48.810	0.029	0.857	0.121
−27.924	50.923	0.031	0.694	0.091
−28.128	49.183	0.032	0.480	0.199
−24.891	46.477	0.032	0.630	0.097
−29.806	46.681	0.036	0.849	0.094
−38.079	38.625	0.060	0.792	0.120
−26.755	40.217	0.039	0.847	0.106
−25.887	37.029	0.041	0.539	0.128
−24.213	36.358	0.039	0.799	0.142
−23.675	38.145	0.037	0.818	0.115
−21.451	37.998	0.035	0.637	0.143
−20.238	37.167	0.034	0.851	0.157
−20.627	38.879	0.034	0.805	0.198
−21.121	43.888	0.031	0.856	0.123
−18.195	39.401	0.031	0.398	0.152
−18.463	38.801	0.032	0.632	0.224
−18.940	37.247	0.033	0.960	0.210
−17.473	37.273	0.031	0.925	0.294
−17.892	44.541	0.029	0.624	0.150
−19.460	46.367	0.029	0.634	0.080
−15.544	45.000	0.027	0.747	0.087
−16.679	43.819	0.028	0.496	0.097
−15.545	42.823	0.028	0.732	0.171
−13.259	45.162	0.025	0.815	0.231
−11.959	44.163	0.025	0.753	0.153
−12.618	43.821	0.026	0.672	0.160
−13.802	42.558	0.027	0.731	0.139

Table 9.15 (*continued*)

x	y	Exposure	% Own Home	% Over 65
−11.201	41.737	0.025	0.730	0.197
−6.841	39.955	0.023	0.467	0.166
−8.644	41.997	0.024	0.769	0.172
−5.825	41.656	0.023	0.709	0.117
−6.325	37.769	0.024	0.581	0.119
−7.852	35.601	0.025	0.754	0.180
−4.732	35.064	0.023	0.893	0.122
−7.625	31.607	0.025	0.793	0.100
−1.213	35.810	0.023	0.709	0.130
−1.369	35.773	0.023	0.750	0.190
1.035	32.848	0.025	0.756	0.156
1.028	32.994	0.025	0.571	0.116
3.692	37.486	0.023	0.764	0.109
−1.368	41.001	0.021	0.756	0.129
−2.432	39.997	0.021	0.946	0.113
−1.698	45.139	0.020	0.825	0.133
0.683	24.737	0.031	0.853	0.101
−7.767	24.012	0.029	0.805	0.116
−14.328	26.250	0.031	0.878	0.050
−20.450	26.646	0.038	0.909	0.100
−10.325	29.876	0.027	0.923	0.104
−12.444	30.194	0.029	0.837	0.131
−15.661	32.754	0.031	0.651	0.200
−19.003	35.414	0.034	0.627	0.267
−28.670	29.259	0.054	0.861	0.106
−28.688	30.852	0.053	0.495	0.152
−35.983	26.866	0.092	0.651	0.191
−34.554	26.419	0.082	0.759	0.110
−24.898	14.560	0.042	0.478	0.107
−19.610	16.637	0.036	0.586	0.083
−10.921	9.999	0.039	0.667	0.098
0.175	13.306	0.047	0.711	0.096
−14.565	−48.845	0.054	0.774	0.104
−29.003	−52.870	0.057	0.731	0.108
−15.798	−68.106	0.422	0.825	0.102
−14.282	−72.352	0.157	0.839	0.076
−22.738	−67.371	0.300	0.492	0.157
−29.470	−69.684	0.097	0.761	0.108
−43.339	−69.836	0.042	0.748	0.067
−30.749	−13.465	1.000	0.732	0.126
−44.146	−15.211	0.072	0.708	0.097
−40.460	−22.936	0.123	0.509	0.110
−43.466	−20.207	0.093	0.739	0.101
−51.912	−24.866	0.086	0.705	0.121
−43.550	−28.728	0.374	0.448	0.164

(*continued overleaf*)

Table 9.15 (*continued*)

x	y	Exposure	% Own Home	% Over 65
−40.564	−27.572	0.276	0.549	0.150
−38.618	−26.765	0.187	0.516	0.092
−39.284	−29.119	0.309	0.105	0.084
−41.395	−29.395	0.618	0.191	0.032
−41.510	−30.601	1.767	0.261	0.074
−42.080	−31.169	3.526	0.238	0.135
−42.878	−30.248	0.908	0.400	0.160
−47.493	−30.821	0.182	0.734	0.127
−40.500	−32.883	0.403	0.563	0.066
−36.439	−33.877	0.159	0.591	0.120
−37.096	−29.876	0.200	0.571	0.149
−34.078	−27.819	0.118	0.611	0.075
−28.790	−23.104	0.113	0.697	0.081
−34.646	−39.355	0.089	0.712	0.102
−51.142	−42.100	0.069	0.747	0.107
−41.960	−24.820	0.164	0.497	0.128
−42.675	−27.313	0.274	0.134	0.065

[a] x and y denote locations of each census tract centroid, "exposure" the inverse distance from the tract centroid to the nearest TCE site (see text), and "% own home" and "% over 65" denote census variables (1980 U.S. Census).

9.4 Using the New York leukemia data, fit both a SAR and a CAR model based on the proximity measure defined in equation (7.6) with $\delta = 15$ km. Do your results differ from those presented in the data break following Section 9.3.3? Do your conclusions change?

9.5 Derive the universal kriging predictor in Section 9.2.3 using the covariances $\text{Cov}(Y(\boldsymbol{s}_i), Y(\boldsymbol{s}_j))$ instead of the semivariogram.

9.6 Clarify the statement in Section 9.4 regarding the difference between the use of σ^2 in Sections 9.1 and 9.2 and its use in Section 9.4.

9.7 Simulate 100 data sets from the final linear regression model (independent errors) for the New York leukemia data set. Compare the observed (transformed) outcome with the histogram of model-based outcomes at each tract. Are there spatial patterns to the local fit?

9.8 Use Poisson regression with the New York leukemia data to model the effects of the three covariates on the leukemia rates. How do your conclusions differ from those discussed in the data breaks following Sections 9.2.3 and 9.3.3?

9.9 Simulate 100 data sets from your final Poisson regression model (independent errors) for the New York leukemia data set. Compare the observed (transformed) outcome with the histogram of model-based outcomes at each tract. Are there spatial patterns to the local fit?

9.10 Redo the analyses in the data break following Section 9.4.3 using the Scottish lip cancer data in Table 2.6. For spatial analyses, use the latitude and longitude coordinates. Do the results of the spatial analyses based on latitude and longitude differ from those discussed in the data break based on the British National Grid projection? Why? Why not?

References

Agresti, A. (1990). *Categorical Data Analysis*. New York: John Wiley & Sons.

Agresti, A., J. G. Booth, J. P. Hobert, and B. Coffo (2000). Random-effects modeling of categorical response data. *Sociological Methodology 30*, 27–80.

Ahrens, C., N. Altman, G. Casella, M. Eaton, J. T. G. Hwang, J. Staudenmayer, and C. Stefanescu (2001). Leukemia clusters in upstate New York: How adding covariates changes the story. *Environmetrics 12*, 659–672.

Aitchison, J. and J. Brown (1957). *The Lognormal Distribution*. London: Cambridge University Press.

Akaike, H. (1974). A new look at statistical model identification. *IEEE Transactions on Automatic Control 19*, 716–723.

Alexander, F. E. and P. Boyle (1996). *Methods for Investigating Localized Clustering of Disease*. IARC Scientific Publication 135. Lyon, France: International Agency for Research on Cancer.

Alexander, F. E, P. A. McKinney, K. C. Moncrieff, and R. A. Cartwright (1992). Residential proximity of children with leukemia and non-Hodgkins lymphoma in 3 areas of northern England. *British Journal of Cancer 65*(2), 583–588.

Alt, K. W. and W. Vach (1991). The reconstruction of "genetic kinship" in prehistoric burial complexes: Problems and statistics. In H.-H. Bock and P. Ihm (Eds.), *Classification, Data Analysis, and Knowledge Organization: Models and Methods with Applications*, pp. 299–310. Berlin: Springer-Verlag.

Anselin, L. (1988). *Spatial Econometrics: Methods and Models*. Dordrecht, The Netherlands: Kluwer Academic.

Anselin, L. (1990). Spatial dependence and spatial structural instability in applied regression analysis. *Journal of Regional Science 30*, 185–207.

Anselin, L. (1993). Discrete space autoregressive models. In M. Goodchild, B. Parks, and L. Steyaert (Eds.), *Environmental Modeling in GIS*, pp. 454–469. New York: Oxford University Press.

Applied Spatial Statistics for Public Health Data, by Lance A. Waller and Carol A. Gotway
ISBN 0-471-38771-1

Anselin, L. (1995). Local indicators of spatial association: LISA. *Geographical Analysis 27*(2), 93–116.

Anselin, L. and R. J. G. M. Florax (1995). Small sample properties of tests for spatial dependence in regression models: Some further results. In L. Anselin and R. J. G. M. Florax (Eds.), *New Directions in Spatial Econometrics*, pp. 21–74. New York: Springer-Verlag.

Anselin, L. and S. Rey (1991). Properties of tests for spatial dependence in linear regression models. *Geographical Analysis 23*, 112–131.

Anselin, L., A. K. Bera, R. Florax, and M. I. Yoon (1996). Simple diagnostic tests for spatial dependence. *Regional Science and Urban Economics 26*, 77–104.

Armstrong, M. (1984). Common problems seen in variograms. *Journal of the International Association for Mathematical Geology 16*, 305–313.

Armstrong, M. (1999). *Basic Linear Geostatistics*. New York: Springer-Verlag.

Armstrong, M. P., G. Rushton, and D. L. Zimmerman (1999). Geographically masking health data to preserve confidentiality. *Statistics in Medicine 18*(5), 497–525.

Arnold, B. C., E. Castillo, and J. M. Sarabia (1999). *Conditional Specification of Statistical Models*. New York: Springer-Verlag.

Assunção, R. M. and E. A. Reis (1999). A new proposal to adjust Moran's *I* for population density. *Statistics in Medicine 18*, 2147–2162.

Baddeley, A. J. and B. W. Silverman (1984). A cautionary example for the use of second order methods for analyzing point patterns. *Biometrics 40*, 1089–1093.

Baddeley, A. J., J. Møller, and R. Waagepetersen (1999). Non- and semiparametric estimation of interaction in inhomogeneous point patterns. *Statistica Neerlandica 54*, 329–350.

Bailey, T. C. and A. C. Gatrell (1995). *Interactive Spatial Data Analysis*. Harlow, Essex, England: Addison Wesley Longman.

Banerjee, S., A. E. Gelfand, and B. P. Carlin (2003). *Hierarchical Modeling and Analysis for Spatial Data*. Boca Raton, FL: Chapman & Hall/CRC.

Barndorff-Neilsen, O. E., W. S. Kendall, and M. N. M. van Lieshout (Eds.) (1999). *Stochastic Geometry: Likelihood and Computation*, Boca Raton, FL: Chapman & Hall/CRC.

Barnett, E., M. L. Casper, J. A. Halverson, G. A. Elmes, V. E. Braham, Z. A. Majeed, A. S. Bloom, and S. Stanley (2001). *Men and Heart Disease: An Atlas of Racial and Ethnic Disparities in Mortality*. Morgantown, WV: Office for Social Environment and Health Research, West Virginia University.

Bartlett, M. S. (1964). The spectral analysis of two-dimensional point processes. *Biometrika 51*, 299–311.

Basu, S., R. F. Gunst, E. A. Guertal, and M. I. Hartfield (1997). The effects of influential observations on sample semivariograms. *Journal of Agricultural, Biological and Environmental Statistics 2*, 490–512.

Beck, L. H., M. H. Rodriguez, S. W. Dister, A. D. Rodriguez, E. Rejmankova, A. Ulloa, R. A. Meza, D. R. Roberts, J. F. Paris, M. A. Spanner, R. Washino, C. Hacker, and L. J. Legters (1994). Remote sensing as a landscape epidemiologic tool to identify villages at high risk for malaria transmission. *American Journal of Tropical Medicine and Hygiene 51*(3), 271–280.

Bennett, R. J. and R. P. Haining (1985). Spatial structure and spatial interaction: Modeling approaches to the statistical analysis of geographical data. *Journal of the Royal Statistical Society, Series A 148*(Part 1), 1–36.

Bernardinelli, L., D. Clayton, C. Pascutto, M. Montomoli, C. Ghislandi, and M. Songini (1995a). Bayesian analysis of space–time variations in disease risk. *Statistics in Medicine 14*, 2433–2443.

Bernardinelli, L., D. Clayton, and C. Montomoli (1995b). Bayesian estimates of disease maps: How important are priors? *Statistics in Medicine 14*, 2411–2431.

Bertin, J. (1983). *Semiology of Graphics: Diagrams, Networks, Maps*. Madison, WI: University of Wisconsin Press.

Besag, J. (1972). Nearest-neighbor systems and the auto-logistic model for binary data. *Journal of the Royal Statistical Society, Series B 34*, 75–83.

Besag, J. (1974). Spatial interaction and the statistical analysis of lattice systems. *Journal of the Royal Statistical Society, Series B 36*, 192–225.

Besag, J. (1975). Statistical analysis of non-lattice data. *The Statistician 24*, 179–195.

Besag, J. (1977). Discussion of "Modeling spatial patterns" by B. D. Ripley. *Journal of the Royal Statistical Society, Series B 39*, 193–195.

Besag, J. and P. J. Diggle (1977). Simple Monte Carlo tests for spatial patterns. *Applied Statistics 26*, 327–333.

Besag, J. and C. Kooperberg (1995). On conditional and intrinsic autoregressions. *Biometrika 82*, 733–746.

Besag, J. and J. Newell (1991). The detection of clusters in rare diseases. *Journal Of the Royal Statistical Society, Series A 154*, 327–333.

Besag, J., J. York, and A. Mollié (1991). Bayesian image restoration, with two applications in spatial statistics (with discussion). *Annals of the Institute of Statistical Mathematics 43*(1), 1–59.

Besag, J., P. Green, D. Higdon, and K. Mengersen (1995). Bayesian computation and stochastic systems (with discussion). *Statistical Science 10*, 3–66.

Best, D. J. and J. C. W. Rayner (1991). Disease clustering in time. *Biometrics 47*, 589–593.

Best, D. J. and J. C. W. Rayner (1992). Response to Tango's comments. *Biometrics 48*, 327.

Best, N. G., R. A. Arnold, A. Thomas, L. A. Waller, and E. M. Conlon (1999). Bayesian models for spatially correlated disease and exposure data. In J. M. Bernardo, J. O. Berger, A. P. Dawid, and A. F. M. Smith (Eds.), *Bayesian Statistics, Vol. 6*, pp. 131–156. Oxford: Oxford University Press.

Best, N. G., K. Ickstadt, and R. L. Wolpert (2000). Spatial Poisson regression for health and exposure data measured at disparate resolutions. *Journal of the American Statistical Association 95*, 1076–1088.

Bickel, P. J. and K. A. Doksum (1977). *Mathematical Statistics: Basic Ideas and Selected Topics*. Oakland, CA: Holden-Day.

Bithell, J. F. (1990). An application of density estimation to geographical epidemiology. *Statistics in Medicine 9*, 691–701.

Bithell, J. F. (1995). The choice of test for detecting raised disease risk near a point source. *Statistics in Medicine 14*, 2309–2322.

Blum, H. F. (1948). Sunlight as a causal factor in cancer of the skin of man. *Journal of the National Cancer Institute 9*, 247–258.

Bogan, K. T. and L. S. Gold (1997). Trichloroethylene cancer risk: Simplified calculation of PBPK-based MCLs for cytotoxic end points. *Regulatory Toxicology and Pharmacology 25*, 26–42.

Bonham-Carter, G. F. (1994). *Geographic Information Systems for Geoscientists: Modelling with GIS*. Tarrytown, NY: Pergamon/Elsevier Science.

Box, G. E. P. and N. R. Draper (1987). *Empirical Model Building and Response Surfaces*. New York: John Wiley & Sons.

Brandsma, A. S. and R. H. Ketellapper (1979). A biparametric approach to spatial autocorrelation. *Environment and Planning A 11*, 51–58.

Breslow, N. E. (1984). Extra-Poisson variation in log-linear models. *Journal of the Royal Statistical Society, Series C 33*, 38–44.

Breslow, N. E. and D. G. Clayton (1993). Approximate inference in generalized linear mixed models. *Journal of the American Statistical Association 88*, 9–25.

Breslow, N. E. and N. E. Day (1975). Indirect standardization and multiplicative models for rates, with reference to the age adjustment of cancer incidence and relative frequency data. *Journal of Chronic Diseases 28*, 289–303.

Breslow, N. E. and N. E. Day (1987). *Statistical Methods in Cancer Research,* Vol. II: *The Design and Analysis of Cohort Studies*. IARC Scientific Publication. Lyon, France: International Agency for Research on Cancer.

Breusch, T. S. (1980). Useful invariance results for generalized regression models. *Journal of Econometrics 13*, 327–340.

Brewer, C. A. (1994). Color use guidelines for mapping and visualization. In A. M. MacEachren and D. R. F. Taylor (Eds.), *Visualization in Modern Cartography*, pp. 123–147. Oxford: Elsevier.

Brewer, C. A. (1999). Color use guidelines for data representation. *Proceedings of the American Statistical Association's Section on Statistical Graphics*, pp. 55–60.

Brewer, C. A., A. M. MacEachren, L. W. Pickle, and D. J. Herrmann (1997). Mapping mortality: Evaluating color schemes for choropleth maps. *Annals of the Association of American Geographers 87*(3), 411–438.

Brillinger, D. R. (1990). Spatial–temporal modelling of spatially aggregate birth data. *Survey Methodology 16*(2), 255–269.

Brillinger, D. R. (1994). Examples of scientific problems and data analyses in demography, neurophysiology, and seismology. *Journal of Computational and Graphical Statistics, 3*, 1–22.

Brix, A. and P. J. Diggle (2001). Spatiotemporal prediction for log-Gaussian Cox processes. *Journal of the Royal Statistical Society, Series B 63*, 823–841.

Brody, H., M. R. Rip, P. Vinten-Johnson, N. Paneth, and S. Rachman (2000). Map-making and myth-making in Broad Street: The London cholera epidemic, 1854. *Lancet 356*, 64–68.

Brunsdon, C. and M. Charlton (1996). Developing an exploratory spatial analysis system in XLisp-Stat. In D. Parker (Ed.), *Innovations in GIS 3*, pp. 135–146. London: Taylor & Francis.

Burrough, P. A. (1986). *Principles of Geographical Information Systems for Land Resources Assessment*. Oxford: Clarendon Press.

Byth, K. (1982). On robust distance-based intensity estimators. *Biometrics 38*, 127–135.

Carlin, B. P. and T. A. Louis (2000). *Bayes and Empirical Bayes Methods for Data Analysis* (2nd ed.). Boca Raton, FL: Chapman & Hall/CRC.

Carr, D. B. (2001). Designing linked micromap plots for states with many counties. *Statistics in Medicine 20*, 1331–1339.

Carr, D. B., A. R. Olsen, J. P. Courbois, S. M. Pierson, and D. A. Carr (1998). Linked micromap plots: Named and described. *Statistical Computing and Graphics Newsletter 9*(1), 24–32.

Carr, D. B., J. F. Wallin, and D. A. Carr (2000). Two new templates for epidemiology applications: Linked micromap plots and conditioned choropleth maps. *Statistics in Medicine 19*(17/18), 2521–2538.

Carroll, R. J. and D. Ruppert (1988). *Transformation and Weighting in Regression*. Boca Raton, FL: Chapman & Hall/CRC.

Casella, G. and E. I. George (1992). Explaining the Gibbs sampler. *American Statistician 46*, 167–174.

Casper, M. L., E. Barnett, J. A. Halverson, G. A. Elmes, V. E. Braham, Z. A. Majeed, A. S. Bloom, and S. Stanley (2000). *Women and Heart Disease: An Atlas of Racial and Ethnic Disparities in Mortality* (2nd ed.). Morgantown, WV: Office for Social Environment and Health Research, West Virginia University.

Centers for Disease Control and Prevention (1998). *Behavioral Risk Factor Surveillance System User's Guide*. Technical report, Atlanta, GA: U.S. Department of Health and Human Services, Centers for Disease Control and Prevention,

Cherry, S., J. Banfield, and W. F. Quimby (1996). An evaluation of a non-parametric method of estimating semi-variograms of isotropic spatial processes. *Journal of Applied Statistics 23*, 435–449.

Chetwynd, A. G. and P. J. Diggle (1998). On estimating the reduced second moment measure of a stationary point process. *Australian and New Zealand Journal of Statistics 40*, 11–15.

Childs, J. E., S. L. McLafferty, R. Sadek, G. L. Miller, A. S. Khan, E. R. DuPree, R. Advani, J. N. Mills, and G. Glass (1998). Epidemiology of rodent bites and prediction of rat infestation in New York City. *American Journal of Epidemiology 148*(1), 78–87.

Chilès, J. P. and P. Delfiner (1999). *Geostatistics: Modeling Spatial Uncertainty*. New York: John Wiley & Sons.

Choynowski, M. (1959). Maps based on probabilities. *Journal of the American Statistical Association 54*, 385–388.

Christakos, G. (1984). On the problem of permissible covariance and variogram models. *Water Resources Research 20*, 385–388.

Christensen, O. F. and R. Waagepetersen (2002). Bayesian prediction of spatial count data using generalized linear mixed models. *Biometrics 58*, 280–286.

Christensen, R., W. Johnson, and L. M. Pearson (1992). Prediction diagnostics for spatial linear models. *Biometrika 79*(3), 583–591.

Clarke, K. C. (2001). *Getting Started with Geographic Information Systems* (3rd ed.). Upper Saddle River, NJ: Prentice Hall.

Clayton, D. G. and L. Bernardinelli (1992). Bayesian methods for disease mapping. In P. Elliott, J. Cuzick, D. English, and R. Stern (Eds.), *Geographical and Environmental Epidemiology*, pp. 205–220. Oxford: Oxford University Press.

Clayton, D. G. and J. Kaldor (1987). Empirical Bayes estimates of age-standardized relative risks for use in disease mapping. *Biometrics 43*, 671–682.

Cleveland, W. S. (1979). Robust locally weighted regression and smoothing scatterplots. *Journal of the American Statistical Association 74*, 829–836.

Cleveland, W. S. (1985). *Elements of Graphing Data*. Monterey, CA: Wadsworth.

Cleveland, W. S. and S. J. Devlin (1988). Locally weighted regression: An approach to regression analysis by local fitting. *Journal of the American Statistical Association 83*, 596–610.

Cliff, A. D. and J. K. Ord (1973). *Spatial Autocorrelation*. London: Pion.

Cliff, A. D. and J. K. Ord (1981). *Spatial Processes: Models and Applications*. London: Pion.

Cline, B. L. (1970). New eyes for epidemiologists: Aerial photography and remote sensing. *American Journal of Epidemiology 92*(2), 85–89.

Cline, G. A. and R. J. Kryscio (1999). Contagion distributions for defining disease clustering in time. *Journal of Statistical Planning and Inference 78*, 325–347.

Congdon, P. (2003). *Applied Bayesian Modelling*. Chichester, West Sussex, England: John Wiley & Sons.

Cook, D. G. and S. J. Pocock (1983). Multiple regression in geographic mortality studies, with allowance for spatially correlated errors. *Biometrics 39*, 361–371.

Cook, D., J. J. Majure, J. Symanzik, and N. Cressie (1996). Dynamic graphics in a GIS: Exploring and analyzing multivariate spatial data using linked software. *Computational Statistics 11*, 467–480.

Cowles, M. K. and B. P. Carlin (1996). Markov chain Monte Carlo convergence diagnostics: A comparative review. *Journal of the American Statistical Association 91*, 883–904.

Cox, D. R. (1955). Some statistical methods related with series of events (with discussion). *Journal of the Royal Statistical Society, Series B 17*, 129–164.

Cox, D. R. and D. V. Hinkley (1974). *Theoretical Statistics*. London: Chapman & Hall.

Cramer, J. S. (1964). Efficient grouping, regression and correlation in Engel curve analysis. *Journal of the American Statistical Association, 59*, 233–250.

Cressie, N. (1984). Towards resistant geostatistics. In G. Verly, M. David, A. G. Journel, and A. Marechal (Eds.), *Geostatistics for Natural Resources Characterization*, pp. 21–44. Dordrecht, The Netherlands: D. Reidel.

Cressie, N. (1985). Fitting variogram models by weighted least squares. *Journal of the International Association for Mathematical Geology 17*, 563–586.

Cressie, N. (1989). The many faces of spatial prediction. In M. Armstrong (Ed.), *Geostatistics*, pp. 163–176. Dordrecht, The Netherlands: Kluwer Academic.

Cressie, N. A. C. (1993). *Statistics for Spatial Data, rev. ed.* New York: John Wiley & Sons.

Cressie, N. (1996). Change of support and the modifiable areal unit problem. *Geographical Systems 3*, 159–180.

Cressie, N. and N. H. Chan (1989). Spatial modeling of regional variables. *Journal of the American Statistical Association 84*, 393–401.

Cressie, N. and D. M. Hawkins (1980). Robust estimation of the variogram: I. *Journal of the International Association for Mathematical Geology 12*, 115–125.

Cressie, N. and S. N. Lahiri (1996). Asymptotics for REML estimation of spatial covariance parameters. *Journal of Statistical Planning and Inference 50*, 327–341.

Cressie, N. and J. J. Majure (1997). Non-point source pollution of surface waters over a watershed. In V. Barnett and K. F. Turkman (Eds.), *Statistics for the Environment,* Vol. 3: *Pollution Assessment and Control*, pp. 210–224. New York: John Wiley & Sons.

Cressie, N. and T. R. C. Read (1989). Spatial data analysis and regional counts. *Biometrical Journal 31*, 699–719.

Cressie, N., C. A. Gotway, and M. O. Grondona (1990). Spatial prediction from networks. *Chemometrics and Intelligent Laboratory Systems 7*, 251–271.

Cromley, E. K. and S. L. McLafferty (2002). *GIS and Public Health*. New York: Guilford Press.

Curriero, F. C. (1996). The use of non-Euclidean distances in geostatistics. Ph.D. dissertation, Department of Statistics, Kansas State University, Manhattan, KS.

Cuzick, J. (1998). Commentary: Clustering of anophthalmia and microphthalmia is not supported by the data. *British Medical Journal 317*(7163), 910.

Cuzick, J. and R. Edwards (1990). Spatial clustering for inhomogeneous populations (with discussion). *Journal of the Royal Statistical Society, Series B 52*(1), 73–104.

David, M. (1988). *Handbook of Applied Advanced Geostatistical Ore Reserve Estimation*. Amsterdam: Elsevier.

Davis, B. M. and L. E. Borgman (1979). Some exact sampling distributions for variogram estimators. *Journal of the International Association for Mathematical Geology 11*, 643–653.

Davis, B. M. and L. E. Borgman (1982). A note on the asymptotic distribution of the sample variogram. *Journal of the International Association for Mathematical Geology 14*, 189–193.

Davis, G. and M. D. Morris (1997). Six factors which affect the condition number of matrices associated with kriging. *Mathematical Geology 29*, 91–98.

Dean, C. B. (1992). Testing for overdispersion in Poisson and binomial regression models. *Journal of the American Statistical Association 87*, 451–457.

Deutsch, C. V. and A. G. Journel (1992). *GSLIB: Geostatistical Software Library and User's Guide*. New York: Oxford University Press.

Devesa, S. S., D. J. Grauman, W. J. Blot, G. A. Pennello, R. N. Hoover, and J. F. Fraumeni (1999). *Atlas of Cancer Mortality in the United States, 1950–1994*. Bethesda, MD: National Institutes of Health, National Cancer Institute.

Devine, O. J., T. A. Louis, and M. E. Halloran (1994). Empirical Bayes methods for stabilizing incidence rates before mapping. *Epidemiology 5*(6), 622–630.

Diggle, P. J. (1983). *Statistical Analysis of Spatial Point Patterns*. London: Academic Press.

Diggle, P. J. (1989). Discussion of "Royal Statistical Society Meeting on Cancer near Nuclear Installations." *Journal of the Royal Statistical Society, Series A 152*, 369–371.

Diggle, P. J. (1990). A point process modeling approach to raised incidence of a rare phenomenon in the vicinity of a prespecified point. *Journal of the Royal Statistical Society, Series A 153*, 349–362.

Diggle, P. J. (2000). Overview of statistical methods for disease mapping and its relationship to cluster detection. In P. Elliott, J. C. Wakefield, N. G. Best, and D. J. Briggs (Eds.), *Spatial Epidemiology: Methods and Applications*. Oxford: Oxford University Press.

Diggle, P. J. and A. G. Chetwynd (1991). Second-order analysis of spatial clustering for inhomogeneous populations. *Biometrics 47*, 1155–1163.

Diggle, P. J. and T. F. Cox (1983). Some distance-based tests of independence for sparsely-sampled multivariate spatial point-patterns. *International Statistical Review 51*, 11–23.

Diggle, P. J., J. A. Tawn, and R. A. Moyeed (1998). Model-based geostatistics. *Applied Statistics 47*, 229–350.

Diggle, P. J., S. E. Morris, and J. C. Wakefield (2000). Point-source modelling using matched case-control data. *Biostatistics 89*, 89–105.

Dobson, A. J. (1990). *An Introduction to Generalized Linear Models*. London: Chapman & Hall.

Dockery, D. W. and C. A. Pope III (1994). Acute respiratory effects of particulate air pollution. *Annual Review of Public Health 15*, 107–132.

Dockerty, J. O., K. S. Sharples, and B. Borman (1999). An assessment of spatial clustering of leukaemias and lymphomas among young people in New Zealand. *Journal of Epidemiology and Community Health 53*(3), 154–158.

Doherr, M. G., R. E. Carpenter, W. D. Wilson, and I. A. Gardner (1999). Evaluation of temporal and spatial clustering of horses with *corynebacterium* pseudotuberculosis infection. *American Journal of Veterinary Research 60*(3), 284–291.

Dolk, H., A. Busby, B. G. Armstrong, and P. H. Walls (1998). Geographic variation in anophthalmia and microphthalmia in England, 1988–94. *British Medical Journal 317*(7163), 905–909.

Dowd, P. A. (1992). A review of recent developments in geostatistics. *Computers & Geosciences 17*, 1481–1500.

Draper, N. R. and H. Smith (1998). *Applied Regression Analysis*. New York: John Wiley & Sons.

Dykes, J. (1996). Dynamic maps for spatial science: A unified approach to cartographic visualization. In D. Parker (Ed.), *Innovations in GIS 3*, pp. 177–188. London: Taylor & Francis.

Ecker, M. D. and A. E. Gelfand (1997). Bayesian variogram modeling for an isotropic spatial process. *Journal of Agricultural, Biological and Environmental Statistics 2*, 347–369.

Ecker, M. D. and A. E. Gelfand (1999). Bayesian modeling and inference for geometrically anisotropic spatial data. *Mathematical Geology 31*, 67–83.

Ederer, F., M. H. Myers, and N. Mantel (1964). A statistical problem in time and space: Do leukemia cases come in clusters? *Biometrics 20*, 626–638.

Elandt-Johnson, R. C. (1975). Definition of rates: Some remarks on their use and misuse. *American Journal of Epidemiology 102*(4), 267–271.

Elliott, P., M. Hills, J. Beresford, I. Kleinschmidt, D. Jolley, and D. Pattenden (1992). Incidence of cancer of the larynx and lung near incinerators of waste solvents and oils in Great Britain. *Lancet 339*, 854–858.

Elliott, P., M. Martuzzi, and G. Shaddick (1995). Spatial statistical methods in environmental epidemiology: A critique. *Statistical Methods in Medical Research 4*, 137–159.

Elliott, P., G. Shaddick, I. Kleinschmidt, D. Jolley, P. Walls, and J. Beresford (1996). Cancer incidence near municipal solid waste incinerators in Great Britain. *British Journal of Cancer 73*, 702–710.

English, P., R. Neutra, R. Scalf, M. Sullivan, L. Waller, and L. Zhu (1999). Examining associations between childhood asthma and traffic flow using a geographic information system. *Environmental Health Perspectives 107*, 761–767.

Environmental Systems Research Institute (1999). *Getting to Know ArcView GIS*. Redlands, CA: ESRI Press.

Eriksson, M. and P. P. Siska (2000). Understanding anisotropy computations. *Mathematical Geology 32*, 683–700.

Ferrándiz, J., A. López, A. Llopis, M. Morales, and J. L. Tejerizo (1995). Spatial interaction between neighboring counties: cancer mortality data in Valencia (Spain). *Biometrics 51*, 665–678.

Fienberg, S. E. and D. H. Kaye (1991). Legal and statistical aspects of some mysterious clusters. *Journal of the Royal Statistical Society, Series A 154*, 61–74.

Finney, D. J. (1971). *Probit Analysis* (3rd ed.). Cambridge: Cambridge University Press.

Firebaugh, G. (1978). A rule for inferring individual-level relationships from aggregate data. *American Sociological Review 43*, 557–572.

Fleiss, J. L. (1981). *Statistical Methods for Rates and Proportions* (2nd ed.). New York: John Wiley & Sons.

Foley, J. E., P. Foley, and J. E. Madigan (2001). Spatial distribution of seropositivity to the causative agent of granulocytic ehrlichiosis in dogs in California. *American Journal of Veterinary Research 62*(10), 1599–1605.

Fotheringham, A. S. (1989). Scale-independent spatial analysis. In M. Goodchild and S. Gopal (Eds.), *The Accuracy of Spatial Data Bases*, pp. 221–228. London: Taylor & Francis.

Fotheringham, A. S. and F. B. Zhan (1996). A comparison of three exploratory methods for cluster detection in spatial point patterns. *Geographical Analysis 28*, 200–218.

Fotheringham, A. S., C. Brunsdon, and M. Charlton (2002). *Geographically Weighted Regression: The Analysis of Spatially Varying Relationships*. New York: John Wiley & Sons.

Freedman, D. A., S. P. Klein, M. Ostland, and M. R. Roberts (1998). On "A solution to the ecological inference problem." *Journal of the American Statistical Association 93*, 1518–1522.

Freeman, D. H. and T. R. Holford (1980). Summary rates. *Biometrics 36*(2), 195–205.

Frerichs, R. (2000). History, maps, and the Internet: UCLA's John Snow site. *Society of Cartographers (SOC) Bulletin 34*(2), 3–7.

Gail, M. H. (1978). The analysis of heterogeneity for indirect standardized mortality ratios. *Journal of the Royal Statistical Society, Series A 141*, 224–234.

Gail, M. H. (1986). Adjusting for covariates that have the same distribution in exposed and unexposed cohorts. In S. H. Moolgavkar and R. L. Prentice (Eds.), *Modern Statistical Methods in Chronic Disease Epidemiology*. New York: John Wiley & Sons.

Gallant, J. C., I. D. Moore, M. F. Hutchinson, and P. Gessler (1994). Estimating fractal dimension of profiles: A comparison of methods. *Mathematical Geology 26*, 455–481.

Gandin, L. S. (1963). *Objective Analysis of Meteorological Fields*. Leningrad: Gidrometeorologicheskoe Izdatel'stvo (GIMIZ). (Translated by Israel Program for Scientific Translations, Jerusalem, 1965.)

Gangnon, R. E. and M. K. Clayton (2000). Bayesian detection and modeling of spatial disease clustering. *Biometrics 56*, 922–935.

Gangnon, R. E. and M. K. Clayton (2001). A weighted average likelihood ratio test for spatial clustering of disease. *Statistics in Medicine 20*(19), 2977–2987.

Geary, R. C. (1954). The contiguity ratio and statistical mapping. *The Incorporated Statistician 5*, 115–145.

Gehlke, C. E. and K. Biehl (1934). Certain effects of grouping upon the size of the correlation coefficient in census tract material. *Journal of the American Statistical Association Supplement 29*, 169–170.

Gelfand, A. E. and A. F. M. Smith (1990). Sampling-based approaches to calculating marginal densities. *Journal of the American Statistical Association 85*, 398–409.

Gelfand, A. E., H.-J. Kim, C. F. Sirmans, and S. Banerjee (2003). Spatial modeling with spatially varying coefficient processes. *Journal of the American Statistical Association 98*, 387–396.

Gelman, A. and P. N. Price (1999). All maps of parameter estimates are misleading. *Statistics in Medicine 18*, 3221–3234.

Gelman, A., P. N. Price, and C. Lin (2000). A method for quantifying artefacts in mapping methods illustrated by application to headbanging. *Statistics in Medicine 19*(17/18), 2309–2320.

Gelman, A., J. B. Carlin, H. S. Stern, and D. B. Rubin (2004). *Bayesian Data Analysis* (2nd ed.). Boca Raton, FL: Chapman & Hall/CRC.

Genton, M. G. (1998). Variogram fitting by generalized least squares using an explicit formula for the covariance structure. *Mathematical Geology 30*, 323–345.

Getis, A. and J. K. Ord (1992). The analysis of spatial association by distance statistics. *Geographical Analysis 24*(3), 189–207.

Getis, A. and J. K. Ord (1996). Local spatial statistics: An overview. In P. Longley and M. Batty (Eds.), *Spatial Analysis: Modelling in a GIS Environment*, pp. 261–277. New York: John Wiley & Sons.

Geyer, C. (1999). Likelihood inference for spatial point processes. In O. E. Barndorff-Neilsen, W. S. Kendall, and M. N. M. van Lieshout (Eds.), *Stochastic Geometry: Likelihood and Computation*, pp. 79–140. Boca Raton, FL: Chapman & Hall/CRC.

Ghosh, M. and J. N. K. Rao (1994). Small area estimation: An appraisal (with discussion). *Statistical Science 9*, 55–93.

Ghosh, M., K. Natarajan, T. W. F. Stroud, and B. P. Carlin (1998). Generalized linear models for small-area estimation. *Journal of the American Statistical Association 93*, 273–282.

Ghosh, M., K. Natarajan, L. A. Waller, and D. Kim (1999). Hierarchical GLMs for the analysis of spatial data: An application to disease mapping. *Journal of Statistical Planning and Inference 75*, 305–318.

Gilbert, R. O. (1997). *Statistical Methods for Environmental Pollution Monitoring*. New York: Van Nostrand Reinhold.

Glaz, J., J. I. Naus, and S. Wallenstein (2001). *Scan Statistics*. New York: Springer-Verlag.

Gong, G. and F. J. Samaniego (1981). Pseudo maximum likelihood estimation: Theory and applications. *Annals of Statistics 9*, 861–869.

Goodman, L. A. (1959). Some alternatives to ecological correlation. *American Journal of Sociology, 64*, 610–625.

Goovaerts, P. (1997). *Geostatistics for Natural Resources Evaluation*. New York: Oxford University Press.

Gotway, C. A. (1994). The use of conditional simulation in nuclear waste site performance assessment (with discussion). *Technometrics 36*, 129–161.

Gotway, C. A. and N. Cressie (1993). Improved multivariate prediction under a general linear model. *Journal of Multivariate Analysis 45*, 56–72.

Gotway, C. A. and G. W. Hergert (1997). Incorporating spatial trends and anisotropy in geostatistical mapping of soil properties. *Soil Science Society of America Journal 61*, 298–309.

Gotway, C. A. and B. M. Rutherford (1994). Stochastic simulation for imaging spatial uncertainty: Comparison and evaluation of available algorithms. In M. Armstrong and P. A. Dowd (Eds.), *Geostatistical Simulations*, pp. 1–16. Dordrecht, The Netherlands: Kluwer Academic.

Gotway, C. A. and W. W. Stroup (1997). A generalized linear model approach to spatial data analysis and prediction. *Journal of Agricultural, Biological and Environmental Statistics 2*, 157–178.

Gotway, C. A. and R. D. Wolfinger (2003). Spatial prediction of counts and rates. *Statistics in Medicine 22*, 1415–1432.

Gotway, C. A. and L. J. Young (2002). Combining incompatible spatial data. *Journal of the American Statistical Association 97*, 632–648.

Gotway, C. A., R. B. Ferguson, G. W. Hergert, and T. A. Peterson (1996). Comparison of kriging and inverse-distance methods for mapping soil parameters. *Soil Science Society of America Journal 60*, 1237–1247.

Gould, P. (1989). Geographic dimension of the AIDS epidemic. *The Professional Geographer 41* (1), 71–78.

Graybill, F. A. (1976). *Theory and Application of the Linear Model*. North Scituate, MA: Duxbury Press.

Green, P. J. (1987). Penalized likelihood for general semi-parametric regression models. *International Statistical Review 55*, 245–259.

Greenland, S. (Ed.) (1987). *Evolution of Epidemiologic Ideas: Annotated Readings on Concepts and Methods*. Chestnut Hill, MA: Epidemiologic Resources.

Greenland, S. (1989). Reader reaction: Confounding in epidemiologic studies. *Biometrics 45*, 1309–1310.

Greenland, S. (1998). Confounding. In P. Armitage and T. Colton (Eds.), *Encyclopedia of Biostatistics*, Vol. 1, pp. 900–907. Chichester, West Sussex, England: John Wiley & Sons.

Greenland, S. and J. M. Robins (1986). Identifiability, exchangeability, and epidemiologic confounding. *International Journal of Epidemiology 15*, 413–419.

Greenland, S. and J. M. Robins (1994). Ecologic studies: Biases, misconceptions, and counterexamples. *American Journal of Epidemiology 139*, 747–760.

Greenland, S., J. M. Robins, and J. Pearl (1999). Confounding and collapsibility in causal inference. *Statistical Science 14*, 29–46.

Gregorio, D. I., M. Kulldorff, L. Barry, H. Samocuik, and K. Zarfos (2001). Geographical differences in primary therapy for early-stage breast cancer. *Annals of Surgical Oncology 8*, 844–849.

Griffith, D. (1992). What is spatial autocorrelation? *L'Espace geographique 21*, 265–280.

Griffith, D. A. (1996). Some guidelines for specifying the geographic weights matrix contained in spatial statistical models. In S. L. Arlinghaus (Ed.), *Practical Handbook of Spatial Statistics*, pp. 65–82. Boca Raton, FL: CRC Press.

Griffith, D. A. and L. J. Layne (1999). *A Casebook for Spatial Statistical Data Analysis: A Compilation of Analyses of Different Thematic Datasets*. New York: Oxford University Press.

Gumpertz, M. L., J. M. Graham, and J. B. Ristaino (1997). Autologistic model of spatial pattern of phytophthora epidemic in bell pepper: Effects of soil variables on disease presence. *Journal of Agricultural, Biological, and Environmental Statistics 2*, 131–156.

Haining, R. (1990). *Spatial Data Analysis in the Social and Environmental Sciences*. Cambridge: Cambridge University Press.

Haining, R. (1994). Diagnostics for regression modeling in spatial econometrics. *Journal of Regional Science 34*(3), 325–341.

Haining, R. P. (1995). Data problems in spatial econometric modeling. In L. Anselin and R. J. G. M. Florax (Eds.), *New Directions in Spatial Econometrics*, pp. 156–171. Berlin: Springer-Verlag.

Haining, R., S. Wise, and J. S. Ma (1996). The design of a software system for interactive spatial statistical analysis linked to a GIS. *Computational Statistics 11*, 449–466.

Haining, R., S. Wise, and J. S. Ma (1998). Exploratory spatial data analysis in a geographic information system environment. *Journal of the Royal Statistical Society, Series D 47*, 457–469.

Hansen, K. M. (1991). Headbanging: Robust smoothing in the plane. *IEEE Transactions on Geoscience and Remote Sensing 29*, 369–378.

Harr, J. (1995). *A Civil Action*. New York: Random House.

Haslett, J. (1998). Residuals for the linear model with general covariance structure. *Journal of the Royal Statistical Society Series B 60*(Part 1), 201–215.

Hastie, T. J. and R. J. Tibshirani (1990). *Generalized Additive Models*. New York: Chapman & Hall.

Hastie, R., O. Hammerle, J. Kerwin, C. M. Croner, and D. J. Herrmann (1996). Human performance reading maps. *Journal of Experimental Psychology: Applied 2*, 3–16.

Hepple, L. W. (1998). Exact testing for spatial autocorrelation among regression residuals. *Environment and Planning A 30*, 85–108.

Herrmann, D. J. and L. W. Pickle (1996). A cognitive subtask model of statistical map reading. *Visual Cognition 3*(2), 165–190.

Hertz-Picciotto, I. (1998). Environmental epidemiology. In K. J. Rothman and S. Greenland (Eds.), *Modern Epidemiology (2nd ed.)*. Philadelphia: Lippincott-Raven.

Hill, E. (2002). General saddlepoint approximations to the null distributions of Moran's I-type measures of spatial autocorrelation. Ph.D. dissertation, Department of Biostatistics, Rollins School of Public Health, Emory University, Atlanta, GA.

Hjalmars, U., M. Kulldorff, Y. Wahlqvist, and B. Lannering (1999). Increased incidence rates but no space-time clustering of childhood astrocytoma in Sweden, 1973–1992: A population-based study of pediatric brain tumors. *Cancer 85*, 2077–2090.

Holland, P. W. (1989). Reader reaction: Confounding in epidemiologic studies. *Biometrics 45*, 1310–1316.

Hook, E. B. and A. D. Carothers (1997). Use of computer simulation to evaluate a putative cluster of genetic or teratologic outcomes: Adjustment for "multiple hypotheses" and application to a reported excess of Down's Syndrome. *Genetic Epidemiology 14*, 133–145.

Horm, J. W., A. J. Asire, J. L. Young Jr., and E. S. Pollack (1984). *SEER Program: Cancer Incidence and Mortality in the United States, 1973–1981*. Technical Report 85-1837. Bethesda, MD: National Institutes of Health.

Howe, G. M. (1989). Historical evolution of disease mapping in general and specifically of cancer mapping. In P. Boyle, C. S. Muir, and E. Grundmann (Eds.), *Cancer Mapping (Recent Results in Cancer Research)*, pp. 1–21. Berlin: Springer-Verlag.

Huffer, F. W. and H. Wu (1998). Markov chain Monte Carlo for autologistic regression models with application to the distribution of plant species. *Biometrics 54*, 509–524.

Ihaka, R. and R. Gentleman (1996). R: A language for data analysis and graphics. *Journal of Computational and Graphical Statistics 5*, 299–314.

Inskip, H. (1998). Standardization methods. In P. Armitage and T. Colton (Eds.), *Encyclopedia of Biostatistics*, pp. 4237–4250. Chichester, West Sussex, England: John Wiley & Sons.

Isaaks, E. H. and R. M. Srivastava (1989). *An Introduction to Applied Geostatistics*. New York: Oxford University Press.

Jacqmin-Gadda, H., D. Commenges, C. Nejjari, and J.-F. Dartigues (1997). Tests of geographical correlation with adjustment for explanatory variables: An application to dyspnoea in the elderly. *Statistics in Medicine 16*, 1283–1297.

Jacquez, G. M. (1994). Cuzick and Edwards test when exact locations are unknown. *American Journal of Epidemiology 140*(1), 58–64.

Jelinski, D. E. and J. Wu (1996). The modifiable areal unit problem and implications for landscape ecology. *Landscape Ecology 11*, 129–140.

Jensen, J. (1996). *Introductory Digital Image Processing: A Remote Sensing Perspective* (2nd ed.). Upper Saddle River, NJ: Prentice Hall.

Joffe, M. M. and S. Greenland (1994). Re: Toward a clearer definition of confounding. *American Journal of Epidemiology 139*, 962.

Johnson, N. L. and S. Kotz (1969). *Discrete Distributions*. New York: John Wiley & Sons.

Johnston, K., J. M. Ver Hoef, K. Krivoruchko, and N. Lucas (2001). *Using ArcGIS Geostatistical Analyst*. Redlands, CA: Environmental Systems Research Institute (ESRI).

Journel, A. G. (1983). Nonparametric estimation of spatial distributions. *Journal of the International Association for Mathematical Geology 15*, 445–468.

Journel, A. G. and C. J. Huijbregts (1978). *Mining Geostatistics*. London: Academic Press.

Judge, G. G., W. E. Griffiths, R. C. Hill, H. Lütkepohl, and T.-C. Lee (1985). *The Theory and Practice of Econometrics*. New York: John Wiley & Sons.

Kafadar, K. (1994). Choosing among two-dimensional smoothers in practice. *Computational Statistics and Data Analysis 18*, 419–439.

Kafadar, K. (1996). Smoothing geographical data, particularly rates of disease. *Statistics in Medicine 15*, 2539–2560.

Kaiser, M. S. and N. Cressie (1997). Modeling Poisson variables with positive spatial dependence. *Statistics and Probability Letters 35*, 423–432.

Kaiser, M. S. and N. Cressie (2000). The construction of multivariate distributions from Markov random fields. *Journal of Multivariate Analysis 73*, 199–220.

Kaluzny, S. P., S. C. Vega, T. P. Cardoso, and A. A. Shelly (1998). *S+SpatialStats*. New York: Springer-Verlag.

Kaufman, P. R., A. T. Herlihy, J. W. Elwood, M. E. Mitch, K. H. Overton, A. J. Kinney, S. J. Christie, D. D. Brown, C. A. Hagly, and H. L. Jager (1988). *Chemical Characteristics of Streams in the Mid-Atlantic and Southeastern United States*, Vol. I: *Population Description and Physico-Chemical Relationships*. Technical Report 600/3-88/021a, Washington, DC: U.S. Environmental Protection Agency.

Kelsall, J. E. and P. J. Diggle (1995a). Kernel estimation of relative risk. *Bernoulli 1*, 3–16.

Kelsall, J. E. and P. J. Diggle (1995b). Non-parametric estimation of spatial variation in relative risk. *Statistics in Medicine 14*, 2335–2342.

Kelsall, J. E. and P. J. Diggle (1998). Spatial variation in risk: A nonparametric binary regression approach. *Statistics in Medicine 47*, 559–573.

Kelsall, J. E. and J. C. Wakefield (1999). Discussion of Best et al. 1999. In J. M. Bernardo, J. O. Berger, A. P. Dawid, and A. F. M. Smith (Eds.), *Bayesian Statistics, Vol. 6*, pp. 151. Oxford: Oxford University Press.

Kemp, I., P. Boyle, M. Smans, and C. Muir (1985). *Atlas of Cancer in Scotland, 1975–1980: Incidence and Epidemiologic Perspective*. IARC Scientific Publication 72. Lyon, France: International Agency for Research on Cancer.

Kenward, M. G. and J. H. Roger (1999). Small sample inference for fixed effects from restricted maximum likelihood. *Biometrics 53*, 983–997.

King, M. L. (1981). A small sample property of the Cliff–Ord test for spatial correlation. *Journal of the Royal Statistical Society, Series B 43*(2), 263–264.

King, G. (1997). *A Solution to the Ecological Inference Problem*. Princeton, NJ: Princeton University Press.

Kleinbaum, D. G., L. L. Kupper, and H. Morgenstern (1982). *Epidemiologic Research: Principles and Quantitative Methods*. New York: Van Nostrand Reinhold.

Knorr-Held, L. and J. Besag (1998). Modelling risk from a disease in time and space. *Statistics in Medicine 17*, 2045–2060.

Knorr-Held, L. and N. G. Best (2001). A shared component model for detecting joint and selective clustering of two diseases. *Journal of the Royal Statistical Society, Series A 164*, 73–85.

Knorr-Held, L. and G. Rasser (2000). Bayesian detection of clusters and discontinuities in disease maps. *Biometrics 56*, 13–21.

Knox, E. G. (1964). The detection of space–time interactions. *Applied Statistics 13*, 25–29.

Korn, E. L. and B. I. Graubard (1999). *Analysis of Health Surveys*. New York: John Wiley & Sons.

Krieger, N. and D. R. Williams (2001). Changing to the 2000 standard million: Are declining racial/ethnic and socioeconomic inequalities in health real progress or statistical illusion? *American Journal of Public Health 91*(8), 1209–1213.

Krieger, N., P. Waterman, K. Lemieux, S. Zierler, and J. W. Hogan (2001). On the wrong side of the tracts? Evaluating the accuracy of geocoding in public health research. *American Journal of Public Health 91*(7), 1114–1116.

Kulldorff, M. (1997). A spatial scan statistic. *Communications in Statistics: Theory and Methods 26*, 1487–1496.

Kulldorff, M. (2001). Prospective time periodic geographical disease surveillance using a scan statistic. *Journal of the Royal Statistical Society, Series A 164*, 61–72.

Kulldorff, M. (2002). Tests for spatial randomness adjusted for an inhomogeneity: A general framework. Unpublished manuscript. Storrs, CT: Division of Biostatistics, Department of Community Medicine, University of Connecticut School of Medicine.

Kulldorff, M. and International Management Services, Inc. (2002). *SaTScan v. 3.0: Software for the Spatial and Space–Time Scan Statistics*. Bethesda, MD: National Cancer Institute.

Kulldorff, M., W. F. Athas, E. J. Feuer, B. A. Miller, and C. R. Key (1998). Evaluating cluster alarms: A space–time statistic and brain cancer in Los Alamos, New Mexico. *American Journal of Public Health 88*, 1377–1380.

Kulldorff, M., T. Tango, and P. J. Park (2003). Power comparisons for disease clustering tests. *Computational Statistics and Data Analysis 42*, 665–684.

Lagakos, S. W., B. J. Wessen, and M. Zelen (1986). An analysis of contaminated water and health effects in Woburn, Massachusetts (with discussion). *Journal of the American Statistical Association 81*, 583–614.

Lancaster, H. O. (1956). Some geographical aspects of the mortality from melanoma in Europeans. *Medical Journal of Australia 1*, 1082–1087.

Lawson, A. B. (1989). Discussion of "Royal Statistical Society Meeting on Cancer near Nuclear Installations." *Journal of the Royal Statistical Society, Series A 152*, 374–375.

Lawson, A. B. (1993). On the analysis of mortality events associated with a prespecified fixed point. *Journal of the Royal Statistical Society, Series A 156*, 363–377.

Lawson, A. B. (2001). *Statistical Methods in Spatial Epidemiology*. Chichester, West Sussex, England: John Wiley & Sons.

Lawson, A. B. and D. G. T. Denison (Eds.) (2002). *Spatial Cluster Modelling.*, Boca Raton, FL: Chapman & Hall/CRC.

Lawson, A. B. and L. A. Waller (1996). A review of point pattern methods for spatial modelling of events around sources of pollution. *Environmetrics 7*, 471–488.

Lawson, A. B. and F. L. R. Williams (1993). Applications of extraction mapping in environmental epidemiology. *Statistics in Medicine 12*, 1249–1258.

Lawson, A. B., A. Biggeri, and E. Dreassi (1999). Edge effects in disease mapping. In A. Lawson, A. Biggeri, D. Böhning, E. Lesaffre, J.-F. Viel, and R. Bertollini (Eds.), *Disease Mapping and Risk Assessment for Public Health*, pp. 85–98. Chichester, West Sussex, England: John Wiley & Sons.

Lazarus, R., K. Kleinman, I. Dashevsky, C. Adams, P. Kludt, A. DeMaria, and R. Platt (2002). Use of automated ambulatory-care encounter records for detection of acute illness clusters, including potential bioterrorism events. *Emerging Infectious Diseases 8*, 753–760.

Lee, Y. and J. A. Nelder (1996). Hierarchical generalized linear models. *Journal of the Royal Statistical Society, Series B 58*, 619–678.

Lee, J. and D. W. S. Wong (2001). *Statistical Analysis with ArcView GIS*. New York: John Wiley & Sons.

Lehmann, E. L. (1994). *Testing Statistical Hypotheses* (2nd ed.). New York: Chapman & Hall.

Leroux, B. G. (2000). Modelling spatial disease rates using maximum likelihood. *Statistics in Medicine 19*, 2321–2332.

Levin, S. A. (1992). The problem of pattern and scale in ecology. *Ecology 73*, 1943–1967.

Levison, M. E. and W. Haddon (1965). The area adjusted map: An epidemiologic device. *Public Health Reports 80*, 55–59.

Lewandowsky, S., J. T. Behrens, L. W. Pickle, D. J. Herrmann, and A. A. White (1993). Perception of clusters in statistical maps. *Applied Cognitive Psychology 7*, 533–551.

Lewis, P. A. W. and G. S. Shedler (1979). Simulation of non-homogeneous Poisson processes by thinning. *Naval Research Logistics Quarterly 26*, 403–413.

Liang, K. Y. and S. L. Zeger (1986). Longitudinal data analysis using generalized linear models. *Biometrika 73*, 13–22.

Lilienfeld, D. E. and P. D. Stolley (1984). *Foundations of Epidemiology (3rd ed.)*. New York: Oxford University Press.

Lindley, D. V. (2002). Seeing and doing: The concept of causation. *International Statistical Review 70*(2), 191–197.

Littell, R. C., G. A. Milliken, W. W. Stroup, and R. D. Wolfinger (1996). *The SAS System for Mixed Models*. Cary, NC: SAS Institute, Inc.

Little, L. S., D. Edwards, and D. E. Porter (1997). Kriging in estuaries: As the crow flies or as the fish swims? *Journal of Experimental Marine Biology 213*, 1–11.

Loader, C. R. (1991). Large-deviation approximations to the distribution of scan statistics. *Advances in Applied Probability 23*, 751–771.

Longley, P. A., M. F. Goodchild, D. J. Maguire, and D. W. Rhind (2001). *Geographic Information Systems and Science*. Chichester, West Sussex, England: John Wiley & Sons.

Lumley, T. (1995). Efficient execution of Stone's likelihood ratio tests for disease clustering. *Computational Statistics and Data Analysis 20*, 499–510.

MacEachren, A. M. (1994). *Some Truth with Maps: A Primer on Symbolization and Design*. Washington, DC: Association of American Geographers.

MacEachren, A. M. (1995). *How Maps Work: Representation, Visualization, and Design*. New York: Guilford Press.

MacMahon, B. and T. F. Pugh (1970). *Epidemiology: Principles and Methods*. Boston: Little, Brown.

Malec, D., J. Sedransk, C. L. Moriarity, and F. B. LeClere (1997). Small area inference for binary variables in the National Health Interview Survey. *Journal of the American Statistical Association 92*, 815–826.

Maling, D. H. (1973). *Coordinate Systems and Map Projections*. London: George Philip and Son.

Mantel, N. (1967). The detection of disease clustering and a generalised regression approach. *Cancer Research 27*, 209–220.

Mantel, N. (1989). Reader reaction: Confounding in epidemiologic studies. *Biometrics 45*, 1317–1318.

Mantel, N. (1990). Reader reaction: Confounders: Correcting superstitions. *Biometrics 46*, 869–870.

Mardia, K. V. and R. J. Marshall (1984). Maximum likelihood estimation of models for residual covariance in spatial regression. *Biometrika 71*, 135–146.

Mariman, E. C. M. (1998). Clustering of anophthalmia and microphthalmia. *British Medical Journal 317*(7163), 895–896.

Marshall, R. J. (1991). Mapping disease and mortality rates using empirical Bayes estimators. *Applied Statistics 40*, 283–294.

Martin, R. J. (1992). Leverage, influence and residuals in regression models when observations are correlated. *Communications in Statistics: Theory and Methods 21*(5), 1183–1212.

Matérn, B. (1960). *Spatial Variation*. Meddelanden fran Statens Skogsforskningsinstitut, Band 49, No. 5; 2nd edition, 1986. Berlin: Springer-Verlag.

Matheron, G. (1963). Principles of geostatistics. *Economic Geology 58*, 1246–1266.

Mausner, J. S. and S. Kramer (1985). *Epidemiology: An Introductory Text*. Philadelphia: W. B. Saunders.

Maxcy, K. F. (1926). An epidemiological study of endemic typhus (Brill's disease) in the Southeastern United States with special reference to the mode of transmission. *Public Health Reports 41*, 2967–2995.

McCullagh, P. and J. A. Nelder (1989). *Generalized Linear Models (2nd ed.)*. New York: Chapman & Hall.

McMaster, R. B. and K. S. Shea (1992). *Generalization in Digital Cartography*. Washington, DC: Association of American Geographers.

McMillen, D. P. (2003). Spatial autocorrelation or model misspecification?, *International Regional Science Review 26*(2), 208–217.

McShane, L. M., P. S. Albert, and M. A. Palmatier (1997). A latent process regression model for spatially correlated count data. *Biometrics 53*, 698–706.

Messina, J. P. and K. A. Crews-Meyer (2000). The integration of remote sensing and medical geography. In D. P. Albert, W. M. Gesler, and B. Levergood (Eds.), *Spatial Analysis, GIS, and Remote Sensing Applications in the Health Sciences*, pp. 147–167. Chelsea, MI: Ann Arbor Press.

Møller, J., A. R. Syversveen, and R. P. Waagepetersen (1998). Log Gaussian Cox processes. *Scandinavian Journal of Statistics 25*, 451–482.

Mollié, A. (1996). Bayesian mapping of disease. In W. R. Gilks, S. Richardson, and D. J. Spiegelhalter (Eds.), *Markov Chain Monte Carlo in Practice*, pp. 360–379. Boca Raton, FL: Chapman & Hall/CRC.

Monmonier, M. (1996). *How to Lie with Maps, (2nd ed.)*. Chicago: University of Chicago Press.

Moore, D. A. (1999). Spatial diffusion of raccoon rabies in Pennsylvania, U.S.A. *Preventive Veterinary Medicine 40*, 19–32.

Moran, P. A. P. (1950). Notes on continuous stochastic phenomena. *Biometrika 37*, 17–23.

Morgenstern, H. (1982). Uses of ecologic analysis in epidemiologic research. *American Journal of Public Health 72*, 1336–1344.

Morris, S. E. and J. C. Wakefield (2000). Assessments of disease risk in relation to a prespecified source. In P. Elliott, J. C. Wakefield, N. G. Best, and D. J. Briggs (Eds.), *Spatial Epidemiology: Methods and Applications*, pp. 153–184. Oxford: Oxford University Press.

Morton-Jones, T., P. Diggle, and P. Elliott (1999). Investigation of excess environmental risk around putative sources: Stone's test with covariate adjustment. *Statistics in Medicine 18*, 189–197.

Morton-Jones, T., P. Diggle, L. Parker, H. O. Dickinson, and K. Binks (2000). Additive isotonic regression models in epidemiology. *Statistics in Medicine 19*, 849–859.

Mostashari, F., M. Kulldorff, J. J. Hartman, J. R. Miller, and V. Kulasekera (2003). Dead bird clusters as an early warning system for West Nile virus activity. *Emerging Infectious Diseases 9*, 641–646.

Mugglin, A. S., B. P. Carlin, L. Zhu, and E. Conlon (1999). Bayesian areal interpolation, estimation, and smoothing: An inferential approach for geographic information systems. *Environment and Planning A 31*, 1337–1352.

Mugglin, A. S., B. P. Carlin, and A. E. Gelfand (2000). Fully model-based approaches for spatially misaligned data. *Journal of the American Statistical Association 95*, 877–887.

Muirhead, C. R. and A. M. Ball (1989). Contribution to discussion of the Royal Statistical Society Meeting on Cancer near Nuclear Installations. *Journal of the Royal Statistical Society, Series A 152*, 376.

Muirhead, C. R. and B. K. Butland (1996). Testing for over-dispersion using an adapted form of the Potthoff–Whittinghill method. In F. E. Alexander and P. Boyle (Eds.), *Methods for Investigating Localized Clustering of Disease*, IARC Scientific Publication, 35 pp. 40–52. Lyon, France: International Agency for Research on Cancer.

Müller, H.-G., U. Stadtmüller, and F. Tabnak (1997). Spatial smoothing of geographically aggregated data, with application to the construction of incidence maps. *Journal of the American Statistical Association 92*, 61–71.

Mungiole, M., L. W. Pickle, and K. H. Simonson (1999). Application of a weighted head-banging algorithm to mortality data maps. *Statistics in Medicine 18*, 3201–3209.

Nagarwalla, N. (1996). A scan statistic with a variable window. *Statistics in Medicine 15*, 845–850.

National Research Council (1997). *Rediscovering Geography: New Relevance for Science and Society*. Washington, DC: National Academy Press.

Neter, J., M. H. Kutner, C. J. Nachtsheim, and W. Wasserman (1996). *Applied Linear Statistical Models* (4th ed.). Boston: WCB McGraw-Hill.

Neutra, R. R. and M. E. Drolette (1978). Estimating exposure-specific disease rates from case–control studies using Bayes' theorem. *American Journal of Epidemiology 108*, 214–222.

New York State Department of Environmental Conservation (1987). *Inactive Hazardous Waste Disposal Sites in New York State*, Vol. 7. Technical report. Albany, NY: New York State.

Neyman, J. (1939). On a new class of "contagious" distributions, applicable in entomology and bacteriology. *Annals of Mathematical Statistics 10*, 35–57.

Neyman, J. and E. L. Scott (1958). Statistical approach to problems of cosmology. *Journal of the Royal Statistical Society, Series B 20*, 1–43.

Oakley, G. P., L. M. James, and L. D. Edmonds (1983). Temporal trends in reported malformation incidence for the United States: Birth Defect Monitoring Program. *Morbidity and Mortality Weekly Report 32*(SS01), 7–8.

O'Brien, L. (1992). *Introducing Quantitative Geography: Measurement, Methods, and Generalised Linear Models*. London: Routledge.

O'Brien, D. J., J. B. Kaneene, A. Getis, J. W. Lloyd, G. M. Swanson, and R. W. Leader (2000). Spatial and temporal comparison of selected cancers in dogs and humans, Michigan, USA, 1964–1994. *Preventive Veterinary Medicine 47*, 187–204.

Oden, N. (1995). Adjusting Moran's *I* for population density. *Statistics in Medicine 14*, 17–26.

Ogata, Y. (1981). On Lewis' simulation method for point processes. *IEEE Transactions on Information Theory IT-27*, 23–31.

Olea, R. A. (1984). Sampling design optimization for spatial functions. *Mathematical Geology 16*, 369–392.

Olea, R. A. (1999). *Geostatistics for Engineers and Earth Scientists*. Norwell, MA: Kluwer Academic.

Olsen, A. R., J. Sedransk, D. Edwards, C. A. Gotway, W. Liggett, S. Rathbun, K. H. Reckhow, J. Young, L. J. Neyman, and E. L. Scott (1999). Statistical issues for monitoring ecological and natural resources in the United States. *Environmental Monitoring and Assessment 54*, 1–45.

Openshaw, S. (1984). *The Modifiable Areal Unit Problem*. Norwich, England: Geo Books.

Openshaw, S. (1990). Automating the search for cancer clusters: A review of problems, progress, and opportunities. In R. W. Thomas (Ed.), *Spatial Epidemiology*, pp. 48–78. London: Pion.

Openshaw, S. and P. J. Taylor (1979). A million or so correlation coefficients: Three experiments on the modifiable areal unit problem. In N. Wrigley (Ed.), *Statistical Applications in the Spatial Sciences*, pp. 127–144. London: Pion.

Openshaw, S., A. W. Craft, M. Charlton, and J. M. Birch (1988). Investigation of leukaemia clusters by use of a geographical analysis machine. *Lancet 1(8580)*, 272–273.

Ord, K. (1975). Estimation methods for models of spatial interaction. *Journal of the American Statistical Association 70*, 120–126.

Ord, K. (1990). Discussion of "Spatial clustering for inhomogeneous populations" by J. Cuzick and R. Edwards. *Journal of the Royal Statistical Society, Series B 52*, 97.

Ord, J. K. and A. Getis (1995). Local spatial autocorrelation statistics: Distributional issues and an application. *Geographical Analysis 27*, 286–306.

Pace, R. K. and J. P. LeSage (2002). Semiparametric maximum likelihood estimates of spatial dependence. *Geographical Analysis 34*(1), 76–90.

Palm, T. A. (1890). The geographical distribution and aetiology of rickets. *Practitioner 45*, 270–279.

Pamuk, E. R. (2001). Cautiously adjusting to the new millennium: Changing to the 2000 population standard. *American Journal of Public Health 91*(8), 1174–1176.

Pardo-Iqúsquiza, E. and P. Dowd (2001). Variance–covariance matrix of the experimental variogram: Assessing variogram uncertainty. *Mathematical Geology 33*, 397–419.

Pearl, J. (2001). *Causality: Models, Reasoning, and Inference*. Cambridge: Cambridge University Press.

Pearl, J. (2002). Comments on seeing and doing. *International Statistical Review 70*(2), 207–209.

Pickle, L. W. (2000). Mapping mortality data in the United States. In P. Elliott, J. C. Wakefield, N. G. Best, and D. J. Briggs (Eds.), *Spatial Epidemiology: Methods and Applications*, pp. 240–252. Oxford: Oxford University Press.

Pickle, L. W. and D. J. Herrmann (1995). *Cognitive Aspects of Statistical Mapping*, pp. 201–208. Working Paper Series 18. Hyattsville, MD: National Center for Health Statistics.

Pickle, L. W. and A. A. White (1995). Effect of the choice of age-adjustment on maps of death rates. *Statistics in Medicine 14*, 615–627.

Pickle, L. W., D. J. Herrmann, J. Kerwin, C. M. Croner, and A. A. White (1994). The impact of statistical graphical design on interpretation of disease rate maps. *Proceedings of the American Statistical Association's Section on Statistical Graphics*, pp. 111–116.

Pickle, L. W., M. Mungiole, G. Jones, and A. A. White (1996). *Atlas of United States Mortality*. Hyattsville, MD: National Center for Health Statistics.

Pocock, S. J., D. G. Cook, and S. A. A. Beresford (1981). Regression of area mortality rates on explanatory variables: What weighting is appropriate? *Applied Statistics 30*, 286–295.

Pocock, S. J., D. G. Cook, and A. G. Shaper (1982). Analysing geographic variation in cardiovascular mortality: Methods and results. *Journal of the Royal Statistical Society, Series A 145*, 313–341.

Potthoff, R. F. and M. Whittinghill (1966a). Testing for homogeneity: I. The binomial and multinomial distributions. *Biometrika 53*, 167–182.

Potthoff, R. F. and M. Whittinghill (1966b). Testing for homogeneity: II. The Poisson distribution. *Biometrika 53*, 183–190.

Prais, S. J. and J. Aitchison (1954). The grouping of observations in regression analysis. *Revue de l'Institut International de Statistique 1*, 1–22.

Prince, M. I., A. Chetwynd, P. Diggle, M. Jarner, J. V. Metcalf, and O. F. W. James (2001). The geographical distribution of primary biliary cirrhosis in a well-defined cohort. *Hepatology 34*(6), 1083–1088.

Rao, C. R. (1973). *Linear Statistical Inference* (2nd ed.). New York: John Wiley & Sons.

Rathbun, S. L. (1998). Kriging estuaries. *Environmetrics 9*, 109–129.

Rayens, M. K. and R. J. Kryscio (1993). Properties of Tango's index for detecting clustering in time. *Statistics in Medicine 12*, 1813–1827.

Richardson, S. (1992). Statistical methods for geographical correlation studies. In P. Elliott, J. Cuzick, D. English, and R. Stern (Eds.), *Geographical and Environmental Epidemiology: Methods for Small Area Studies*, pp. 181–204. New York: Oxford University Press.

Richardson, S., C. Guihenneuc, and V. Lasserre (1992). Spatial linear models with autocorrelated error structure. *The Statistician 41*, 539–557.

Ripley, B. D. (1976). The second-order analysis of stationary point patterns. *Journal of Applied Probability 13*, 255–266.

Ripley, B. D. (1977). Modeling spatial patterns (with discussion). *Journal of the Royal Statistical Society, Series B 39*, 172–212.

Ripley, B. D. (1981). *Spatial Statistics*. New York: John Wiley & Sons.

Ripley, B. D. (1987). *Stochastic Simulation*. Chichester, West Sussex, England: John Wiley & Sons.

Ripley, B. D. (1988). *Statistical Inference for Spatial Processes*. Cambridge: Cambridge University Press.

Rivoirard, J. (1994). *Introduction to Disjunctive Kriging and Nonlinear Geostatistics*. Oxford: Clarendon Press.

Robinson, W. S. (1950). Ecological correlations and the behavior of individuals. *American Sociological Review 15*, 351–357.

Robinson, A. H. (1952). *The Look of Maps*. Madison, WI: University of Wisconsin Press.

Robinson, A. H. (1956). The necessity of weighting values in correlation analysis of areal data. *Annals of the Association of American Geographers 46*, 233–236.

Rogers, J. F., S. J. Thompson, C. L. Addy, R. E. McKeown, D. J. Cowen, and P. DeCoulfé (2000). The association of very low birthweight with exposures to environmental sulfur dioxide and total suspended particulates. *American Journal of Epidemiology 151* (6), 602–613.

Rogerson, P. A. (1999). The detection of clusters using a spatial version of the chi-square goodness-of-fit statistic. *Geographical Analysis 31* (1), 130–147.

Rogerson, P. A. (2001). Monitoring point patterns for the development of space–time clusters. *Journal of the Royal Statistical Society, Series A 164*, 87–96.

Rothman, K. J. (1986). *Modern Epidemiology*. Boston: Little, Brown.

Rothman, K. J. and S. Greenland (1998). *Modern Epidemiology (2nd ed.)*. Philadelphia: Lippincott-Raven.

Rudd, R. A. (2001). The geography of power: A cautionary example for tests of spatial patterns of disease. Master's thesis, Department of Biostatistics, Rollins School of Public Health, Emory University, Atlanta, GA.

Rushton, G. and P. Lolonis (1996). Exploratory spatial analysis of birth defect rates in an urban population. *Statistics in Medicine 15*, 717–726.

Sackrowitz, H. and E. Samuel-Cahn (1999). p-Values as random variables: Expected p values. *American Statistician 53* (4), 326–331.

Sahu, S. K., R. B. Bendel, and C. P. Sison (1993). Effect of relative risk and cluster configuration on the power of the one-dimensional scan statistic. *Statistics in Medicine 12*, 1853–1865.

Sankoh, O. A., Y. Ye, R. Sauerborn, O. Muller, and H. Becker (2001). Clustering of childhood mortality in rural Burkina Faso. *International Journal of Epidemiology 30*, 485–492.

Schaible, W. L. (Ed.) (1996). *Indirect Estimators in U.S. Federal Programs*. Lecture Notes in Statistics 108. New York: Springer-Verlag.

Schlattman, P. and D. Böhning (1993). Mixture models and disease mapping. *Statistics in Medicine 12*, 1943–1950.

Schulman, J., S. Selvin, and D. W. Merrill (1988). Density equalized map projections: A method for analysing clustering around a fixed point. *Statistics in Medicine 7*, 491–505.

Scott, D. W. (1992). *Multivariate Density Estimation: Theory, Practice, and Visualization*. New York: John Wiley & Sons.

Searle, S. R., G. Casella, and C. E. McCulloch (1992). *Variance Components*. New York: John Wiley & Sons.

Seber, G. A. F. (1986). A review of estimating animal abundance. *Biometrics 42*, 267–292.

Seber, G. A. F. and C. J. Wild (1989). *Nonlinear Regression*. New York: John Wiley & Sons.

Self, S. G. and K. Y. Liang (1987). Asymptotic properties of maximum likelihood estimators and likelihood ratio tests under nonstandard conditions. *Journal of the American Statistical Association 82*, 605–610.

Selvin, H. C. (1958). Durkheim's "suicide" and problems of empirical research. *American Journal of Sociology 63*, 607–619.

Selvin, S. (1991). *Statistical Analysis of Epidemiologic Data*. New York: Oxford University Press.

Selvin, S., G. Shaw, J. Schulman, and D. W. Merrill (1987). Spatial distribution of disease: Three case studies. *Journal of the National Cancer Institute 79*, 417–423.

Selvin, S., D. W. Merrill, J. Schulman, S. Sacks, L. Bedell, and L. Wong (1988). Transformations of maps to investigate clusters of disease. *Social Science and Medicine 26*, 215–221.

Shapiro, A. and J. D. Botha (1991). Variogram fitting with a general class of conditionally nonnegative definite functions. *Computational Statistics and Data Analysis 11*, 87–96.

Silverman, B. W. (1986). *Density Estimation for Statistics and Data Analysis*. Boca Raton, FL: Chapman & Hall/CRC.

Singer, R. S., J. T. Case, T. E. Carpenter, R. L. Walker, and D. C. Hirsh (1998). Assessment of spatial and temporal clustering of ampicillin- and tetracycline-resistant strains of *pasteurella multocida* and *p. haemolytica* isolated from cattle in California. *Journal of the American Veterinary Medical Association 212*(7), 1001–1005.

Skellam, J. G. (1952). Studies in statistical ecology: I. spatial pattern. *Biometrika 39*, 346–362.

Slocum, T. A. (1999). *Thematic Cartography and Visualization*. Upper Saddle River, NJ: Prentice Hall.

Smith, J. R. (1997). *Introduction to Geodesy: The History and Concepts of Modern Geodesy*. New York: John Wiley & Sons.

Snow, J. (1855). *On the Mode of Communication of Cholera*. London: John Churchill.

Snow, J. (1936). *Snow on Cholera*. London: Oxford University Press.

Snyder, J. P. (1997). *Flattening the Earth: Two Thousand Years of Map Projections*. Chicago: University of Chicago Press.

Somes, G. W. and K. F. O'Brien (1985). Odds ratio estimators. In S. Kotz and N. L. Johnson (Eds.), *Encyclopedia of Statistical Sciences,* Vol. 6, pp. 407–410. New York: John Wiley & Sons.

Spiegelhalter, D. J., A. Thomas, and N. G. Best (1999). *WinBUGS Version 1.2 User's Manual*. Technical report. Cambridge: MRC Biostatistics Unit, Cambridge University.

Stehman, S. V. and W. S. Overton (1994). Environmental sampling and monitoring. In G. P. Patil and C. R. Rao (Eds.), *Handbook of Statistics,* Vol. 12, pp. 263–306. Amsterdam: Elsevier Science.

Stehman, S. V. and W. S. Overton (1996). Spatial sampling. In S. L. Arlinghaus (Ed.), *Practical Handbook of Spatial Statistics*, pp. 31–63. Boca Raton, FL: CRC Press.

Stein, M. L. (1999). *Interpolation of Spatial Data: Some Theory for Kriging*. New York: Springer-Verlag.

Stevens, D. L. Jr. (1994). Implementation of a national environmental monitoring program. *Journal of Environmental Management 42*, 1–29.

Stone, R. A. (1988). Investigations of excess environmental risks around putative sources: Statistical problems and a proposed test. *Statistics in Medicine 7*, 649–660.

Stoyan, D., W. S. Kendall, and J. Mecke (1995). *Stochastic Geometry and Its Applications*. Chichester, West Sussex, England: John Wiley & Sons.

Stroup, N. E., M. M. Zack, and M. Wharton (1994). Sources of routinely collected data for surveillance. In S. M. Teutsch and R. E. Churchill (Eds.), *Principles and Practice of Public Health Surveillance*, pp. 31–85. New York: Oxford University Press.

Sullivan, J. (1984). Conditional recovery estimation through probability kriging: Theory and practice. In G. Verly, M. David, A. Journel, and A. Marechal (Eds.), *Geostatistics for Natural Resources Characterization*, pp. 365–384. Dordrecht, The Netherlands: D. Reidel.

Sun, D., R. K. Tsutakawa, and P. L. Speckman (1999). Posterior distribution of hierarchical models using CAR(1) distributions. *Biometrika 86*, 341–350.

Symanzik, J., T. Kötter, S. Schmelzer, S. Klinke, D. Cook, and D. F. Swayne (1998). Spatial data analysis in the dynamically linked Arc-View/XGobi/XploRe environment. *Computing Science and Statistics 29*, 561–569.

Takatsuka, M. and M. Gahegan (2002). GeoVISTA Studio: A codeless visual programming environment for geoscientific data analysis and visualization. *Computers and Geosciences 28*, 1131–1144.

Talbot, T. O., M. Kulldorff, S. P. Forand, and V. B. Haley (2000). Evaluation of spatial filters to create smoothed maps of health data. *Statistics in Medicine 19*, 2399–2408.

Tango, T. (1984). The detection of disease clustering in time. *Biometrics 40*, 15–26.

Tango, T. (1990a). Asymptotic distribution of an index for disease clustering. *Biometrics 46*, 351–357.

Tango, T. (1990b). An index for cancer clustering. *Environmental Health Perspectives 87*, 157–162.

Tango, T. (1992). Letter regarding Best and Rayner's (1991) "Disease clustering in time." *Biometrics 48*, 326–327.

Tango, T. (1995). A class of tests for detecting "general" and "focused" clustering of rare diseases. *Statistics in Medicine 14*, 2323–2334.

Thomas, E. N. and D. L. Anderson (1965). Additional comments on weighting values in correlation analysis of areal data. *Annals of the Association of American Geographers 55*, 492–505.

Tiefelsdorf, M. (1998). Some practical applications of Moran's I's exact conditional distribution. *Papers in Regional Science 77*(2), 101–129.

Tiefelsdorf, M. (2000). *Modelling Spatial Processes: The Identification and Analysis of Spatial Relationships in Regression Residuals by Means of Moran's I*. Berlin: Springer-Verlag.

Tiefelsdorf, M. (2002). The saddlepoint approximation of Moran's I's and local Moran's I's reference distribution and their numerical evaluation. *Geographical Analysis 34*(3), 187–206.

Tiefelsdorf, M. and B. Boots (1995). The exact distribution of Moran's I. *Environment and Planning A 27*, 985–999.

Tiefelsdorf, M. and B. Boots (1996). Letter to the editor: The exact distribution of Moran's I. *Environment and Planning A 28*, 1900.

Tobler, W. (1970). A computer movie simulating urban growth in the Detroit region. *Economic Geography 46*, 234–240.

Tobler, W. (1979). Smooth pycnophylactic interpolation for geographical regions (with discussion). *Journal of the American Statistical Association, 74*, 519–536.

Tobler, W. (1989). Frame independent spatial analysis. In M. Goodchild and S. Gopal (Eds.), *The Accuracy of Spatial Data Bases*, pp. 115–122. London: Taylor & Francis.

Tukey, J. W. (1977). *Exploratory Data Analysis.* Reading, MA: Addison-Wesley.

Tukey, J. W. (1988). Statistical mapping: What should not be mapped. In *Collected Works of John W. Tukey*, pp. 109–121. Belmont, CA: Wadsworth.

Tukey, P. A. and J. W. Tukey (1981). Graphical display of data sets in 3 or more dimensions. In V. Barnett (Ed.), *Interpreting Multivariate Data*, pp. 189–275. Chichester, West Sussex, England: John Wiley & Sons.

Turnbull, B. W., E. J. Iwano, W. S. Burnett, H. L. Howe, and L. C. Clark (1990). Monitoring for clusters of disease: Application to leukemia incidence in upstate New York. *American Journal of Epidemiology 132, suppl.*, S136–S143.

Turner, M. G., R. V. O'Neill, R. H. Gardner, and B. T. Milne (1989). Effects of changing spatial scale on the analysis of landscape pattern. *Landscape Ecology 3*, 153–162.

Upton, G. J. G. and B. Fingleton (1985). *Spatial Data Analysis by Example,* Vol. I: *Point Pattern and Quantitative Data.* New York: John Wiley & Sons.

van Lieshout, M. N. M. (2000). *Markov Point Processes and Their Applications.* London: Imperial College Press/World Scientific.

van Lieshout, M. N. M. and A. J. Baddeley (1996). A non-parametric measure of spatial interaction in point patterns. *Statistica Neerlandica 50*, 344–361.

van Lieshout, M. N. M. and A. J. Baddeley (1999). Indices of dependence between types in multivariate point patterns. *Scandinavian Journal of Statistics 26*, 511–532.

Velleman, P. and D. Hoaglin (1981). *The ABCs of EDA: Applications, Basics, and Computing of Exploratory Data Analysis.* Boston: Duxbury Press.

Ver Hoef, J. M. and R. P. Barry (1996). Blackbox kriging: Spatial prediction without specifying variogram models. *Journal of Agricultural, Biological and Environmental Statistics 1*, 297–322.

Viel, J. F., P. Arveux, J. Baverel, and J. Y. Cahn (2000). Soft-tissue sarcoma and non-Hodgkin's lymphoma clusters around a municipal solid waste incinerator with high dioxin emissions level. *American Journal of Epidemiology 152*, 13–19.

Wackernagel, H. (1995). *Multivariate Geostatistics.* Berlin: Springer-Verlag.

Wahba, G. (1983). Bayesian "confidence intervals" for the cross-validated smoothing spline. *Journal of the Royal Statistical Society, Series B 45*, 133–150.

Wahba, G. (1990). *Spline Models for Observational Data.* Philadelphia: SIAM.

Wakefield, J. C., N. G. Best, and L. A. Waller (2000a). Bayesian approaches to disease mapping. In P. Elliott, J. C. Wakefield, N. G. Best, and D. G. Briggs (Eds.), *Spatial Epidemiology: Methods and Applications*, pp. 106–127. Oxford: Oxford University Press.

Wakefield, J. C., J. E. Kelsall, and S. E. Morris (2000b). Clustering, cluster detection, and spatial variation in risk. In P. Elliott, J. C. Wakefield, N. G. Best, and D. Briggs (Eds.), *Spatial Epidemiology: Methods and Applications*, pp. 128–152. Oxford: Oxford University Press.

Waldhör, T. (1996). The spatial autocorrelation coefficient Moran's *I* under heteroscedasticity. *Statistics in Medicine 15*, 887–892.

Wallenstein, S. (1980). A test for detection of clustering over time. *American Journal of Epidemiology 111*, 367–372.

Wallenstein, S., J. Naus, and J. Glaz (1993). Power of the scan statistic for detection of clustering. *Statistics in Medicine 12*, 1829–1843.

Waller, L. A. (1996). Statistical power and design of focused clustering studies. *Statistics in Medicine 15*, 765–782.

Waller, L. A. and G. M. Jacquez (1995). Disease models implicit in statistical tests of disease clustering. *Epidemiology 6*, 584–590.

Waller, L. A. and A. B. Lawson (1995). The power of focused score tests to detect disease clustering. *Statistics in Medicine 14*, 2291–2308.

Waller, L. A. and R. B. McMaster (1997). Incorporating indirect standardization in tests for disease clustering in a GIS environment. *Geographical Systems 4*, 327–342.

Waller, L. A. and C. A. Poquette (1999). The power of focused score tests under misspecified cluster models. In A. Lawson, A. Biggeri, D. Böhning, E. Lesaffre, J.-F. Viel, and R. Bertollini (Eds.), *Disease Mapping and Risk Assessment for Public Health*, pp. 257–269. Chichester, West Sussex, England: John Wiley & Sons.

Waller, L. A. and B. W. Turnbull (1993). The effects of scale on tests for disease clustering. *Statistics in Medicine 12*, 1869–1884.

Waller, L. A., B. W. Turnbull, L. C. Clark, and P. Nasca (1992). Chronic disease surveillance and testing of clustering of disease and exposure: Application to leukemia incidence and TCE-contaminated dumpsites in upstate New York. *Environmetrics 3*, 281–300.

Waller, L. A., B. W. Turnbull, L. C. Clark, and P. Nasca (1994). Spatial pattern analysis to detect rare disease clusters. In N. Lange, L. Ryan, L. Billard, D. Brillinger, L. Conquest, and J. Greenhouse (Eds.), *Case Studies in Biometry*, pp. 3–23. New York: John Wiley & Sons.

Waller, L. A., B. P. Carlin, H. Xia, and A. E. Gelfand (1997). Hierarchical spatio-temporal mapping of disease rates. *Journal of the American Statistical Association 92*, 607–617.

Waller, L. A., D. Smith, J. E. Childs, and L. A. Real (2003). Monte Carlo assessments of goodness of fit for ecological simulation models. *Ecological Modelling 164*, 49–63.

Walter, S. D. and S. E. Birnie (1991). Mapping mortality and morbidity patterns: An international comparison. *International Journal of Epidemiology 20*, 678–689.

Walter, S. D. (1992a). The analysis of regional patterns in health data: I. Distributional considerations. *American Journal of Epidemiology 136*(6), 730–741.

Walter, S. D. (1992b). The analysis of regional patterns in health data: II. The power to detect environmental effects. *American Journal of Epidemiology 136*(6), 742–759.

Walter, S. D. (2000). Disease mapping: A historical perspective. In P. Elliott, J. C. Wakefield, N. G. Best, and D. Briggs (Eds.), *Spatial Epidemiology: Methods and Applications*, pp. 223–239. Oxford: Oxford University Press.

Wand, M. P. and M. C. Jones (1995). *Kernel Smoothing*. Boca Raton, FL: Chapman & Hall/CRC.

Wartenberg, D. and M. Greenberg (1990). Detecting disease clusters: The importance of statistical power. *American Journal of Epidemiology 132, suppl.*, S156–S166.

Washino, R. and B. L. Wood (1994). Application of remote sensing to arthropod vector surveillance and control. *American Journal of Tropical Medicine and Hygiene 50*(6), 134–144.

Weber, D. D. and E. J. Englund (1992). Evaluation and comparison of spatial interpolators. *Mathematical Geology 24*, 381–391.

Webster, R. and A. B. McBratney (1989). On the Akaike information criterion for choosing models for variograms of soil properties. *Journal of Soil Science 40*, 493–496.

Webster, R. and M. A. Oliver (2001). *Geostatistics for Environmental Scientists*. Chichester, West Sussex, England: John Wiley & Sons.

Wedderburn, R. W. M. (1974). Quasi-likelihood functions, generalized linear models and the Gauss–Newton Method. *Biometrika 61*, 439–447.

Weinberg, C. (1993). Toward a clearer definition of confounding. *American Journal of Epidemiology 137*, 1–8.

Weinberg, C. (1994). Response to "Re: Toward a clearer definition of confounding." *American Journal of Epidemiology 139*, 962–963.

Whittemore, A. and J. B. Keller (1986). On Tango's index for disease clustering in time. *Biometrics 42*, 218.

Whittemore, A. S., N. Friend, B. W. Brown, and E. A. Holly (1987). A test to detect clusters of disease. *Biometrika 74*, 631–635.

Whittle, P. (1954). On stationary processes in the plane. *Biometrika 41*, 434–449.

Wickramaratne, P. J. and T. R. Holford (1987). Confounding in epidemiologic studies: The adequacy of the control group as a measure of confounding. *Biometrics 43*, 751–765.

Wickramaratne, P. J. and T. R. Holford (1989). Response to reader reaction: "Confounding in epidemiologic studies." *Biometrics 45*, 1319–1322.

Wickramaratne, P. J. and T. R. Holford (1990). Response to reader reaction: "Confounders: Correcting superstitions". *Biometrics 45*, 870–872.

Wiggins, L. (Ed.) (2002). *Using Geographic Information Systems Technology in the Collection, Analysis, and Presentation of Cancer Registry Data: Introduction to Basic Practices. Draft report.* Springfield, IL: North American Association of Cancer Registries.

Wise, S., R. Haining, and P. Signoretta (1999). Scientific visualization and the exploratory analysis of area data. *Environmental and Planning A 31* (10), 1825–1838.

Wolfinger, R. D. and M. O'Connell (1993). Generalized linear mixed models: A pseudo-likelihood approach. *Journal of Statistical Computing and Simulation 48*, 233–243.

Wollenhaupt, N., D. Mulla, and C. A. Gotway (1997). Soil sampling and interpolation techniques for mapping spatial variability of soil parameters. In F. e. a. Pierce (Ed.), *The Site-Specific Management for Agricultural Systems*, pp. 19–53. Madison, WI: American Society of Agronomy.

Wolpert, R. L. and K. Ickstadt (1998). Poisson/gamma random field models for spatial statistics. *Biometrika 85*, 251–267.

Wong, D. W. S. (1996). Aggregation effects in geo-referenced data. In D. Griffiths (Ed.), *Advanced Spatial Statistics*, pp. 83–106. Boca Raton, FL: CRC Press.

Xia, H. and B. P. Carlin (1998). Spatio-temporal models with errors in covariates: Mapping Ohio lung cancer mortality. *Statistics in Medicine 17*, 2025–2043.

Xiang, H., J. R. Nuckols, and L. Stallones (2000). A geographic information assessment of birth weight and crop production patterns around mother's residence. *Environmental Research 82*, 160–167.

Yasui, Y. and S. Lele (1997). A regression method for spatial disease rates: An estimating function approach. *Journal of the American Statistical Association 92*, 21–32.

Yule, G. U. and M. G. Kendall (1950). *An Introduction to the Theory of Statistics*. (14th ed.). London: Griffin.

Zeger, S. L. (1988). A regression model for time series of counts. *Biometrika 75*, 621–629.

Zeger, S. L. and K. Y. Liang (1986). Longitudinal data analysis for discrete and continuous outcomes. *Biometrics 42*, 121–130.

Zhang, H. (2002). On estimation and prediction for spatial generalized linear mixed models. *Biometrics 58*, 129–136.

Zidek, J. V., W. Sun, and N. D. Le (2000). Designing and integrating composite networks for monitoring multivariate Gaussian pollution fields. *Applied Statistics 49*, 63–79.

Zimmerman, D. L. (1989). Computationally efficient restricted maximum likelihood estimation of generalized covariance functions. *Mathematical Geology 21*, 655–672.

Zimmerman, D. L. (1993). Another look at anisotropy in geostatistics. *Mathematical Geology 25*, 453–470.

Zimmerman, D. L. and M. B. Zimmerman (1991). A comparison of spatial semivariogram estimators and corresponding ordinary kriging predictors. *Technometrics 33*, 77–92.

Zimmerman, D., C. Pavlik, A. Ruggles, and M. P. Armstrong (1999). An experimental comparison of ordinary and universal kriging and inverse distance weighting. *Mathematical Geology 31*, 375–389.

Zirschky, J. H. and D. J. Harris (1986). Geostatistical analysis of hazardous waste site data. *Journal of Environmental Engineering, ASCE 112*, 770–784.

Author Index

Applied Spatial Statistics for Public Health Data, by Lance A. Waller and Carol A. Gotway
ISBN 0-471-38771-1

Subject Index

Applied Spatial Statistics for Public Health Data, by Lance A. Waller and Carol A. Gotway
ISBN 0-471-38771-1

WILEY SERIES IN PROBABILITY AND STATISTICS

ESTABLISHED BY WALTER A. SHEWHART AND SAMUEL S. WILKS

The ***Wiley Series in Probability and Statistics*** is well established and authoritative. It covers many topics of current research interest in both pure and applied statistics and probability theory. Written by leading statisticians and institutions, the titles span both state-of-the-art developments in the field and classical methods.

Reflecting the wide range of current research in statistics, the series encompasses applied, methodological and theoretical statistics, ranging from applications and new techniques made possible by advances in computerized practice to rigorous treatment of theoretical approaches.

This series provides essential and invaluable reading for all statisticians, whether in academia, industry, government, or research.

ABRAHAM and LEDOLTER · Statistical Methods for Forecasting
AGRESTI · Analysis of Ordinal Categorical Data
AGRESTI · An Introduction to Categorical Data Analysis
AGRESTI · Categorical Data Analysis, *Second Edition*
ALTMAN, GILL, and McDONALD · Numerical Issues in Statistical Computing for the Social Scientist
AMARATUNGA and CABRERA · Exploration and Analysis of DNA Microarray and Protein Array Data
ANDĚL · Mathematics of Chance
ANDERSON · An Introduction to Multivariate Statistical Analysis, *Third Edition*
*ANDERSON · The Statistical Analysis of Time Series
ANDERSON, AUQUIER, HAUCK, OAKES, VANDAELE, and WEISBERG · Statistical Methods for Comparative Studies
ANDERSON and LOYNES · The Teaching of Practical Statistics
ARMITAGE and DAVID (editors) · Advances in Biometry
ARNOLD, BALAKRISHNAN, and NAGARAJA · Records
*ARTHANARI and DODGE · Mathematical Programming in Statistics
*BAILEY · The Elements of Stochastic Processes with Applications to the Natural Sciences
BALAKRISHNAN and KOUTRAS · Runs and Scans with Applications
BARNETT · Comparative Statistical Inference, *Third Edition*
BARNETT and LEWIS · Outliers in Statistical Data, *Third Edition*
BARTOSZYNSKI and NIEWIADOMSKA-BUGAJ · Probability and Statistical Inference
BASILEVSKY · Statistical Factor Analysis and Related Methods: Theory and Applications
BASU and RIGDON · Statistical Methods for the Reliability of Repairable Systems
BATES and WATTS · Nonlinear Regression Analysis and Its Applications
BECHHOFER, SANTNER, and GOLDSMAN · Design and Analysis of Experiments for Statistical Selection, Screening, and Multiple Comparisons
BELSLEY · Conditioning Diagnostics: Collinearity and Weak Data in Regression

*Now available in a lower priced paperback edition in the Wiley Classics Library.

BELSLEY, KUH, and WELSCH · Regression Diagnostics: Identifying Influential Data and Sources of Collinearity
BENDAT and PIERSOL · Random Data: Analysis and Measurement Procedures, *Third Edition*
BERRY, CHALONER, and GEWEKE · Bayesian Analysis in Statistics and Econometrics: Essays in Honor of Arnold Zellner
BERNARDO and SMITH · Bayesian Theory
BHAT and MILLER · Elements of Applied Stochastic Processes, *Third Edition*
BHATTACHARYA and WAYMIRE · Stochastic Processes with Applications
BILLINGSLEY · Convergence of Probability Measures, *Second Edition*
BILLINGSLEY · Probability and Measure, *Third Edition*
BIRKES and DODGE · Alternative Methods of Regression
BLISCHKE AND MURTHY (editors) · Case Studies in Reliability and Maintenance
BLISCHKE AND MURTHY · Reliability: Modeling, Prediction, and Optimization
BLOOMFIELD · Fourier Analysis of Time Series: An Introduction, *Second Edition*
BOLLEN · Structural Equations with Latent Variables
BOROVKOV · Ergodicity and Stability of Stochastic Processes
BOULEAU · Numerical Methods for Stochastic Processes
BOX · Bayesian Inference in Statistical Analysis
BOX · R. A. Fisher, the Life of a Scientist
BOX and DRAPER · Empirical Model-Building and Response Surfaces
*BOX and DRAPER · Evolutionary Operation: A Statistical Method for Process Improvement
BOX, HUNTER, and HUNTER · Statistics for Experimenters: An Introduction to Design, Data Analysis, and Model Building
BOX and LUCEÑO · Statistical Control by Monitoring and Feedback Adjustment
BRANDIMARTE · Numerical Methods in Finance: A MATLAB-Based Introduction
BROWN and HOLLANDER · Statistics: A Biomedical Introduction
BRUNNER, DOMHOF, and LANGER · Nonparametric Analysis of Longitudinal Data in Factorial Experiments
BUCKLEW · Large Deviation Techniques in Decision, Simulation, and Estimation
CAIROLI and DALANG · Sequential Stochastic Optimization
CHAN · Time Series: Applications to Finance
CHATTERJEE and HADI · Sensitivity Analysis in Linear Regression
CHATTERJEE and PRICE · Regression Analysis by Example, *Third Edition*
CHERNICK · Bootstrap Methods: A Practitioner's Guide
CHERNICK and FRIIS · Introductory Biostatistics for the Health Sciences
CHILÈS and DELFINER · Geostatistics: Modeling Spatial Uncertainty
CHOW and LIU · Design and Analysis of Clinical Trials: Concepts and Methodologies, *Second Edition*
CLARKE and DISNEY · Probability and Random Processes: A First Course with Applications, *Second Edition*
*COCHRAN and COX · Experimental Designs, *Second Edition*
CONGDON · Applied Bayesian Modelling
CONGDON · Bayesian Statistical Modelling
CONOVER · Practical Nonparametric Statistics, *Third Edition*
COOK · Regression Graphics
COOK and WEISBERG · Applied Regression Including Computing and Graphics
COOK and WEISBERG · An Introduction to Regression Graphics
CORNELL · Experiments with Mixtures, Designs, Models, and the Analysis of Mixture Data, *Third Edition*
COVER and THOMAS · Elements of Information Theory
COX · A Handbook of Introductory Statistical Methods

*Now available in a lower priced paperback edition in the Wiley Classics Library.

*COX · Planning of Experiments
CRESSIE · Statistics for Spatial Data, *Revised Edition*
CSÖRGŐ and HORVÁTH · Limit Theorems in Change Point Analysis
DANIEL · Applications of Statistics to Industrial Experimentation
DANIEL · Biostatistics: A Foundation for Analysis in the Health Sciences, *Eighth Edition*
*DANIEL · Fitting Equations to Data: Computer Analysis of Multifactor Data, *Second Edition*
DASU and JOHNSON · Exploratory Data Mining and Data Cleaning
DAVID and NAGARAJA · Order Statistics, *Third Edition*
*DEGROOT, FIENBERG, and KADANE · Statistics and the Law
DEL CASTILLO · Statistical Process Adjustment for Quality Control
DeMARIS · Regression with Social Data: Modeling Continuous and Limited Response Variables
DEMIDENKO · Mixed Models: Theory and Applications
DENISON, HOLMES, MALLICK and SMITH · Bayesian Methods for Nonlinear Classification and Regression
DETTE and STUDDEN · The Theory of Canonical Moments with Applications in Statistics, Probability, and Analysis
DEY and MUKERJEE · Fractional Factorial Plans
DILLON and GOLDSTEIN · Multivariate Analysis: Methods and Applications
DODGE · Alternative Methods of Regression
*DODGE and ROMIG · Sampling Inspection Tables, *Second Edition*
*DOOB · Stochastic Processes
DOWDY, WEARDEN, and CHILKO · Statistics for Research, *Third Edition*
DRAPER and SMITH · Applied Regression Analysis, *Third Edition*
DRYDEN and MARDIA · Statistical Shape Analysis
DUDEWICZ and MISHRA · Modern Mathematical Statistics
DUNN and CLARK · Basic Statistics: A Primer for the Biomedical Sciences, *Third Edition*
DUPUIS and ELLIS · A Weak Convergence Approach to the Theory of Large Deviations
*ELANDT-JOHNSON and JOHNSON · Survival Models and Data Analysis
ENDERS · Applied Econometric Time Series
ETHIER and KURTZ · Markov Processes: Characterization and Convergence
EVANS, HASTINGS, and PEACOCK · Statistical Distributions, *Third Edition*
FELLER · An Introduction to Probability Theory and Its Applications, Volume I, *Third Edition,* Revised; Volume II, *Second Edition*
FISHER and VAN BELLE · Biostatistics: A Methodology for the Health Sciences
FITZMAURICE, LAIRD, and WARE · Applied Longitudinal Analysis
*FLEISS · The Design and Analysis of Clinical Experiments
FLEISS · Statistical Methods for Rates and Proportions, *Third Edition*
FLEMING and HARRINGTON · Counting Processes and Survival Analysis
FULLER · Introduction to Statistical Time Series, *Second Edition*
FULLER · Measurement Error Models
GALLANT · Nonlinear Statistical Models
GHOSH, MUKHOPADHYAY, and SEN · Sequential Estimation
GIESBRECHT and GUMPERTZ · Planning, Construction, and Statistical Analysis of Comparative Experiments
GIFI · Nonlinear Multivariate Analysis
GLASSERMAN and YAO · Monotone Structure in Discrete-Event Systems
GNANADESIKAN · Methods for Statistical Data Analysis of Multivariate Observations, *Second Edition*
GOLDSTEIN and LEWIS · Assessment: Problems, Development, and Statistical Issues
GREENWOOD and NIKULIN · A Guide to Chi-Squared Testing

*Now available in a lower priced paperback edition in the Wiley Classics Library.

GROSS and HARRIS · Fundamentals of Queueing Theory, *Third Edition*
*HAHN and SHAPIRO · Statistical Models in Engineering
HAHN and MEEKER · Statistical Intervals: A Guide for Practitioners
HALD · A History of Probability and Statistics and their Applications Before 1750
HALD · A History of Mathematical Statistics from 1750 to 1930
HAMPEL · Robust Statistics: The Approach Based on Influence Functions
HANNAN and DEISTLER · The Statistical Theory of Linear Systems
HEIBERGER · Computation for the Analysis of Designed Experiments
HEDAYAT and SINHA · Design and Inference in Finite Population Sampling
HELLER · MACSYMA for Statisticians
HINKELMAN and KEMPTHORNE: · Design and Analysis of Experiments, Volume 1: Introduction to Experimental Design
HOAGLIN, MOSTELLER, and TUKEY · Exploratory Approach to Analysis of Variance
HOAGLIN, MOSTELLER, and TUKEY · Exploring Data Tables, Trends and Shapes
*HOAGLIN, MOSTELLER, and TUKEY · Understanding Robust and Exploratory Data Analysis
HOCHBERG and TAMHANE · Multiple Comparison Procedures
HOCKING · Methods and Applications of Linear Models: Regression and the Analysis of Variance, *Second Edition*
HOEL · Introduction to Mathematical Statistics, *Fifth Edition*
HOGG and KLUGMAN · Loss Distributions
HOLLANDER and WOLFE · Nonparametric Statistical Methods, *Second Edition*
HOSMER and LEMESHOW · Applied Logistic Regression, *Second Edition*
HOSMER and LEMESHOW · Applied Survival Analysis: Regression Modeling of Time to Event Data
HUBER · Robust Statistics
HUBERTY · Applied Discriminant Analysis
HUNT and KENNEDY · Financial Derivatives in Theory and Practice
HUSKOVA, BERAN, and DUPAC · Collected Works of Jaroslav Hajek—with Commentary
HUZURBAZAR · Flowgraph Models for Multistate Time-to-Event Data
IMAN and CONOVER · A Modern Approach to Statistics
JACKSON · A User's Guide to Principle Components
JOHN · Statistical Methods in Engineering and Quality Assurance
JOHNSON · Multivariate Statistical Simulation
JOHNSON and BALAKRISHNAN · Advances in the Theory and Practice of Statistics: A Volume in Honor of Samuel Kotz
JOHNSON and BHATTACHARYYA · Statistics: Principles and Methods, *Fifth Edition*
JOHNSON and KOTZ · Distributions in Statistics
JOHNSON and KOTZ (editors) · Leading Personalities in Statistical Sciences: From the Seventeenth Century to the Present
JOHNSON, KOTZ, and BALAKRISHNAN · Continuous Univariate Distributions, Volume 1, *Second Edition*
JOHNSON, KOTZ, and BALAKRISHNAN · Continuous Univariate Distributions, Volume 2, *Second Edition*
JOHNSON, KOTZ, and BALAKRISHNAN · Discrete Multivariate Distributions
JOHNSON, KOTZ, and KEMP · Univariate Discrete Distributions, *Second Edition*
JUDGE, GRIFFITHS, HILL, LÜTKEPOHL, and LEE · The Theory and Practice of Econometrics, *Second Edition*
JUREČKOVÁ and SEN · Robust Statistical Procedures: Aymptotics and Interrelations
JUREK and MASON · Operator-Limit Distributions in Probability Theory
KADANE · Bayesian Methods and Ethics in a Clinical Trial Design

*Now available in a lower priced paperback edition in the Wiley Classics Library.

KADANE AND SCHUM · A Probabilistic Analysis of the Sacco and Vanzetti Evidence
KALBFLEISCH and PRENTICE · The Statistical Analysis of Failure Time Data, *Second Edition*
KASS and VOS · Geometrical Foundations of Asymptotic Inference
KAUFMAN and ROUSSEEUW · Finding Groups in Data: An Introduction to Cluster Analysis
KEDEM and FOKIANOS · Regression Models for Time Series Analysis
KENDALL, BARDEN, CARNE, and LE · Shape and Shape Theory
KHURI · Advanced Calculus with Applications in Statistics, *Second Edition*
KHURI, MATHEW, and SINHA · Statistical Tests for Mixed Linear Models
KLEIBER and KOTZ · Statistical Size Distributions in Economics and Actuarial Sciences
KLUGMAN, PANJER, and WILLMOT · Loss Models: From Data to Decisions
KLUGMAN, PANJER, and WILLMOT · Solutions Manual to Accompany Loss Models: From Data to Decisions
KOTZ, BALAKRISHNAN, and JOHNSON · Continuous Multivariate Distributions, Volume 1, *Second Edition*
KOTZ and JOHNSON (editors) · Encyclopedia of Statistical Sciences: Volumes 1 to 9 with Index
KOTZ and JOHNSON (editors) · Encyclopedia of Statistical Sciences: Supplement Volume
KOTZ, READ, and BANKS (editors) · Encyclopedia of Statistical Sciences: Update Volume 1
KOTZ, READ, and BANKS (editors) · Encyclopedia of Statistical Sciences: Update Volume 2
KOVALENKO, KUZNETZOV, and PEGG · Mathematical Theory of Reliability of Time-Dependent Systems with Practical Applications
LACHIN · Biostatistical Methods: The Assessment of Relative Risks
LAD · Operational Subjective Statistical Methods: A Mathematical, Philosophical, and Historical Introduction
LAMPERTI · Probability: A Survey of the Mathematical Theory, *Second Edition*
LANGE, RYAN, BILLARD, BRILLINGER, CONQUEST, and GREENHOUSE · Case Studies in Biometry
LARSON · Introduction to Probability Theory and Statistical Inference, *Third Edition*
LAWLESS · Statistical Models and Methods for Lifetime Data, *Second Edition*
LAWSON · Statistical Methods in Spatial Epidemiology
LE · Applied Categorical Data Analysis
LE · Applied Survival Analysis
LEE and WANG · Statistical Methods for Survival Data Analysis, *Third Edition*
LePAGE and BILLARD · Exploring the Limits of Bootstrap
LEYLAND and GOLDSTEIN (editors) · Multilevel Modelling of Health Statistics
LIAO · Statistical Group Comparison
LINDVALL · Lectures on the Coupling Method
LINHART and ZUCCHINI · Model Selection
LITTLE and RUBIN · Statistical Analysis with Missing Data, *Second Edition*
LLOYD · The Statistical Analysis of Categorical Data
MAGNUS and NEUDECKER · Matrix Differential Calculus with Applications in Statistics and Econometrics, *Revised Edition*
MALLER and ZHOU · Survival Analysis with Long Term Survivors
MALLOWS · Design, Data, and Analysis by Some Friends of Cuthbert Daniel
MANN, SCHAFER, and SINGPURWALLA · Methods for Statistical Analysis of Reliability and Life Data
MANTON, WOODBURY, and TOLLEY · Statistical Applications Using Fuzzy Sets
MARCHETTE · Random Graphs for Statistical Pattern Recognition
MARDIA and JUPP · Directional Statistics

*Now available in a lower priced paperback edition in the Wiley Classics Library.

MASON, GUNST, and HESS · Statistical Design and Analysis of Experiments with Applications to Engineering and Science, *Second Edition*
McCULLOCH and SEARLE · Generalized, Linear, and Mixed Models
McFADDEN · Management of Data in Clinical Trials
McLACHLAN · Discriminant Analysis and Statistical Pattern Recognition
McLACHLAN and KRISHNAN · The EM Algorithm and Extensions
McLACHLAN and PEEL · Finite Mixture Models
McNEIL · Epidemiological Research Methods
MEEKER and ESCOBAR · Statistical Methods for Reliability Data
MEERSCHAERT and SCHEFFLER · Limit Distributions for Sums of Independent Random Vectors: Heavy Tails in Theory and Practice
MICKEY, DUNN, and CLARK · Applied Statistics: Analysis of Variance and Regression, *Third Edition*
*MILLER · Survival Analysis, *Second Edition*
MONTGOMERY, PECK, and VINING · Introduction to Linear Regression Analysis, *Third Edition*
MORGENTHALER and TUKEY · Configural Polysampling: A Route to Practical Robustness
MUIRHEAD · Aspects of Multivariate Statistical Theory
MULLER and STOYAN · Comparison Methods for Stochastic Models and Risks
MURRAY · X-STAT 2.0 Statistical Experimentation, Design Data Analysis, and Nonlinear Optimization
MURTHY, XIE, and JIANG · Weibull Models
MYERS and MONTGOMERY · Response Surface Methodology: Process and Product Optimization Using Designed Experiments, *Second Edition*
MYERS, MONTGOMERY, and VINING · Generalized Linear Models. With Applications in Engineering and the Sciences
NELSON · Accelerated Testing, Statistical Models, Test Plans, and Data Analyses
NELSON · Applied Life Data Analysis
NEWMAN · Biostatistical Methods in Epidemiology
OCHI · Applied Probability and Stochastic Processes in Engineering and Physical Sciences
OKABE, BOOTS, SUGIHARA, and CHIU · Spatial Tesselations: Concepts and Applications of Voronoi Diagrams, *Second Edition*
OLIVER and SMITH · Influence Diagrams, Belief Nets and Decision Analysis
PALTA · Quantitative Methods in Population Health: Extensions of Ordinary Regressions
PANKRATZ · Forecasting with Dynamic Regression Models
PANKRATZ · Forecasting with Univariate Box-Jenkins Models: Concepts and Cases
*PARZEN · Modern Probability Theory and Its Applications
PEÑA, TIAO, and TSAY · A Course in Time Series Analysis
PIANTADOSI · Clinical Trials: A Methodologic Perspective
PORT · Theoretical Probability for Applications
POURAHMADI · Foundations of Time Series Analysis and Prediction Theory
PRESS · Bayesian Statistics: Principles, Models, and Applications
PRESS · Subjective and Objective Bayesian Statistics, *Second Edition*
PRESS and TANUR · The Subjectivity of Scientists and the Bayesian Approach
PUKELSHEIM · Optimal Experimental Design
PURI, VILAPLANA, and WERTZ · New Perspectives in Theoretical and Applied Statistics
PUTERMAN · Markov Decision Processes: Discrete Stochastic Dynamic Programming
*RAO · Linear Statistical Inference and Its Applications, *Second Edition*
RAUSAND and HØYLAND · System Reliability Theory: Models, Statistical Methods, and Applications, *Second Edition*
RENCHER · Linear Models in Statistics